Wendy Gammon

Introduction to
physiological and pathological
CHEMISTRY

INTRODUCTION TO

physiological and pathological chemistry

L. EARLE ARNOW, PhG, BS, PhD, MB, MD

Senior Scientific Consultant, Warner-Lambert Research Institute, Morris Plains, N. J.; formerly President, Warner-Lambert Research Institute and Vice President, Warner-Lambert Co., Morris Plains, N. J.; formerly Vice President, Merck Sharp & Dohme Research Laboratories Division, and Executive Director, Merck Institute for Therapeutic Research, Merck & Co., Inc., West Point, Pa., and Rahway, N. J.; formerly Professor of Chemistry, Bryn Mawr College Summer School of Nursing, Bryn Mawr, Pa.; formerly Assistant Professor of Physiological Chemistry, University of Minnesota Medical School, and Lecturer in Physiological Chemistry, University of Minnesota School of Nursing, Minneapolis, Minn.

With an introduction by

KATHARINE DENSFORD DREVES, RN, BA, MA, DSc, LLD

Professor and Director Emeritus, University of Minnesota School of Nursing, Minneapolis, Minn.

EIGHTH EDITION

With 197 illustrations

The C. V. Mosby Company

SAINT LOUIS 1972

EIGHTH EDITION

Printed in the United States of America

International Standard Book Number 0-8016-0345-5

Library of Congress Catalog Card Number 70-174157

Distributed in Great Britain by Henry Kimpton, London

To

JENNIE AND PETE

Who have encouraged me anew many times
during the writing of this book

Preface

Knowledge of biochemistry and its relationship to human disease continues to increase at a rapid pace. I have tried to include in this edition the most important of these advances without increasing materially the length of the book. Obviously this necessitated deletion of some of the material in older editions, either because it was outmoded or because I believed it to be less useful and interesting than the new material. Many older illustrations have been omitted and some new, fresh ones have been added.

Numerous references to diseases of enzymic defect are scattered throughout the later chapters, usually presented in fine print. I do not, of course, believe that young students should be familiar with the details of such diseases, but rather I wish to emphasize their importance on two counts. First, they are caused by absent or defective enzymes and thus truly are diseases of abnormal biochemistry. Second, many new ones are discovered each year and their importance in clinical medicine will increase rapidly as physicians learn to recognize them. Probably there are at least 100,000 genes, many responsible for the synthesis of enzymes in the human body. If any one of these is absent or defective, a biochemical disease will result. If this deficiency does not prevent fertilization or cause intrauterine death, it will result in overt disease. Obviously, if a new disease results when more than one gene is involved, the number of potential diseases is increased enormously. Fortunately most of these diseases of enzymic defect so far recognized are rare, but their number makes them important. Moreover, some common diseases, such as diabetes mellitus, may be caused by biochemical lesions of this type.

In previous editions, much of the discussion of the nature and properties of chemical bonds was included along with the discussion of ionization. In this edition, this material has been separated out into a new chapter. Some additional information on the quantum mechanical picture of chemical bonding is given in this chapter, which includes also a brief discussion of the theory of resonance.

In this age of rapid communication and travel, it is desirable that all of us have a greater familiarity with the metric system of measurement, adopted by many countries, and its relationship to the English system, still largely used in this country. I have included a table illustrating some of these relationships in Chapter 2 as well as questions that will give the student practice in using them.

Some teachers who have used this text have suggested that a discussion of the quantum mechanical concept of atomic structure be included. Of course the medical applications of biochemistry can be understood without this information, but this concept is a basic cornerstone of chemical theory and, if told in simple language, can be interesting and informative. I hope my brief presentation of this subject meets this objective. Needless to say, my treatment is not mathematical!

A brief discussion of new techniques of diagnosis involving radioactive isotopes is included as is a short account of the use of heavy subatomic particles in therapy. Much of the chapter on enzymes has been rewritten and some information about cyclic AMP is included in it. A more modern account of lipid transport and metabolism has replaced a part of the older discussion. An account of genetic repressors and an up-to-date table of the codons of the genetic code will be found in Chapter 27. Lactose intolerance and gluten enteropathy are two diseases of biochemical origin that frequently are recognized now and they are described in Chapter 28.

Some of my fellow scientists told me a couple of decades ago that they did not expect many important advances in the field of nutrition in the foreseeable future. How wrong they were! New information has increased rapidly and I have concluded with regret that much of it cannot be included in this book. But I have given brief descriptions of the syndromes now recognized as caused by deficiencies of zinc, magnesium, and copper. Much of the chapter on vitamins has been rewritten and the chapter on nutrition includes modern diet plans for reducing and for attempting to control the level of triglycerides and cholesterol in the plasma.

The cascade theory of blood clotting, as well as new information about the more conventional theory, have been included in Chapter 30. Current ideas about the role of blood platelets in arterial disease are presented briefly. New information about lipoproteins and immunoglobulins will be found.

The hormone of the thymus gland has been established as an entity and the role of this gland and its hormone in immunological processes in the body is summarized. The hormones now known to be made by the hypothalamus are listed and their functions are described.

I am grateful to Dr. Donald Clausen, who made many useful suggestions for improving this book. He has used it as a text and thus his comments were particularly relevant. I am also grateful to my wife, Jennie M. Arnow, for acting as a "listening post" and for her cheerful acceptance of my need to hide away in a library or in my study for hours at a time during the revision of this book.

L. EARLE ARNOW

Contents

part one
Introduction to chemical science

CHAPTER 1

Introduction

Katharine Densford Dreves*
RN, BA, MA, DSc, LLD

"I've taken chemistry and chemistry and chemistry two years and more in the University, and this is the first time I've ever really understood it."

"I have memorized formulas upon formulas, but never before have I grasped their meaning."

"I have studied valence over and over again, but not until today has it been clear."

"Chemistry is so easy!"

"Chemistry is so interesting!"

So spoke nursing students of the introductory course in physiological chemistry that was taught twice a year for more than seven years in the University of Minnesota School of Nursing by Dr. L. Earle Arnow.

RECOMMENDED METHOD OF STUDY

For some unknown reason most persons approaching the study of chemistry do so with fear. We all are, I am sure, familiar with the story of the dervish and his meeting with Cholera. "Where are you going?" inquired the dervish. "To Baghdad," replied Cholera, "to kill 10,000 people." When later the dervish encountered Cholera, he said, "I thought you were going to Baghdad to kill 10,000 people, but 20,000 died." To this Cholera responded, "I killed but 10,000. Fear killed the others." The study of chemistry should be approached with the same ease and confidence that we use in acquiring a knowledge of other subjects. Fear inhibits learning in chemistry in just the same way as it inhibits the learning of a skill like swimming.

Most of you who read this textbook are just beginning your study of nursing. It is quite probable that some of you will have had no previous

*Professor and Director Emeritus, University of Minnesota School of Nursing, Minneapolis, Minn.

instruction in chemistry at all, that others will have had a course in this subject in high school and that a few may have had college chemistry. This text will make it possible for all of you to approach the study of chemistry as applied to nursing in a new way; it will help you to organize your knowledge of chemistry so as to see the principles involved. Proper use of the text will enable you to avoid beginning your study by the mere process of memorization, for to do this is to foredoom yourself to an unhappy period of study, if not to failure. It has been my experience that students who have learned their chemistry by rote are those of whom instructors in nursing say later: "But they know no chemistry. They don't know what it means."

Initially, it may seem easier to think in terms of individual reactions and not in terms of those reactions as governed by principles, but not even the instructor can remember the compilation of details of all individual reactions. If the principles that form the foundation and lie at the very center of chemistry are clearly understood, then the details involved can be reasoned; and this will make unnecessary the memorization of large amounts of material.

To understand, not memorize! That is the thesis of Dr. Arnow's teaching of chemistry.

DEFINITIONS

Perhaps we should look here at some of Dr. Arnow's definitions: "chemistry concerns itself with all of the many things around us . . . the chemist attempts to discover the nature of these things – their composition and the millions of changes in composition that they undergo. Physiological chemistry, or biochemistry, is the chemistry of living things in health, and pathological chemistry is the chemistry of living things in disease."

Shall we think, then, of the human body as a marvelous chemical laboratory to which we are being introduced? We might consider it a group of chemical compounds with reactions going on all the time. Certainly it is the most interesting chemical aggregate we know.

WHY DO WE STUDY CHEMISTRY

Now, what are some of the motives for studying chemistry? For what are we going to use it? Dr. Arnow has suggested five reasons for studying chemistry:

HEALTH. Our primary concern is to keep people well, and, if they must be ill, to get them well. Health depends much upon the food we eat. The vital importance to health of an adequate diet is recognized in every phase of health work. Indeed, doctors very often prescribe various foods as a means of preventing illness as well as of treating actual disease. Food, as we all know, in order to be utilized in our bodies must undergo important chemical changes, changes that are considered in detail in a course in physiological chemistry. How important, then, is it that nurses know something of the chemistry of digestion? An acquaintance with the nature of the chemical processes involved in the digestion and absorption of food is basic to an understanding of how the body functions; this knowledge cannot help but make for better patient care and for more alert nursing service. Perhaps such an acquaintance might make us better able to interpret to others the relation of nutrition and health, a service greatly needed at all times by all people.

DISEASE. So long as reactions in the body take place normally, we remain strong and healthy, but as soon as abnormal reactions set in we become weak and diseased. "To treat disease, the physician may use chemicals, called drugs, in the attempt to change the chemical reactions so that they will become normal again; or, he may follow some procedure (for example, the application of heat) that will assist the body's own chemical defense mechanisms to bring about the desired change; or, he may remove, surgically, the area of the body in which the abnormal changes are taking place." The nurse will not only function better in helping the physician treat disease, but she will also find her duties more fascinating if her training has prepared her to understand why any one or all of these various procedures may be chosen. Is not intelligent nursing a precaution to ensure safe patient care? A nurse alert to the needs of her patient (whether well or ill) should have at least a knowledge of the fundamental principles of chemistry.

SUPERSTITIONS. Some of us will care for patients with rabbits' feet suspended on cords about their necks to keep away the evil spirits of disease. Others will have patients carrying charms against toothache, accidents, etc. Still others will meet with persons who wear odorous asafetida, or camphor, thinking the objectionable odor will prevent illness from coming their way. The belief that a splinter must not be removed from a finger with a pin (no matter how well sterilized) because "it isn't made of steel" is not uncommon. Even the idea that milk and fish are harmful will be encountered occasionally. These are harmless superstitions, but others are not. The intelligent and well-trained nurse can do much toward combating injurious beliefs.

CHANGE. Probably no field of human endeavor is changing faster than that of medical science and its related spheres, one of which is nursing. Truisms of today become the untruths of tomorrow.

If we are to keep abreast of these changes, many of which involve chemistry, we must be informed in the field. We must read our own and related professional journals, and to do so intelligently requires a basic knowledge of the chemistry involved in the change.

PREREQUISITE TO OTHER COURSES. So much of the prevention and treatment of disease rests upon chemistry as a base that it is almost trite to say it should form a prerequisite to advanced work. To understand rightly the normal functioning of the body and the variations from that norm as discussed in such fields as nutrition, pharmacology, pathology, diet therapy, and the treatment of any type of illness it is necessary to know chemistry, and because an understanding of chemical principles is basic to this and to other knowledge, chemistry is essential for safe and intelligent nursing care.

THE SCIENTIFIC METHOD

Perhaps the best definition of the scientific method is that it is the way in which scientists go about their daily work. In general, it consists of the following four steps:

1. The scientist studies experimental data that he has collected either in the library or in the laboratory.

2. He chooses certain of these data that seem to him to be related to each other. The ability to make a proper choice is the hallmark of the competent scientist.
3. From the relationship he has postulated exists among these facts, the scientist sets up a scientific guess, or *hypothesis,* that can serve as a basis for making deductions (predictions) as to the outcome of future experiments. The ability to formulate significant hypotheses has been the hallmark of the scientific genius.
4. Finally, he tests the deduction, and hence the hypothesis leading to it, by experimentation.

How did Einstein go about formulating his theory of relativity? First he made a careful study of the observations and theories of other scientists. He concluded that either the theories then in vogue were wrong or the observations had been inaccurate. He assumed that the older theories were not correct, and set up a hypothesis (the special theory of relativity) that did explain the observations that had been made. This hypothesis, or scientific guess, made it possible for Einstein and other scientists to predict the outcome of experiments, and experiments have been carried out over the years that have shown the predictions to be correct. This, of course, has strengthened our belief in the usefulness of the theory of relativity. There is no real doubt in my mind, however, that observations that are not consistent with this theory will be found in the future. When that happens, some genius, perhaps as yet unborn, will formulate a new hypothesis that will lead to still other verifiable predictions.

It is obvious that there are very few scientific truths. Instead, science progresses from one hypothesis to another. Of course, some hypotheses have persisted so long, and seem so obvious to us, that we are willing to accept them as laws of nature—and, in fact, are willing to believe in their absolute truth. For example, we cannot prove that an apple will fall in the direction of the earth if we shake it from its tree—but nobody really doubts that it will. Pouring a solution of sodium chloride into a solution of silver nitrate *may not* result in the formation of a white precipitate of silver chloride—but every chemist *knows* it will!

CHAPTER 2

Metric system

In the United States we are accustomed in our everyday lives to measure lengths in terms of yards, feet, and inches; weights in pounds and ounces; volumes in quarts and pints; and to express temperature in Fahrenheit degrees. In science, however, another system of weights and measures, known as the *metric system,* is employed. The scientific unit of temperature is the *centigrade degree.*

CENTIGRADE TEMPERATURE SCALE

On the familiar Fahrenheit temperature scale the freezing point of water is 32° F and its boiling point is 212° F. On the centigrade scale these values are 0° C for the freezing point and 100° C for the boiling point. The average body temperature of a normal individual is 98.6° F or 37° C. Because it was Anders Celsius, a Swedish astronomer, who in 1742 invented the thermometer whose scale has 100 degrees between the ice and steam points, in a number of countries the word Celsius is used instead of centigrade. The General Conference on Weights and Measures, representing 33 nations, adopted the name Celsius for the centigrade temperature scale in 1948. The editorial policy of the National Bureau of Standards of the United States is to use the name Celsius in all of its scientific publications. Some journals have used the word Celsius followed by the word centigrade in parentheses: 37° Celsius (centigrade).*

UNITS OF LENGTH

The standard unit of length is called the *meter.* For many years the meter was defined as the distance between two scratches on a platinum-iridium bar that is kept at the International Bureau of Weights and Measures in France. Since the length of the bar is not quite the same for differ-

*The kelvin temperature scale can be defined as C° + 273.16. Absolute zero, the temperature at which all atomic and molecular motion ceases (the absolute minimum temperature) is −273.16° C. Hence, 273.16 K (Kelvin)—the word "degree" and its abbreviation are omitted in using this notation—is 0° C.

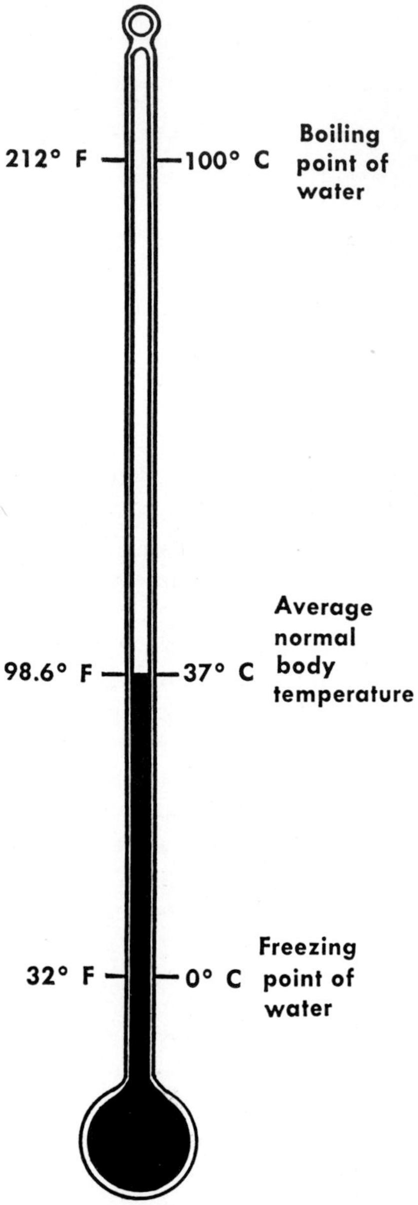

Fig. 2-1. Comparison of centigrade and Fahrenheit temperature scales. To convert degrees centigrade to degrees Fahrenheit, add 40, multiply by $^{9}/_{5}$, and subtract 40 from the result. To convert degrees Fahrenheit to degrees centigrade, add 40, multiply by $^{5}/_{9}$, and subtract 40 from the result. Convert 70° F to degrees centigrade; and 25° C to degrees Fahrenheit.

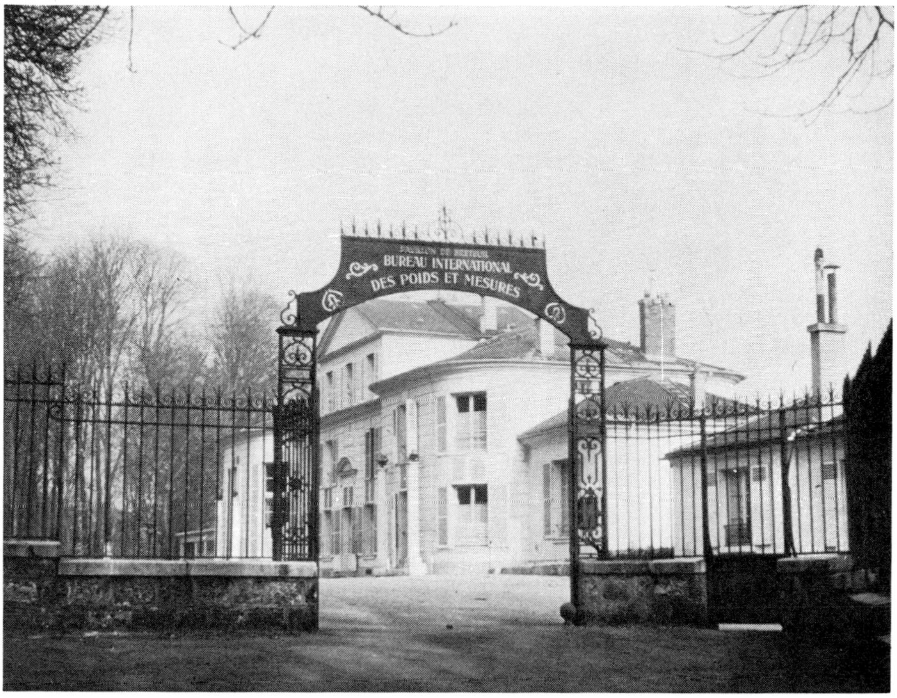

Fig. 2-2. The International Bureau of Weights and Measures, Sèvres, France. What is the standard unit of length? (Courtesy National Bureau of Standards.)

ent temperatures, the length was always measured at 0° C. This length was originally meant to be one ten-millionth the distance from the equator to the North Pole, but it was later found that the first measurements of this distance were not accurate. The Eleventh General Conference on Weights and Measures, meeting in Paris in 1960, adopted a new international standard of length based on a specific wavelength of light. The meter now is defined as 1,650,763.73 wavelengths of the orange-red line of the element krypton 86 (^{86}Kr) (see pages 15 and 113). The meter is equivalent to 39.37 inches and is, therefore, a little longer than a yard. It is interesting to note that our yard is defined in terms of the meter. The abbreviation for meter is m.

The *centimeter* is one-hundredth the length of the meter. There are about 30 centimeters in 1 foot, or about 2.5 centimeters in 1 inch. The *millimeter* is one-tenth the length of the centimeter. The abbreviations for these units of length are cm (centimeter) and mm (millimeter).

In summary, we may say that the units of length are related to each other as follows: 1 m = 100 cm = 1,000 mm.

UNITS OF WEIGHT

The *kilogram* (abbreviated kg) is the standard unit of weight. This is defined as the weight of a block of platinum-iridium kept at the International Bureau of Weights and Measures. One kilogram weighs approxi-

Table 2-1. Metric system of weights and measures

Number	Length (meters)	Weight (grams)	Volume (liters)
1,000,000,000,000	1 terameter (Tm)	1 teragram (Tg)	1 teraliter (Tl)
1,000,000,000	1 gigameter (Gm)	1 gigagram (Gg)	1 gigaliter (Gl)
1,000,000	1 megameter (Mm)	1 megagram (Mg)	1 megaliter (Ml)
1,000	1 kilometer (km or Km)*	1 kilogram (kg or Kg)*	1 kiloliter (kl or Kl)*
100	1 hectometer (hm or Hm)*	1 hectogram (hg or Hg)*	1 hectoliter (hl or Hl)*
10	1 dekameter (dkm or Dm)*	1 dekagram (dkg or Dg)*	1 dekaliter (dkl or Dl)*
1	1 meter (m or M)*	1 gram (g or gm)*	1 liter (l or L)*
0.1	1 decimeter (dm)	1 decigram (dg)	1 deciliter (dl)
0.01	1 centimeter (cm)	1 centigram (cg)	1 centiliter (cl)
0.001	1 millimeter (mm)	1 milligram (mg)	1 milliliter (ml)
0.000,001	1 micron (μ)	1 microgram (μg or mcg) or 1 gamma (γ)	1 microliter (μl or λ)
0.000,000,001	1 nanometer (nm)	1 nanogram (ng)	1 nanoliter (nl)
0.000,000,000,001	1 picometer (pm)	1 picogram (pg)	1 picoliter (pl)

*The abbreviation given first is that used by the National Bureau of Standards.

Table 2-2. Some measurement relationships

Unit	Exact conversion figure	Approximate conversion figure
1 millimeter	0.03937 inch	0.04 inch
1 centimeter	0.3937 inch	0.4 inch
1 meter	39.37 inches	39 inches
1 meter	1.09361 yards	1.1 yards
1 kilometer	0.6214 mile	0.6 mile
1 inch	2.540 centimeters	2.5 centimeters
1 foot	30.480 centimeters	30 centimeters
1 foot	0.3048 meter	0.3 meter
1 yard	0.9144 meter	0.9 meter
1 mile	1.6093 kilometers	1.6 kilometers
1 square meter	1.196 square yards	1.2 square yards
1 milliliter	0.06102 cubic inches	0.06 cubic inches
1 cubic inch	16.387 milliliters	16 milliliters
1 fluidounce	29.573 milliliters	30 milliliters
1 pint	473.166 milliliters	500 milliliters
1 gallon	3.785 liters	4 liters
1 gram	15.432 grains	15 grains
1 ounce	26.3495 grams	28 grams
1 pound	453.5924 grams	450 grams

STUDY QUESTIONS

1. Define the following: kilogram, liter, centimeter, gram, milliliter, meter.
2. Give the abbreviations for the weights and measures mentioned in question 1.
3. What is the average normal body tempera ture expressed in centigrade degrees? In Fahrenheit degrees?
4. Does 37° Celcius have the same meaning as 37° centigrade? Explain your answer.
5. Assuming that there are 8 fluidounces in one measuring cup, about how many milliliters are there in a fluidounce?
6. If a room is 15 feet long, what is its length in meters?
7. If a bandage pad measures 4 inches on each side, how many square centimeters does it contain?
8. What is the length in centimeters of an incision that has a length of 5 inches?
9. If a circular birthmark has a diameter of 1/4 inch, what is its radius in millimeters?
10. Is the 100 meter dash run in the Olympics shorter or longer than the 100 yard dash? How much?
11. If your car's speedometer indicates you are driving at a speed of 50 miles per hour, what is your speed in kilometers per hour?
12. A car is traveling on an autobahn in Germany at a speed of 120 kilometers per hour. What is its speed in miles per hour?
13. A patient has a height of 5 feet 2 inches. What is her height in meters?
14. Two hospitals are separated by a distance of 5 miles. What is this distance in kilometers?
15. How many milliliters will an 8-fluidounce medicine bottle contain?
16. How many fluidounces are there in 2 liters?
17. How many liters are there in 2 1/2 quarts of milk?
18. What is the weight in milligrams of 15 grains of aspirin?
18. How many kilograms does 3 pounds of butter weigh?
20. If a person has a body surface area of 1.5 square meters, what is his body surface area in square yards? In square inches?
21. A capsule used to induce sleep contains 100 milligrams of powder. What is the weight of this powder in grains?
22. What is the weight in kilograms of a patient whose weight is 150 pounds?

CHAPTER 3

Chemical substances

In our everyday conversation we use the word "substance" to refer to any tangible thing that seems to have individuality. Wood, concrete, steel, paper, cloth – all these are substances from this point of view. In chemistry, however, "substance" is defined in another way. A *chemical substance* is something that cannot be changed into anything simpler except by changing its chemical composition. Cold cream, for example, is not a chemical substance because it is made by mixing wax, spermaceti (a waxlike substance obtained from sperm whales), oil of almond, sodium borate, and perfume. It is also true that not even the wax, the spermaceti, the oil of almond, or the perfume is a chemical substance. Each of these materials can be separated into simpler things. The sodium borate, on the other hand, cannot be made simpler without destroying its chemical nature and is thus a true chemical substance. Other examples of chemical substances are sodium chloride (table salt), sucrose (cane sugar), iron, mercury, carbon, and gold. None of these substances can be made less complex without destroying its chemical structure.

Just as no two people are exactly alike, no two chemical substances are identical in appearance and chemical behavior. A substance has its own particular color, odor, and taste. It always melts at the same temperature if it is a solid or boils at the same temperature if it is a liquid. It always behaves in the same way when it is mixed with some other substance. A knowledge of the specific properties of a substance allows us to distinguish it from all other substances. *Specific properties* are properties that are characteristic of the particular substance under consideration; all of these properties in the same combination will not be characteristic of any other substance.

Materials that are made up of two or more substances mixed together are called *mixtures*. The individual substances present in a mixture are called *components* of the mixture. Mixtures are characterized by the fact that the components can be separated by physical methods; that is, separation can be effected without changing the chemical identities of the various substances that are present.

PHYSICAL AND CHEMICAL CHANGES

All of the various changes that substances can undergo can be classified under one of two groups: physical change or chemical change. *Physical changes* affect the state or condition of a substance without affecting its chemical composition. Suppose some table salt, which is a true chemical substance, is dissolved in water. The solid, salt, has been transformed into something that is no longer a solid. Nevertheless, the composition of the salt has not been affected as can be proved by heating the solution until the water is boiled off, in which case the salt remains behind—again the familiar solid. As another example, when ice is heated it becomes water. This involves a change in physical state, but no change in composition has occurred.

Chemical changes, on the other hand, are changes in which an alteration in the composition of the substance has taken place. Such changes, in contrast to physical changes, can be reversed only by some other chemical change. If iron is left in moist air some of it unites with another substance, oxygen, to form the red compound we call rust. The composition of this rust is not the same as that of the original iron. Consequently, a chemical change has taken place. Chemical changes can be recognized by the fact that the new substances formed have properties that are different from the properties of the substances that were present before the change took place.

SIMPLE AND COMPOUND SUBSTANCES

Certain substances are called *simple substances* because they cannot be made simpler even by chemical methods. One hundred five such substances are known. Examples are gold, platinum, iodine, oxygen, neon, lead, and arsenic. It frequently happens that two or more of these simple substances unite with each other to form *compound substances*. These compound substances can be made to separate again into the original simple substances by a suitable procedure. If an electric current is passed through water the water is changed to oxygen and hydrogen. The liquid, water, is a compound substance; the passage of the electric current has separated it into the gases, hydrogen and oxygen, which are simple substances. If the red compound substance known as mercuric oxide is heated, the simple substances mercury and oxygen are produced.

When simple substances unite with each other to form compound substances they always do so in a very particular way. Every compound substance always contains a definite proportion by weight of each of the simple substances of which it is composed. This law is often called the *law of definite weight proportions*. Eighteen grams of water *always* contains 2 grams of hydrogen and 16 grams of oxygen. Forty-four grams of carbon dioxide gas *always* contains 12 grams of carbon and 32 grams of oxygen.

ELEMENTS AND COMPOUNDS

The chemist refers to the simple substances mentioned above as *elements*. The compound substances are called *compounds*. In nonchemical conversations we often use the word element to refer to such things as wind, rain, and snow. Wind, which is air in motion, is not a *chemical element,* however, since air is a mixture of both elements and compounds.

The elements that we find in the earth are the same elements present in our bodies. In weight percentage, the body contains oxygen, 65 percent; carbon, 18 percent; hydrogen, 10 percent; nitrogen, 3 percent; calcium, 1.5 percent; and phosphorus, 1 percent. Other elements (including chlorine, silicon, iron, sodium, potassium, magnesium, and traces of gold and silver) make up the additional 1.5 percent. One scientist has estimated that the approximate value of the chemicals in one human body in 1969 was $3.50.

Certain elements have the peculiar ability to change spontaneously into other elements. These elements are called *radioactive elements.* The best known of them is radium. When radium breaks down to form other elements energy is released. We make use of this energy in treating cancer and certain other diseases.

FACTORS INFLUENCING THE ACTIVITIES OF SUBSTANCES

The *chemical activity* of a substance is defined as the tendency of the substance to react with another substance to form one or more new substances. When two elements react with each other they combine, or join together, to form a compound. When compounds react with each other or with elements, the elements of which they are composed rearrange themselves to form new combinations of elements. This results in the formation of new substances.

Almost any compound can be made to react with other substances if the experimental conditions are properly adjusted. Under certain other conditions, however, many compounds are said to be *chemically stable.* This means that they maintain their individual compositions even when mixed with other substances. Water exists all around us. We can dissolve many different substances in it without changing the composition of the water. In other words, under ordinary conditions, water is a stable compound.

We are able to make use of the stability and instability of compounds in many ways. By mixing unstable compounds we can make stable ones that are of great importance in modern civilization. Such things are Cellophane, rayon, Bakelite, and many synthetic drugs are made in this way. On the other hand it is equally fortunate that not all compounds are unstable. If all substances reacted rapidly with all other substances, the world as we know it could not exist. Water, steel, wood, and our own bodies, all of which actually do undergo slow but continuous chemical changes, would transform rapidly to other materials. The new materials thus formed would in turn quickly be converted to new substances, and the universe would be reduced to chaos.

FACTORS AFFECTING THE SPEED OF CHEMICAL REACTIONS

Most of the reactions that are familiar to us will occur only very slowly unless something is done to touch off or start the reaction. A loaded shotgun shell, for instance, does not explode until the percussion cap is struck. The ordinary agencies used to bring about chemical change include heat, light, electricity, concussion, vibration, pressure, and solution. We apply heat to a candle to start it burning. Hydrogen and chlorine gases react so slowly in the dark that we do not really regard the reaction as occurring at all, but these same gases do combine, often explosively, when exposed to sunlight. If an electric current is passed through water the water decomposes to form hydrogen and oxygen. If the compound known as mercury fulminate is allowed to explode, air vibrations are set up that will cause acetylene gas to decompose to form carbon and hydrogen. Lead and sulfur ordinarily do not unite at an appreciable rate when they are mixed together, but if the mixture is subjected to great pressure, lead sulfide is formed. Citric acid, a solid obtained from citrus fruits, apparently does not react with solid sodium bicarbonate, but if these compounds are dissolved in water, chemical union takes place as signified by the rapid evolution of carbon dioxide gas.

Some reactions take place with appreciable speed only in the presence of small quantities of another substance; this latter substance, however, apparently remaining unchanged. Such a substance, which changes the rate of a chemical reaction without itself being permanently altered, is called a *catalyst*. Hydrogen and oxygen gases combine with each other to form water almost instantly in the presence of a small amount of finely divided platinum. Liquid vegetable oils unite with hydrogen to form solid fats if nickel is present. Many of our common cooking fats are made in this way. When starch is mixed with yeast, alcohol and carbon dioxide gas are formed. The yeast contains a mixture of substances known as zymase that acts as a catalyst for this reaction. Catalysts may also slow down the rate of a chemical change: for example, those mixed with iron to slow down its reaction with oxygen, thereby preventing rust formation.

Catalysts that are formed by living cells are called *enzymes*. Enzymes are very important because they influence the rate of most of the thousands of reactions always going on in our bodies. For instance, most foods when we ingest them are not very soluble in water. In order for the body to make use of the nutrients in the food, digestion must take place in the intestinal tract. *Digestion* means that chemical changes occur so that the foods are converted to substances that are soluble and can be absorbed from the intestinal tract into the blood- and lymph streams. The digestive reactions are catalyzed by enzymes.

STUDY QUESTIONS

1. What is a chemical substance?
2. Name some of the properties of table salt (sodium chloride).
3. What is a mixture? A component?
4. Explain the difference between a physical and a chemical change, and give some examples of each that are not given in the book.
5. What is the chemist's name for simple substances? For compound substances?
6. How many elements are known?
7. What is the law of definite weight proportions?
8. Name ten elements found in the earth.
9. Name ten elements found in the body.
10. What is a radioactive element? For what purpose is radium used in medicine?
11. Explain what is meant by the phrase, "certain compounds are chemically stable."
12. Why is the stability and instability of chemical compounds of importance to us?
13. Name eight factors that affect the speed of chemical reactions.
14. What is a catalyst? An enzyme?
15. What is meant by digestion?

CHAPTER 4

Atoms and molecules

ATOMIC THEORY

When elements unite with each other to form a compound, a definite weight of each element always combines with definite weights of the other elements. This is another way of stating the law of definite weight proportions. Early in the last century, John Dalton, an Englishman, advanced a hypothesis, or scientific guess, to explain this fact. This hypothesis has stood the test of time and is now known as the *atomic theory*. This theory assumes, first, that all elements are composed of small invisible particles called *atoms*. An atom is, therefore, the smallest unit of an element. It is further assumed that all the atoms of the same element have the same properties and the same weight, and that they differ in these respects from the atoms of all other elements. These atoms are capable, under the proper conditions, of uniting or *combining with* other atoms to form tiny particles, or molecules, of compounds. In doing so, however, the weight of the individual atoms does not change.

Atoms may be regarded, then, as the units of matter—the smallest particles that can combine to form chemical compounds.

MASS AND WEIGHT

Matter is anything that has mass and occupies space. *Mass* describes the tendency of an object in motion to continue moving or to remain at rest if it is stationary. The mass of an object is constant and can be determined by comparing its weight with that of a known mass, as is done when a chemical balance is used. *Weight* on the earth is a measure of the force exerted by gravity on a given mass. Since the gravitational force varies at different points on the earth, the weight of an object also varies, although its mass remains constant. An object on the moon has a weight much less than that of the same object on the earth, because the gravitational force on the moon is much lower than that on the earth. Its mass, of course, is the same in both locations.

In the following discussion the terms, *atomic weight* and *atomic mass*, have the same meaning, since the numbers with which we shall be concerned are relative numbers; that is, numbers related to the weight of a standard. Most chemists use the phrase "atomic weight" rather than "atomic mass."

ATOMIC WEIGHT

Since atoms are so very minute (there are about 36,000,000,000,000,000,000,000,000 atoms in a pound of cane sugar) it is not possible for us to weigh just one of them. It has proved possible, however, to find the *relative* weights of the atoms in terms of some standard. We can say whether a certain atom is heavier or lighter than some other atom and, in fact, we can determine how much heavier or lighter the first atom is than the second. Chemists have agreed to use the most abundant natural form of *carbon* as the standard reference element and have agreed to specify that the atomic weight of this form of carbon (symbolized ^{12}C) is exactly 12. The oxygen atom is $^{16}/_{12}$ as heavy as the carbon atom, and the atomic weight of oxygen is 16. Since the sulfur atom is $^{32}/_{12}$ as heavy as the carbon atom, the atomic weight of sulfur is 32. A complete table of atomic weights will be found on page 474.

Atomic weights, then, are numbers representing the relative weights of the atoms of different elements, the atomic weight of carbon (^{12}C) arbitrarily being fixed at 12 as the standard.

ATOMIC NUMBERS

If the 105 elements are arranged in the order of their atomic weights, it is possible to assign a number, called the *atomic number,* to each element. Hydrogen is the lightest element and its atomic number is 1. The next lightest element is helium; it has an atomic number of 2. Oxygen is the eighth member of the series and its atomic number is 8. The heaviest *naturally* occurring element is uranium, which has an atomic number of 92.

MOLECULES

When 2 or more elements unite to form a compound the atomic theory assumes that a definite number of atoms of each element unite to form a small particle of the compound. This means simply that every small particle of a compound contains the same number of atoms of each of the elements that form the compound. For example, every small particle of water contains 2 atoms of hydrogen and 1 atom of oxygen. Every small particle of cane sugar contains 12 atoms of carbon, 22 atoms of hydrogen, and 11 atoms of oxygen.

These small particles that are made up of atoms are called *molecules.* The smallest particles of a chemical compound are molecules.

Some of the *elements,* particularly those that are gases at room temperature (oxygen, hydrogen, nitrogen, chlorine, and fluorine), exist as molecules, each molecule containing 2 atoms of the element.

MOLECULAR WEIGHT

The sum of all the atomic weights of all the atoms present in one molecule of a compound is called the *molecular weight* of the compound. A molecule of sulfur trioxide contains 1 atom of sulfur and 3 atoms of oxygen. Since the atomic weight of sulfur is approximately 32 and the atomic weight of oxygen is approximately 16, the molecular weight of sulfur trioxide is $32 + 16 + 16 + 16 = 80$. Each atom of oxygen has a weight of its own, and thus the atomic weight of oxygen occurs three times in the above calculation. A molecule of sulfuric acid contains 2 atoms of hy-

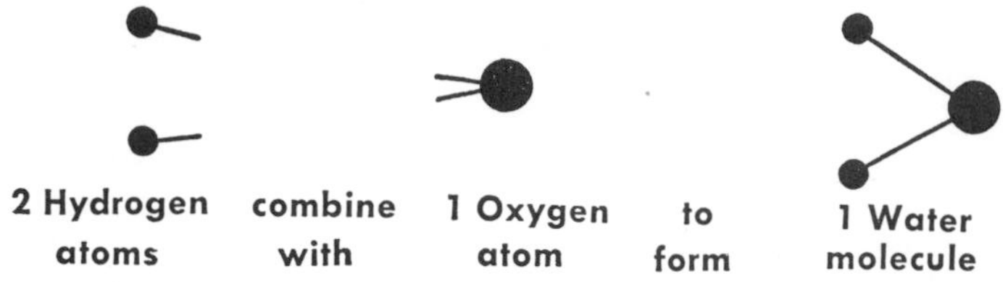

Fig. 4-1. Diagram to show the difference between atoms and molecules. Does a molecule ever contain less than 2 atoms?

drogen, 1 atom of sulfur, and 4 atoms of oxygen. The atomic weight of hydrogen is approximately 1, and the molecular weight of sulfuric acid is $1 + 1 + 32 + 16 + 16 + 16 + 16 = 98$.

The atomic weight of an element expressed in grams is called the *gram-atomic weight* of the element. The molecular weight of a compound expressed in grams is called the *gram-molecular weight* of the compound and is the sum of the gram atomic weights of all the atoms present in the molecule. We observe, then, that the gram-molecular weight of sulfur trioxide is 80 grams. The gram-molecular weight of sulfuric acid is 98 grams. It is known that *a gram-molecular weight of any compound contains the same number of molecules as a gram-molecular weight of any other compound.* Likewise, *gram-atomic weights of the elements contain equal numbers of atoms.* Thus, 80 grams of sulfur trioxide contains the same number of molecules as 98 grams of sulfuric acid. We often refer to this fact as *Avogadro's law*, after the scientist who first stated it.

When 2 molecules react with each other the reaction consists in a rearrangement of the individual atoms so that new molecules are formed. We cannot see the individual molecules, of course, but when large numbers of them react with each other at one time we can observe the results because large numbers of new molecules are formed. When a solution of magnesium sulfate is mixed with a solution of barium chloride, one of the new compounds formed is a white, insoluble powder called barium sulfate. We cannot actually see the molecules of magnesium sulfate reacting with those of barium chloride to produce the molecules of barium sulfate, but we know that they must have reacted in this manner because we can see the barium sulfate that has been formed by the reaction.

SUBATOMIC PARTICLES

For many years it was thought that the atom represented the smallest particle of matter. It is evident today, however, that a number of particles of subatomic size exist. For convenience, physicists classify these particles as *baryons* (heavy particles), *mesons* (particles of intermediate weight), and *leptons* (light particles). Protons and neutrons are baryons; electrons are leptons. Under ordinary conditions atoms probably consist almost entirely of protons, neutrons, and electrons. Most of the other subatomic particles exist only for short periods of time and are formed when atoms are "excited" or disintegrated in some way.

In 1964, it was possible to write down a list of more than 100 subatomic particles, and some scientists believed that very few more, if any, would be

Table 4-1. Stable subatomic particles*

Class	Particle	Mass (MeV)†	Life (seconds)
Photon	γ	0	∞
Leptons	ν_0	2×10^{-4}	∞
	ν_μ	4	∞
	e (electron)	0.511006	∞
	μ	105.059	2.2001×10^{-6}
Mesons	$\pi^\pm$	139.60	2.551×10^{-8}
	π^0	135.01	1.80×10^{-16}
	$K^\pm$	493.8	1.229×10^{-10}
	$K_1{}^0$	498.0	0.92×10^{-10}
	$K_2{}^0$	498.0	5.62×10^{-8}
	η	548.7	
Baryons	p (proton)	938.256	∞
	n (neutron)	939.550	1.01×10^3
	Λ^0	1115.40	2.62×10^{-10}
	Σ^+	1189.41	0.788×10^{-10}
	Σ^0	1192.3	1×10^{-14}
	Σ^-	1197.08	1.58×10^{-10}
	Ξ^0	1314.3	3.06×10^{-10}
	Ξ^-	1320.8	1.74×10^{-10}
	Ω^-	1675	0.7×10^{-10}

*Arbitrarily defined as subatomic particles with a life exceeding 10^{-16} second. The other known subatomic particles have lifetimes less than 10^{-23} second and are believed to be higher energy states of the stable mesons and baryons.
†We know today that mass (weight) and energy can be converted into one another. In other words, every particle of matter that has a mass also has a potential amount of energy into which it can be converted under suitable conditions. A good example is the atomic bomb, in which large amounts of energy are released as a result of converting matter to energy. The figures given in the table are measured in *million electron volts*, which is a measurement of energy rather than a measurement of mass. It is possible, however, to convert these figures into units of weight. For example, if this is done the weight of the electron is approximately 9×10^{-28} g. The other figures can be converted by using this conversion factor.

discovered. However, since that time new ones have been identified and studied, and the end is not in sight.

Some of these particles are electrically neutral, but most of them have either a positive or a negative charge. The *amount* of electrical charge present in each of the charged particles is exactly the same. For example, protons and positrons each have the same amount of charge even though protons weight about 1,840 times as much as do positrons. Electrons and positrons have approximately the same weight and have exactly the same amount of electric charge, although in this case the *sign* of the charge is different. (Electrons carry a negative charge; positrons are positively charged.)

ANTI-PARTICLES. By using cosmic rays and billion-volt accelerators it has been possible to identify a certain number of anti-particles—that is, particles opposite in electric charge to those of our normal universe. For example, an anti-proton having a negative charge but otherwise identical with a proton has been observed. The positron is exactly like the electron except that it has a positive charge. When a given particle and its anti-particle collide, both are annihilated; that is, they are converted to radiant energy. It is interesting to speculate that somewhere in our vast universe there may exist a world in which the "abnormal" anti-particles of our world are the normal ones. On such a world an atom of hydrogen would consist of a negatively charged anti-proton around which would revolve a positron. If such a world collided with our own, the two would annihilate each other, with the creation of an unimaginable quantity of energy.

THE BOHR STRUCTURE OF THE ATOM

In 1913 the Danish physicist, Niels Bohr, suggested a structure for the atom that accounted for its known properties. Although the Bohr theory now has been supplanted by the more modern theory of quantum mechanics, it still is useful, especially for the beginning student, in explaining many of the properties and chemical reactions of atoms.

According to this theory, each atom consists of a *nucleus* or group of subatomic particles, around which electrons revolve. We may compare the nucleus of an atom with the sun; and the earth, which revolves around the sun, may be compared with an electron revolving around its nucleus. The weight of the atom is due almost entirely to its nucleus because all the heavy subatomic particles are located in it. The exact structure of the nucleus of the atom is not known, but most scientists believe that it contains only protons and neutrons bound together in some way by mesons.*

Many experiments have shown that atoms have the same number of both negative and positive electrical charges. If this were not true, we would be unable to touch any of the objects around us without receiving a severe electrical shock. Now, as we have seen, the particles revolving around the nucleus are all *electrons*. Since each of these electrons has a negative charge, we come to the conclusion that the nucleus contains *positive charges*. Furthermore, it must be true that *the number of positive charges in the nucleus is exactly equal to the number of electrons revolving around the nucleus*. For example, the oxygen atom has 8 electrons revolving around its nucleus. Since an atom is electrically neutral (that is, contains the same number of positive and negative charges) we know that the nucleus of the oxygen atom must have 8 positive charges. In other words, the oxygen atomic nucleus has a charge† of 8+.

The electrons that revolve around the atomic nucleus are called *planetary electrons. The number of planetary electrons that an atom has is equal to the atomic number of the atom.* It must also be true, then, that *the positive charge of the atomic nucleus is numerically equal to the atomic number of the atom.* For example, suppose we are told that the

*Since like electric charges repel each other, there is a great tendency for the positively charged protons in the nucleus to fly apart. This repulsive force is believed to be overcome by a nuclear force created by the continuous creation and destruction within the nucleus of heavy mesons. The nuclear force thus created is about 100 times as strong as the repulsive force. Without the mesons, then, our universe probably would consist largely of one vast cloud of protons!

†We shall define the *charge* of the nucleus as the number of positive charges present. If only protons and neutrons are present in the nucleus, the number of positive charges in the nucleus is identical with the number of protons present.

atomic number of carbon is 6. We can deduce at once that the carbon atom has 6 planetary electrons, and that the charge on the nucleus of the carbon atom is 6+.

One more fact is needed before we can picture the Bohr structure of the atom. We need to know *how* the planetary electrons are grouped around thc nucleus. In a farily large atom where there are many planetary electrons these electrons are pictured as revolving around the nucleus in groups. The group that is closest to the nucleus is said to belong to the *first electron shell* of the atom.* The group that is next closest to the nucleus belongs to the *second shell*. The next closest group belongs to the *third shell*, and so on. The first electron shell cannot contain more than 2 planetary electrons. If, for example, a given atom has 3 planetary electrons, 2 of them will be in the first shell, but the third electron will be in the second shell. The second electron shell is filled when it contains 8 electrons. The structures of the remaining electron shells are more complicated: for our purposes it will be unnecessary to describe them.

The foregoing statements can be made clearer by means of examples. Suppose we represent the nucleus of the atom by means of a circle, the planetary electrons by means of dots, and the electron shells by means of circles around the nucleus. What will a diagram of the hydrogen atom look like? We start by drawing a circle to represent the nucleus (Fig. 4-2, *A*). Since the atomic weight of hydrogen is 1, we know that only one heavy particle is present in the nucleus.† Its *atomic number* is also 1; this tells us that the charge of the nucleus is 1+ (Fig. 4-2, *B*), and that one planetary electron is revolving around this nucleus (Fig. 4-2, *C*). The hydrogen atom is thus pictured as having one planetary electron revolving around a nucleus whose charge is 1+.

Suppose we now draw a diagram of a more complicated atom – the oxygen atom. We are told that the atomic weight of oxygen is 16 and that its atomic number is 8. A knowledge of the atomic weight allows us to state that the nucleus contains 16 heavy subatomic particles. Again we begin our diagram by drawing a circle to represent the nucleus (Fig. 4-3, *A*). The charge of this nucleus will be 8+ (Fig. 4-3, *B*), and the number of planetary electrons will be 8 (Fig. 4-3, *C*), since the atomic number is 8. We must remember that the first electron shell can hold only 2 electrons. The remaining electrons must be placed in the second shell. The completed diagram shows that the nucleus of the oxygen atom has a charge of 8+, and that 8 planetary electrons (2 in the first shell and 6 in the second) revolve around this nucleus.

*The electron shells also are identified by capital letters: K for the first shell, L for the second, M for the third, and so on.

†If we remember that practically all the *weight* of an atom is due to the heavy subatomic particles in the nucleus of an atom of the element, we realize that the *atomic weight* of an element must be proportional to the number of heavy particles. Hydrogen has an atomic weight that is approximately 1, and the hydrogen atom has 1 heavy particle in its nucleus. Oxygen has an atomic weight of approximately 16, and oxygen atoms have 16 heavy particles in their nuclei.

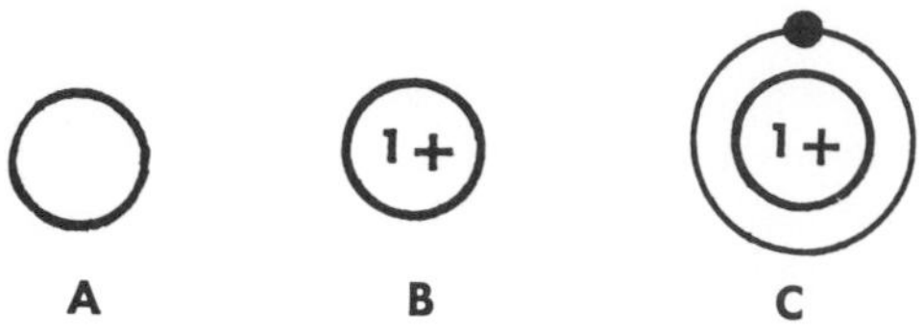

Fig. 4-2. Steps in drawing a diagram of the hydrogen atom. What is a planetary electron?

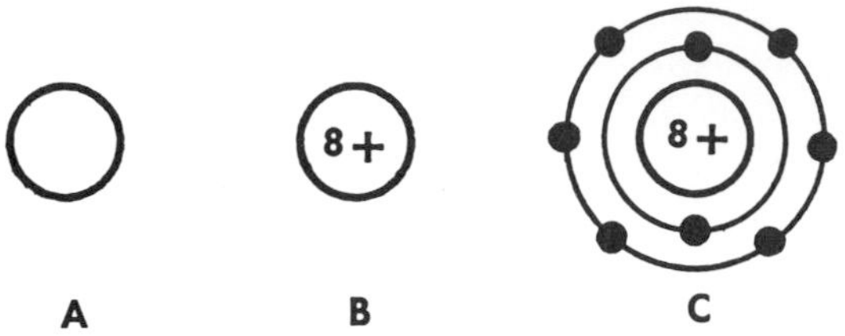

Fig. 4-3. Steps in drawing a diagram of the oxygen atom. Are all atoms electrically neutral?

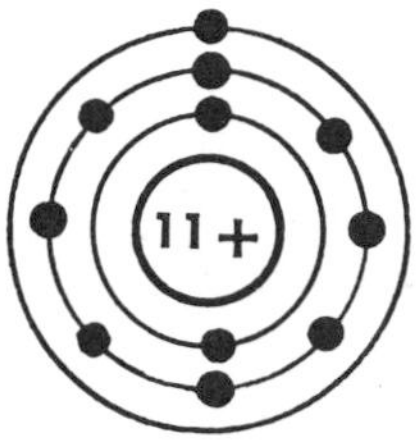

Fig. 4-4. Diagram of the sodium atom. Why is it necessary to know the atomic number before an atomic diagram can be constructed?

The sodium atom has an atomic weight of 23 and an atomic number of 11. Remembering that the second electron shell can contain only 8 electrons and proceeding as we did in the above examples, we see that the sodium atom can be represented as shown in Fig. 4-4. Since the atomic weight is 23 we know that the nucleus contains 23 heavy subatomic particles.

THE QUANTUM MECHANICAL CONCEPT OF ATOMIC STRUCTURE

As already mentioned, the model of the atom as a nucleus surrounded by electrons revolving in orbit was suggested by a 27-year-old Danish physicist, Niels Bohr, in 1913. Since the 1920s, however, scientists have agreed that a different model is more useful in predicting the properties of atoms. Fortunately, the relatively simple Bohr model still is highly useful, both to the practicing chemist and to the student. As a matter of fact, it is not possible to draw or to describe exactly how an atom would look if it could be seen. The diagrams used by chemists are only aids to understanding and predicting the properties of atoms.

In both models the major portion of the mass of the atom is located in an exceedingly tiny nucleus. Electrons are distributed around this positively charged nucleus; most of the time they are to be found at enormous distances (on the size scale of electrons and nuclei) away from it. For example, the radii of atoms are about 10,000 to 100,000 times the radii of their nuclei. To put these figures into perspective, suppose we make a dot whose radius is 1 mm at the bottom of a wall on the first floor of a modern office building. This dot symbolizes the nucleus of an atom. The so-called "outer boundary" of this symbolic atom then would be located somewhere between the fourth floor and the thirty-first floor of the building.

Studies based largely on investigations of the radiant energy (visible light, ultraviolet radiation, infrared radiation, and so on) emitted when atoms are "excited" led to the foundations of the quantum theory. Atoms are capable of existing only in certain energy (see Chapter 7) states. Stated differently, atoms can absorb or emit energy only in definite quanta (discrete "bundles" of energy).

It requires energy to move an electron farther away from the nucleus of the atom. This is so because the positively charged nucleus attracts the negatively charged electron and resists increasing the distance between them. When an electron is so moved, the atom is said to be *excited*. That is, it has gained energy. If it returns to a position closer to the nucleus, energy is released in the form of photons (quantized packets of radiant energy).

According to the Heisenberg uncertainty principle, the position of an electron in an atom at any given instant of time cannot be specified exactly. It is possible, however, to define mathematically a region of space in relation to the nucleus in which the electron will be present most (say, 95 percent) of the time. The probability is 1 (certainty; 100 percent) that the electron is *somewhere* in space. It is highly probable, of course, that it is relatively close to the nucleus.

Each solution of the mathematical equations used in calculating these probabilities contains a set of values for 4 numbers, called quantum numbers. These numbers, represented by n, l, m, and n, can have the following possible values:

$n = 1, 2, 3, 4, 5, \ldots$, any whole number

$l = 0, 1, 2, 3, 4, \ldots, n - 1$

$m = +1, (l - 1), (l - 2), \ldots, 0, \ldots, (-l + 2), (-l + 1), -1$

$s = +1/2, -1/2$

Each energy state permitted by the quantum theory is described by a set of values for these 4 quantum numbers.

The number n is known as the *main quantum number*. It determines, at least to a large extent, the energy corresponding to an allowed quantum state. A value of $n - 1$ represents the lowest permitted energy state of the electron. The number l is related to the distance from the nucleus. The larger the value of l, the higher the probability that the electron will be at a distance far from the nucleus. The number m has to do with the direction in space in which an electron would most probably be located, especially if it were exposed to a magnet. The number s is called the *spin quantum number*. Electrons can be thought of as spinning around an axis. In each energy level, s has a value of $+1/2$ or $-1/2$, indicating that the electron is spinning in a clockwise direction or in a counterclockwise direction.

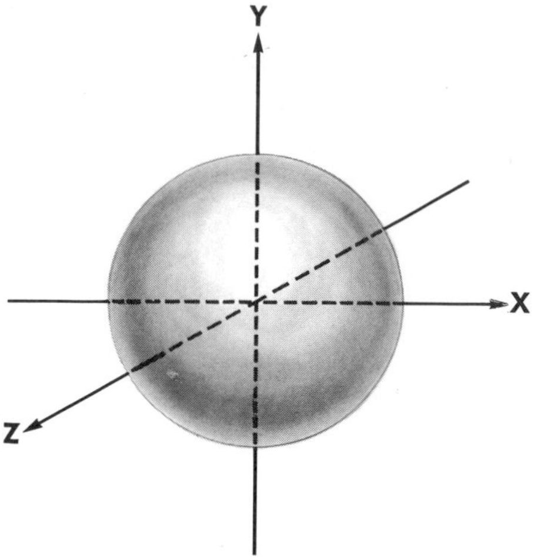

Fig. 4-5. Diagram of the hydrogen atom. An electron charge cloud is shown. It depicts the region in which there is a high probability that the electron is located at any given time. The *most probable* location in the cloud (that is, the region most often occupied by the electron) turns out to be the surface of a sphere that is the exact distance from the nucleus as the first electron shell in the Bohr model. This diagram serves equally well to indicate the shape of an *s* orbital, since the hydrogen atom has only a single *s* orbital in its resting state. Could you construct a diagram of a region in space in which there is a 100 percent probability that the electron will be at all times located?

For each value of the main quantum number n there are a number of sets of values for the 4 quantum numbers: 2 for $n = 1$; 8 for $n = 2$; 18 for $n = 3$; 32 for $n = 4$; and so on. These are exactly the numbers of electrons required to fill the shells of atoms in their stable states as pictured in the Bohr theory.

The lowest electron energy state of the simplest atom (hydrogen, which has only 1 electron) is represented by $1s$. (The 1 is the value for n; m and l are 0.) We can calculate the probability that an electron in this state will be inside of a certain region of space most (say, 95 percent) of the time. This space can be represented pictorially as shown in Fig. 4-5. For the hydrogen atom in its lowest energy state, the space (often called an *electron charge cloud*) is a sphere surrounding the nucleus. This diagram is not a *quantitative* one. Assuming the nucleus to be represented in such a diagram as a tiny dot, the "actual" cloud would be enormously larger than the one depicted. The drawing does illustrate the shape of the space, however.

It is customary to denote energy levels for which l has a value of 0 as *s;* for $l = 1$, the level is *p;* for $l = 2$, the level is *d;* and for $l = 3$, the level is *f.** The value for n is given by a whole number (1, 2, 3, 4, and so on). Thus the lowest energy state is $1s$. The energy state for which $n = 2$ and

*The letters *s, p, d,* and *f* are the first letters of the words sharp, principal, diffuse, and fundamental. These words were used to describe spectral patterns of radiant energy emitted when atoms were "excited" by elevated temperatures.

$l = 1$ is a higher energy state designated as $2p$. Similarly, an energy state for which $n = 3$ and $l = 0$ is $3s$; if $n = 3$ and $l = 2$, the energy state is $3d$; if $n = 4$ and $l = 3$, the level is $4f$; and so on.

Theoretically the electron in a hydrogen atom can exist at any possible energy level. Of course it is necessary for the atom to absorb energy to move the electron from the $1s$ level to higher levels; this absorbed energy is released, in part or altogether, as quanta (photons) of radiant energy (energies of permitted wavelengths) when the electron "falls back" to lower energy levels.

The term *electron shell* is defined in quantum mechanics as the collection of all sets of values for the 4 quantum numbers with a given value of n. This means that the first electron shell includes all energy states for which $n = 1$; the second shell includes states for $n = 2$; and so on. There is no theoretical limit for the value of n, but the highest value is 7 for the most stable states of atoms of atomic number 87 and above.*

An important law of quantum mechanics, the *Pauli exclusion principle*, states that, in a given atom, no 2 electrons can have the same set of values for the 4 quantum numbers. This rule really establishes the maximal number of electrons that can occupy the various electron shells (2, 8, 18, 32, and so on).

The *electron subshell* denotes the sets of values of the 4 quantum numbers that correspond to the same values for both n and l. Thus the $2s$ energy state ($n = 2$ and $l = 0$) forms the $2s$ subshell; the $2p$ energy state ($n = 2$ and $l = 1$) forms the $2p$ subshell. Each s subshell has a capacity of 2 electrons; each p subshell can contain 6 electrons; each d subshell can contain 10 electrons; and each f subshell can have 14 electrons. s Subshells occur in all of the 7 shells found in atoms of atomic number 87 and above; p subshells occur in shells 2 through 6; d subshells are present in shells 3 through 6; and f subshells occur only in shells 4 and 5.

The term *electron orbital* applies to each pair of sets of values for the 4 quantum numbers where the values for n, l, and m are the same. They differ only in that the value for s for one set is $+1/2$ and for the other set is $-1/2$. Thus electrons occupying the same orbitals will differ from each other only in having opposite spins. In agreement with the Pauli exclusion principle, no more than 2 electrons can occupy a single orbital. An orbital thus can contain 0, 1, or 2 electrons. Each s subshell contains 1 orbital; each p subshell contains 3 orbitals located at right angles to each other in space (p_x, p_y, and p_z, where x, y, and z are the usual coordinates of three-dimensional space); each d subshell contains 5 orbitals; and each f subshell has 7 orbitals.

Hund's rule states that, in a given atom, electrons in the same subshell will occupy orbitals with different values of m and their spins will not pair up unless the number of available orbitals of the same energy level requires that 2 electrons occupy a single orbital. This rule can be illustrated by noting

*The shells also are identified, as in the Bohr model, by the capital letters K (first shell), L (second shell), M (third shell), and so on.

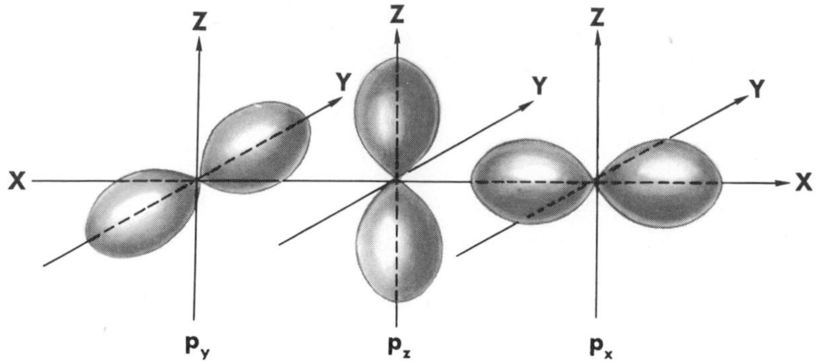

Fig. 4-6. Electron charge cloud for electrons in the three *p* orbitals. The x, y, and z indicate the usual axes of 3-dimensional space. How many electrons can occupy a single *p* orbital?

the arrangement of the 8 electrons in the most stable state of an oxygen atom. The 1*s* orbital contains 2 electrons; the 2*s* orbital contains 2. There are 3 2*p* orbitals, which must contain the remaining 4 electrons. The $2p_x$ orbital thus contains 2 electrons; there is 1 electron in the $2p_y$ orbital; and 1 electron occupies the $2p_z$ orbital. The last two electrons, then, did not occupy a single orbital, because there was an empty orbital of the same subshell available for each of them. The 2*p* orbitals have different orientations in space and, hence, different *m* values. The $2p_y$ and $2p_z$ orbitals of the oxygen atom contain only 1 electron each and can participate in chemical bonding (see page 95).

Electron charge cloud diagrams indicating the shapes and spatial relationships of some of the orbitals for different energy levels of the hydrogen atom are illustrated in Figs. 4-5, 4-6, and 4-7. Remember that these clouds represent the shapes of the volumes in space in which the electrons will be located most (say, 95 percent) of the time.

The *exact* shapes of the orbitals of atoms of the other elements have not been worked out mathematically, but approximations have been made. Probably the orbitals calculated for hydrogen are very similar in shape to those of the other elements.

ISOTOPES

If we look at the table of atomic weights (page 474) we find that the atomic weight of chlorine is 35.453. How many heavy subatomic particles occur in the nucleus of this atom? Should this number be taken as 35 or as 36? Scientists have found that there are really two different kinds of chlorine atoms. One kind contains 35 large particles and another kind contains 37. Ordinarily, both kinds of atoms, *which have nearly identical chemical properties*, are present in a given sample of chlorine in proportions such that the *average* number of heavy particles per atom is 35.453. These two kinds of chlorine atoms are called *isotopes*. Probably all of the elements exist in the form of isotopes.

The hydrogen atom, as we have seen, usually contains 1 heavy particle in its nucleus. Every sample of hydrogen, however, contains a few

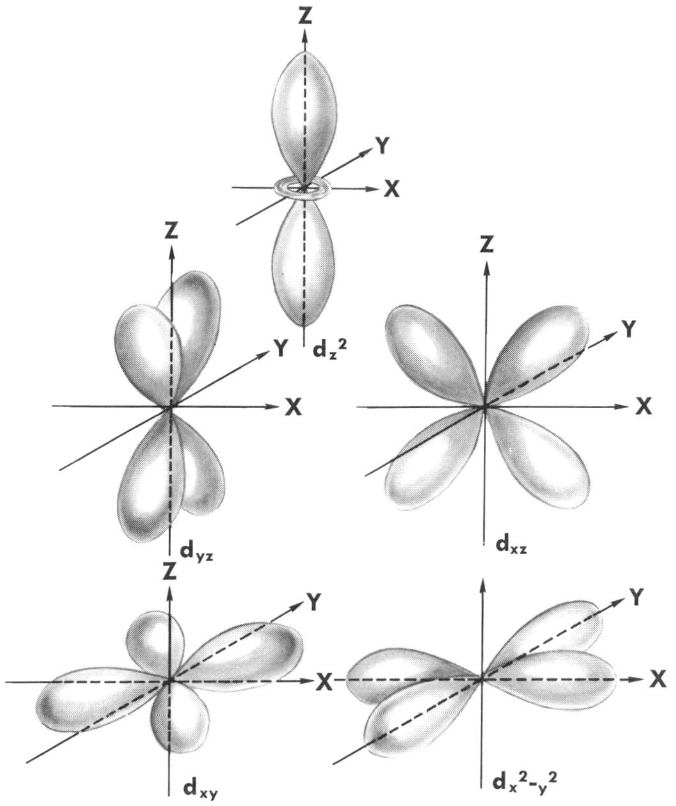

Fig. 4-7. Electron charge clouds for electrons in the five *d* orbitals. How many electrons are required to fill all five *d* orbitals?

hydrogen atoms that have 2 heavy particles in their nuclei. This "heavy hydrogen" is known as *deuterium* and its nucleus is spoken of as a *deuteron*. Water containing heavy hydrogen as a part of its molecule is called "heavy water," or deuterium oxide. Any sample of water collected at random contains extremely small amounts of deuterium oxide.

A heavy isotope of nitrogen, having an atomic weight of 15 (^{15}N) instead of the common atomic weight of 14 (^{14}N), is used in labeling or tagging chemical compounds so that they can be used in biochemical experimentation. (See page 95 for a discussion of the experimental use of isotopes.)

VAN DER WAALS FORCES

As we have seen, molecules contain negative and positive charges distributed in and around themselves in space. When molecules come very close together they exhibit a weak attraction for each other. This is caused by the fact that the negative charges of one molecule attract the positive charges of the other, and vice versa. This attraction is said to be caused by *van der Waals* forces. This name is used because the Dutch physicist, J. D. van der Waals (1837–1923), first gave a thorough discussion of the importance of these forces in explaining the behavior of gases and liquids.

The temperature to which a liquid must be raised to cause its molecules

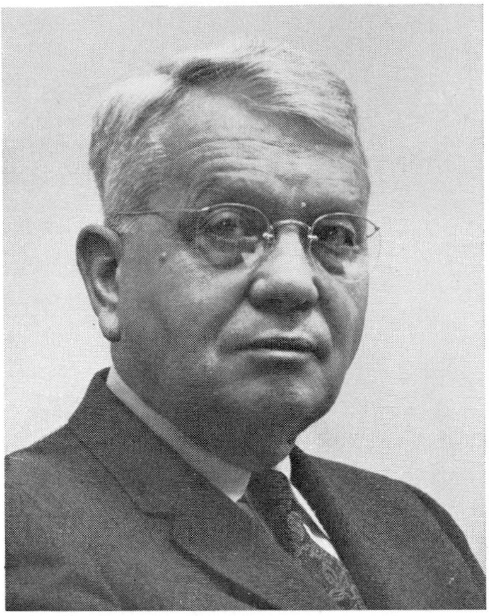

Fig. 4-8. Dr. H. C. Urey, who was awarded the Nobel Prize in 1934 for his work in separating heavy water from naturally occurring water. What is the molecular weight of heavy water?

to fly apart (that is, to cause the liquid to boil) is a measure of the strength of the van der Waals forces, since these tend to hold the molecules close to each other. In general, the van der Waals forces increase in proportion to the number of electrons per molecule. Hence, heavy molecules ordinarily attract one another more strongly than do lighter ones. As a rule, compounds of high molecular weight have high boiling temperatures, and compounds of low molecular weight have low ones.

The van der Waals forces are quite weak—much weaker than the forces uniting the atoms in molecules (see pages 34 and 90). Occasionally a molecule will become agitated enough to fly away from its neighbors. These free molecules make up the vapor that always occurs in the vicinity of a liquid—and to a lesser extent in the vicinity of a solid. This explains how substances can evaporate even at temperatures far below the boiling point.

STUDY QUESTIONS

1. State three assumptions of the atomic theory.
2. Who first advanced the atomic theory?
3. What is an atom? A molecule?
4. Explain how mass differs from weight.
5. What element has been adopted as a standard in computing atomic weights? What is its atomic weight?
6. The nitrogen atom is $7/8$ as heavy as the oxygen atom. What is the atomic weight of nitrogen?
7. Name five gases that exist as molecules containing 2 atoms each.
8. Carbon dioxide molecules contain 1 atom of carbon and 2 atoms of oxygen. What is the molecular weight of carbon dioxide?
9. What is Avogadro's law?
10. Carbon has an atomic weight of 12 and an atomic number of 6. Draw a diagram of the carbon atom. How many heavy subatomic particles are in its nucleus?
11. Phosphorus has an atomic weight of 31 and

an atomic number of 15. Draw a diagram of the phosphorus atom. How many heavy subatomic particles are in its nucleus?

12. What letters are used to designate the 4 quantum numbers?
13. What numerical value can each of the quantum numbers have?
14. What does quantum number *n* determine?
15. Which quantum number has a relationship to direction in space?
16. To what quantity is quantum number *l* related? Quantum number *s*?
17. What is the "electron charge cloud"?
18. What is the significance of the letters *s*, *p*, *d*, and *f*?
19. How is the *electron shell* defined in quantum mechanics?
20. State the Pauli exclusion principle. State Hund's rule and explain it.
21. What is an electron subshell?
22. Define electron orbital.
23. Why can the electron charge cloud for the hydrogen atom be used to illustrate the *s* orbital?
24. What are isotopes?
25. How does deuterium oxide differ from ordinary water?
26. What is meant by an anti-particle?
27. Explain in your own words the meaning of van der Waals forces.

CHAPTER 5

Chemical shorthand and the concept of valence

ATOMIC SYMBOL

Chemists use symbols to represent the various elements. In some cases the symbol is merely the first letter of the element's name. The symbol for hydrogen is H, for sulfur it is S, for oxygen it is O, and for carbon it is C. It is obvious that not all elements can be abbreviated by the first letter of their names since there are 105 elements and only 26 letters in the alphabet. No symbol, however, is longer than two letters. The symbol for chlorine is Cl; Br is the symbol for bromine; Mn is the symbol for manganese. Some symbols are derived from the Latin names of the elements. *Argentum* is the Latin name for silver, and the symbol for silver is Ag. The symbol for mercury is Hg, the Latin name of this element being *hydrargyrum.* Fe, an abbreviation of the Latin word *ferrum,* is the symbol for iron. Notice that the first letter of each symbol is written as a capital letter. If a second letter is present it is written as a small letter.

These symbols are known as *atomic symbols.* The atomic symbol is more than an abbreviation for the element. H means hydrogen, of course, but it also means 1 *atom* of hydrogen. Ag means 1 atom of silver. Sometimes the chemists use this symbol to mean *1 gram-atomic weight* of silver. If we desire to indicate 2 *atoms* of silver we write 2 Ag; 3 Fe means 3 atoms of iron, or 3 *gram-atomic weights* of iron. *The number 1 is never written in chemical shorthand.*

The atomic symbols for some of the common elements are given in Table 5-1. All the information given in this table *must* be memorized by the student.

FORMULA FOR THE COMPOUND

Suppose we are told that 1 molecule of water contains 2 atoms of hydrogen and 1 atom of oxygen. What will be the chemical shorthand symbol that gives this information? The symbol for *1 molecule of water* is H_2O. The small subscript 2 that *follows* the H indicates that there are 2 atoms of

Table 5-1. Symbols and valences of some elements and radicals

Name	Symbol	Usual valence
Metals		
Aluminum	Al	3+
Barium	Ba	2+
Calcium	Ca	2+
Copper	Cu	1+ or 2+
Iron	Fe	2+ or 3+
Lead	Pb	2+
Magnesium	Mg	2+
Mercury	Hg	1+ or 2+
Potassium	K	1+
Silver	Ag	1+
Sodium	Na	1+
Zinc	Zn	2+
Nonmetals		
Bromine	Br	1−
Chlorine	Cl	1−
Hydrogen	H	1+
Iodine	I	1−
Oxygen	O	2−
Sulfur	S	2−, 4+, or 6+
Radicals		
Ammonium	NH_4	1+
Bicarbonate	HCO_3	1−
Carbonate	CO_3	2−
Hydroxyl	OH	1−
Nitrate	NO_3	1−
Nitrite	NO_2	1−
Phosphate	PO_4	3−
Sulfate	SO_4	2−
Sulfite	SO_3	2−

hydrogen in each molecule of water. Since there is only 1 oxygen atom in each molecule we do not need to place a subscript after the O. As we have seen, when no number is written before or after a symbol, the number 1 is understood. Stated completely in words, then, H_2O means "1 molecule of water made up of 2 atoms of hydrogen and 1 atom of oxygen." This same symbol is also used to mean "1 gram-molecular weight of water that contains 2 gram-atomic weights of hydrogen and 1 gram-atomic weight of oxygen." The formula for sucrose, or cane sugar, is $C_{12}H_{22}O_{11}$. This means "1 molecule of sucrose made up of 12 atoms of carbon, 22 atoms of hydrogen, and 11 atoms of oxygen," or it may mean "1 gram-molecular weight of sucrose that contains 12 gram-atomic weights of carbon, 22 gram-atomic weights of hydrogen, and 11 gram-atomic weights of oxygen." Notice again that the small subscript numbers are written *after* the atomic symbols to which they belong. Remember that these numbers indicate the number of atoms in *1 molecule* of the compound, or the number of gram-atomic weights in *1 gram-molecular weight* of the compound.

The expression 2 $C_{12}H_{22}O_{11}$ means 2 *molecules* of sucrose. The formula

3 H_2O means *3 molecules* of water. The number, then, that is written in front of the formula for the compound tells us how many molecules, or gram-molecular weights, are indicated. *Do not confuse the small subscript numbers with the larger numbers written in front of the formulas, which indicate the number of molecules.*

CONCEPT OF VALENCE

There is a difference in the number of atoms that can combine in molecules of different compounds. Let us consider the following chemical compounds:

HCl	H_2O	NH_3	CH_4
Hydrochloric acid	Water	Ammonia	Methane

It is evident that 1 atom of chlorine is capable of combining with 1 atom of hydrogen; 1 atom of oxygen can combine with 2 hydrogen atoms; 1 atom of nitrogen can combine with 3 hydrogen atoms; and 1 atom of carbon can unite with 4 hydrogen atoms. If an element will combine with hydrogen *the maximal number of hydrogen atoms that will combine with 1 atom of the element is said to be the valence of the element.* In the foregoing examples the valence of chlorine is 1; of oxygen, 2; of nitrogen, 3; and of carbon, 4. The valence of hydrogen is 1.

Hydrogen will not combine with all other elements. Ordinarily it will not, for example, combine with sodium. How are we to determine the valence of sodium? Both sodium and hydrogen will combine with certain elements, for instance, with chlorine.

$NaCl$	HCl
Sodium chloride	Hydrochloric acid

We see by inspecting the above formulas that 1 sodium atom can combine with 1 chlorine atom. One hydrogen atom also combines with 1 chlorine atom. In other words, the combining power, or valence, of sodium is the same as that of hydrogen. Since we know that hydrogen has a valence of 1, sodium must also have a valence of 1. Calcium chloride has the formula $CaCl_2$. Since the calcium atom can combine with twice as many chlorine atoms as the hydrogen atom can, we know that the valence of calcium is 2.

The elements can be divided into two groups as respects their valence. *Elements that combine with hydrogen are said to have negative valence; hydrogen and the elements that ordinarily do not combine with hydrogen are said to have positive valence.* In the preceding examples hydrogen, sodium, and calcium have positive valence. Chlorine, oxygen, nitrogen, and carbon have negative valence.

Metals are elements characterized by their luster and by their ability to conduct heat and electricity well. Many of the metals, such as iron, copper, silver, gold, and tin, are well known to all of us. In general, hydrogen and the metals have positive valence. The other elements, called nonmetals, usually have negative valence. *When an element is not combined with any other element it is considered to have zero valence.*

The number of positive valences in a given compound must equal the number of negative ones. This rule is of great assistance in writing the formulas of compounds. The valence of aluminum is 3+, and the valence of chlorine is 1−. Three chlorine atoms will combine with 1 aluminum atom to form aluminum chloride, which has the formula $AlCl_3$. We cannot write $AlCl_2$ as the formula for aluminum chloride because this formula contains 3 positive valences (the valence of aluminum is 3) and only 2 negative valences (the valence of each chlorine atom is 1). We *must* write $AlCl_3$.

It is customary in writing formulas to write the symbol of the element having positive valence first.

Some of the elements commonly have more than one valence. Mercury forms two compounds with chlorine. HgCl is called mercurous chloride, or calomel, and the mercury in this compound has a valence of 1+. $HgCl_2$ is mercuric chloride, or bichloride of mercury; here the mercury has a valence of 2+. Iron commonly has a valence of 2+ or 3+. $FeCl_2$ is ferrous chloride and $FeCl_3$ is ferric chloride.

STRUCTURAL FORMULA

So far the formulas we have considered have been *empirical formulas*. They have indicated the kind and number of atoms present in a molecule of the compound, but they have not indicated how these atoms are joined together. Chemists also make use of the *structural formula*. This type of shorthand gives all the information the empirical formula does but, as the name implies, it also illustrates the *structure* of the molecule—it indicates the way in which the various atoms are connected with each other. The valence is indicated by means of a short straight line called a *bond*. The number of bonds leaving, or connected with, each atom is equal to the valence of the atom. Each bond must be connected with 2 atoms; that is, there must be no free bonds left over.

NaCl Sodium chloride (Empirical formula)	Na—Cl Sodium chloride (Structural formula)
H_2O Water (Empirical formula)	H—O—H Water (Structural formula)
FeI_3 Ferric iodide (Empirical formula)	I—Fe—I │ I Ferric iodide (Structural formula)

CHEMICAL EQUATION

The chemical equation is a symbolic way of expressing what happens when chemical substances react to form new substances. It tells us what atoms or molecules are reacting with each other. The number of atoms or molecules concerned is indicated. If we like we can regard the reaction as taking place between gram-atomic weights and gram-molecular weights instead of between single atoms and molecules. This allows us to compute the number of grams of new substances that will be formed from known weights of the reacting substances.

The method of writing an equation can best be indicated by means of an example. Suppose we assemble the equation that represents the reaction between silver fluoride and barium chloride to form barium fluoride and silver chloride.

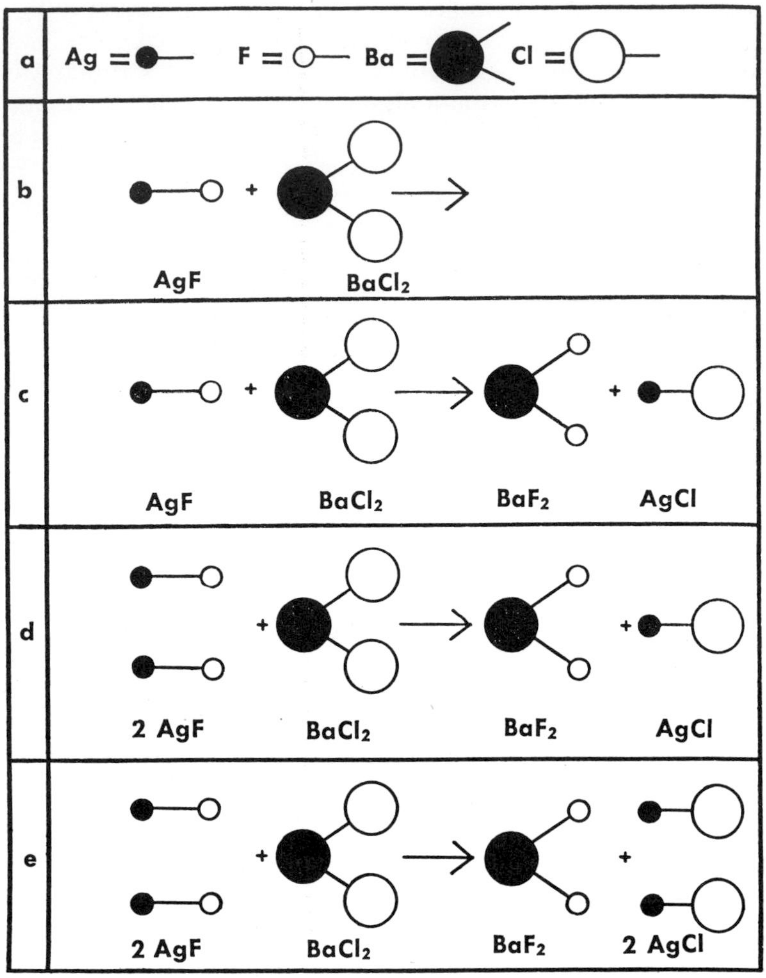

Fig. 5-1. Diagram illustrating the steps in writing and balancing a chemical equation. Why must the equation be balanced?

Step 1. As the left-hand member of the equation, write down the formulas for silver fluoride and barium chloride, separating them by a + sign. After the barium chloride, we draw an arrow to indicate that the remainder of the equation refers to the products that are formed by the reaction (Fig. 5-1, *a* and *b*).

AgF		$BaCl_2$	
(Silver fluoride)	+	(Barium chloride)	→
126.87*		208.25	

*The numbers written beneath the formulas of the various compounds are molecular weights (see table of atomic weights on page 38). In writing equations it is unnecessary to indicate molecular weights unless special calculations are planned (see page 38).

Step 2. As the right-hand member of the equation write down the formulas for barium fluoride and silver chloride, again separating them by + symbols (Fig. 5-1, *c*).

$$\begin{array}{ccccccc} AgF & + & BaCl_2 & \rightarrow & BaF_2 & + & AgCl \\ 126.85 & & 208.25 & & \text{(Barium fluoride)} & & \text{(Silver chloride)} \\ & & & & 175.34 & & 143.32 \end{array}$$

Step 3. A very important chemical law, known as the *law of conservation of matter*, states that matter (that is, atoms or anything composed of them) can neither be created nor destroyed by a chemical reaction. This means that when a chemical reaction occurs, the number and kind of atoms in the reacting substances must be the same as the number and kind of atoms in the substances formed by the reaction. In other words, the number of each kind of atom must be the same on both the left and the right side of the arrow. As the third step, then, we must *balance* the equation. Looking at our equation as it now exists, we see that there is 1 fluorine atom on the left of the arrow and 2 fluorine atoms on the right. The law of conservation of matter tells us that we cannot create a fluorine atom. The only way 2 fluorine atoms could be present when the reaction is over is for 2 such atoms to have been present before the reaction occurred. Before the preceding reaction can occur, therefore, we must have 2 *molecules* of silver fluoride. Since each molecule of this compound contains 1 fluorine atom 2 molecules will contain 2 fluorine atoms. Accordingly, we change our equation to read (Fig. 5-1, *d*):

$$\begin{array}{ccccccc} 2\ AgF & + & BaCl_2 & \rightarrow & BaF_2 & + & AgCl \\ 253.70 & & 208.25 & & 175.34 & & 143.32 \\ (2 \times 126.87) & & & & & & \end{array}$$

Now we observe that, by starting with 2 molecules of silver fluoride instead of 1, we have arranged matters so that the number of fluorine atoms is the same on both sides of the arrow. Inspection shows us, however, that we have 2 chlorine atoms on the left-hand side of the equation and only 1 on the right-hand side. If we start out with 2 atoms of chlorine, we must end up with 2 of them. This means that 2 *molecules* of silver chloride must have been formed, since each molecule contains only 1 chlorine atom. Again we modify our equation to read (Fig. 5-1, *e*):

$$\begin{array}{ccccccc} 2\ AgF & + & BaCl_2 & \rightarrow & BaF_2 & + & 2\ AgCl \\ 253.70 & & 208.25 & & 175.34 & & 286.64 \\ & & & & & & (2 \times 143.32) \end{array}$$

Now we see that the number of each kind of atom is the same on both sides of the equation. That is, the equation is *balanced.*

Many beginning students attempt to balance equations by changing the small subscript numbers used to indicate the number of atoms *in a single molecule*. For example, it might appear at first thought that the unbalanced equation,

$$AgF + BaCl_2 \rightarrow BaF_2 + AgCl$$

could be balanced by changing it to read,

$$AgF_2 + BaCl_2 \rightarrow BaF_2 + AgCl_2$$

This cannot under any circumstances be done, however, because AgF_2 is *not* the correct formula for silver fluroide (since it represents a molecule containing 1 positive valence and 2 negative valences), nor is $AgCl_2$ the correct formula for silver chloride. The correct formulas for these two compounds are AgF and AgCl, respectively. In other words, the only correct procedure to be used in balancing an equation, assuming that all formulas have been written correctly, is to vary the numbers of molecules indicated until the number of atoms of each element are equal on both sides of the arrow. Remember that the large number written in front of each molecular formula indicates the minimal number of molecules taking part in the reaction (except that the number 1 never is written in chemical shorthand). Keep in mind also the fact that the number of molecules of any one compound required in an equation is not known until the equation is balanced correctly.

The finished equation gives other information of great value to the chemist. By using molecular weights he can predict the amount of new compound that can be formed from a given weight of starting compound. In the case of the above reaction he can predict that 253.70 g of silver fluoride will react with exactly 208.25 g of barium chloride to yield exactly 175.34 g of barium fluoride and 286.64 g of silver chloride. Notice that the molecular weights of silver fluoride and of silver chloride have been doubled, since the equation indicates that 2 molecules (or 2 gram-molecular weights) of each are required for the reaction. Since only 1 molecule of barium chloride and 1 of barium fluoride occur in the equation the molecular weights of these compounds have *not* been doubled.

By using simple arithmetic, other similar calculations can be made. For example, suppose a chemist wishes to prepare 10 g of silver chloride, using the above reaction. How much barium chloride will be required? Since 10 g is $^{10}/_{286.64}$ of the amount of silver chloride present in the 2 gram-molecular weights indicated in the preceding equation, then $^{10}/_{286.64} \times 208.25\text{ g} = 7.27\text{ g}$ of barium chloride will be necessary. It will be noted that 208.25 is the molecular weight of barium chloride. Similarly $^{10}/_{286.64} \times 253.70$ (twice the molecular weight of AgF) = the amount of silver fluoride necessary.

RADICALS

Groups of atoms that cling together and act in chemical reactions as though they were really only 1 atom are called *radicals*. Sulfuric acid has the formula H_2SO_4. If we allow it to react with calcium chloride,

$CaCl_2$	+	H_2SO_4	→	$CaSO_4$	+	2 HCl
Calcium chloride		Sulfuric acid		Calcium sulfate		Hydrochloric acid

we see that the SO_4 group of atoms has traded hydrogen atoms for a calcium atom. The SO_4 group of atoms is called the *sulfate radical*. Other examples of radicals include the hydroxyl radical (OH), the nitrate radical (NO_3), the ammonium radical (NH_4), the sulfite radical (SO_3), and the nitrite radical (NO_2). From the preceding formula we see that 1 sulfate radical can combine with 2 hydrogen atoms. The valence of this radical must therefore be 2− since the valence of hydrogen is 1+. We can determine the valence of a radical in another way. The valence of oxygen is 2− and the valence of hydrogen is 1+. The valence of the OH radical will be 1− because there is only 1 hydrogen atom present and this atom can neutralize only 1 of the 2 negative valences of the oxygen atom. This leaves 1 negative valence unbalanced by a positive one.

In a chemical formula when there are 2 or more of the same radical in a molecule, parentheses are placed around the radical symbol, and the number of radicals present in the molecule is indicated by a subscript

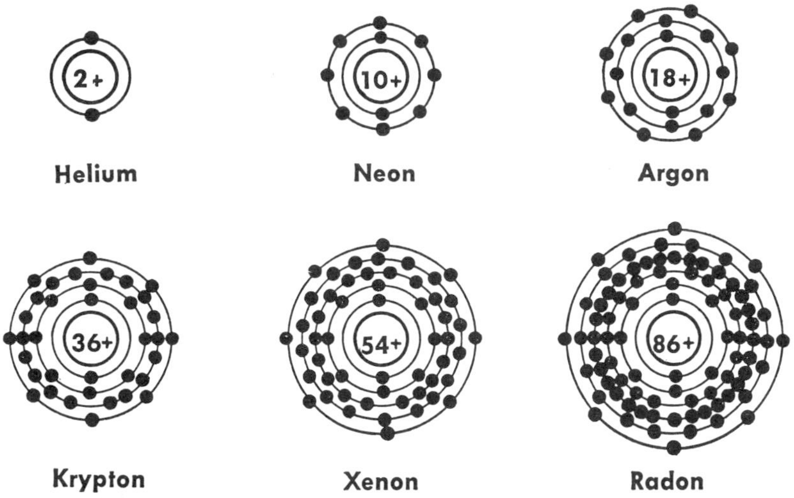

Fig. 5-2. Diagrams of the atomic structures of the rare gases. How many electrons are there in the outer electron shells of each of these atoms?

number written *after* the parentheses. The formula for ammonium sulfate is $(NH_4)_2SO_4$. This compound contains 2 ammonium radicals, which is indicated by placing parentheses around the NH_4 and writing the subscript 2. Since only 1 sulfate radical is present we do not have to place parentheses around the SO_4.

PREDICTION OF THE PRODUCTS OF REACTION

In the foregoing discussion it has been assumed that the products of the reactions mentioned were known. Frequently we are able to predict in advance what these products will be. Suppose potassium iodide (KI) reacts with silver nitrate ($AgNO_3$). What will be the products of the reaction? We recall that there must be both positive and negative valences in a molecule of a compound. Therefore, potassium, which has positive valence, must react with something that has negative valence. In this example we know that potassium will unite with the nitrate radical, NO_3, to form potassium nitrate, KNO_3, because the silver has positive valence. For the same reason the silver will unite with the iodine to form silver iodide, AgI.

RELATIONSHIP BETWEEN VALENCE AND ATOMIC STRUCTURE

Atoms are most stable chemically when the outer electron shell is completely filled. Certain of the elements, known as the rare gases, have their outer shells filled, and these elements are so stable that it is difficult to make them react with other elements; indeed, until recent years it was thought that they were completely nonreactive (Fig. 5-2). The rare gases are helium, neon, argon, krypton, xenon, and radon. Notice that all of these gases have 8 electrons in the outer electron shell.* Since these are the most stable of all the atoms, we conclude that *an atom is in its most stable state when its outer electron shell contains 8 electrons.*

*Helium has only 2 electrons; it will be remembered that the first electron shell can contain only 2 electrons.

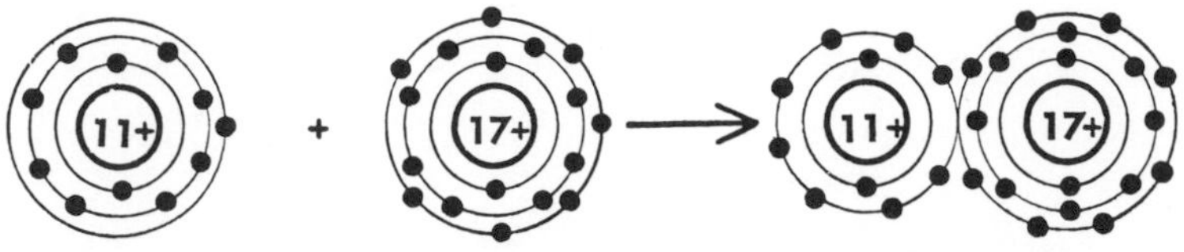

Fig. 5-3. Diagram of the reaction of a sodium atom with a chlorine atom to form a sodium chloride molecule. Why is the sodium atom said to have zero valence before the reaction and a valence of 1+ after the reaction has taken place?

The most probable valence of an atom is determined, then, by the number of planetary electrons in its outer shell. The sodium atom has 1 electron in its outer shell; the chlorine atom has 7. When sodium reacts with chlorine to form sodium chloride, the sodium atom contributes its outer electron to the chlorine as illustrated by Fig. 5-3. Since the sodium atom has lost 1 electron it is left with a positive charge, and we say the sodium atom has a valence of 1+. The chlorine atom has gained 1 electron and the valence of chlorine is 1−; the two atoms are held together by electrostatic attraction.*

The outer shell of the sulfur atom contains 6 electrons. If sulfur gained 2 electrons its outer shell would be filled. The outer shell could also lose all 6 electrons; the outer shell remaining would then be filled. We guess, then, that the valence of sulfur is either 2− or 6+. As a matter of fact, sulfur has both of these valences. The most probable valence, however, is 2− since usually it is easier for the sulfur atom to gain 2 new electrons than to lose 6 of them.

Na_2S	SO_3
Sodium sulfide	Sulfur trioxide
Valence of sulfur is 2−	Valence of sulfur is 6+

The outer shell of the calcium atom contains 2 electrons. The most probable valence of calcium is 2+ because the calcium atom could complete its outer shell by losing 2 electrons. Theoretically, calcium might also gain 6 more electrons and have a valence of 6−, but compounds of calcium with this valence are not known.

*Opposite charges of electricity attract each other. This attractive force is referred to as *electrostatic attraction.*

STUDY QUESTIONS

1. Write the shorthand expression for "four atoms of calcium."
2. A molecule of aluminum oxide contains 2 atoms of aluminum and 3 atoms of oxygen. What is the formula for aluminum oxide?
3. What is the shorthand expression for "one gram-molecular weight of water"?
4. What kind of elements usually have positive valence? Negative valence?
5. What is a metal?
6. The valence of aluminum is 3+ and the valence of sulfur is 2−. What is the formula for aluminum sulfide (which is composed of aluminum and sulfur)?
7. What kind of elements are usually written first in chemical formulas?
8. Write the structural formulas for the following compounds: CaI_2, Na_2O, AlF_3.

9. Balance the following equations:

   $Cu + O_2 \rightarrow CuO$

   $Na_2CO_3 + CaCl_2 \rightarrow CaCO_3 + NaCl.$

10. Complete and balance the following equations:

    $BaBr_2 + H_2SO_4 \rightarrow$

    $NH_4Cl + Al(NO_3)_3 \rightarrow$

11. What is a radical?
12. Nitrogen contains 5 electrons in its outer shell. What is the most likely valence of nitrogen?
13. Carbon contains 4 electrons in its outer shell. What is the valence of carbon?
14. How many g of $CaCl_2$ will be required to prepare 10 g of HCl?

CHAPTER 6

Oxygen

OCCURRENCE

Oxygen is the most abundant element in the earth's surface. Eight-ninths by weight of water is oxygen. The element is a constituent of sand and rocks. All living organisms, both plant and animal, contain large amounts of oxygen, chiefly in combined form. About 21 percent of the volume of the air is free molecular oxygen. It will be recalled that oxygen gas exists as molecules, each containing 2 atoms of oxygen; the formula of free oxygen (oxygen not combined with another element) is thus O_2. The air also contains about 1 percent argon and about 78 percent nitrogen. Traces of other gases are present. Small amounts of molecular oxygen are dissolved in blood, tissue fluids, plant juices, and water.

DISCOVERY OF OXYGEN

Karl Scheele, a Swedish pharmacist, made oxygen in 1771 by heating manganese dioxide (MnO_2) and potassium nitrate (KNO_3). He did not tell the world about his discovery until six years later. In the meantime, in 1774, Joseph Priestley, an English chemist, prepared oxygen by heating mercuric oxide (HgO). Since he published his discovery at once, many people credit Priestley with the actual discovery. In 1777 Antoine Lavoisier, a Frenchman, showed that oxygen plays a vital part in respiration and in the chemical reactions that occur in living tissues.

PREPARATION

In the laboratory oxygen is usually prepared by heating potassium chlorate ($KClO_3$). If a little manganese dioxide is added, the speed of the reaction is increased. Manganese dioxide is not changed by the reaction and is, therefore, a *catalyst*.

$2\ KClO_3$	$\rightarrow$	$2\ KCl$	$+$	$3\ O_2$
Potassium chlorate		Potassium chloride		Oxygen

It must be remembered that free oxygen exists as O_2. For this reason we cannot write the equation in such a way as to suggest that oxygen *atoms*

Table 6-1. Composition of clean, dry air near sea level*

Component	Content (percent by volume)	Molecular or atomic wt
Nitrogen	78.084	28.0134
Oxygen	20.9476	31.9988
Argon	0.934	39.948
Carbon dioxide	0.0314	44.00995
Neon	0.001818	20.183
Helium	0.000524	4.0026
Krypton	0.000114	83.80
Xenon	0.0000087	131.30
Hydrogen	0.00005	2.01594
Methane	0.0002	16.04303
Nitrous oxide	0.00005	44.0128
Ozone	Summer: 0 to 0.000007	47.9982
	Winter: 0 to 0.000002	
Sulfur dioxide	0 to 0.0001	64.0628
Nitrogen dioxide	0 to 0.000002	46.0055
Ammonia	0 to trace	17.03061
Carbon monoxide	0 to trace	28.01055
Iodine	0 to 0.000001	253.8088

*From Chemical & Engineering News **44**:20A, 1966.

are produced. In other words, the following equation *is incorrect and cannot be written:*

$$KClO_3 \rightarrow KCl + 3\ O$$

Oxygen can also be prepared by Priestley's method: that is, by heating the red powder called mercuric oxide.

$$\underset{\text{Mercuric oxide}}{2\ HgO} \rightarrow \underset{\text{Mercury}}{2\ Hg} + \underset{\text{Oxygen}}{O_2}$$

When air is subjected to a sufficiently low temperature and a sufficiently high pressure it liquefies. This liquid is called liquid air. Oxygen usually is prepared commercially by allowing the more volatile nitrogen to evaporate, leaving the oxygen behind as liquid oxygen. Such oxygen is not entirely pure because traces of other gases present in air remain with it.

Another commercial method of preparing oxygen is by *electrolysis*. If an electric current is passed through water, oxygen forms at the positive electrical pole (called the *anode*) and hydrogen forms at the negative electrical pole (called the *cathode*). Since each molecule of water contains 2 atoms of hydrogen and only 1 atom of oxygen, the volume of hydrogen produced is twice the volume of oxygen produced.

PROPERTIES

Oxygen is a colorless, odorless gas. It is slightly heavier than air. It has no taste and is perfectly transparent. It is soluble enough in water to support aquatic life, and to diffuse from the bloodstream to the tissue cells in animals.

At ordinary temperatures the gas is not particularly active chemically, although it will combine rapidly with certain elements (such as phosphorus, sodium, and potassium) under these circumstances. It is very reactive, however, at higher temperatures, uniting directly with almost all the other elements. Oxygen unites readily with many compounds in plant and animal tissues, and these reactions are catalyzed by *enzymes*. It combines slowly with iron at ordinary temperatures, particularly in the presence of moisture, to form rust (ferric oxide, Fe_2O_3).

VITAL IMPORTANCE

Oxygen is absolutely necessary for life. People have lived for several weeks without food and for several days without water, but no one can live more than a few minutes without oxygen. In the presence of enzymes oxygen unites with many substances found in the cells to produce new tissue and change old tissue into substances that can be eliminated from the body. The energy required to make muscles contract, glands secrete, and nerves conduct impulses comes from reactions involving oxygen.

Many substances in the body contain carbon and hydrogen. When these elements unite with oxygen, water (H_2O) and carbon dioxide (CO_2) are formed. Carbon dioxide is eliminated in the expired air, and water is eliminated through the lungs, the skin (perspiration), and by the kidneys (urine).

BURNING

We frequently say that many substances are "burned" in the body. We mean by this that these substances unite with oxygen in the tissues. Burning also is used to mean any chemical reaction in which sufficient heat is produced to cause the products of the reaction to vaporize and to emit light. This mixture of hot gases that is emitting light is the *flame*. Burning usually takes place when oxygen is one of the reacting substances, but reactions involving burning are known in which this element is not present. Hydrogen will burn in the presence of chlorine to form hydrogen chloride (HCl). When hydrogen chloride, which is a gas, is dissolved in water it forms hydrochloric acid.

KINDLING TEMPERATURE

As we have seen, oxygen does not unite readily with most substances at room temperature. The temperature to which a substance must be raised before it begins to burn, or combine rapidly with oxygen, is called the *kindling temperature*. A burning match will light a cigarette simply because the heat produced by the reaction between the wood of the match and oxygen yields sufficient heat to raise the temperature of the tobacco in the cigarette to its kindling temperature. Substances like ether and gasoline, that have low kindling temperatures, are said to be *inflammable*. A *noninflammable substance* is one that either has combined already with all the oxygen possible for it or whose kindling temperature is too high to be reached under ordinary circumstances. Stone and asbestos are examples of noninflammable materials.

Fire hazards are produced when materials with low kindling temperatures are not sufficiently protected from temperature changes. The hay in a farmer's barn is always uniting slowly with oxygen. If the heat produced does not escape readily, the hay may become heated to such an extent that the entire pile catches fire.

EXTINGUISHING FIRES

Fires can be extinguished either by separating the material that is burning from oxygen or by lowering the temperature to a value below the kindling temperature of the burning material. Water puts out fires by lowering the temperature. Many fire extinguishers contain chemicals that react to produce carbon dioxide (CO_2) gas, which is heavier than air and settles down over the burning material, separating it from its oxygen supply. Some extinguishers contain a liquid known as carbon tetrachloride (CCl_4). When carbon tetrachloride is thrown on the fire, the heat vaporizes it, and the resulting gas, which is heavier than air, surrounds the fire and prevents contact with oxygen. Gasoline fires cannot be extinguished with water because the gasoline, being lighter than water, floats on the surface and unites so violently with oxygen that the water beneath it is unable to lower the temperature to below the kindling temperature. If chemicals are not available, gasoline fires can often be extinguished by covering the burning fluid with sand. This separates the gasoline and oxygen.

IMPORTANCE OF OXYGEN GAS IN EVERYDAY LIFE

The union of oxygen with various partner substances is very important in our everyday lives. We burn wood, coal, gas, kerosene, and other fuels to heat our homes and public buildings and to cook our food. Engines are made to run by burning gasoline and other substances. If electric lights are not available, we burn candles, lamps, or gas to furnish light. Dead plants and animals, under the influence of enzymes produced by bacteria, unite with oxygen, or *decay*. Oxygen acts to some extent as a water purifier, since it oxidizes and renders harmless many forms of putrid matter that contaminate our sources of drinking water.

COMMERCIAL USES OF OXYGEN

When oxygen is mixed with hydrogen or acetylene gas and the mixture is ignited, an intense heat is produced. This type of blowtorch is used in cutting metals. Oxygen in combined form is found in most of the dyes and other synthetic compounds used in industry. The commercial supplies of oxygen have enabled men and women to climb high mountains, to explore the stratosphere, and to examine the bottom of the ocean.

USE OF OXYGEN IN THERAPY

When we inspire (breathe in), oxygen enters the blood and unites loosely with *hemoglobin*, the red pigment of the blood. Hemoglobin takes the oxygen to the blood capillaries, where it splits off and diffuses through the tissue fluids to the tissue cells. When the gas reacts with foods and waste products in the cells, one of the waste products formed is carbon dioxide gas (CO_2). When we expire (breathe out), this gas is eliminated from the body through the lungs.

When an individual has been exposed to gases other than oxygen, or has been exposed to smoke, or has been immersed in water for several minutes, he becomes unconscious and may die because of the resulting *asphyxiation* (lack of oxygen). Such patients are treated by forcing them to breathe pure oxygen in the attempt to get oxygen to the cells as quickly as possible. Carbon monoxide gas (CO), which is usually present in automobile exhaust gas and in the gas used for cooking and heating purposes, is poisonous because it unites with hemoglobin and prevents this pigment from uniting with oxygen. Carbon monoxide poisoning is also treated with oxygen. Patients who have various lung diseases, such as pneumonia, often do not have enough normal lung tissue left to absorb sufficient oxygen from the air. These patients may be able to live until the disease condition

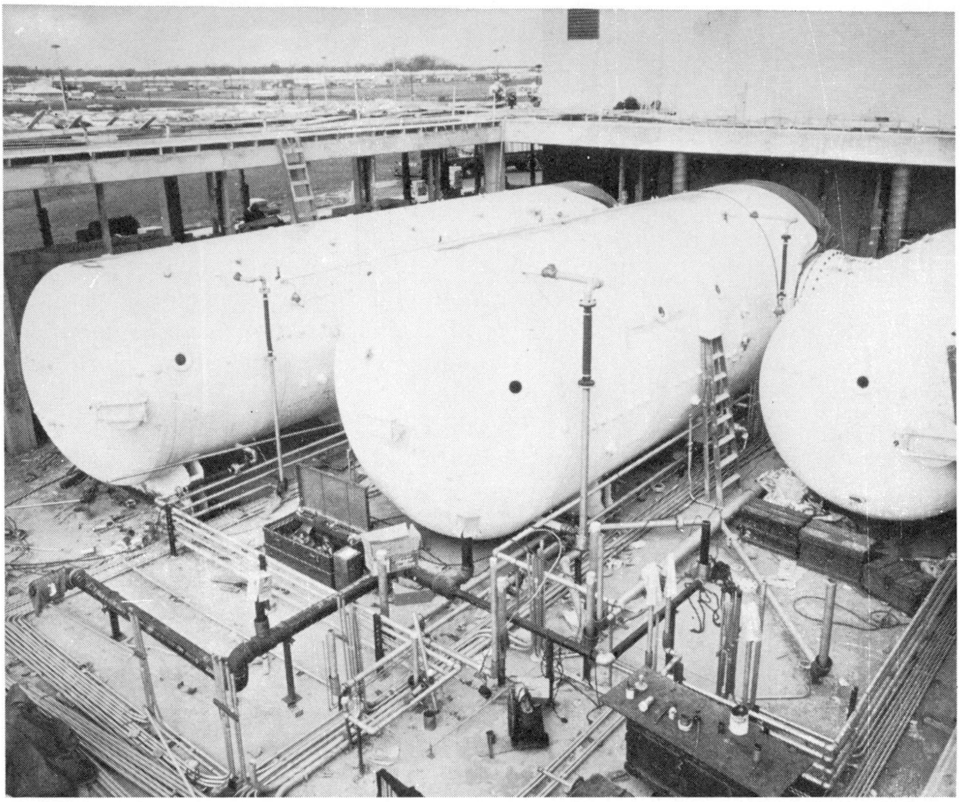

Fig. 6-1. The huge hyperbaric, or high pressure, oxygen "room" at Lutheran General Hospital, Park Ridge, Illinois. Name some diseases for which this chamber might be useful therapeutically. (Courtesy Dr. Herbert O. Sieker.)

is healed if they breathe oxygen instead of air. Oxygen has to be administered along with some of the gas anesthetics, such as nitrous oxide (N_2O, "laughting gas") and ethylene, in order to supply the patient with it while the gas anesthetic is breathed.

Hyperbaric, or high pressure, oxygen "rooms" are being used for therapeutic purposes in some hospitals. Patients with such diseases as gas gangrene (caused by microorganisms that cannot grow in an oxygen atmosphere), carbon monoxide poisoning, heart disease, and shock are placed in such rooms. They are useful rooms in which to perform certain operations on the heart. Such a room was used in a futile attempt to save the life of the late President Kennedy's baby son in 1963.

PROBLEM OF THE RUSTING OF IRON

Steel is made by melting iron and dissolving small amounts of carbon (and, sometimes, traces of other elements) in it. When iron or steel is exposed to air, particularly moist air, it combines with oxygen to form rust, of ferric oxide (Fe_2O_3). The rust is soft and crumbly as compared with the original iron. The problem of the rusting of iron is very important to us because many of our large buildings, automobiles, engines, ships, airplanes and various forms of commercial apparatus are made from iron and steel. Rust formation is prevented in two ways. The iron may be covered with watertight and airtight coatings, such as metals or paints, to prevent contact with moisture and oxygen, or catalysts, which greatly *slow down* the reaction of the iron and oxygen, can be mixed with the iron. Small amounts of the metals chromium, nickel, and copper frequently are used for this purpose. All of us are familiar with *stainless steel* that contains such catalysts.

OXIDES When oxygen combines with an element or radical having *positive valence* the resulting compound is called an *oxide*. Oxides are named by giving the name of the element or radical having positive valence and adding the word oxide.

Na_2O	CaO	Al_2O_3
Sodium oxide	Calcium oxide	Aluminum oxide

STUDY QUESTIONS

1. What is the formula of oxygen gas?
2. What percentage, by weight, of water is oxygen?
3. What is the composition of air? Is air an element, a compound, or a mixture?
4. Name two men who played a part in discovering oxygen. Who first pointed out the vital importance of oxygen?
5. Write equations showing how oxygen can be prepared in the laboratory.
6. What are the commercial methods for preparing oxygen?
7. What is the anode? The cathode?
8. List some physical and chemical properties of oxygen.
9. Why is oxygen necessary for life?
10. How can an inflammable substance be made to burn? What is the flame?
11. Is oxygen necessary for burning?
12. What causes fire hazards?
13. How does water extinguish a fire?
14. Name some other methods of extinguishing fires.
15. How do we use oxygen in our everyday lives?
16. Name some commercial uses of oxygen not listed in the book.
17. What substance in the blood takes oxygen to the cells?
18. How is oxygen used in therapy?
19. What is steel?
20. Write an equation showing what happens when iron rusts.
21. How can iron or steel be prevented from rusting?
22. Name the following compounds: MgO, K_2O.

CHAPTER 7

Energy transformations

DEFINITION

Energy exists in many forms and it is difficult to formulate a definition that includes all of these forms. In general, however, we may say that energy is anything that can be made to do work, or to change the rate of motion of substances. If a test tube is lifted from a table, work has been done because the test tube, which was at rest before it was lifted, has been moved to another position. When gasoline explodes in an automobile engine, energy is released, and the automobile wheels are made to turn. When muscles contract, various parts of our bodies move; the energy for this motion comes from chemical reactions that take place within the muscle cells.

ENERGY CONVERSIONS

An important law, known as the *law of conservation of energy,* states that energy can neither be created nor destroyed (although under certain circumstances, it can be converted to matter and vice versa; see page 122). However, we are often able to convert one form of energy into another form. When radiant energy from the sun strikes the skin, it is converted to heat energy, and the skin feels warmer. When electrical energy passes through the filament of an electric light bulb, it is converted to heat and to radiant energy (light). When the terminals of a storage battery are connected to a suitable electric motor, the chemical energy stored in the battery is converted to electrical energy, which, in turn, is converted to mechanical energy. When foods are united with oxygen in the cells, the chemical energy contained in the foods is converted to heat and to mechanical energy.

MEASUREMENT OF ENERGY

In medicine and dentistry energy is usually measured by converting it into heat energy and then measuring the heat energy. Heat cannot be converted completely into other forms of energy, but all other forms of energy *can* be converted entirely into heat.

The unit of heat is the *calorie*. It is defined as the amount of heat required to raise the temperature of 1 gram of water 1° C. The abbreviation for calorie is cal. The *large calorie* is 1,000 small calories. Its abbreviation is Cal. The large calorie is nearly always used in medical and dental energy measurements, and in nutritional and medical literature the word "calorie" always refers to the large calorie.

It is important that we understand the difference between heat and temperature. Except at absolute zero,* molecules and atoms are in constant motion. Temperature is a measure of the relative speed with which they are moving. The average speed of motion of the molecules in a glass of water is less at 20° C than it is at 30° C. The heat energy of the moving particles is due to their motion. Temperature measures, then, the average heat energy of the molecules or atoms.

The total heat, which we measure in calories, will be the sum of the heat energies of all the molecules or atoms present. A bathtub filled with water at 25° C has a lower temperature than a teaspoonful of water at 95° C, but the total amount of heat energy is much greater in the tub. A molecule in the teaspoonful of water has more energy than a molecule in the tub, but there are many more molecules in the latter.

CHEMICAL ENERGY

Whenever chemical changes occur, energy changes occur also. Every chemical compound has a definite amount of chemical energy. This means that a given chemical compound when it reacts with a given substance will always release or absorb the same amount of energy if the same amounts of reacting substances are used. Chemical energy is important because it can be converted into other kinds of energy that are useful to us. When coal burns, chemical energy contained in the coal and in the oxygen is converted to heat and light. When a candy bar is eaten, the chemical energy contained in it can be changed in the tissues into heat and mechanical energy.

It is also true that other forms of energy can be converted to chemical energy. The chemical energy of a storage battery is increased if an electric current is passed through it in the correct way. Plants contain a green pigment called chlorophyll. This pigment absorbs light, and the plant uses the energy obtained to make starch from carbon dioxide and water. This reaction is known as the *photosynthesis reaction*. It is one of the most important of all natural chemical reactions because animals cannot make starch and have to depend on plants for their supplies of it. When animals eat these plants, the chemical energy stored in the starch is released as heat and mechanical energy when the starch is combined with oxygen in the tissues.

ENERGY PRODUCTION FROM FOODS

The principal types of food are grouped as carbohydrates, fats, and proteins. All of these substances release energy when they react with oxygen. Carbohydrates are converted principally into a sugar called glucose in the body, fats are changed into fatty acids, and proteins are transformed into acids called amino acids. When glucose, fatty acids, and amino acids unite

*Absolute zero is the temperature at which all atomic and molecular motion ceases. Its value is approximately −273° C.

with oxygen in the cells, they are changed chiefly to carbon dioxide and water. The energy released by these reactions furnishes us with heat, which we use to maintain body temperature; energy is also utilized for muscular movement, gland secretion, and nerve conduction. For each volume of oxygen used in these reactions, 1 volume of CO_2 is produced from glucose, about 0.7 volume of CO_2 from fatty acids, and about 0.8 volume of CO_2 from amino acids.

STUDY QUESTIONS

1. Name five forms of energy.
2. What is the law of conservation of energy?
3. What is the unit of heat energy? How is it defined?
4. What is a large calorie?
5. How many large calories of heat are required to raise the temperature of 1 kg of water from 30° C to 37° C?
6. Explain the difference between temperature and heat.
7. Why is chemical energy important to us?
8. Do energy changes always occur when chemical changes occur?
9. Give two examples showing the conversion of chemical energy to other forms of energy.
10. Give two examples showing the conversion of other forms of energy to chemical energy.
11. What products are formed when glucose, fatty acids, or amino acids react with oxygen?
12. One liter of oxygen is used in burning a certain amount of fatty acid, glucose, or amino acid. How much CO_2 is produced in each case?

CHAPTER 8

Water

COMPOSITION

One molecule of water contains 2 atoms of hydrogen and 1 atom of oxygen. If water is decomposed by passing an electric current through it, 2 volumes of hydrogen are produced for each volume of oxygen. The oxygen atom is about 16 times as heavy as the hydrogen atom, and water by weight is therefore eight-ninths oxygen and one-ninth hydrogen.

OCCURRENCE

Water is the most common of all chemical compounds. Nearly three-fourths of the earth's surface is covered by it. Many of the lower organisms are more than 90 percent water. Most plants are made up of more than 50 percent of it. Approximately two-thirds, or 67 percent, of the weight of the human body is water. Plants could not live if the soil did not contain large amounts of this compound. We know that the atmosphere contains water because it often condenses and falls to the earth as rain or snow.

PHYSICAL PROPERTIES OF BIOLOGICAL IMPORTANCE

Water, when it is pure, is transparent and practically tasteless. The familiar taste of naturally occurring water results from the presence of dissolved gases. If these gases are removed by boiling, the water tastes "flat." In thin layers water has no color, but most large bodies of water look blue. If water is cooled it contracts, or decreases in volume, until a temperature of 4° C is reached. Below this temperature it expands again. When 0° C is reached, the water freezes, and in doing so expands by nearly one-tenth of its volume. This explains why water pipes often burst when water freezes in them. Ice, or solid water, is lighter than liquid water and floats in the latter. If it were not for this property, aquatic life in northern climates would be impossible, since lakes and rivers would freeze solid in the winter. The top layers of the lakes freeze first, and because ice is lighter than water, this layer of ice actually protects the lower levels of water from the cold.

More substances will dissolve in water than in any other liquid. The components of the cells of our bodies are kept in solution by water, and this

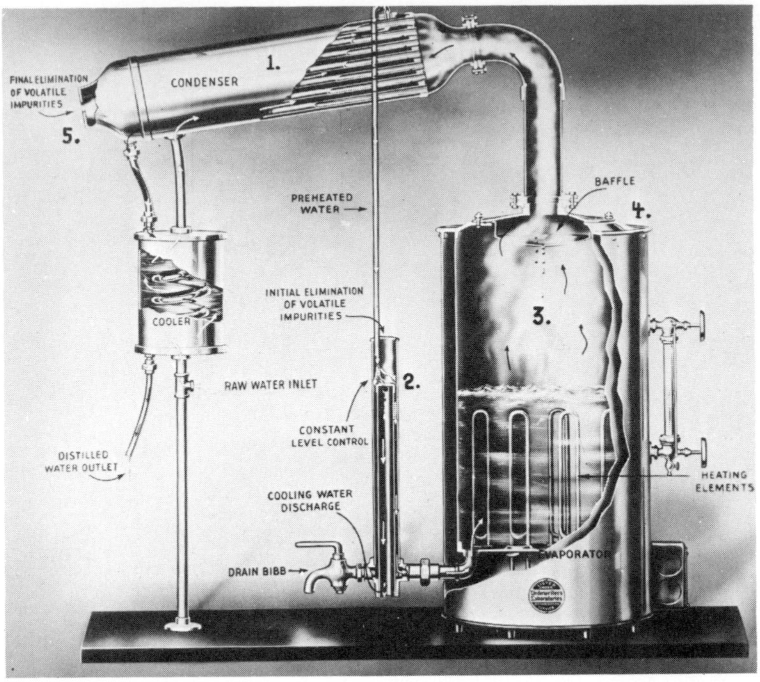

Fig. 8-1. A still used to prepare distilled water for laboratory use. This is a common method of purifying water. Why does distilled water taste "flat"? (Courtesy Barnstead Still and Sterilizer Co., Inc.)

makes it possible for chemical changes to take place. Water is the most important of all catalysts, and most of the reactions that take place in the tissues will not take place in its absence. Water maintains the proper degree of dilution in the tissue fluids that bathe the cells; it provides a fluid medium for transporting food materials to and waste materials away from the tissues. Water is necessary for the proper excretion of waste materials, many of which are excreted in solution in the urine. It is largely responsible for the heat regulation of the body because it equalizes the temperature in the various parts of the body by acting as a circulating fluid. When 1 gram of water evaporates from the skin it takes about 580 small calories of heat with it. This explains why perspiration cools the skin. Water is the principal component of the secretions of glands and is essential for the proper functioning of these glands.

REACTION WITH METALS

Water reacts with certain metals to form hydroxides (compounds containing the OH radical) and hydrogen gas.

$$2\,Na + 2\,H_2O \rightarrow 2\,NaOH + H_2$$

Notice that hydrogen, like oxygen, always exists when not combined with other elements as molecules, each containing 2 hydrogen atoms. Not all the metals react with water in this way. In fact, the metals can be arranged in a list in the order of their activity so that each metal will be found to displace from its compounds any metal below it in the series. Hydrogen is included in this series, and all the metals above this element displace it from dilute acids (compounds containing hydrogen in a form that is chemically reactive) and from water, while those below it in the series do not. The order of activity of some of the common metals is: K, Na, Ca, Mg, Al, Zn, Fe, Pb, H, Bi, Cu, Pt (platinum), Au (gold). This series is known as the *electromotive series*. The series does not tell us, however, how *rapidly* the metals above hydrogen will replace it from water. Potassium and sodium react with water with such violence that heat and light are produced, while iron and lead react so slowly that they do not appear to react at all for hours. Bismuth, copper, platinum, and gold are below hydrogen in the series and will not react with water no matter how long they remain in contact with it.

The ability of a metal high on the electromotive series list to replace a metal of lower activity can be utilized to clean silver rapidly. The discolored silverware should be placed in an aluminum vessel and covered with water. One heaping tablespoonful of washing soda (Na_2CO_3) or scouring powder containing trisodium phosphate (Na_3PO_4) should be added for each quart of water. If these agents are not available, use two heaping tablespoonfuls of ordinary baking soda [$NaHCO_3$] for each quart of water.) Heat until the water is boiling, stirring to dissolve the added powder. In approximately two minutes, the tarnish on the silverware will have vanished. A high gloss can be obtained by rubbing the silver with chamois.

The dark-colored material on the tarnished silver is silver sulfide, Ag_2S. This compound results from a slow reaction between silver and hydrogen sulfide, H_2S, a gas formed in small amounts during the cooking or decomposition of foods. The procedure just described for removing the tarnish illustrates the replacement of the silver from silver sulfide by sodium, as illustrated by the following equation:

$$3\ Ag_2S + 2\ Al + 3\ Na_2CO_3 \rightarrow 6\ Ag + 3\ Na_2S + Al_2(CO_3)_3$$

Stainless steel also can be cleaned in this way, but it should be removed from the boiling solution within a minute or two, since otherwise it might undergo slight corrosion.

REACTION WITH OXIDES

Metal oxides are compounds that are composed of a metal combined with oxygen. Water reacts with some metal oxides to form compounds containing OH radicals.

$$\underset{\text{Potassium oxide}}{K_2O} + H_2O \rightarrow \underset{\text{Potassium hydroxide}}{2\ KOH}$$

Compounds of nonmetals with oxygen are called *nonmetal oxides*. Some of these react with water to form acids, which are compounds containing hydrogen in chemically reactive form.

$$\underset{\text{Sulfur trioxide}}{SO_2} + H_2O \rightarrow \underset{\text{Sulfuric acid}}{H_2SO_4}$$

HYDRATES

Many *crystals* (particles of matter having definite geometrical shape) contain water. Some crystals will give up definite amounts of water when they are heated or exposed to air at ordinary temperatures. This water is called *water of crystallization* or *water of hydration* and is written separately in a formula to show its loose chemical attachment. Crystalline copper sulfate is $CuSO_4 \cdot 5H_2O$. This means that 1 molecule of copper sulfate has combined loosely with 5 molecules of water to form crystalline copper sulfate.

Substances that hold water of crystallization are known as *hydrates*. When such substances have lost their water of crystallization they are said to be *anhydrous*. Substances that *give up* water of crystallization on exposure to air at ordinary temperatures are said to be *efflorescent*, and those that *take up* water at ordinary temperatures are called *hygroscopic*. A solid that is so hygroscopic that it finally dissolves in the water it has taken up is said to be *deliquescent*.

A substance much used in making surgical casts is *plaster of Paris*. This substance is calcium sulfate from which part of the water of crystallization has been removed. Its formula is $(CaSO_4)_2 \cdot H_2O$. This formula indicates that 2 molecules of calcium sulfate ($CaSO_4$) have combined loosely with 1 molecule of water. When plaster of Paris is mixed with water and allowed to "set," it increases its water of crystallization to form a hard substance known as *gypsum*.

$$\underset{\text{Plaster of Paris}}{(CaSO_4)_2 \cdot H_2O} + 3\,H_2O \rightarrow \underset{\text{Gypsum}}{2\,(CaSO_4 \cdot 2H_2O)}$$

HYDROLYSIS

A reaction in which water reacts with some other substance is called *hydrolysis*. A compound that is made of a metal or of a radical with positive valence combined with some other elements or radical (other than OH) is called a *salt*. Water reacts to a slight extent with many salts to form small amounts of hydroxide and acid.

$$\underset{\text{Ammonium chloride}}{NH_4Cl} + H_2O \rightleftarrows \underset{\text{Ammonium hydroxide}}{NH_4OH} + \underset{\text{Hydrochloric acid}}{HCl}$$

The double arrow indicates that only a small amount of the ammonium chloride present actually reacts in this way with the water. Many salts will not react with water at all.

The reactions that take place when food is digested in the intestinal tract are hydrolytic reactions. Complex carbohydrates unite with water to form *simple sugars*. For example, cane sugar (sucrose) hydrolyzes to form glucose and fructose.

$$\underset{\text{Sucrose}}{C_{12}H_{22}O_{11}} + H_2O \rightarrow \underset{\text{Glucose}}{C_6H_{12}O_6} + \underset{\text{Fructose}}{C_6H_{12}O_6}$$

Glucose and fructose have the same empirical formulas, but differ in their structural formulas. Fats are hydrolyzed in the intestinal tract to *glycerol* and *fatty acids*. Proteins react with water to form *amino acids*.

STUDY QUESTIONS

1. How much oxygen is present in 100 g of water?
2. Fifty milliliters of oxygen were produced by decomposing a certain amount of water. How many milliliters of hydrogen were produced?
3. What percentage of the human body is water?
4. At what temperature does water have the least volume for a given weight?
5. What is the biological importance of the fact that ice is lighter than water?
6. Name four physiological functions of water.

7. Write an equation showing the reaction of potassium with water.
8. Would you expect aluminum to react with calcium chloride? Why?
9. Would you expect magnesium to react with zinc chloride? Why?
10. Write equations showing: (a) the reaction between Na_2O and H_2O and (b) the reaction between CO_2 and H_2O.
11. What is the formula for crystalline copper sulfate? For anhydrous copper sulfate?
12. Define: efflorescent, hygroscopic, deliquescent, water of crystallization, hydrate.
13. Write an equation showing what happens when plaster of Paris hardens.
14. Write an equation showing the reaction between NH_4NO_3 (ammonium nitrate) and water.
15. What type of reaction occurs when foods are digested? List the digestive products of carbohydrates, fats, and proteins.

CHAPTER 9

Solutions

MEANING OF THE TERM "SOLUTION"

If we place a lump of sugar in a glass of water, the billions of sugar molecules that make up the lump separate from each other and become uniformly distributed among the water molecules. We have formed a mixture in which all the particles present are of molecular size. Mixtures composed entirely of individual molecules or atoms mixed together are called *solutions*. When we recall that matter can exist in different physical states (solid, liquid, gas) we realize that many different types of solution are possible. When sugar is dissolved in water, the solution is made by dissolving a solid in a liquid; if liquid mercury is rubbed on solid gold, the solution formed consists of a liquid dissolved in a solid. The air we breathe is a solution composed entirely of gases. We dissolve carbon dioxide gas in water to make the solution called carbonated water. Mixtures of alcohol (a liquid) and water are used to sterilize the skin. Amalgams, several of which are used in dentistry as fillings for carious (decayed) teeth, are solutions made by dissolving one or more metals in another metal.

SOLVENT AND SOLUTE

In the case of a cane sugar solution, the water is said to be the *solvent and the sugar is called the solute*. In other words, the solute is the substance that is dissolved and the solvent is the substance in which the molecules of solute are dispersed.

SOLUTIONS WITH LIQUID SOLVENTS

The most important class of solutions is that class in which some liquid is used as the solvent, and the most important of the liquid solvents is water. All the foods and waste products that enter and leave the cells of our bodies are carried as water solutions. Even such insoluble substances as marble and iron will dissolve to a slight extent in water. Carbon tetrachloride, a liquid, is an exdellent solvent for grease; most paints dissolve readily in turpentine; and fingernail polish is easily removed with amyl acetate.

FACTORS INFLENC-ING SOLU-BILITY

The factors that influence solubility are the nature of the solute and of the solvent, temperature, and pressure.

NATURE OF THE SOLUTE AND OF THE SOLVENT. One hundred milliliters of water at a temperature of 18° C will dissolve about 204 g of zinc chloride ($ZnCl_2$), 36 g of sodium chloride ($NaCl$), or 0.0013 g of silver chloride ($AgCl$). In other words, all solutes are not soluble to the same extent in a common solvent. The solubility of a substance is dependent also on the chemical nature of the solvent. Fatty substances are nearly insoluble in water, but most of them dissolve in ether, gasoline, or benzene. Serum albumin, a protein found in the bloodstream, readily dissolves in water, but will not dissolve at all in alcohol.

TEMPERATURE. Most solid solutes become more soluble as the temperature of a solution is raised. Thirteen grams of potassium nitrate (KNO_3) will dissolve in 100 ml of water at 0° C; 247 g will dissolve in the same amount of water at 100° C. There are some exceptions to this general rule. Calcium hydroxide ($Ca(OH)_2$) becomes slightly less soluble as the temperature rises. Calcium hydroxide solution is often called *limewater*. Gases, in contrast to most solids, become less soluble if the temperature is increased. When a warm bottle of ginger ale is opened, the foam that spouts from the bottle is caused by the escape of carbon dioxide gas. If a cold bottle is opened, however, only a little gas escapes because the carbon dioxide is more soluble at the lower temperature.

PRESSURE. Pressure increases the solubility of gases, although it has little effect on the solubility of solids or liquids. Carbonated water is made by dissolving carbon dioxide gas in water under pressure. When this pressure is released, some of the gas leaves the solution and the carbonated water becomes filled with bubbles of escaping gas.

TYPES OF SOLUTION

A solution that contains all the solute it is capable of holding under the given conditions is called a *saturated* solution. If less than this amount of solute is present, the solution is *unsaturated*. *Concentrated* solutions are either saturated or are nearly so. *Dilute* solutions contain only a small fraction of the total amount of solute that could be made to dissolve in the solvent. Sometimes, if we make a saturated solution at a high temperature and then carefully lower the temperature, we may, if we do not jar the solution, get a solution that contains more solute than ordinarily is possible at the given temperature. Such a solution, which can exist only a short while as such, is called a *supersaturated solution*.

FREEZING AND BOILING POINTS OF SOLUTIONS

The freezing point of a solution is always lower than the freezing point of the pure solvent; the boiling point is always higher. Alcohol, ethylene glycol, and other substances are mixed with the water in automobile radiators in the winter to prevent freezing. It is more difficult to freeze a carbonated beverage than it is to freeze a noncarbonated one because the former contains carbon dioxide in solution.

METHODS OF EXPRESSING CONCEN-TRATION

A common way to describe the concentration of a solution is to indicate the number of grams of solute in 100 ml of the solution. If the solvent is water, 100 ml of the solution probably will weigh about 100 g, unless the solution contains a large amount of solute, since 1 ml of water weighs 1 g.

For this reason it is customary in medicine and dentistry to indicate the number of grams of solute in 100 ml of water solution by writing down this number and following it by the word "percent." For example, if 1 g of sodium chloride is dissolved in 100 ml of solution, the solution is called a "1 percent solution of sodium chloride." Liquids usually are measured by volume rather than by weight, and the expression "5 percent solution of alcohol" indicates that each 100 ml of alcohol solution contains 5 ml of alcohol.

Chemists often indicate the concentration of solutions by giving the number of *moles* (gram-molecular weights) of the solute contained in 1 liter of solution. A solution containing 1 mole (17.031 g) of ammonia gas (NH_3) in a liter of solution is a 1 molar (1 M) solution of ammonia. If 25.546 g of NH_3 were present in 1 liter of the solution, the solution would contain 1.5 moles per liter and would thus be a 1.5 M solution. This method of expressing concentration is very useful because it enables the chemist to obtain the number of moles of substance he requires simply by measuring a volume, a procedure much simpler than weighing the substance on a chemical balance.

NORMAL SOLUTIONS. The *equivalent weight*, or *gram-equivalent weight*, of a substance (element or compound) is that weight that will furnish, react with, or displace 1 gram-atomic weight (1.008 g) of hydrogen. Methods for calculating equivalent weights are described briefly as follows.

Equivalent weights of elements. The valence of combined hydrogen is unity (1+). Therefore, 1 gram-atomic weight of hydrogen will combine with, or will be displaced by, exactly 1 gram-atomic weight of other elements whose valence is 1. Elements whose valence is 2 can combine with, or displace, exactly 2 gram-atomic weights of hydrogen, and so on. Therefore, the equivalent weight of an element can be calculated by *dividing its gram-atomic weight by its valence.* For example, the atomic weight of iodine is 126.90. Since the valence of combined iodine is 1−, the gram-equivalent weight of iodine is 126.90 g. Calcium has an atomic weight of 40.08 and a valence of 2+; thus, its equivalent weight is 20.04 g. The equivalent weight of aluminum, which has an atomic weight of 26.98 and a valence of 3+, is 8.99 g.

Equivalent weights of acids. All acids contain replaceable hydrogen; that is, hydrogen that can be replaced by some other element in the course of a chemical reaction. The equivalent weight of an acid is calculated by *dividing the gram-molecular weight of the acid by the number of replaceable gram-atomic weights of hydrogen.* Hydrochloric acid (HCl) has 1 replaceable hydrogen atom; thus the equivalent weight of HCl is the same as its molecular weight (36.46 g). Sulfuric acid (H_2SO_4), which has 2 replaceable hydrogen atoms in each molecule and a molecular weight of 99.08, has an equivalent weight of 49.54 g.

Equivalent weights of bases. Bases contain OH radicals in their molecules. Since the valence of this radical is 1−, the equivalent weight of a base is calculated by *dividing its gram-molecular weight by the number of OH groups in each molecule.* Sodium hydroxide (NaOH) has a molecular weight of 40.0; its equivalent weight, therefore, is 40.0 g. Barium hydroxide, $Ba(OH)_2$, has a molecular weight of 171.35 and an equivalent weight of 85.68 g.

Equivalent weights of salts. Most salts contain neither replaceable hydrogen atoms nor hydroxyl radicals in their molecules. All of them, however, contain a radical or atom of positive valence combined with a radical or atom of negative valence. The equivalent weight of a salt can be computed by *dividing the gram-molecular weight by the valence of the positive radical (radicals) or atom (atoms).*

The ammonium radical (NH_4) has a valence of 1+; hence the equivalent weight of ammonium chloride (NH_4Cl) is 53.49 g, since the molecular weight of this salt is 53.49. Calcium sulfate ($CaSO_4$), because the calcium has a valence of 2+, has a molecular weight of 136.14 and an equivalent weight of 68.07 g. Each sodium atom in a molecule of sodium carbonate (Na_2CO_3) has a valence of 1+. However, the *total positive valence* of the molecule is 2+, and the equivalent weight (52.99 g) of sodium carbonate is found by dividing its molecular weight (105.99) by 2.

Equivalent weights of oxidizing agents (see page 99). When an oxidation occurs, at least 1 of the atoms present in the molecule of the oxidizing agent gains electrons (that is, loses positive valence). In the reaction

$$2\,K\overset{7+}{Mn}O_4 + 5\,CaC_2O_4 + 8\,H_2SO_4 \rightarrow K_2SO_4 + 2\,\overset{2+}{Mn}SO_4 + 5\,CaSO_4 + 10\,CO_2 + 8\,H_2O,$$

each of the manganese atoms present in a molecule of the oxidizing agent (potassium permanganate) gains 5 electrons; that is, loses 5 positive valences. Since hydrogen is able to gain or lose only 1 electron when it takes part in an oxidation-reduction reaction, the equivalent weight of potassium permanganate (31.61 g) is determined by dividing its molecular weight (158.04) by 5.

A solution that contains 1 gram-equivalent weight of substance in 1 liter of solution is called a *normal (1 N) solution.* A 0.1 N solution of sulfuric acid thus contains 4.95 g of H_2SO_4 per liter. A 0.05 N solution of potassium permanganate contains 1.58 g of $KMnO_4$ per liter, and so on.

Normal solutions are particularly useful to the chemist because *equal volumes of solutions of equal normality will react exactly with each other* (provided, of course, the substances in the solutions are capable of undergoing reaction). For example, 10 ml of 0.05 N sodium hydroxide will neutralize *exactly* 10 ml of 0.05 N sulfuric acid. When the normalities of the reacting solutions are not identical, the amounts of solution required can be calculated readily if the normalities are known. Suppose we wish to neutralize 100 ml of 0.1 N barium hydroxide solution with 0.2 N hydrochloric acid. Since the normality of the hydrochloric acid is twice that of the barium hydroxide, only one-half as much of the acid solution (50 ml) will be required for exact neutralization.

SURFACE TENSION

Molecules attract each other just as the sun attracts the earth and the earth attracts the moon. A molecule in the middle of a glass of water is completely surrounded by other water molecules and is thus attracted in all directions at once. The result of this is that the molecule has little tendency to move in any particular direction; the force that tries to pull it up is neutralized by the force that tries to pull it down, and the forces that try to pull it to one side are balanced by the forces that try to pull it in the opposite direction. The situation is different, however, for a molecule at the *surface* of the water. Here the molecule is pulled downward by the attractive forces of the molecules below it. It is not attracted upward very much because there are not nearly as many molecules in the air above the water surface as there are in the water below. Suppose several balloons are floating on the surface of a lake. We shall imagine that each balloon has a string tied around its neck and that the other ends of these strings are hanging down in the water. Now, if a skillful swimmer dives beneath the balloons, grasps the strings that are hanging down in the water, and pulls them down toward the bottom of the lake, the balloons on the surface will be jammed, or packed, closely together. This is what happens to molecules at the surface of a glass of water; they are packed tightly together to form a *surface film.* This film is strong enough so that a steel needle will

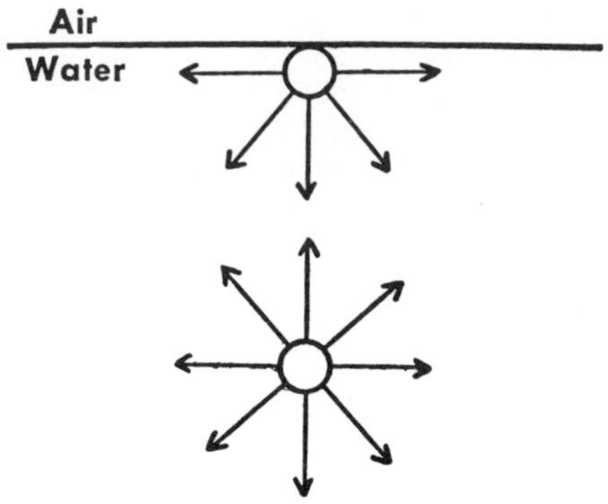

Fig. 9-1. Diagram illustrating surface tension. The arrows indicate the direction in which the water molecules (the circles) are attracted by other molecules. Notice that molecules away from the surface are attracted equally in all directions, but molecules at the surface are attracted only downward and sideways. This unequal attraction causes the surface molecules to pack together and form a surface film. How would you define surface tension?

float on water if we are careful not to break the film in placing the needle on the surface. The tension, or force, necessary to break this film is called the *surface tension* of the liquid. All liquids exhibit surface tension, but water has a higher surface tension than most other liquids.

INTERFACIAL TENSION

If we place some mineral oil and some water together in a test tube, the two liquids soon separate; the mineral oil, which is the lighter of the two liquids, will float on top of the water. Water molecules at the surface are pulled downward by the water molecules below them and upward by the oil molecules above. We have already discovered, however, that the surface tension of water is higher than that of most other liquids. This means that the water molecules will be pulled downward harder than they are pulled upward. This causes the water molecules at the surface to pack together, just as they did when no oil was present, but the film that is formed at this "water-oil interface" will not be as strong as the film at the "water-air interface." The force necessary to break the film existing between two liquids, or between a liquid and a solid, is called *interfacial tension.*

SURFACE-ACTIVE SUBSTANCES

Certain substances when dissolved in water tend to collect at the surface, so that the number of molecules of these substances in a given volume in the surface is much greater than elsewhere in the solution. These substances, which are said to be *surface-active,* lower the surface tension of the water, just as the mineral oil lowered it in the example given in the preceding paragraph. Surface-active substances lower both interfacial tensions and surface tensions.

EMULSIONS

If we add a few drops of some oil (for example, linseed oil) to water and shake the mixture, the oil, being insoluble in water, can be made to separate into tiny drops. The mixture formed when tiny drops of oil are suspended in water is called an *emulsion.* Emulsions made as just described are not permanent because the oil drops quickly separate out, and the oil

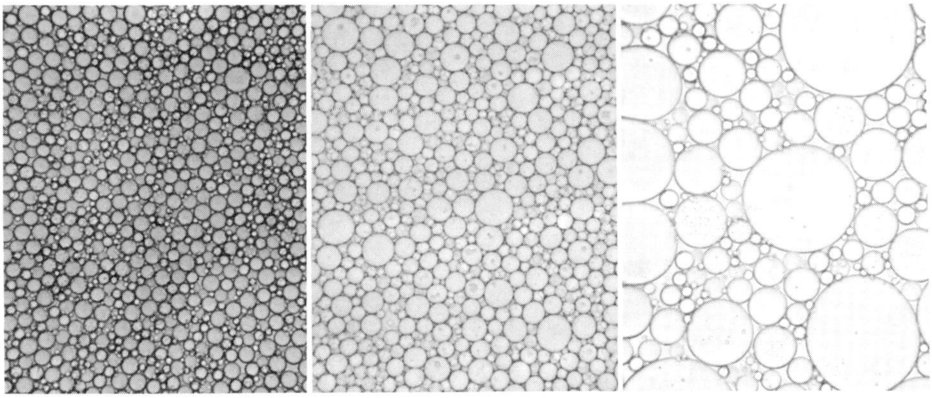

Fig. 9-2. Photomicrographs (photographs taken through a microscope) of emulsions. Which of these 3 emulsions would be most rapidly digested in the intestinal tract, assuming that the suspended droplets were digestible fat? (Courtesy Dr. Thomas Simon, Warner-Lambert Research Institute.)

is soon floating on top of the water. Suppose we imagine that a flexible rubber sheet is stretched parallel to the floor. Suppose a steel marble is placed on the sheet. The rubber, which has elasticity, will stretch slightly; that is, the part beneath the marble will be under tension. If now a second steel marble is placed somewhere else on the rubber sheet, the tension of the rubber will cause the two marbles to move toward each other until finally they touch. That is what happens to the oil drops suspended in the water. The water has a higher surface tension than the oil drops, and this tension causes the drops to move toward each other until finally all the drops collect into one big drop that separates out and floats on the water. We see at once, then, that substances that lower the surface tension of water (surface-active substances) will help to prevent the separation of the oil from the water. Indeed, if we succeed in lowering the surface tension of the water until it equals that of the oil, there will be no appreciable tendency for the oil drops to approach each other, and the emulsion will be permanent and stable. Surface-active substances that are used to make emulsions more stable are called *emulsifying agents.* Gums (acacia, tragacanth) and soaps are commonly used as emulsifying agents. Compounds found in bile, called *bile salts,* are excellent emulsifying agents; as we shall see later, bile salts are very important in the digestion of fats. Fats cannot be digested properly until they are emulsified.

OSMOTIC PRESSURE

Suppose a container is separated into two equal halves by means of a thin metal sheet that is perforated with a number of holes. We shall imagine that a solution of cane sugar is placed on one side (compartment A) of the metal sheet and that pure water is placed on the other side (compartment B). It will be remembered that all molecules are in constant motion, except when the temperature is zero on the absolute temperature scale (−273° C). Because of this molecular motion some of the water molecules

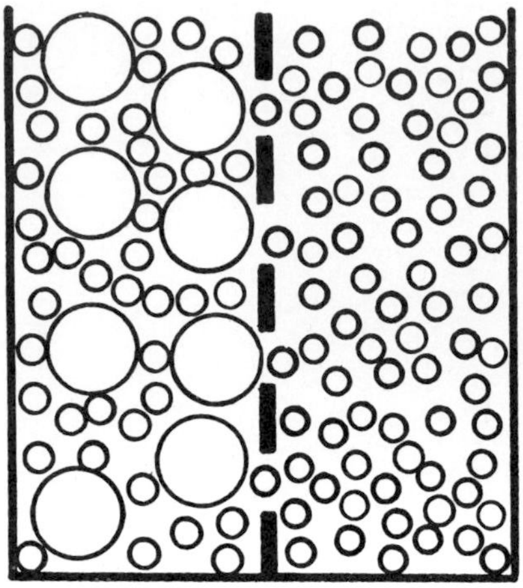

Fig. 9-3. Diagram illustrating osmotic pressure. Compartment **A** contains both sugar molecules (large circles) and water molecules (small circles). Compartment **B** contains only water molecules. Notice that the sugar molecules are too large to pass through the pores in the membrane separating the two compartments. Why do more water molecules diffuse from compartment **B** into compartment **A** than from compartment **A** into compartment **B**?

and sugar molecules will pass through the holes in the metal membrane and will enter compartment B. Some of the water molecules in compartment B will enter compartment A for the same reason. After a time the number of sugar and water molecules will be the same on both sides of the membrane; that is, the sugar concentration will be the same in both compartments.

Now, suppose the above experiment is repeated, except that this time the holes in the metal membrane are large enough to allow passage of water molecules but are too small to permit the passage of sugar molecules. The holes on the B side of the membranes will be bombarded only by water molecules, while the holes on the A side will be bombarded by both water molecules and sugar molecules. Because more water molecules strike the holes on the B side than on the A side, water will pass from compartment B into compartment A more rapidly than it passes in the reverse direction. This means, as we watch the experiment proceed, that the volume in compartment A will gradually *increase* and the volume in compartment B will gradually *decrease*. Finally, however, the volume of solution in compartment A ceases to increase because the weight of the solution in this compartment becomes enough greater than the weight of the water in compartment B to prevent the passage of any more water into A. This extra weight of water in compartment A means that the mechanical pressure is greater on the A side of the membrane than it is on the B side. This extra pressure is equal to what we call the *osmotic pressure of the sugar solution.*

A membrane that allows water molecules to pass through but that does not allow the passage of other kinds of molecules is called a *semipermeable membrane*. If one solution is separated from another solution of different concentration by means of a semipermeable membrane, we may regard the osmotic pressure as a force that causes water molecules to pass *from the solution of lower concentration of the solute into the solution of higher concentration of the solute.*

COLLOIDAL DISPERSIONS

As we have already seen, when very small particles, such as sodium chloride molecules, are suspended in water, the resulting mixture is called a solution. The particles suspended in a true solution are small enough to pass through most animal membranes and will never settle out of solution. On the other hand, if we shake clay with water, the particles of clay, which are much larger than sodium chloride molecules, will remain suspended for a time, but eventually they will settle out of solution. The type of mixture that results from shaking clay with water is called a *suspension*. A third type of mixture, often encountered in animal and plant tissue, is called a *colloidal dispersion*. The particles of a colloidal dispersion are larger than the particles of a true solution, but they are smaller than those of a suspension. In general, particles in colloidal dispersion are too large to pass through most animal membranes, but they are small enough so they do not settle out of solution. Particles in true solution are always of about the same size, but in many cases the particles of a colloidal dispersion are of many different sizes. Colloidal dispersions look slightly cloudy when viewed at right angles to a beam of light that passes through them. The particles present in most kinds of colloidal dispersion consist of clumps of molecules, but this is not always true. Protein molecules, for example, are so large that even when single molecules are suspended in water, the resulting mixture is a colloidal dispersion.

DIALYSIS

A membrane that will allow water molecules and particles in true solution to pass through but that will not allow particles in colloidal dispersion to pass through is called a *dialyzing membrane*. Most animal membranes can be regarded as dialyzing membranes. Dialyzing membranes can be used as filters to separate particles in true solution and water molecules from particles in colloidal dispersion, and this method of separation is called *dialysis*. Particles in colloidal dispersion frequently cannot enter or leave cells in the body because most of the membranes that surround cells are dialyzing membranes.

COLLOID OSMOTIC PRESSURE

If a colloidal dispersion is separated from a true solution, or from water, by a dialyzing membrane, water will tend to flow across the membrane in the direction of the colloidal dispersion. In other words, colloidal particles act just like particles in true solution in causing osmotic pressure. Particles in true solution will not have much effect on osmotic pressure if the membrane we are using is a dialyzing one because they can easily diffuse through the membrane, and their concentration on both sides soon will be the same.

Colloid osmotic pressure is extremely important in physiology and medicine. This importance can be illustrated by means of an example. Suppose we consider the role of colloid osmotic pressure in the regulation of the exchange of water across the membranes that constitute the walls of the blood capillaries (see Fig. 30-3, page 357). Two different kinds of pressure act to cause a flow of water across capillary membranes. One of these pressures is the blood pressure, which tends to cause water to move across the membrane from the inside of the capillary to the tissue spaces. The other pressure is the colloid osmotic presure,* which tends to cause water to leave the tissue spaces and pass across the capillary membrane into the inside of the capillary. At the arterial end of the capillary (the end connected to an artery by means of an arteriole) the blood pressure is higher than the colloid osmotic pressure, and water will, therefore, leave the capillary, entering the tissue spaces. At the venous end of the capillary (the end connected to a vein by means of a venule) the blood pressure is lower than the colloidal osmotic pressure; at this end most of the water that left the arterial end of the capillary returns again to the bloodstream. In conditions like nephrosis, where the concentration of colloid in the plasma is reduced, the colloid osmotic pressure is also reduced. When this occurs, the amount of water that leaves the capillary will be greater than the amount that returns to it, and water will collect in the tissue spaces. The patient thus becomes "waterlogged." The medical name for this waterlogged condition is *edema*.

ADSORPTION

Particles in colloidal dispersion or in suspension have a very large total surface. Molecules in true solution that touch the surface of one of these particles tend to stick to it, and so are removed from solution. In other words, colloidal dispersions and suspensions, because of their large amount of surface, tend to *adsorb* molecules. Powdered charcoal, which also has a large surface, is placed in gas masks to adsorb poisonous gases. Charcoal sometimes is administered to patients to adsorb gases in the intestinal tract. The colloidal dispersions in cells adsorb molecules from the tissue fluids around them.

It will be recalled that substances that lower surface tension collect at surfaces. This kind of substance is most readily adsorbed by colloidal particles since a large amount of it will be present at the interface between the particle and the solution. Many dyes, such as methylene blue, are easily removed from solution by colloidal dispersions, or by powdered charcoal. Such dyes are surface active. Surface-active dyes are often used to dye cloth.

CHROMATOGRAPHY

The Russian botanist Michael Tswett (Mikhail Semenovich Tsvett, 1872–1919) invented chromatography, a procedure widely used in chemical laboratories today. The following translation from his article published in the *Berichte der deutschen botanischen Gesellschaft* in 1906 describes his observation in a very clear manner:

*The principal particles in colloidal dispersion in the blood plasma are the molecules of proteins, called plasma proteins. About 7 g of protein are present in each 100 ml of blood plasma. The net colloidal osmotic pressure from the plasma proteins sometimes is referred to as oncotic pressure.

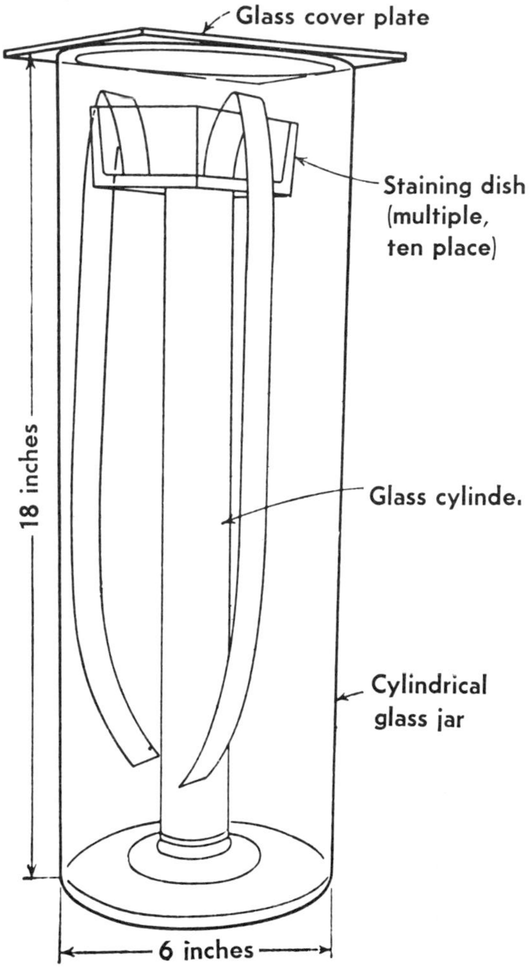

Fig. 9-4. Simple assembly for development of paper-strip chromatograms with descending solvent flow. Who first discovered chromatography? (Courtesy Dr. C. L. Comar.)

There exists a certain adsorption sequence, according to which substances are able to replace one another. The following application is based on this law. If a petroleum ether solution of chlorophyll is filtered through a column of adsorbent (I use mainly calcium carbonate which is stamped firmly into a narrow glass tube), then the pigments, according to the adsorption sequence, are resolved from top to bottom into various colored zones, since the stronger adsorbed pigments displace the weaker adsorbed ones and force them farther downward. This separation becomes practically complete if, after the pigment solution has flowed through, one passes a stream of pure solvent through the adsorbent column. Like light rays in the spectrum, so the different components of a pigment mixture are resolved on the calcium carbonate column according to a law and can be estimated on it qualitatively and quantitatively. Such a preparation I term a chromatogram and the corresponding method, the chromatographic method. It is self-evident that the adsorption phenomena described are not restricted to the chlorophyll pigments, and one must assume that all kinds of colored and colorless chemical compounds are subject to the same laws.

Many variations of Tswett's original method are used today. Colorless substances often can be identified by causing them to react with chemicals to produce a new colored substance. In some cases they can be detected with the aid of ultraviolet radiant energy. When a strip or sheet of filter paper is used as the adsorbent (that is, instead of Tswett's column of calcium carbonate) the procedure is known as *paper chromatography*.

STUDY QUESTIONS

1. What is a solution? Name several kinds of solution, giving an example of each kind.
2. Explain what is meant by the terms solvent and solute.
3. What solvent would you use to remove a grease spot from a dress? Why cannot fingernail polish be removed with water?
4. Name three factors that influence solubility. Try to list illustrative examples not given in the book.
5. Define the following terms: saturated solution; concentrated solution; unsaturated solution; supersaturated solution; dilute solution.
6. How do the freezing and boiling points of a cane sugar solution differ from the freezing and boiling points of water?
7. How many grams of calcium chloride are there in 300 ml of a 5 percent solution of calcium chloride? How many milliliters of acetone are there in 100 ml of 7 percent acetone solution?
8. How many grams of sodium hydroxide (NaOH) will be required to make 1 liter of 1 M solution of sodium hydroxide (refer to table of atomic weights on page 474)?
9. Explain, in your own words, what is meant by "surface tension." What is "interfacial tension"? What is meant by "surface-active substance"? What is the effect of surface-active substances on surface tension?
10. Name several emulsions that you have seen in your home.
11. How do surface-active substances (emulsifying agents) stabilize emulsions?
12. Explain, in your own words, what is meant by "osmotic pressure."
13. Define the following terms: semipermeable membrane; dialyzing membrane; dialysis.
14. How do colloidal dispersions differ from true solutions and from suspensions?
15. Explain how colloid osmotic pressure helps to regulate water exchanges between the bloodstream and the tissue fluids.
16. What is meant by "adsorption"? Explain the difference between adsorption and absorption (use any good dictionary). Give several examples of adsorption.
17. Make up your own definition of chromatography.
18. What is meant by "paper chromatography"?

CHAPTER 10

Acids, bases, and salts

INORGANIC AND ORGANIC COMPOUNDS

Compounds that contain carbon are much more numerous than all other compounds combined. It has been estimated that the total number of compounds now known to be present in the universe is in the millions. The overwhelming majority of these contain carbon. It is convenient, therefore, to divide chemical compounds into two groups: (1) those that do not contain carbon (inorganic compounds) and (2) those that do contain carbon (organic compounds). There are a few organic compounds, however, that are so similar in chemical behavior to typical inorganic ones that they may be considered for all practical pruposes as inorganic. Carbon itself, carbon monoxide (CO), carbon dioxide (CO_2), compounds containing the carbonate radical (CO_3), compounds containing the bicarbonate radical (HCO_3), and compounds containing the cyanide radical (CN) act like typical inorganic compounds and usually are included in discussions of inorganic chemistry.

DEFINITIONS

Acids are compounds made up of *hydrogen* combined with some other element or with a radical. Bases are compounds containing a metal or the ammonium radical combined with the *hydroxyl* (OH) radical. In a more general sense, any compound that will neutralize acids is regarded as a base. The word alkali often is used as a synonym for base. Salts are compounds formed by replacing the hydrogen of an acid by a metal or by the ammonium radical. Water, which contains both hydrogen and the hydroxyl radical, ordinarily is not included in any of the above three groups. Oxides, which may be thought of as compounds in which all the hydrogen of water has been replaced by a metal, usually are listed as a separate group of compounds. Since oxides can neutralize acids, they are often called alkalies in medicine.

The foregoing definitions apply to inorganic compounds. As we shall see later, acids, bases, and salts also are found among organic compounds.

Compounds that exhibit one color in the presence of acids and another color in the presence of bases are called *indicators*. Most of these compounds are organic. A few typical ones are given in Table 10-2.

INDICATORS

If a piece of filter paper is dipped in a solution of litmus, the paper becomes stained with the indicator and is called *litmus paper;* when a piece of it is dipped into a solution containing acid, it turns red. Bases turn litmus paper blue. *Phenolphthalein* is a white, tasteless powder, used in medicine both as an indicator and as a mild laxative. The chemical name for phenol red is *phenolsulfonphthalein*. The medical abbreviation of this term is PSP. In addition to its use as an indicator, this substance is used to find out whether or not the kidneys are functioning properly. When it is injected into the bloodstream of people whose kidneys are normal, 50 to 70 percent of it is eliminated in the urine in two hours. If the amount eliminated in the two-hour period is less than this, the physician assumes that the patient's kidneys are not functioning in a normal manner.

Table 10-1. Typical acids, bases, salts, and oxides

Acids	Bases	Salts	Oxides
HCl Hydrochloric acid	$NaOH$ Sodium hydroxide	$NaCl$ Sodium chloride	Na_2O Sodium oxide
HNO_3 Nitric acid	NH_4OH Ammonium hydroxide	NH_4NO_3 Ammonium nitrate	Ammonium oxide does not exist
H_2SO_4 Sulfuric acid	KOH Potassium hydroxide	K_2SO_4 Potassium sulfate	K_2O Potassium oxide
HCN Hydrocyanic acid	$AgOH$ Silver hydroxide	$AgCN$ Silver cyanide	Ag_2O Silver oxide
HNO_2 Nitrous acid	$Ca(OH)_2$ Calcium hydroxide	$Ca(NO_2)_2$ Calcium nitrite	CaO Calcium oxide
H_3PO_4 Phosphoric acid	$Mg(OH)_2$ Magnesium hydroxide	$Mg_3(PO_4)_2$ Magnesium phosphate	MgO Magnesium oxide
H_2CO_3 Carbonic acid	$Zn(OH)_2$ Zinc hydroxide $Pb(OH)_2$ Lead hydroxide	$ZnCO_3$ Zinc carbonate $Pb(HCO_3)_2$ Lead bicarbonate	ZnO Zinc oxide PbO Lead oxide

Table 10-2. Some common indicators

Indicator	Color with acids	Color with bases
Litmus	Red	Blue
Phenolphthalein	Colorless	Red
Phenol red	Yellow	Red
Methyl red	Red	Yellow

ACIDS

GENERAL PROPERTIES OF ACIDS

All acids possess certain characteristic properties and generally react with other substances in a definite manner. Following are the general properties of acids.

1. *All acid solutions taste sour.* Vinegar tastes sour, for example, because it contains a small amount (3 to 5 percent) of an organic acid called acetic acid.

2. *Many acids damage and destroy tissue.* Acids that destroy tissue and are very reactive chemically are called *strong acids.** Acids that damage tissue only slightly or not at all, and that react only slowly with other kinds of chemical compounds are called *weak acids.* Hydrochloric acid (HCl), sulfuric acid (H_2SO_4), and nitric acid (HNO_3) are strong acids commonly used in chemical laboratories. Phosphoric acid (H_3PO_4) is a weaker inorganic acid. In general, organic acids are weak acids. Acetic acid, found in vinegar, and lactic acid, found in sour milk and in many animal tissues, are weak organic acids.

3. *Acids react with most metals to form hydrogen gas and salts.*

Zn	+ 2 HCl	→	$H_2\uparrow$	+ $ZnCl_2$
Metal	Acid		Hydrogen	Salt
Fe	+ H_2SO_4	→	$H_2\uparrow$	+ $FeSO_4$
Metal	Acid		Hydrogen	Salt

The small vertical arrow written after H_2 indicates that this product is a gas. The *noble* metals (platinum, gold, silver) do not react with most acids. Acids should never be stored in metal containers, nor should metal surgical or dental instruments be cleaned with acids. Chemists ordinarily use glass vessels in experiments involving acids. If the type of experiment renders this impossible (if, for example, the temperature at which the reaction is to be carried out is high enough to melt glass), platinum vessels often are used.

4. *Acids react with oxides to form water and salts.*

CaO	+ 2 HNO_3	→	H_2O	+ $Ca(NO_3)_2$
Oxide	Acid		Water	Salt
MgO	+ 2 HCl	→	H_2O	+ $MgCl_2$
Oxide	Acid		Water	Salt

When this type of reaction is completed, acid is no longer present. In other words, oxides destroy, or *neutralize*, acids. A neutral solution is one that contains neither acid nor base. Oxides often are regarded as alkalies, or bases, because they have the ability to neutralize acids.

Normal gastric juice (the digestive fluid secreted by the stomach) contains small amounts (about 0.5 percent) of hydrochloric acid (HCl). Sometimes the stomach secretes too much hydrochloric acid (hyperacidity). Since this is a strong acid, too much of it in the stomach causes unpleasant symptoms, and the physician may give magnesium oxide (MgO), a harmless oxide, to the patient in order to neutralize the excess acid. Excessive

*A more scientific definition will be given later (see page 81).

amounts of hydrochloric acid are present in the stomach in simple hyperacidity (acid indigestion), ulceration of the duodenum, and gastritis (inflammation of the lining of the stomach). Hydrochloric acid is absent from the gastric juice of many old people and from patients who have the disease known as pernicious anemia. It is usually absent, or reduced in amount, in cases of cancer of the stomach.

5. *Acids react with bases to form water and salts.*

H_2SO_4 +	$2\,NaOH$	→	$2\,H_2O$ +	Na_2SO_4
Acid	Base		Water	Salt
HCl +	NH_4OH	→	H_2O +	NH_4Cl
Acid	Base		Water	Salt

When this type of reaction is completed, the acid and the base have both been neutralized. The reaction of an acid with a base to form water and a salt is called a *neutralization reaction.*

Acid burns are treated by flooding the burned area with water, after which a weak alkaline solution should be applied to neutralize any acid that still remains. It is important to wash the area first with water because acids are soluble in water and can be quickly removed with it. Dilute ammonia water (containing ammonium hydroxide, NH_4OH) or limewater (containing calcium hydroxide, $Ca(OH)_2$) may be applied without injury to tissue. Sodium bicarbonate ($NaHCO_3$, known also as baking soda) is not a true base, since it does not contain the OH radical, but it neutralizes acids and can be used in the emergency treatment of acid burns. If it is necessary to use a strong base, such as sodium hydroxide or potassium hydroxide, *it must be used in very dilute solution.*

Alkali burns are treated by preliminary flooding of the area with water, with subsequent application of a solution of a weak acid or of a dilute solution of a strong acid. Vinegar (which contains acetic acid) or boric acid solution is usually available, even in the home. If a strong acid is used, *it must be greatly diluted* to avoid injury to the patient. *Lye,* which is impure sodium hydroxide, is a frequent cause of alkali burns.

6. *Acids react with carbonates and bicarbonates to form carbon dioxide gas (CO_2), water, and salts.*

H_2SO_4 +	K_2CO_3	→	$CO_2\uparrow$ +	H_2O +	K_2SO_4
Acid	Carbonate		Carbon	Water	Salt
HCl +	$NaHCO_3$	→	$CO_2\uparrow$ +	H_2O +	$NaCl$
Acid	Bicarbonate		Carbon dioxide	Water	Salt

Sodium bicarbonate ($NaHCO_3$), ordinary baking soda, often is employed to neutralize excess acid in the stomach. Sodium carbonate (Na_2CO_3), or washing soda, is irritating to the lining of the alimentary tract and is not used to treat hyperacidity. We are familiar with calcium carbonate ($CaCO_3$) as *chalk* and as *marble.* This compound is frequently administered to patients for the purpose of removing excess hydrochloric acid from the stomach contents.

7. *Acids react with many salts to form new acids and new salts.*

$$\underset{\text{Acid}}{H_2SO_4} + \underset{\text{Salt}}{BaCl_2} \rightarrow 2\ \underset{\text{Acid}}{HCl} + \underset{\text{Salt}}{BaSO_4}\downarrow$$

The small arrow pointing downward indicates that barium sulfate, $BaSO_4$, is insoluble in water and therefore precipitates during the reaction. Soluble barium salts, like barium chloride ($BaCl_2$), are poisonous, but barium sulfate ($BaSO_4$) is too insoluble to be absorbed from the alimentary tract and can be administered to patients. This compound stops x-rays much better than does tissue and is often used in obtaining x-ray photographs of the intestinal tract. The intestinal tract, which contains the barium sulfate, shows up as a light area on the developed film.

Reactions of acids with salts are used in making many of the compounds used as drugs in medicine.

PHYSICAL PROPERTIES OF ACIDS Acids exist in all of the three physical states of matter. Boric acid, citric acid, and salicylic acid are examples of acids that are solids. Sulfuric acid and phosphoric acid are liquids. Hydrochloric acid, when it is not dissolved in water, is a gas and is usually called hydrogen chloride gas. None of the acids are very reactive, however, unless they are in solution.

RULES FOR NAMING ACIDS Acids containing only two elements are called *binary acids*. The name of a binary acid always begins with the prefix *hydro-*, and ends with the suffix *-ic*.

HCl	HBr	HF
*Hydro*chlor*ic* acid	*Hydro*brom*ic* acid	*Hydro*fluor*ic* acid

Ternary acids are composed of hydrogen, oxygen, and some third element. As a general rule, ternary acids are named after the third element (that is, the element present in addition to hydrogen and oxygen), and the most common ending employed is the suffix *-ic*.

H_2SO_4	H_3PO_4	H_2CO_3	HNO_3
Sulfuric acid	Phosphoric acid	Carbonic acid	Nitric acid

In some cases, however, more than one ternary acid that is made up of the same three elements exists. In this case the name of the acid with the greatest number of oxygen atoms per molecule ends in *-ic;* the name of the acid with the least number of oxygen atoms per molecule ends in *-ous*.

H_2SO_4 – sulfur*ic* acid	HNO_3 – nitr*ic* acid
H_2SO_3 – sulfur*ous* acid	HNO_2 – nitr*ous* acid

We may regard ternary acids as compounds formed by the union of hydrogen with radicals containing oxygen. Thus, sulfuric acid contains hydrogen united with the sulfate radical; sulfurous acid contains hydrogen united with the sulfite radical. This gives us another rule for naming ternary acids, provided we know the name of the radical that is united with hydrogen. If the name of the radical ends in *-ate*, the name of the acid will end in *-ic*. If the name of the radical ends in *-ite*, the name of the acid ends in *-ous*. Compare these rules with the examples given above. It will help to review the names of common radicals given in Table 5-1 (page 33).

BASES

GENERAL PROPERTIES OF BASES

Characteristic properties of bases and their reactions with other compounds are as follows.

1. *Solutions containing bases feel slippery. Such solutions have a bitter, somewhat metallic taste.* It is not safe to taste basic solutions unless they are very dilute.

2. *Strong bases damage and destroy tissue.* Sodium hydroxide (NaOH, lye) and potassium hydroxide (KOH, potash) are examples of strong bases. Ammonium hydroxide (NH_4OH) is weaker and will damage tissue only when it is in concentrated solution. Ammonium hydroxide is made by dissolving ammonia gas (NH_3) in water.

$$\underset{\text{Ammonia}}{NH_3} + \underset{\text{Water}}{H_2O} \rightarrow \underset{\text{Ammonium hydroxide}}{NH_4OH}$$

Calcium hydroxide ($Ca(OH)_2$) is a weak base. A solution of this compound is known as *limewater.*

The emergency treatment of burns caused by bases already has been described.

3. *Some bases react with metals of low atomic weight (for example, Na and K) to form new bases and metals.*

$$\underset{\text{Metal}}{2\,K} + \underset{\text{Base}}{Ca(OH)_2} \rightarrow \underset{\text{Base}}{2\,KOH} + \underset{\text{Metal}}{Ca}$$

This is a method of preparing certain metals. Most surgical and dental instruments and apparatus, however, are made of heavy metals that do not react with the bases commonly used in laboratories. Ammonia water, containing NH_4OH, often is used to clean such instruments, and grease or blood stains can be removed from them with dilute sodium hydroxide (NaOH) solution.

4. *Bases react with acids to form water and salts.*

$$\underset{\text{Acid}}{HNO_3} + \underset{\text{Base}}{KOH} \rightarrow \underset{\text{Water}}{H_2O} + \underset{\text{Salt}}{KNO_3}$$

This reaction, called *neutralization,* already has been discussed.

5. *Bases react with many salts to form other bases and other salts.* This reaction frequently is used to prepare bases.

$$\underset{\text{Salt}}{MgSO_4} + \underset{\text{Base}}{2\,NaOH} \rightarrow \underset{\text{Salt}}{Na_2SO_4} + \underset{\text{Base}}{Mg(OH)_2}\downarrow$$

Magnesium sulfate ($MgSO_4$), often called Epsom salt, and sodium sulfate (Na_2SO_4), also called Glauber's salt, are used in medicine as laxatives. Magnesium hydroxide ($Mg(OH)_2$) is insoluble, but it forms a milky suspension, known as milk of magnesia, when it is mixed with water. Milk of magnesia is used as an antacid (that is, a drug that will neutralize acids) and as a laxative. The reaction just preceding can be used to make milk of magnesia.

PHYSICAL PROPERTIES OF BASES

All common bases that can be isolated in pure form are solids at room temperature. (It has not yet been possible to separate ammonium hydroxide from water; that is, this base apparently does not exist except in solution.) In general, bases are reactive only when they are in solution.

RULE FOR NAMING BASES

Bases that are composed of a metal and the hydroxyl radical (OH) are named by giving the name of the metal and following this with the word *hydroxide*.

$NaOH$	$Ca(OH)_2$	$Al(OH)_3$
Sodium hydroxide	Calcium hydroxide	Aluminum hydroxide

KOH
Potassium hydroxide

Ammonium hydroxide is the name given to NH_4OH; it does not contain a metal.

SALTS

GENERAL PROPERTIES OF SALTS

Characteristic properties of salts and their reactions with other compounds are as follows.

1. *There is no general rule concerning the taste of salts.* Some taste sour; some, bitter; some, salty; some, metallic; and some, sweet. Many salts are poisons, and unknown salt solutions should be tasted only if the salt is in dilute solution.

2. *Under certain conditions a salt will react with a metal to form another salt and another metal.* If an iron nail is dipped into a solution of copper sulfate ($CuSO_4$), metallic copper will be deposited on the nail.

$$\underset{\text{Metal}}{Fe} + \underset{\text{Salt}}{CuSO_4} \rightarrow \underset{\text{Salt}}{FeSO_4} + \underset{\text{Metal}}{Cu}$$

Whether this type of reaction will occur or not depends upon the relative positions of the two metals in the electromotive series (review this; see page 53). Iron is above copper in this series and will therefore replace it from its salt. The preceding equation teaches us that it would not be wise to place copper sulfate solutions in containers made of iron, since some of the copper sulfate would thereby be changed to metallic copper and ferrous sulfate ($FeSO_4$).

3. *When salts react with each other, new salts are formed.* This type of reaction is utilized in making many salts employed in medicine and dentistry. Barium sulfate, which is used in taking x-ray photographs of the gastrointestinal tract, can be prepared by the following reaction.

$$Na_2SO_4 + BaCl_2 \rightarrow 2\ NaCl + BaSO_4\downarrow$$

4. *Some salts react with water to form small amounts of acids and bases* (see page 54). *Hydrolysis* is the name given to a reaction in which water is one of the reacting compounds. Hydrolysis in the case of salts may be regarded as the reverse of neutralization (review the equations illustrating neutralization, page 70).

$$\underset{\text{Salt}}{Na_2CO_3} + \underset{\text{Water}}{2\ H_2O} \rightleftarrows \underset{\text{Base}}{2\ NaOH} + \underset{\text{Acid}}{H_2CO_3}$$

The double arrow is used to indicate that this reaction takes place in both directions at once. The reaction is fastest when it is proceeding toward the left (when salt and water are being formed). This means that only small amounts of acid and base will be present at any particular time. In the example given above, the sodium hydroxide (NaOH) formed is much stronger as a base than carbonic acid (H_2CO_3) is as an acid. For this reason a solution of sodium carbonate (Na_2CO_3) acts like a solution of a weak base, and will turn litmus blue. We may regard Na_2CO_3 as a salt that has been made from the strong base NaOH and the weak acid H_2CO_3.

Ammonium chloride (NH_4Cl) is the salt of a strong acid (hydrochloric acid, HCl) and a weak base (ammonium hydroxide, NH_4OH). When NH_4Cl is dissolved in water it acts like the solution of a weak acid, since the small amount of HCl formed is many times more reactive than the NH_4OH that is also formed.

$$\underset{\text{Salt}}{NH_4Cl} + \underset{\text{Water}}{H_2O} \rightleftarrows \underset{\text{Acid}}{HCl} + \underset{\text{Base}}{NH_4OH}$$

Salts made by the reaction of a strong acid and a strong base will not hydrolyze (that is, they will not react with water). For example, potassium chloride (KCl), made by allowing a strong acid (HCl) to react with a strong base (KOH), will not hydrolyze.

5. *Salts react with acids and bases to form other acids and salts, and bases and salts.* Reactions of salts with acids and bases have been discussed.

SALTS RESPONSIBLE FOR HARD WATER

Water containing small amounts of calcium and magnesium salts is called *hard water*. Such salts are present in rocks and in soil, from which they are dissolved by water. If ordinary soap is added to hard water, the soap is converted to calcium soap (or magnesium soap), which is insoluble and precipitates out of solution.

$$\underset{\substack{\text{Calcium}\\\text{chloride}}}{CaCl_2} + \underset{\substack{\text{Sodium stearate}\\\text{(a soluble soap)}}}{2\,C_{17}H_{35}COONa} \rightarrow \underset{\substack{\text{Sodium}\\\text{chloride}}}{2\,NaCl} + \underset{\substack{\text{Calcium stearate}\\\text{(an insoluble soap)}}}{(C_{17}H_{35}COO)_2Ca\downarrow}$$

For this reason soap will not lather well in hard water. The situation is made worse by the fact that sodium chloride (NaCl, used as table salt) also is formed in the reaction, and soaps are not very soluble in NaCl solutions. For example, ordinary soap will not lather in sea water, which contains, in addition to calcium and magnesium salts, a considerable amount of NaCl.

The removal of the calcium and magnesium salts from hard water is said to *soften* the water. Water containing calcium and magnesium bicarbonates is called *temporary hard water*. Temporary hard water can be softened by boiling. This procedure converts the calcium and magnesium bicarbonates (which are soluble) to calcium and magnesium carbonates, which are insoluble, and which therefore precipitate from solution.

$$\underset{\substack{\text{Calcium}\\\text{bicarbonate}}}{Ca(HCO_3)_2} + \xrightarrow{\Delta} \underset{\substack{\text{Calcium}\\\text{carbonate}}}{CaCO_3\downarrow} + \underset{\text{Water}}{H_2O} + \underset{\substack{\text{Carbon}\\\text{dioxide}}}{CO_2\uparrow}$$

$Mg(HCO_3)_2$ +	$\xrightarrow{\Delta}$	$MgCO_3 \downarrow$	+ H_2O	+ $CO_2 \downarrow$
Magnesium bicarbonate		Magnesium carbonate	Water	Carbon dioxide

The small triangle indicates that heat has been used to cause the reaction to occur. If the hardness of the water is caused by other salts of calcium and magnesium, the condition is called *permanent hardness*. Permanent hard water can be softened by adding some compound that will convert the soluble calcium and magnesium salts to insoluble salts. Sodium carbonate (Na_2CO_3 washing soda) often is used for this purpose.

$$CaCl_2 + Na_2CO_3 \rightarrow CaCO_3 \downarrow + 2\ NaCl$$

Some sodium chloride also is formed in this reaction, but the amount formed is small and does not interfere very much with the solubility of the soap. Another compound used to soften water is *permutite* ($Na_2Al_2Si_2O_8$), which forms insoluble compounds with Ca and Mg.

ACID SALTS

It will be recalled that salts are compounds formed when the hydrogen of an acid is replaced by a metal or by the ammonium radical. It is sometimes possible to replace only a part of the hydrogen so that the resulting salt contains one or more of the hydrogen atoms (per molecule) that were present in a molecule of the acid.

H_2CO_3	+	NaOH	→	$NaHCO_3$	+	H_2O
Carbonic acid		Sodium hydroxide		Sodium bicarbonate		Water

Carbonic acid molecules contain 2 hydrogen atoms. If just the right amount of sodium hydroxide is added to carbonic acid, only 1 of these hydrogen atoms will be replaced by Na, and sodium bicarbonate will be formed. Salts that still contain a part of the hydrogen originally present in the acid are called *acid salts*. Sodium bicarbonate ($NaHCO_3$), potassium bisulfate ($KHSO_4$), and ammonium bisulfite (NH_4HSO_3) are examples of acid salts. If an alkali is added to an acid salt the hydrogen of the acid salt will be replaced by the metal of the alkali.

$NaHCO_3$	+	NaOH	→	Na_2CO_3	+	H_2O
Sodium bicarbonate		Sodium hydroxide		Sodium carbonate		Water

The salt formed (in this case, Na_2CO_3) does not have any of the hydrogen of the acid. Salts that do not contain in their molecules any of the reactive hydrogen atoms of the acids from which they are made are called *normal salts*. In the example just given, Na_2CO_3 is a normal salt. As the equation shows, acid salts can react with alkalies to form normal salts and water.

RULES FOR NAMING SALTS

The names of normal salts containing only 2 elements begin with the name of the metal (or ammonium radical) and end with the suffix *-ide*.

NaCl	NH_4Br	CaI_2	AlF_3
Sodium chloride	Ammonium bromide	Calcium iodide	Aluminum fluoride

In some cases the metal of this type of salt can have more than one valence. When this occurs, the endings *-ous* and *-ic* are added to the name of the metal, the former (-ous) indicating that the metal has its lower valence and the latter (-ic) indicating that the metal has its higher valence. Often the Latin name of the metal is used in naming this type of salt.

$HgCl$ —mercur*ous* chloride (valence of Hg here is 1+)
$HgCl_2$ —mercur*ic* chloride (valence of Hg here is 2+)

FeI_2 —ferr*ous* iodide (valence of Fe here is 2+)
FeI_3 —ferr*ic* iodide (valence of Fe here is 3+)
Latin name of iron is *ferrum.*

$CuBr$ —cupr*ous* bromide (valence of Cu here is 1+)
$CuBr_2$ —cupr*ic* bromide (valence of Cu here is 2+)
Latin name of copper is *cuprum.*

Mercurous chloride (calomel) is used in small doses as a laxative. Mercuric chloride (bichloride of mercury, corrosive sublimate) is used in dilute solution as a germicide (agent for killing germs). Both of these salts are poisonous if taken by mouth in too large doses.

The rules just given apply also to the naming of oxides, which, as we have seen, ordinarily are not regarded as salts.

Cu_2O	CuO	Na_2O	CaO	BaO
Cuprous oxide	Cupric oxide	Sodium oxide	Calcium oxide	Barium oxide

Normal salts, consisting of a metal (or ammonium radical) combined with a radical, are named by writing the name of the metal (or ammonium radical) and following it by the name of the radical.

Na_2CO_3	NH_4NO_3	$ZnSO_4$	$CaSO_3$	K_3PO_4
Sodium carbonate	Ammonium nitrate	Zinc sulfate	Calcium sulfite	Potassium phosphate

This type of salt also can be named by recalling the name of the acid from which the salt is derived. If the name of the acid ends in *-ic*, the name of the salt will end in *-ate;* if the acid name ends in *-ous*, the salt name will end in *-ite*.

H_2SO_4—sulfur*ic* acid	Na_2SO_4—sodium sulf*ate*
H_2SO_3—sulfur*ous* acid	Na_2SO_3—sodium sulf*ite*
HNO_3—nitr*ic* acid	KNO_3—potassium nitr*ate*
HNO_2—nitr*ous* acid	KNO_2—potassium nitr*ite*

If the metal of the salt has more than one valence, the rules already given above apply.

Hg_2SO_4	$HgSO_4$	Cu_2SO_3	$CuSO_3$
Mercurous sulfate	Mercuric sulfate	Cuprous sulfite	Cupric sulfite

The rules for naming normal salts also apply to acid salts, except that the prefix *bi-*, the word *acid,* or the word *hydrogen,* precedes the name of the radical.

$NaHCO_3$—sodium *bi*carbonate, sodium *acid* carbonate, or sodium *hydrogen* carbonate
NH_4HSO_3—ammonium *bi*sulfite, ammonium *acid* sulfite, or ammonium *hydrogen* sulfite

STUDY QUESTIONS

1. What is the essential difference between organic and inorganic compounds?
2. Name some compounds containing carbon that usually are discussed in inorganic chemistry.
3. Define: acid, base, salt, oxide, alkali. Why are oxides sometimes called alkalies?
4. What is an indicator? Name four indicators, listing the color of each in acid and in alkaline solution.

5. What substance, used as an indicator in chemistry, is used as a laxative in medicine?
6. What is the medical abbreviation for phenolsulfonphthalein? What is its use in medicine?
7. List seven general properties or reactions of acids. Illustrate the reactions by means of equations.
8. Why do vinegar and sour milk have a sour taste? What acid is present in vinegar? In sour milk?
9. Many baking powders contain sodium bicarbonate and a weak acid. When the baking powder is mixed with dough, carbon dioxide gas is formed and this causes the dough to rise. Explain. Explain why sour milk and baking soda can be substituted for baking powder.
10. Outline the emergency treatment for acid burns and for alkali burns. What impure substance is a frequent cause of alkali burns?
11. How do strong acids or bases differ from weak acids or bases? Give examples.
12. Name three metals that do not react with most acids.
13. Why should not surgical and dental instruments be cleaned with acids?
14. What acid is found in the stomach? In what conditions is too much of this acid present? In what conditions is too little present?
15. Name two compounds used in medicine to treat hyperacidity.
16. Define: neutralization, acid salt, normal salt, ternary acid, binary acid.
17. What is chalk? Marble?
18. Barium chloride is poisonous, but barium sulfate is not. Explain. For what purpose is barium sulfate used in medicine?
19. Name an acid that exists as a gas; as a solid; as a liquid.
20. Name the following compounds:

HCl	Na_3PO_4	$Ca(HCO_3)_2$	$Zn(OH)_2$
H_2SO_3	KBr	$Ba(HSO_4)_2$	$Fe(OH)_3$
HNO_3	$Pb(NO_2)_2$	NH_4HSO_3	$Fe(OH)_2$
$HgCl$	$HgCl_2$	Ag_2O	Fe_2O_3

21. List five general properties of bases. Illustrate reactions with equations.
22. Is it safe to wash metal surgical instruments with alkalies?
23. What is the chemical name of Epsom salt? Of Glauber's salt? For what purpose are they used in medicine? What is milk of magnesia?
24. List four general properties of salts. Illustrate reactions with equations.
25. Write an equation illustrating the hydrolysis of ammonium sulfate ($(NH_4)_2SO_4$). What color would an ammonium sulfate solution turn litmus paper?
26. Why should a copper sulfate solution, intended for use as an eye wash, not be stored in an iron container? Write an equation to illustrate.
27. What type of salt does not undergo hydrolysis?
28. What is the difference between temporary hardness and permanent hardness of water? What happens if a soap solution is added to hard water? Why is this a disadvantage?
29. Write equations illustrating the methods of softening water.
30. What is washing soda? Why is it useful in the laundry?

CHAPTER 11

Ionization

ELECTROLYTES AND NONELECTROLYTES

Some water solutions will conduct an electric current and others will not. Suppose we assemble the apparatus shown in Fig. 11-1. A battery, *B*, is connected by means of copper wires, *1* and *2*, to a solution contained in a beaker, *A*. An ordinary electric light bulb, *L*, is placed in the electrical circuit so hat if the solution in the beaker conducts the current the bulb lights up. Wire 1 is connected to the positive terminal of the battery and is called the *anode*. Wire 2, which is connected to the negative terminal, is the *cathode*. With this apparatus we find that solutions of acids, bases, and salts will conduct the current, but solutions of most other kinds of compounds will not. For example, solutions of hydrochloric acid, sodium hydroxide, and potassium sulfate when placed in the beaker cause the bulb to glow; solutions of cane sugar, alcohol, and glycerol produce no visible effect. Compounds whose solutions will conduct an electric current are called *electrolytes*. *Nonelectrolytes* are compounds whose solutions do not conduct the current. As the above examples illustrate, acids, bases, and salts are electrolytes; in general, other types of compounds are nonelectrolytes.

STRONG AND WEAK ELECTROLYTES

Some electrolytes in solution conduct the electric current well and are called *strong* electrolytes. Electrolytes that conduct the current poorly are termed *weak* electrolytes. Strong acids, strong bases, and salts are strong electrolytes. Solutions of hydrochloric acid, sodium hydroxide, or sodium chloride, when placed in the beaker, cause the light bulb to glow brightly. Weak acids and bases are weak electrolytes. Solutions of acetic acid and ammonium hydroxide cause the light to glow feebly.

OSMOTIC PRESSURE OF ELECTROLYTES

It will be recalled that the osmotic pressure of a solution depends on the number of dissolved particles in a given volume of solvent. A solution containing 1,000 particles dissolved in a small volume of water has twice the osmotic pressure of a solution containing only 500 particles in the same volume. The size of the particles has no effect on the osmotic pressure; the

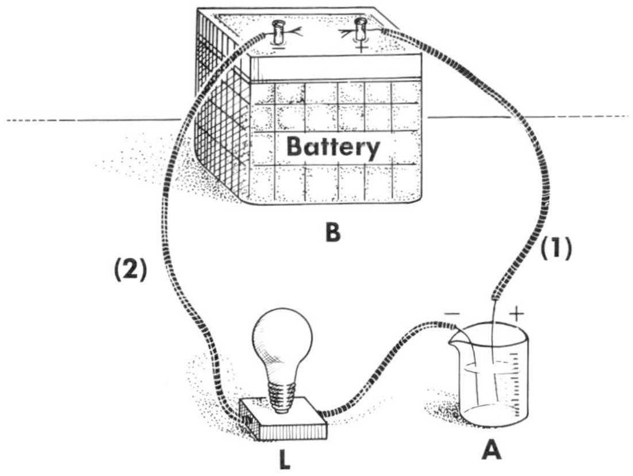

Fig. 11-1. Diagram illustrating the apparatus used in demonstrating electrolysis. What is the purpose of the electric light bulb?

number of particles, regardless of individual size in a given volume of solvent, is the determining factor. Avogadro's law (see page 20) tells us that gram-molecular weights of compounds contain the same number of molecules. Suppose we dissolve a gram-molecular weight of cane sugar in enough water to make a volume of 1 liter. We make another solution by dissolving a gram-molecular weight of alcohol in enough water to make 1 liter. It is to be expected that the osmotic pressures of the two solutions will be the same since they contain the same number of dissolved molecules in a liter of solution. If we measure the osmotic pressure of the solutions we find that this expectation is a fact: the value is the same for both solutions.

The experiment just described and many others similar to it show that solutions containing gram-molecular weights of *nonelectrolytes* in the same volumes of solution all have the same osmotic pressure. But if we dissolve a gram-molecular weight of sodium chloride in a given volume of water, we find that the osmotic pressure of the solution is about twice as great as it was in the case of nonelectrolytes. In the case of all electrolytes, strong or weak, the osmotic pressure is greater than we would predict. Since gram-molecular weights of electrolytes contain the same number of molecules as gram-molecular weights of nonelectrolytes, we are forced to the conclusion that some of the electrolyte molecules *must split into smaller particles in solution*. When we remember that the osmotic pressure depends only on the *number* of particles present in a given volume, it becomes clear that there must be more particles in a gram-molecular weight of an electrolyte in solution than there are in a gram-molecular weight of a nonelectrolyte in solution, in spite of the fact that the same number of *molecules* are present in both cases.

In the case of sodium chloride the osmotic pressure is nearly twice what we would expect. We can assume, then, that almost all of the sodium chloride molecules have split into 2 particles. Potassium sulfate molecules appear to split into 3 particles in solution; sodium phosphate molecules, into 4. If we examine these molecules, we find that we can account for the number of particles formed in solution by supposing that the individual atoms and radicals that make up the molecule have separated from each other: NaCl molecules contain 2 atoms; K_2SO_4 molecules contain 2 K atoms and 1 SO_4 radical; and Na_3PO_4 molecules contain 3 Na atoms and 1 PO_4 radical.

THEORY OF IONIZATION

In 1887 Svante Arrhenius, a Swedish chemist, advanced a theory to account for the fact that electrolytes in solution conduct the electric current and have high osmotic pressures. He assumed that some of the molecules in solution split into separate particles. These particles were assumed to be the atoms and radicals that made up the molecules, *except that these atoms and radicals, in separating from each other, were assumed to become electrically charged.* The charge that each atom or radical gained was thought to be equal to its *valence* both numerically and as to its positive or negative character. These electrically charged atoms and radicals are called *ions.*

When a sodium chloride molecule is dissolved in water it *ionizes,* or *dissociates,* to form a sodium ion and a chloride ion.* Since the valence of Na is 1+, the charge on the sodium ion is 1+. The chloride ion has a charge of 1− since in the case of binary salts the valence of chlorine is 1−. The ionization of NaCl may be written in the form of an equation:

$$\underset{\text{Sodium chloride molecule}}{NaCl} \rightleftarrows \underset{\text{Sodium ion}}{Na^+} + \underset{\text{Chloride ion}}{Cl^-}$$

Notice that the symbol for an ion is the same as the symbol for the atom (or radical) except that the value of the charge (which is equal to the valence) is also indicated. The double arrow indicates that some of the ions formed combine again with each other to form NaCl molecules. At any one time, then, both molecules and ions will be present in the solution.

The ionization of ammonium sulfate is illustrated by the following equation:

$$\underset{\text{Ammonium sulfate molecule}}{(NH_4)_2SO_4} \rightleftarrows \underset{\text{Ammonium ion}}{NH_4^+} + \underset{\text{Ammonium ion}}{NH_4^+} + \underset{\text{Sulfate ion}}{SO_4^{--}}$$

In other words, the 3 radicals (2 ammonium radicals and 1 sulfate radical) that make up the ammonium sulfate molecule separate from one another in solution. In so doing each radical acquires a charge that is equal to its valence (1+ for each ammonium ion and 2− for the sulfate ion) and thus becomes an *ion.* The individual atoms that make up the radical *do not separate from each other;* instead, the radical acts here as it does in all chemical reactions—as if it were a single atom. It would be wrong to say that

*It is customary to name ions after the molecule from which they are formed. Thus sodium ions and chloride (instead of chlorine) ions are formed from sodium chloride. Ions that are formed from radicals are named after the radical. Phosphoric acid (H_3PO_4) and sodium phosphate (Na_3PO_4) both form phosphate ions in solutions because both contain the phosphate radical.

ammonium sulfate ionizes to form hydrogen, nitrogen, sulfur, and oxygen ions. All of these atoms are present, but the atoms of a radical stick together in ionization. In writing ionization equations it is a useful check to remember that electrolytes *never form oxygen or nitrogen ions in solution.* If either of these ions appear in an equation we know at once that the equation is incorrect.

CONDUCTION OF AN ELECTRIC CURRENT BY ELECTROLYTE SOLUTIONS

Electrolyte solutions can conduct an electric current because electrically charged particles (ions) are present in the solution. Let us refer to Fig. 11-1. The flow of an electric current through a wire results from the passage of electrons through the wire. Under the influence of the battery (*B* in the diagram) electrons flow from the anode (wire 1) into the battery; and electrons flow from the battery to the cathode (wire 2). The anode loses negative charges and becomes positively charged; the cathode becomes negatively charged because it gains electrons. Suppose a solution of HCl is placed in beaker *A*. Because this compound is an electrolyte, it ionizes to form hydrogen ions and chloride ions:

$$HCl \rightleftarrows H^+ + Cl^-$$

The hydrogen ions have positive charge and are attracted to the cathode, which is negatively charged. Every time a hydrogen ion touches the cathode, the ion takes an electron from the wire and thereby becomes a hydrogen atom. (Remember that a hydrogen ion is a hydrogen atom that has lost 1 electron.) The hydrogen atoms (H) unite with each other to become hydrogen molecules (H_2), and hydrogen gas is formed at the cathode. This is one method of making hydrogen gas. The negatively charged chloride ions are attracted to the positively charged anode. Whenever a chloride ion touches the anode, the ion gives up an electron and becomes a chlorine atom. (Recall that a chloride ion is a chlorine atom that has gained an electron.) The chlorine atoms (Cl) thus formed unite with each other to form chlorine molecules (Cl_2), and chlorine gas is seen leaving the solution at the anode.

From what has been said, it is evident that electrolyte solutions such as HCl solutions give up electrons at the anode and take up electrons at the cathode. This enables a continuous stream of electrons to flow through the wires. It is this stream of electrons that causes the light bulb to glow and that we call the electric current.

Negatively charged ions, attracted to the anode, are called *anions.* Positively charged ions are called *cations* because they are attracted to the cathode.

ACIDS AND BASES IN WATER SOLUTION

It is now possible to define acids and bases in terms of the kinds of ion they produce in water solution. *Acids produce hydrogen ions, and bases produce hydroxyl (OH) ions in water.*

HCl	$\rightleftarrows$	H^+	+	Cl^-
Hydrochloric acid		Hydrogen ion		Chloride ion
$NaOH$	$\rightleftarrows$	Na^+	+	OH^-
Sodium hydroxide		Sodium ion		Hydroxyl ion

The chemical properties of acids and bases, explained in Chapter 10, are largely the chemical properties of the hydrogen and hydroxyl ions formed when the compounds containing them are dissolved in water. Strong acids and bases are highly ionized in solution. That is, most of the molecules in solution split apart to form ions. Only a small fraction of the molecules of a weak acid or base are ionized in water. We can drink vinegar, which contains about 4 percent acetic acid, without injuring our tissues, but an equal number of hydrochloric acid molecules in the same volume of solution is very destructive to tissue. This is true because the solution of hydrochloric acid contains many times more *hydrogen ions* than are present in the acetic acid solution.

The percentage of molecules that ionize in solution is determined partly by the concentration of the solution. A concentrated solution of sulfuric acid, for example is not nearly as reactive chemically as a more dilute solution. As the concentrated solution is diluted more and more, the percentage of molecules that split into ions increases until all the molecules finally are dissociated. Further dilution after this point is reached cannot, of course, cause the formation of any more ions. This effect of dilution on the degree of ionization applies equally to all electrolytes. We can say, in general, that chemical reactions take place most rapidly in solutions that are relatively dilute.

It will be recalled that the hydrogen atom is composed of a proton and an electron. Hydrogen ions have lost the electrons present in the original hydrogen atoms and hence really are protons (see page 24). Many modern chemists define an acid as something that donates, or gives up, a proton (hydrogen ion) to something else. From this point of view a base is something that accepts protons from an acid. For example, in the reaction*

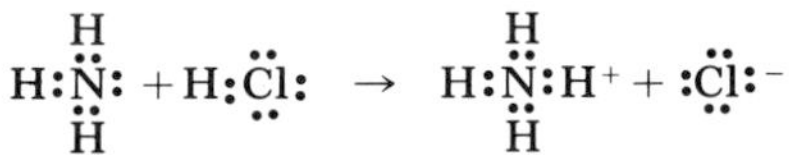

ammonia (NH_3) acts as a base, since it accepts a proton (H^+). The acid, of course, is HCl, since this compound donates a proton to the ammonia. Water is considered to act as a base when it comes in contact with a strong acid, since some of the water molecules accept protons, thus forming *hydronium ions* (H_3O^+).

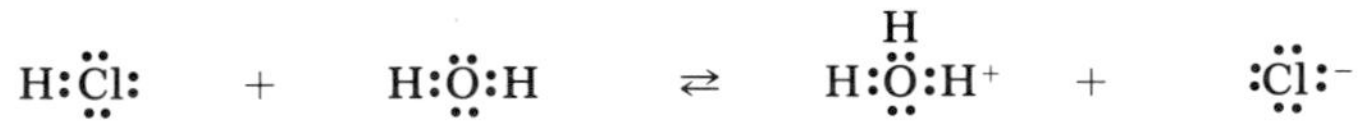

Acid (proton donor) | Base (proton acceptor) | Acid (proton donor) | Base (proton acceptor)

Note that this is a reversible reaction; when it proceeds to the left the hydronium ion (H_3O^+) acts as an acid (proton donor) and the chloride ion (Cl^-) acts as a base (proton acceptor).

SALTS IN WATER SOLUTION

Most of the salts soluble in water act as strong electrolytes. A solution of a salt, then is really in the main a solution of *ions*. When sodium chloride is dissolved in water the resulting solution is one of sodium ions (Na^+) and chloride ions (Cl^-), and only a very few undissociated molecules will be present.

*The dots represent the electrons in the outer electron shells of the atoms.

PHYSIOLOGICAL IMPORTANCE OF IONS

Ions are so important to the life and functioning of the tissues of the body that a special chapter largely devoted to this subject will be found in a later section of this book (Chapter 29). Correct osmotic pressure relations in the body are regulated largely by ions. Chemical reactions involving building new tissue and destroying and eliminating worn out tissue require ions in addition to carbohydrates, proteins, and fats, which form the bulk of the solid portion of living cells. Muscles cannot contract and nerves cannot conduct impulses except in the presence of certain necessary ions. Carbohydrates cannot pass from the intestinal tract to the bloodstream, nor from the bloodstream to the muscles without the assistance of phosphate ions. Calcium, magnesium, phosphate, and carbonate ions must combine with each other in proper proportions in order that bones be formed. The correct balance between hydroxyl and hydrogen ions in the various body fluids is necessary for life itself. The reactions that foods must undergo before it is possible for them to enter the body can take place only if the ratio of hydrogen and hydroxyl ions in the gastric and intestinal fluids is correct. Hemoglobin, the red pigment contained in the red blood cells, whose function it is to take oxygen from the lungs to the tissues, can be made only if ferrous (Fe^{++}) ions are available. Blood will not clot, nor will milk clot in the stomachs of infants, without calcium ions. In short, all that marvelous group of chemical reactions that we call life cannot take place without the intimate and active participation of *ions*.

EQUILIBRIUM IN ELECTROLYTE SOLUTIONS

A state of equilibrium is said to be reached when the number of ions and of undissociated molecules in the solution remains constant. Since molecules do not dissociate until they are in solution, it follows that none of the molecules are dissociated at the very instant they are placed in water. However, as time goes on, more and more molecules disintegrate to form ions. At the same time, as oppositely charged ions collide with each other, molecules are being re-formed. It is apparent that at first ions will be formed more rapidly than molecules because the number of ions present will be too small to allow frequent collisions. (Remember that molecules are formed when oppositely charged ions collide in solution.) As the number of ions in solution increases, the chance for collision increases, and the speed with which molecules are formed increases. Finally, there must come a time when the speed with which molecules dissociate to form ions exactly equals the speed with which new molecules are formed from the ions already present. When this *state of equilibrium* is reached, the number of ions and of molecules in solution will not change as time goes on because, on the average, as each new molecule is formed in solution another molecule splits into ions. As we have already observed, in writing ionization equations, a double arrow is used to indicate the simultaneous formation and dissociation of molecules.

Equilibrium can exist only if certain essential conditions are met: no molecules or ions must be added to or removed from the solution, and the temperature and pressure must remain constant.

1. Equilibrium cannot be reached if either molecules or ions are added to or removed from the solution. For example, if insoluble molecules are

formed when ions collide, these molecules will precipitate and equilibrium will not be reached, since the reaction will continue in only one direction until all possible insoluble molecules have thus been formed. Suppose, for example, that sodium chloride is added to water. It will ionize as indicated by the following equation.

$$NaCl \rightleftarrows Na^+ + Cl^-$$

If silver nitrate is added to another sample of water, it also ionizes:

$$AgNO_3 \rightleftarrows Ag^+ + NO_3^-$$

Now, if these two solutions are mixed, we shall have for a very short time a solution containing four different kinds of ion: Na^+, Cl^-, Ag^+, NO_3^-. Every time a silver ion collides with a chloride ion, however, an insoluble molecule of silver chloride (AgCl) is formed and precipitates from solution. This means that silver and chloride ions are removed permanently from solution; since this reaction is irreversible, it can proceed in only one direction.

$$Na^+ + Cl^- + Ag^+ + NO_3^- \rightarrow AgCl\downarrow + Na^+ + NO_3^-$$

Notice that we use only a single arrow in the above equation. Equilibrium between silver chloride and the ions that unite to form it (Ag^+ and Cl^-) is not possible, then, because *the silver chloride does not remain in solution and therefore cannot dissociate again into ions.*

2. Equilibrium cannot be reached unless the temperature and, to a lesser extent, the pressure exerted on the solution remain constant. When the temperature is changed the speed with which molecules dissociate to form ions changes, as does also the speed with which molecules are formed. Since these speeds are constantly changing as the temperature changes, equilibrium cannot be attained.

WATER AS AN ELECTROLYTE

Water is an extremely poor electrolyte since only 1 out of about 550,000,000 water molecules is ionized at ordinary temperatures.

$$H_2O \rightleftarrows H^+ + OH^-$$

The hydrogen and hydroxyl ions that water produces, however, are of great importance to living organisms. All body fluids contain a large proportion of water, and therefore all body fluids contain both hydrogen and hydroxyl ions. Even a solution of an acid, such as gastric juice, will contain hydroxyl as well as hydrogen ions, although in this case the latter (H^+) will far outnumber the former (OH^-).

The concentration of hydrogen ions in solution can be measured in several ways. Electrical methods, which require equipment too elaborate to be described here, give most accurate results. A simpler method consists in using indicators. As we have seen, indicators change color as the relative concentrations of hydrogen and hydroxyl ions change; that is, as the solution becomes more acid or more alkaline. No two indicators change color at exactly the same hydrogen ion concentration. Therefore, by using a series of different indicators and by observing which ones change color when they are added to a given solution, we can make a rough measurement of the concentration of hydrogen ions. If we desire to know the concentration of hydroxyl ions, we can then compute it by means of the following relation, which has been found to be true by experiment: $cH \times cOH = 10^{-14}$ (at 25° C). In this equation cH means concentration of hydrogen ions; cOH means concentration of hydroxyl ions. cH is measured as gram-atomic weights of hydrogen ions per liter of solution. Since the atomic weight of hydrogen is approximately 1, cH equals 1 when the solution contains about 1 gram of H^+ per liter. Similarly, cOH equals 1 when the solution contains about 17 (1 + 16) grams of OH^- per liter.

If the cH of a water solution is *greater* than the cOH, the solution has an *acid* reaction; if cH *equals* cOH the reaction is *neutral;* if cH is less than cOH the reaction is *basic* (alkaline).

PH NOTATION

The concentration of hydrogen ions in a neutral solution at 25° C is approximately 0.0000001 g per liter. In order to avoid having to write so many numbers scientists usually employ a notation known as the pH notation. The pH* of a neutral solution is 7. The pH of alkaline solutions is greater than 7, and the pH of acid solutions is less than 7. The following comparison will illustrate the relationship between cH, pH, and cOH:

If cH = 1.0, pH = 0, and cOH = 0.00000000000001.
If cH = 0.1, pH = 1, and cOH = 0.0000000000001.
If cH = 0.01, pH = 2, and cOH = 0.000000000001.
If cH = 0.001, pH = 3, and cOH = 0.00000000001.
If cH = 0.0001, pH = 4, and cOH = 0.0000000001.
If cH = 0.00001, pH = 5, and cOH = 0.000000001.
If cH = 0.000001, pH = 6, and cOH = 0.00000001.
The above pH values represent *acid* solutions.

If cH = 0.0000001, pH = 7, and cOH = 0.0000001.
This pH value (7) represents a *neutral* solution.

If cH = 0.00000001, pH = 8, and cOH = 0.000001.
If cH = 0.000000001, pH = 9, and cOH = 0.00001.
If cH = 0.0000000001, pH = 10, and cOH = 0.0001.
If cH = 0.00000000001, pH = 11, and cOH = 0.001.
If cH = 0.000000000001, pH = 12, and cOH = 0.01.
If cH = 0.0000000000001, pH = 13, and cOH = 0.1.
If cH = 0.00000000000001, pH = 14, and cOH = 1.0.
The above values represent *basic* (alkaline) solutions.

Notice that a change of one unit on the pH scale represents a change of 10 times in hydrogen ion concentration. For example, the concentration of hydrogen ions is 10 times as high at pH 5 as is the case at pH 6. If the pH of a solution is *lowered* from pH 6 to pH 4, the concentration of hydrogen ions increases 100 (10 × 10) times. Conversely, when the pH is *raised* from 6 to 8 the hydrogen ion concentration is lowered to one-hundredth (0.1 × 0.1) of its former value.

*The pH can be defined by the mathematical expression, $pH = \log \frac{1}{cH}$. Since the cH of a neutral solution at 25° C is 0.0000001, the $pH = \log \frac{1}{0.0000001} = \log 10000000 = 7$.

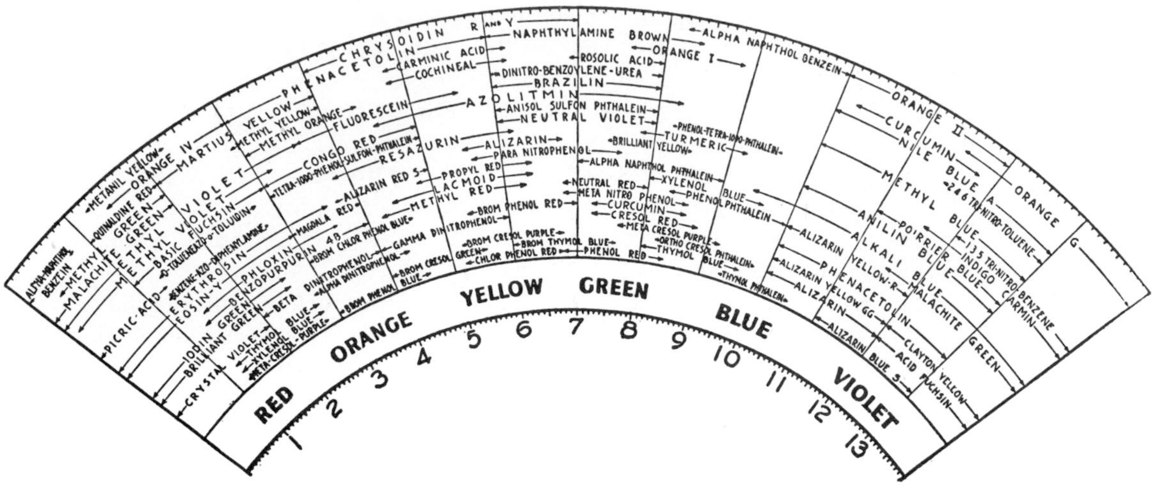

Fig. 11-2. Diagram showing a number of indicators and the pH values between which they change color. The numbers indicate pH. How could these indicators be used to measure the pH of a sample of urine? (Courtesy Hartman-Leddon Co.)

The concentration of hydrogen ions is said to be 1 when the solution contains an equivalent weight (1.008 g, see page 58) of hydrogen ions per liter. The concentration of hydroxide ions is 1 when the solution contains 17.01 g of hydroxide ions per liter, since the equivalent weight of the OH radical is 17.01. The figure 10^{-14} in the relation on page 85 refers to gram-equivalent weights.

In the special case where $[H^+] = [OH^-]$ we may write:

$$[H^+]^2 = 10^{-14}, \text{ or } [H^+] = 10^{-7}$$

In other words, a neutral solution (that is, a solution in which $[H^+] = [OH^-]$) contains 10^{-7} gram-equivalent weights of hydrogen ions per liter.

The term pH, an abbreviation for "power function of $[H^+]$," is defined by the equation

$$[H^+] = 10^{-pH}$$

Since the hydrogen ion concentration of a neutral solution is 10^{-7}, we say that *the pH of a neutral solution is* 7. In acid solutions $[H^+]$ is always greater than 10^{-7}, and the pH is always *less than* 7. For example, the concentration of hydrogen ions in a 0.01 N solution of HCl is approximately 0.01 (10^{-2}), and the pH is approximately 2. In basic (alkaline) solutions $[H^+]$ always is less than 10^{-7} and the pH is *greater than* 7. A 0.01 N solution of NaOH contains approximately 10^{-2} gram equivalents of hydroxide ions per liter. Since $[H^+] \times [OH^-] = 10^{-14}$, the hydrogen ion concentration of the solution will be 10^{-12}, and the pH will be 12.

IMPORTANCE OF pH CONTROL

The normal pH of the blood is about 7.4. The blood is thus very slightly alkaline in reaction. If the pH of the blood rises above 7.8 or falls below 7.0, death follows. The pH of freshly secreted gastric juice is about 1; gastric juice cannot perform its digestive functions if the pH is too high (as it

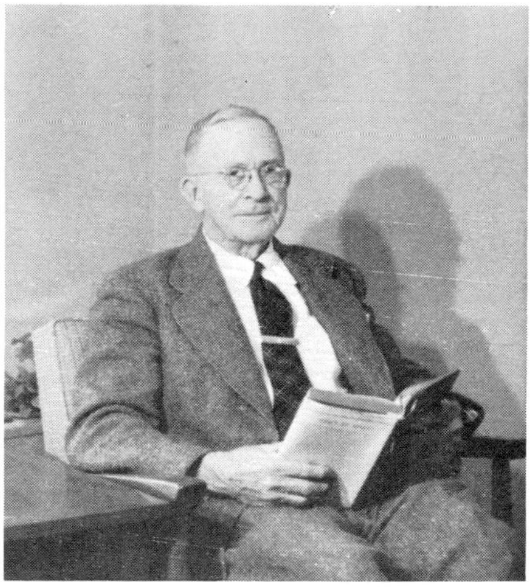

Fig. 11-3. Dr. Jesse Francis McClendon was one of the first scientists in the United States to recognize the importance of the control of pH in biochemical and biological experimentation. He and his students proved that the pH of the small intestine was not above 7, as had been supposed (see page 329), by swallowing electrodes and making actual measurements of the intestinal pH. Early in his scientific career, Dr. McClendon constructed one of the first workable microdissection instruments. He has done a great deal of work on the physiology of the thyroid gland (see page 390), and long before the use of fluoride in inhibiting dental decay, he suggested that the remaining enamel of sound teeth probably contained more fluoride than did the enamel of decayed teeth; one of his graduate students proved that this was true. He produced fluorine deficiency in the rat by feeding a diet composed of vegetables grown in fluoride-free solutions. He produced true osteoporosis in the rat and explained how it differed anatomically and etiologically from rickets (see page 439). He demonstrated also that calcium salts, if give in large amounts over a long period of time, could reverse osteoporosis in the rat. He has made numerous other contributions in the fields of nutrition and biochemistry. Why do you think it is important to control pH in a biological experiment?

may be, for example, after taking a teaspoonful of baking soda, an amount sufficient to neutralize all the hydrochloric acid in the average normal stomach). Pancreatic juice has a pH of about 8 and is, therefore, slightly alkaline. The pancreatic enzymes do their work best in slightly alkaline solutions. Normal saliva is nearly neutral (pH 7) in reaction; if the pH of this fluid falls below 4, the enamel of the teeth begins to dissolve.

The pH is important in all the fields of medical and biological science. The bacteriologist has found that bacteria do not grow unless the pH of the culture medium is carefully adjusted. Bacteria are more easily killed at certain pH values than at others. Indeed, a slight alteration of the pH of a bacterial culture is often sufficient to destroy the living microorganisms. The physiologist knows that muscles and nerves cannot be maintained alive outside the body unless they are contained in solutions whose pH values are those of the body fluids. Histologists and pathologists have discovered that tissues can only be stained for microscopic examination when the pH of the stain solution is proper. Certain drugs injected into the veins of patients become useless, or even deadly poisons, if the pH of their solutions is incorrectly adjusted.

BUFFERS Certain compounds have the ability to neutralize acids or bases and in this way prevent large changes in pH. Such compounds, called *buffers,* are found in all body fluids, and are responsible for maintaining the proper pH of each such fluid. Suppose a weak solution of hydrochloric acid (and even a weak solution of a strong acid has a much lower pH than the blood) is injected into the bloodstream. The following reactions immediately occur:

$$HCl + NaHCO_3 \rightarrow NaCl + H_2CO_3$$
$$H_2CO_3 \downarrow H_2O + CO_2\uparrow$$

The carbon dioxide (CO_2) formed is eliminated in the lungs. The sodium bicarbonate, a normal component of the blood, has neutralized the hydrochloric acid, and by so doing has prevented a fatal alteration of the blood pH. Sodium bicarbonate is one of the principal buffers of the alkaline body fluids. If weak sodium hydroxide is injected into a vein, carbonic acid, another blood buffer, neutralizes it:

$$NaOH + H_2CO_3 \rightarrow H_2O + NaHCO_3$$

Other important buffers of the blood include the phosphates and proteins.

Many procedures carried out in scientific laboratories and in hospital laboratories require the use of buffered solutions (solutions that resist a change in pH). Suitable buffer solutions usually are prepared by mixing together two chemicals, one of which is more acidic than the other. Depending on the pH value desired, one or both of these compounds has the ability to combine with hydrogen or hydroxyl ions that might find their way into the solution. They thus tend to prevent a large change in pH. A buffer solution suitable for the range of pH from 5.3 to 8.0 is made by dissolving appropriate quantities of KH_2PO_4 and Na_2HPO_4 in water. If hydrogen ions enter the solution, the Na_2HPO_4 combines with them:

$$Na_2HPO_4 + HCl \rightarrow NaH_2PO_4 + NaCl$$

Similarly, if hydroxyl ions enter, the KH_2PO_4 will undergo a reaction:

$$KH_2PO_4 + KOH \rightarrow K_2HPO_4 + H_2O$$

These reactions tend to minimize changes in pH, because the new compounds formed (NaH_2PO_4 and K_2HPO_4 in the above examples) do not appreciably increase the acidity or alkalinity of the solution. The quantity of strong acid required to change the pH of a phosphate buffer by 0.3 of a pH unit would, if added to unbuffered pure water, change the pH value by 5.7 pH units.

Other buffers frequently used are boric acid–sodium acetate (pH 3.6 to 5.6), sodium citrate–hydrochloric acid (pH 1.0 to 3.5), acetic acid–sodium acetate (pH 3.6 to 5.6), and glycine*–sodium hydroxide (pH 8.5 to 13.0).

*Glycine is an amino acid; see page 270.

STUDY QUESTIONS

1. What is the anode? The cathode?
2. Define electrolyte. What is the distinction between strong and weak electrolytes?
3. What is the effect of the size of dissolved particles on osmotic pressure?
4. State Avogadro's law.

5. Explain why the osmotic pressure of a K_2SO_4 solution is about three times as great as the osmotic pressure of an alcohol solution containing an equal number of molecules.
6. Who was Arrhenius? What theory did he advocate to explain the difference between electrolytes and nonelectrolytes?
7. How do you account for the fact that the charge an ion has is equal numerically to its valence?
8. How does an ion differ from an atom? From a radical?
9. Write ionization equations for the following electrolytes: H_2SO_4, $Ca(OH)_2$, $MgBr_2$, $NaHCO_3$, NH_4Cl.
10. Why do not the atoms that form radicals separate from each other in solution?
11. What is the electric ourrent that passes along a wire? Through a solution?
12. What would be formed at the cathode and at the anode if an electric current passes through a solution of NaCl?
13. Define acids, bases, and salts in terms of the type of ions they produce in water solution.
14. Which would you expect would react most rapidly with zinc: concentrated sulfuric acid or dilute sulfuric acid? Why?
15. List 10 reasons why ions are important in physiology and medicine.
16. What is meant by equilibrium in electrolyte solutions? What conditions are necessary in order that such an equilibrium can be reached?
17. Write the ionization equation for water. What ions are present in pure water?
18. Describe a method for measuring the concentration of hydrogen ions. In what units is the concentration of hydrogen ions usually measured?
19. What is the pH of a neutral solution?
20. How many times more hydrogen ions are present in a liter of solution of pH 3 than are present in a liter of solution of pH 5?
21. Give reasons why pH control is important in medicine.
22. Would the pH of vinegar be more or less than 7? The pH of limewater? Explain.
23. How do buffers work? Name some important buffers found in the blood.

CHAPTER 12

Chemical bonds

ELECTROVALENCE AND THE NATURE OF IONS The sodium atom contains 1 electron in its outer electron shell; the chlorine atom has 7. When Na reacts with Cl to form NaCl, the Na atom *gives* its 1 electron to the Cl atom. This completes the outer electron shells of both atoms. Both atoms were electrically neutral (that is, they had the same number of positive and negative charges) before the reaction. Cl now gains an electron from Na, however, and becomes charged 1−. Na, since it has lost a charge of 1− (an electron), becomes charged 1+. The negatively charged Cl is now a chloride *ion,* and the positively charged Na is a sodium *ion.* Because opposite electrical charges attract each other, the Na ion and the Cl ion stick to each other to form a molecule of NaCl (see Fig. 5-3, page 40). In short, molecules of NaC1 (and of nearly all electrolytes) may be regarded as consisting of ions. Since molecules are electrically neutral (we do not get an electric shock when we touch NaCl) the number of + charges on the ions in a molecule equals the number of − charges present. When an electrolyte is dissolved in water, some of its molecules simply separate into the individual ions of which the molecule is composed. The number of + ionic charges produced by ionization will always equal the number of − ionic charges. This must be true because + and − charges are equal in number in the original molecule.

The type of valence in which the forces that hold the atoms (or radicals) of a molecule together result from attractions between oppositely charged ions is called *electrovalence.* Only molecules having electrovalence can form ions in water. Electrovalence is thus characteristic of electrolytes.

COVALENCE The type of valence holding the atoms of nonelectrolyte molecules together is called *covalence.* Some water molecules possess electrovalence, but most water molecules contain only covalent linkages. We may picture a water molecule as shown in Fig. 12-1. We see that each hydrogen atom is *sharing* its electron with the oxygen atom. In turn the oxygen atom is *sharing* 1 electron with each hydrogen atom. Each hydrogen atom thus

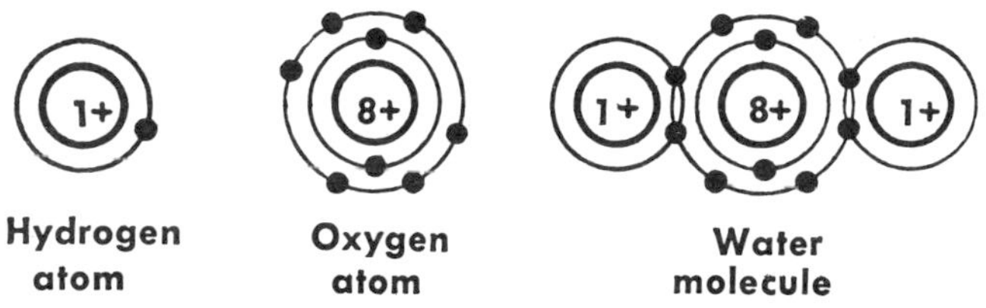

Fig. 12-1. Diagrams of the hydrogen atom, the oxygen atom, and the water molecule. How does covalence differ from electrovalence?

becomes associated with 2 electrons, which fills its outer shell (remember that the first electron shell is filled by 2 electrons). The oxygen atom has completed its outer electron shell by sharing the electrons of the hydrogen atoms. This type of molecule does not possess ions and will not ionize in water.

The atoms of a radical are held together by covalence. This explains why radicals do not split apart into individual atoms in ionization. For example, the molecule of NaOH may be pictured diagrammatically as follows:

$$Na \xrightarrow[\text{bond}]{+\ \text{electrovalent}\ -} O \xrightarrow[\text{bond}]{\text{covalent}} H$$

When this molecule is placed in water only the electrovalent bond can break, and NaOH ionizes to form Na^+ and OH^-.

$$NaOH \rightleftarrows Na^+ + OH^-$$

Coordinate covalence. When ammonia gas, NH_3, is bubbled into a solution containing hydrogen ions and chloride ions (that is, into a solution of hydrochloric acid) the NH_3 promptly unites with a hydrogen ion to form the ammonium ion NH_4^+.

Ordinary equation: $NH_3 + HCl \rightarrow NH_4Cl$
Ionic equation: $NH_3 + H^+ + Cl^- \rightarrow NH_4^+ + Cl^-$

How are we to account for this union of a hydrogen ion with an ammonia molecule? Since neither the ammonia molecule nor the hydrogen ion has given away an electron, it cannot be electrovalence. It cannot be ordinary covalence either because an ion of hydrogen has no electron to share with the ammonia. Suppose we write the ionic equation in another way, using small dots to indicate the electrons in the *outer* electron shells of the atoms and ions.

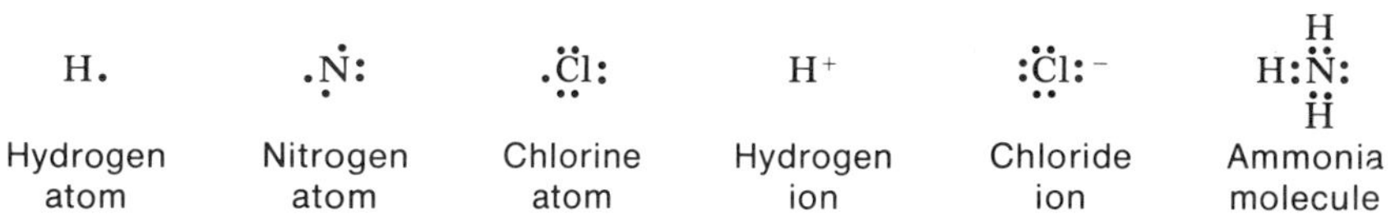

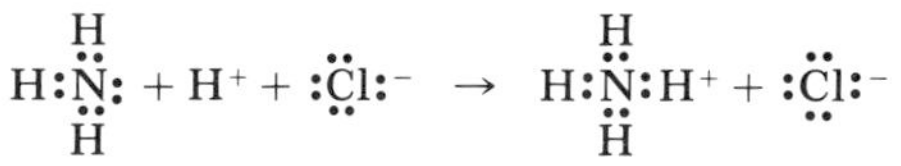

What has happened? We notice that before the reaction takes place, the nitrogen atom in the ammonia molecule has 2 electrons that *it is not sharing with anything*, and that the hydrogen ion *has no electrons*. The nitrogen of the ammonia molecule shares its 2 extra electrons with the hydrogen ion to form an ammonium ion. In doing so it completes the outer shell of hydrogen (which now contains 2 electrons), and the outer shell of the nitrogen still is complete (since it still contains 8 electrons). This type of linkage is known as *coordinate covalence*, or *semipolar valence*. It differs from covalence because in covalence each reacting particle shares *one* of its electrons with the other particle; in coordinate covalence *each of the 2 shared electrons is donated by one of the reacting particles, the other particle (in our example, the hydrogen ion) contributing no electron to the linkage.*

HYDROGEN BOND The structure of hydrogen fluoride (hydrofluoric acid when in solution) ordinarily is written HF. However, it has been found that other compounds containing only hydrogen and fluorine exist. Some of them have the following molecular formulas: H_2F_2, H_3F_3, H_4F_4, H_5F_5, H_6F_6. This suggests that molecules of HF tend to unite with each other. What is the nature of the chemical bond that holds them together? In order to answer this question, let us write the structure of HF in such a way that the electrons in the outer shell of fluorine are indicated by dots.

$$H^+{:}\ddot{\underset{\cdot\cdot}{F}}{:}^-$$

The H^+ is simply a proton (hydrogen atom minus its electron) that has a unit positive charge. The fluoride portion of the molecule has a unit negative charge because it has acquired one electron from the hydrogen atom. If two HF molecules approach each other, the positively charged hydrogen of one will attract the negatively charged fluoride of the other, and there will be a tendency for the two molecules to stick together, as illustrated by the following formula:

$$H^+{:}\ddot{\underset{\cdot\cdot}{F}}{:}^-H^+{:}\ddot{\underset{\cdot\cdot}{F}}{:}^-$$

Evidently the force holding the two molecules together is the mutual attraction of the two negatively charged fluorine atoms for the positively charged hydrogen atom (proton) between them. This type of bond in which two negatively charged ions are bound together by a proton is called a *hydrogen bond*. The various forms of hydrogen fluoride can be illustrated by the following diagrams:

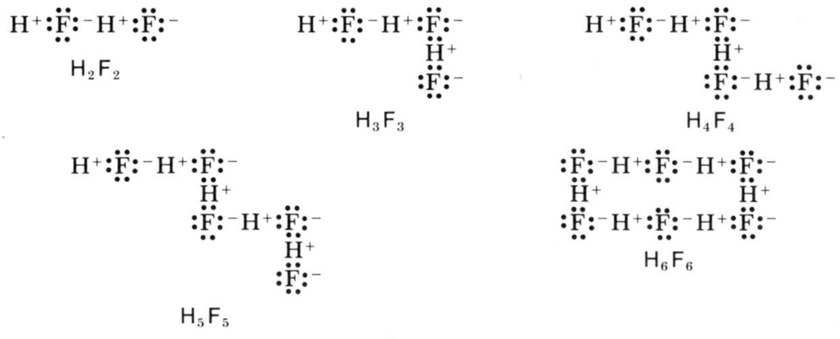

The hydrogen bond is weaker than ordinary ionic or covalent bonds, but is stronger than ordinary van der Waals forces (see page 29).

In writing structural formulas hydrogen bonds usually are indicated by dotted lines. For example, the structural formula of H_2F_2 can be written

$$F^-—H^+ \ldots\ldots F^-—H^+$$

Only the most electronegative atoms form hydrogen bonds. The only elements involved (aside from hydrogen) in most cases are fluorine, oxygen, and nitrogen.

Water molecules contain two hydrogen ions attached to an oxygen possessing two unshared pairs of electrons.

$$H^{+-}:\ddot{\underset{\cdot\cdot}{O}}:^-H^+$$

Hence, there is the possibility of having four hydrogen bonds formed for each water molecule (one for each H^+ and one for each unshared electron pair). This leads to the characteristic crystal structure of ice in which each H_2O molecule is surrounded by four other H_2O molecules.

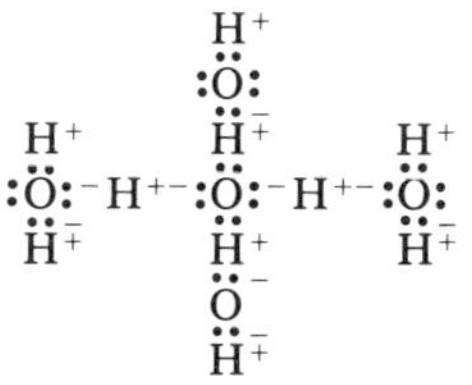

This is a rather "open" structure (that is, it contains many "holes"), with

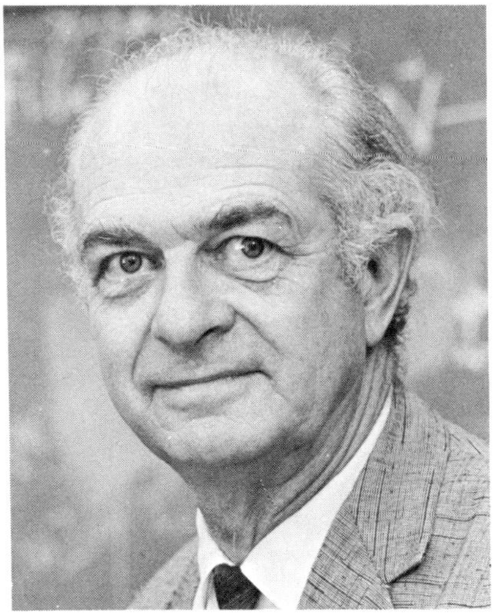

Fig. 12-2. Dr. Linus C. Pauling, then Chairman of the Division of Chemistry and Chemical Engineering at the California Institute of Technology, was awarded the Nobel Prize in chemistry in 1954 for his work on the nature of the chemical bond. In 1963 he had the remarkable distinction of receiving a second Nobel Prize, this one the Nobel Peace Prize. How does a semipolar bond differ from a hydrogen bond?

the result that ice actually is lighter than is liquid water. At the freezing point of water this structure is partly destroyed, but many hydrogen bonds remain. As the temperature is raised, more and more hydrogen bonds are disrupted, causing a further increase in the density of the water. Finally, at 4° C, where water has its maximal density, the normal expansion (separation of molecules from each other) due to increased molecular motion caused by an increase in temperature overcomes this effect. Above 4° C the density of the water decreases with increasing temperature.

Hydrogen bonds, usually between nitrogen and oxygen atoms, occur in the structures of proteins and nucleic acids (see pages 273 and 299).

RESONANCE BONDING

In a relatively few cases it is not possible to arrange the valence electrons in a molecule in such a way that the octet rule (8 electrons in the outer shell of each combined atom) and the rule that valence electrons between atoms in the molecule generally are paired (one pair for a single bond, 2 pairs for a double bond, and 3 pairs for a triple bond) are satisfied. One compound that illustrates this difficulty is sulfur dioxide, SO_2. Both S and O in the uncombined state have 6 electrons in their outer shells.

One structure that would at first glance appear to obey the rules is this:

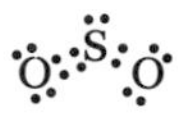

But this specifies a molecule in which one of the bonds between S and O is a double bond (4 shared electrons) and the other is a single bond (2 shared electons). However, careful physical measurements have shown that a double bond is shorter than a single bond. Equally careful measurements prove that both of the bonds in the SO_2 molecule are equal in length, and so the above structure is ruled out.

There are some compounds in which it is necessary to assume that unpaired electrons occur in the molecule. A common example is O_2. (Try to draw dot diagrams of this molecule.) However, all such compounds are *paramagnetic;* that is, they are weakly attracted to magnets. A diagram for SO_2 in which unpaired electrons occur is as follows:

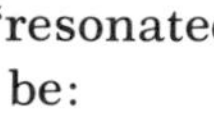

SO_2 is *not* paramagnetic and thus this structure is ruled out also.

Resonance is a word introduced into the nomenclature of chemistry to describe the situation in which *no single electronic configuration satisfies both the octet rule and observed properties.* Probably the word resonance was chosen because chemists at first thought that such molecules existed in 2 forms that rapidly "resonated" back and forth between each other. The 2 forms of SO_2 might be:

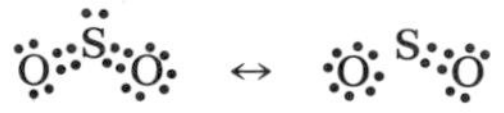

However, chemists believe today that compounds such as SO_2 that exhibit resonance really have only one electronic structure. This single structure is called a *resonance hybrid*—perhaps in a far-fetched sense like the hybrid roses that result from crossing different varieties with each other. The problem, then, is that we simply do not know how to draw the "correct" electronic structure for resonance bonds.

THE QUANTUM MECHANICAL PICTURE OF THE CHEMICAL BOND

(*Review Quantum mechanical concept of atomic structure,* page 24.) One of the principles of the branch of physics known as quantum mechanics is the *uncertainty principle.* It states, among other things, that it is impossible to describe the *exact* motions or orbit of even a single planetary electron. It is possible, however, to calculate the probability (chance) that a given electron will occupy a given point in space at a given time. Physically, the electron, then, can be pictured as occupying a "cloud," the density of which varies from place to place—the greater the probability of occupancy by the electron, the greater the density of the cloud.

The electron cloud is known as an *orbital,* and can be thought of as the electron's region of influence. Another principle of quantum mechanics—the exclusion principle—says that a single orbital can be occupied by 1 or by 2 electrons. If 2 are present, they must be spinning in opposite directions.

The orbitals of an atom are identified by 2 quantum numbers. The first of these (n) is simply the number of the electron shell (1, 2, 3, 4, and so on). The first electron shell has only 1 orbital, identified as 1*s*. The second electron shell has 2 subshells, designated 2*s* and 2*p*. The 2*s* subshell has a single orbital; it can contain 0, 1, or 2 electrons. The 2*p* subshell has 3 orbitals; each can contain 0, 1, or 2 electrons. Thus the second electron shell can contain a total of 8 electrons, as we have learned already. The exclusion principle does not allow any 2 orbitals in a given subshell to have the same direction in space. Hence the 3 orbitals of the 2*p* subshell are at right angles to each other; that is, they lie along the x, y, and z axes of three-dimensional space.

Other shells are more complicated. They contain *s* and *p* subshells as well as new ones identified with the quantum numbers *d* and *f*. Each *d* subshell has 5 orbitals; *f* subshells have 7 orbitals.

Quantum mechanics pictures the chemical bond as the overlapping of two orbitals, each containing only a single electron. Orbitals containing 2 electrons cannot form chemical bonds, and actually repel each other. The strength of the bond depends on the amount of overlap: the greater the overlap, the stronger the bond. In this new picture of valence, electrovalence and covalence are not really separate types of structure. If each of the electrons involved spends all of its time near one of the nuclei of a molecule, the bond will be ionic (electrovalent); if the 2 electrons divide their time equally between the two nuclei, the bond is covalent. In many cases the bond is somewhere between these extremes. For example, the principal bonding in water is covalent, but some of the bonds at any given time are ionic (electrovalent), as proved by the fact that hydrogen ions and hydroxyl ions occur in low concentrations in water.

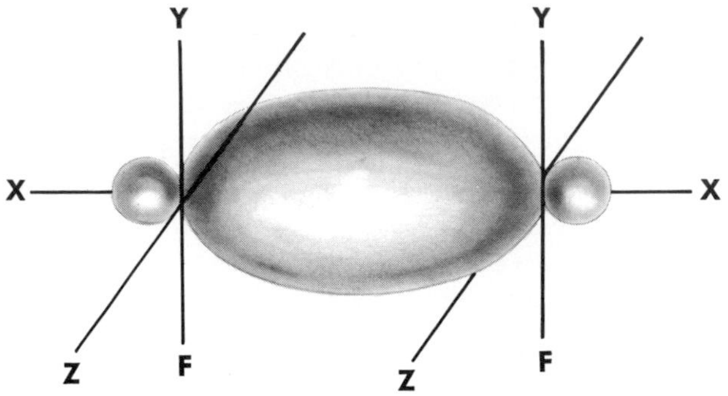

Fig. 12-3. Electron charge cloud representing the electron-pair bond (covalent bond) involving the overlap of two *p* orbitals in the F_2 molecule. Is there distortion of the overlapping *p* orbitals (see Fig. 4-6, page 28)?

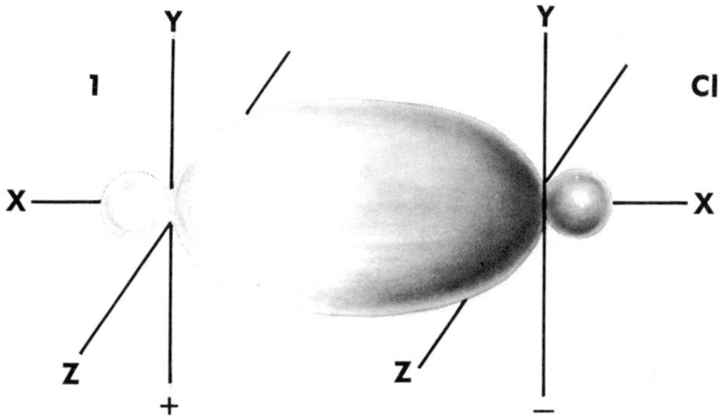

Fig. 12-4. Electron charge cloud representing the overlap of the valence orbitals of Cl and I to form the ClI molecule. Why is the resulting charge distribution unequal?

When 2 atoms of a single element combine with each other, the chemical bond is covalent and the electron charge cloud resulting from the interaction of the valence electrons (overlapping of valence orbitals) is symmetrical. The fluorine atom, for example, contains 9 electrons: 2 in the 1*s* orbital; 2 in the 2*s* orbital; 2 in two of the three 2*p* orbitals; and 1 in the remaining 2*p* orbital. When 2 fluorine atoms combine to form F_2, the 2*p* orbitals containing only one electron overlap symmetrically to form the covalent bond—(Fig. 12-3).

Iodine atoms have 53 electrons, located in 5 electron shells. Chlorine atoms have only 17 electrons in 3 shells. When these 2 atoms combine to form ClI, the electrons in the overlapping orbitals (a 3*p* orbital of chlorine and a 5*p* orbital of iodine) are pushed toward the chlorine atom by the repulsive force of the large number of iodine electrons. Thus the electron charge cloud is displaced toward the Cl (Fig. 12-4). This type of bond often is referred to as a *polar covalent bond.*

Strong electrolytes, in which the atoms are held together by electrovalence, really do not exist as discrete molecules. Instead, when they are

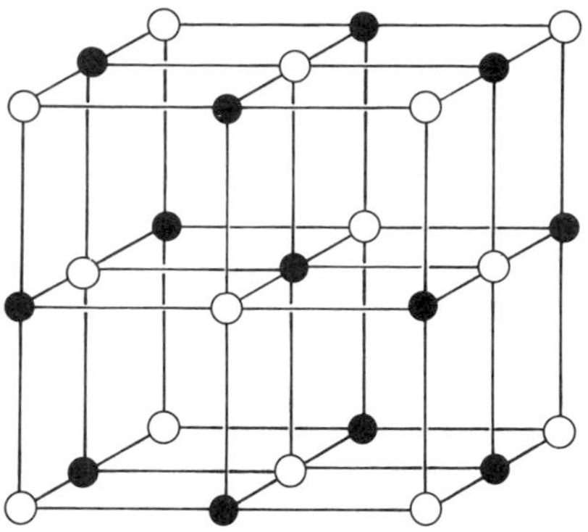

Fig. 12-5. Diagram of the crystalline structure of NaCl. Dark circles represent Na^+; light circles represent Cl^-. What happens when a crystal of NaCl is dissolved in water?

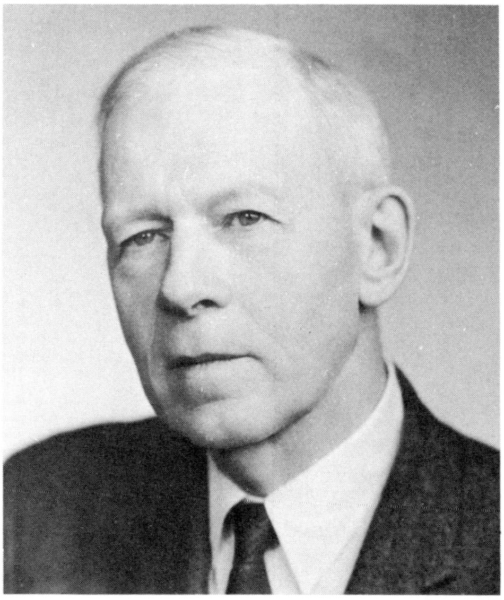

Fig. 12-6. Dr. Robert Sanderson Mulliken of the University of Chicago won the Nobel Prize in Chemistry in 1966 for his "fundamental work concerning chemical bonds and the electronic structure of molecules by the molecular orbital method." What do you think is meant by the term molecular orbital?

dissolved in water, ions are formed. In the solid state, these same ions form crystals in which there is a regular arrangement of negative and positive ions. In the case of NaCl, each Cl^- in the crystal is surrounded by 6 equidistant Na^+ ions and each Na^+ ion is surrounded by 6 equidistant Cl^- ions. A regular arrangement of ions in a crystal occurs even when one ion is formed from a radical. Thus solid Na_2CO_3 consists of a crystalline lattice composed of Na^+ ions and CO_3^{--} ions.

STUDY QUESTIONS

1. Explain what is meant by the term electrovalence.
2. Why is it reasonable to suppose that electrovalence is characteristic of electrolytes?
3. How does covalence differ from electrovalence?
4. Explain why the binding of a hydrogen ion by an ammonia molecule to form an ammonium ion cannot be electrovalence or covalence.
5. Define coordinate covalence; semipolar valence.
6. What is a hydrogen bond?
7. Name 2 types of biologically important compounds that contain hydrogen bonds.
8. In your own words, explain the concept of resonance valence.
9. What is a resonance hybrid?
10. State the uncertainty principle.
11. What is an orbital?
12. How many quantum numbers identify an orbital?
13. What is a chemical bond in terms of the theory of quantum mechanics?
14. What is a polar covalent bond?
15. Do strong electrolytes really exist as individual molecules in the solid state? Explain.

CHAPTER 13

Oxidation and reduction

OXIDATION-REDUCTION REACTIONS

When a change in valence occurs as the result of a chemical reaction, the reaction is called an *oxidation-reduction reaction*. Metallic sodium has a valence of 0 since it is not combined with another element. If sodium is added to water, a violent reaction takes place in which the valence of the sodium changes from 0 to 1+.

$$2\ \overset{0}{Na} + 2\ \overset{1+}{H_2}\overset{2-}{O} \rightarrow 2\ \overset{1+}{Na}\overset{2-}{O}\overset{1+}{H} + \overset{0}{H_2}$$

Notice, also, that the valence of hydrogen has changed from 1+ to 0. The sodium has *gained* and the hydrogen has *lost* positive valence. A gain in positive valence, or a loss in negative valence, is called *oxidation*. A loss in positive valence, or a gain in negative valence, is called *reduction*. Therefore, in the above example sodium has been *oxidized* and hydrogen has been *reduced*.

Mercurous chloride (HgCl, often called calomel, used in small doses as a purgative), can be made to react with chlorine gas to form the poisonous substance mercuric chloride ($HgCl_2$, also known as bichloride of mercury or corrosive sublimate). This is an oxidation-reduction reaction since the mercury has gained positive valence (oxidation) and the chlorine gas has gained negative valence (reduction):

$$2\ \overset{1+}{Hg}\overset{1-}{Cl} + \overset{0}{Cl_2} \rightarrow 2\ \overset{2-}{Hg}\overset{1-}{Cl_2}$$

METATHETIC REACTIONS

Reactions that do not involve a change in valence are called *metathetic reactions*. The following equations illustrate this type of change:

$$\overset{2+}{Mg}\overset{2-}{SO_4} + \overset{2+}{Ba}\overset{1-}{Cl_2} \rightarrow \overset{2+}{Mg}\overset{1-}{Cl_2} + \overset{2+}{Ba}\overset{2-}{SO_4}$$

$$\overset{1+}{Na}\overset{1-}{I} + \overset{1+}{Ag}\overset{1-}{NO_3} \rightarrow \overset{1+}{Na}\overset{1-}{NO_3} + \overset{1+}{Ag}\overset{1-}{I}$$

ELECTRON TRANSFERS IN OXIDATION-REDUCTION REACTIONS

We have already learned that valence is determined by the number of planetary electrons in the outer electron shells of atoms (see page 40). Let us consider what happens when zinc reacts with hydrochloric acid. In the following equation the electrons in the outer shells of the atoms are indicated by small dots:

$$\cdot Zn\cdot + 2\,H{:}\underset{\cdot\cdot}{\overset{\cdot\cdot}{Cl}}{:} \rightarrow {:}\underset{\cdot\cdot}{\overset{\cdot\cdot}{Cl}}{:}Zn{:}\underset{\cdot\cdot}{\overset{\cdot\cdot}{Cl}}{:} + H{:}H$$

Before the reaction takes place Zn has 2 electrons in its outer shell. Since it has not yet lost these electrons by combining chemically with some other atom or radical, the valence of the zinc is 0. Hydrogen has completed its outer shell by giving its 1 electron to chlorine, and its valence is therefore 1+. The valence of chlorine is 1− because it has completed its outer shell by taking an electron from hydrogen. (Remember that an uncombined chlorine atom has 7 electrons in its outer electron shell.) What is the situation after the reaction is completed? Now we find that Zn has given its 2 outer electrons to Cl; its valence has thus changed from 0 to 2+. The Cl atoms have lost the electrons that H had given them, but they have each gained an electron from Zn. The valence of Cl, therefore, is still 1−, as it was before the reaction took place. The H atoms, which had given their electrons to Cl, have regained them, and the valence of the hydrogen gas (H_2) bubbling from the reaction solution is 0. Zinc that has been oxidized has lost electrons. Hydrogen that has been reduced has gained electrons.

Oxidation involves a loss of electrons. Reduction involves a gain of electrons. Since electrons cannot be given away unless some other atom or radical gains them, it is apparent that *oxidation cannot occur without a simultaneous reduction.*

OXIDIZING AND REDUCING AGENTS

Substances receiving electrons in chemical reactions are called *oxidizing agents* since they cause the substance with which they react to be oxidized (that is, to lose electrons). *Reducing agents,* which lose electrons easily, cause other substances to be reduced.

Hydrogen unites with oxygen to form water. Hydrogen is oxidized and oxygen is reduced when this occurs. It is evident, then, that oxygen is an oxidizing agent and hydrogen is a reducing agent. Any substance that combines with oxygen is oxidized; any substance that combines with hydrogen is reduced.

If an electric current is passed through water, hydrogen and oxygen are formed, as the following equation indicates:

$$2\,H_2O \rightarrow 2\,H_2\uparrow + O_2\uparrow$$

Here, oxygen has been oxidized and hydrogen has been reduced. It follows that the removal of oxygen from a compound causes reduction, and the removal of hydrogen from a compound causes oxidation.

Many of the reactions that take place in the tissues involve the loss or gain of hydrogen and oxygen. The following rules will be of great assistance when such reactions are described later in this book:

1. *Any substance that has gained oxygen or lost hydrogen has been oxidized.*

2. *Any substance that has lost oxygen or gained hydrogen has been reduced.*

IMPORTANCE OF OXIDATION-REDUCTION REACTIONS IN MEDICINE

The foods we eat are used either to build or repair tissue, or are changed in such a way as to yield energy. This energy is used to heat the body, to contract muscles, to transmit nerve impulses, to make glands secrete, to build new cells—in short, to carry on all the activities of life. All the reactions that result in energy production in living cells are oxidation-reduction reactions. Many diseases result from the fact that oxidations and reductions cannot be properly or completely carried out in the tissues, with a resultant production of harmful substances. In diabetes mellitus, for example, carbohydrates are not oxidized properly, and harmful acids accumulate in the blood. This disease often is treated by injecting insulin, a protein substance necessary for the oxidation of carbohydrate in the body.

Many antiseptics (substances that can kill bacteria) are oxidizing agents. Potassium permanganate ($KMnO_4$) in dilute solution is used locally in treating infections of the bladder and urethra, and is sometimes used in the attempt to destroy, by oxidation, the irritating principles of poison ivy and poison oak. Potassium chlorate ($KClO_3$) is employed occasionally in the treatment of sore throat. Iodine, both in the form of an alcohol solution (tincture of iodine) and as a water solution (Lugol's solution), is a useful antiseptic for minor cuts and for application to the skin prior to surgical procedures. Hydrogen peroxide (H_2O_2) in 3 percent solution is a mild oxidizing antiseptic. This solution is also used to soften earwax and to assist in cleansing infected wounds. Dakin's solution, once used in the treatment of wounds, infections in the peritoneal cavity, and infections in the thoracic cavity, owes its activity to the presence of the oxidizing agent sodium hypochlorite (NaOCl). Bleaching powder, which is mainly calcium hypochlorite ($Ca(OCl)_2$), is often employed in hospitals to destroy odors and to disinfect floors, toilets, etc.

Sulfur dioxide (SO_2) readily combines with oxygen to form sulfur trioxide (SO_3) and is, therefore, a reducing agent:

$$2\ SO_2 + O_2 \rightarrow 2\ SO_3$$

SO_2 is a colorless gas having a pungent odor and can be made by burning sulfur:

$$S + O_2 \rightarrow SO_2 \uparrow$$

Sulfur candles are sometimes burned in rooms in which patients with contagious diseases have been cared for. The sulfur dioxide gas, if present in high enough concentration in the air, kills bacteria by reduction of some of the substances that make up the bacterial tissue.

BLEACHING AGENTS.* Many stains that are difficult or impossible to remove with

*A valuable pamphlet entitled *Stain Removal from Fabrics, Home Methods* can be obtained at a cost of twenty cents from the Superintendent of Documents, U. S. Government Printing Office, Washington, D. C. 20402. Another pamphlet entitled *How to Prevent and Remove Mildew,* priced at ten cents, can be obtained from the same source.

solvents can be bleached with a suitable oxidizing or reducing agent. Such chemicals will often remove the color of the fabric as well as the stain, however, and must be used carefully. They are particularly useful in bleaching stains on white uniforms. After the stain has been decolorized, the chemical should be removed from the cloth with water; if this is not done, the fabric may be weakened. The commonest bleaching agents are *Javelle water* (Labarraque's solution), *sodium thiosulfate* (hypo), *oxalic acid, hydrogen peroxide,* and *potassium permanganate.*

Javelle water is a solution of sodium hypochlorite ($NaOCl$). This compound is an oxidizing agent. It should not be used on fabrics made from animal proteins, such as wool or silk. It should not be allowed to remain in contact with linen or cotton materials for too long a time, and after its use any excess should be neutralized by washing with a dilute solution of sodium thiosulfate and acetic acid. Some common stains that can often be bleached with Javelle water include:

Chocolate	Ink (except India ink)	Prepared mustard	Shoe polish
Cocoa	Jam	Indelible pencil	Tea
Dyes and stains	Medicine	Perspiration	Tobacco
Fruit	Mildew	Preserves	Walnut

Sodium thiosulfate ($Na_2S_2O_3$) is a reducing agent. It is most effective in removing iodine stains:

$$2\,Na_2S_2O_3 + I_2 \rightarrow 2\,NaI + Na_2S_4O_6$$

Stains caused by silver compounds (silver nitrate, argyrol, protargol) can often be bleached with this substance. Silver nitrate stains on the skin also can be removed by the following procedure: cover the stain with tincture of iodine to convert the silver to silver iodide, AgI; the new stain thus formed can now be dissolved with a solution of ammonia and sodium thiosulfate. Sodium thiosulfate is the ordinary "hypo" used in photography and is usually to be found in photographic and x-ray developing rooms.

Oxalic acid $(COOH)_2$ is a reducing agent particularly useful in bleaching potassium permanganate stains. Saturated solutions of this substance can often be used to remove iron rust, fruit, and ink stains (except India ink), and mildew.

Hydrogen peroxide (H_2O_2) is a weak oxidizing agent. Commercial solutions are usually slightly acid, and enough ammonia water to make the peroxide solution slightly alkaline should be added before attempting to bleach a stain. This substance should not be allowed to remain in contact with cotton or linen fabrics too long, and its use should be followed by rinsing with water. It is useful in removing the following common stains:

Blood	Perspiration
Dyes (on white wool or silk)	Scorch
	Urine

Potassium permanganate ($KMnO_4$) is a powerful oxidizing agent. It can be used on almost all white fabrics except those made from synthetic fibers. If the stain is on a colored material, a small unexposed piece of the cloth should be treated with potassium permanganate to see whether or not the dye is affected by the oxidizing agent; if the dye is altered, some other bleaching agent must be employed. After destruction of the stain with potassium permanganate, any pink or brown stain that is left (left by the permanganate itself) can be removed by treatment with oxalic acid, or with an acid solution of hydrogen peroxide. The following stains can be removed with dilute potassium permanganate solution:

Coffee	Mildew	Preserves
Fruit	Prepared mustard	Shoe polish
Ink (except India ink)	Indelible pencil	Tea
Leather	Perspiration	Tobacco

MATCHES. The head of an ordinary "strike anywhere" match contains phosphorus sesquisulfide (P_4S_3), a substance having a low kindling temperature (see page 44). Present also are an oxidizing agent (usually potassium chlorate, $KClO_3$), a material that burns readily (for example, paraffin), powdered glass, an adhesive, and inert fillers and binders. When the match is "struck," friction between the powdered glass and the rough striking surface generates sufficient heat to raise the temperature to the kindling temperature of the P_4S_3. As this substance burns, the easily combustible material present ignites, and this in turn eventually ignites the wood of the matchstick. The $KClO_3$ furnishes oxygen to support the initial oxidation reactions.

The head of the common safety match contains an oxidizing agent (usually potassium chromate, $K_2Cr_2O_7$, and potassium chlorate, $KClO_3$), antimony sulfide, Sb_2S_3, or sulfur, and an adhesive. The special striking surface on the matchbox or book contains red phosphorus, glue, and powdered glass, The reactions that occur when this type of match is struck are similar to those just described for the household match.

STUDY QUESTIONS

1. Write three equations not given in the text illustrating oxidation-reduction reactions.
2. Define: oxidation, reduction, metathetic reaction.
3. Can oxidation occur in the absence of oxygen? Explain.
4. Define and give examples of: oxidizing agent, reducing agent.
5. Has a compound that has reacted with oxygen been oxidized or reduced? Explain.
6. Has a compound that has reacted with hydrogen been oxidized or reduced? Explain.
7. Give some examples to show the importance of oxidation-reduction reactions in medicine and physiology.
8. Name four antiseptics that are oxidizing agents.
9. Name a reducing agent that is an antiseptic.
10. List five common bleaching agents. Which of them are oxidizing agents? Which are reducing agents? Name two common stains each of them will bleach.
11. What bleaching agent should never be used on wool or silk? Which one should not be used on rayon?

CHAPTER 14

Periodic table and some important elements

PERIODICITY OF THE ELEMENTS

During the latter half of the nineteenth century many chemists attempted to devise some rational system of classifying the chemical elements. Obviously, certain elements resembled each other very closely in their chemical properties, at the same time differing markedly from other groups of related elements. For example, sodium and potassium were metals with a valence of 1+. On the other hand chlorine and bromine certainly were not metallic in nature and usually had a valence of 1− when they were combined with other elements. The most successful attempt to work out a practical classification was made by the Russian chemist Dmitri I. Mendéleeff, who published his *periodic table* in 1861. His final modification of this table was used by chemists essentially in the form in which he presented it until recent years, when improved modifications have become available.

Mendeléeff found that when the elements were listed in order of their atomic weights, most of them then known fell into a pattern such that elements having the same valence recurred every eighth time. In cases where there were apparent gaps he postulated that elements as yet undiscovered must exist, and actually he predicted the existence (and even the properties!) of six elements that later were isolated. The so-called rare gases were incorporated into his table after their discovery a few years before his death.

In order to understand Mendeleeff's idea, let us make a periodic table, using ele-

Usual valence	1+	2+	3+	4+ or 4−	3−	2−	1−	0
Element	Li	Be	B	C	N	O	F	Ne
Atomic number	3	4	5	6	7	8	9	10
Element	Na	Mg	Al	Si	P	S	Cl	A
Atomic number	11	12	13	14	15	16	17	18

ments with atomic numbers 3 to 18 inclusive. (Hydrogen and helium, the two lightest elements, are omitted for reasons that will be apparent later.)

The elements in each of the vertical columns closely resemble each other in chemical properties. For example, lithium (Li) and sodium (Na) are metals with a valence of 1+. Both of them react violently with H_2O, with the production of a hydroxide and hydrogen. Neon (Ne) and argon (A), on the other hand, are gases and are so nonreactive that very few compounds containing them are known. The elements in the other six vertical columns of the table likewise have similar chemical properties. Mendeleeff's table had 9 groups, or periods.

MODERN PERIODIC TABLE

It is apparent to modern chemists that the true cause of the periodicity of the chemical elements is not valence; rather it is to be found in the number and arrangement of the electrons present in an atom of the element. It will be recalled that the hydrogen atom has a single electron; helium, the next lightest atom, contains two electrons in each atom (see page 39). Moreover, since the first electron shell can contain only two electrons, helium is very stable and has zero valence. The *first period* of the modern periodic table thus consists not of 8 elements but of only 2—the gases hydrogen and helium (see Fig. 14-1). The second period ends when we next encounter an element having its outer electron shell filled (see Fig. 5-2 on page 39). It therefore includes the elements lithium through neon. Again, the last element of the second period (neon) is a gas with zero valence. The third period also contains 8 elements and ends with an inert gas, argon. The fourth and fifth periods contain 18 elements instead of 8. Certain of them agree closely in chemical properties with those of the first three periods, whereas others are not so obviously related. Note that the modern periodic table (Fig. 14-1) takes this into account by increasing the number of vertical columns. The fourth and fifth periods end with the stable gases krypton and xenon. The sixth period is a long one, having 32 elements and ending with the chemically nonreactive gas radon. In order to compress all of these elements into the table, certain of them, known as the *lanthanide series* or as the *rare-earth metals,* have been listed to the side of the main body of the table. The last, or seventh, period, a portion of which is known as the *actinide series,* is complete and contains the 17 remaining elements. The last 13 of these were created by man and have not been found in nature (see page 119).* It would not be surprising if additional elements are created in the future. It is natural to predict also that the seventh period, if ever completed, will contain 32 elements, the last of which will be a gas with zero valence. In the table the elements of the actinide series are listed below those elements of the lanthanide series that resemble them in chemical properties.

HYDROGEN

Hydrogen, the lightest element, is the first member of the periodic table. In fact it is an exception to the periodic rule since it differs in most of its chemical properties from the other elements in the first vertical column. It is the most abundant element in nature. When it is not combined with other elements, it is a tasteless, colorless, odorless gas.

*Four lighter elements were also created by man. They are element 43 (technetium), element 61 (promethium), element 85 (astatine), and element 87 (franicum).

PERIODIC CHART OF THE ELEMENTS

Category		Representative Elements							
Periods	Subshells	s		p					
	Electrons*	1	2	1	2	3	4	5	6
1	1s	1 H 1.00797							2 He 4.0026
2	2s	3 Li 6.939	4 Be 9.0122						
2	2p			5 B 10.811	6 C 12.01115	7 N 14.0067	8 O 15.9994	9 F 18.9984	10 Ne 20.183
3	3s	11 Na 22.9898	12 Mg 24.312						
3	3p			13 Al 26.9815	14 Si 28.086	15 P 30.9738	16 S 32.064	17 Cl 35.453	18 Ar 39.948
4	4s	19 K 39.102	20 Ca 40.08						
4	4p			31 Ga 69.72	32 Ge 72.59	33 As 74.9216	34 Se 78.96	35 Br 79 909	36 Kr 83.80
5	5s	37 Rb 85.47	38 Sr 87.62						
5	5p			49 In 114.82	50 Sn 118.69	51 Sb 121.75	52 Te 127.60	53 I 126.9044	54 Xe 131.30
6	6s	55 Cs 132.905	56 Ba 137.34						
6	6p			81 Tl 204.37	82 Pb 207.19	83 Bi 208.980	84 Po (209)	85 At (210)	86 Rn (222)
7	7s	87 Fr (223)	88 Ra (226)						

Category		Transition Elements									
Periods	Subshells	d									
	Electrons*	1	2	3	4	5	6	7	8	9	10
4	3d	21 Sc 44.956	22 Ti 47.90	23 V 50.942	24 Cr 51.996	25 Mn 54.9380	26 Fe 55.847	27 Co 58.9332	28 Ni 58.71	29 Cu 63.54	30 Zn 65.37
5	4d	39 Y 88.905	40 Zr 91.22	41 Nb 92.906	42 Mo 95.94	43 Tc (97)	44 Ru 101.07	45 Rh 102.905	46 Pd 106.4	47 Ag 107.870	48 Cd 112.40
6		57 La 138.91									
6	5d		72 Hf 178.49	73 Ta 180.948	74 W 183.85	75 Re 186.2	76 Os 190.2	77 Ir 192.2	78 Pt 195.09	79 Au 196.967	80 Hg 200.59
7	6d	89 Ac (227)									

Category		Inner Transition Elements													
Periods	Subshells	f													
	Electrons*	1	2	3	4	5	6	7	8	9	10	11	12	13	14
6	4f (Lanthanides)	58 Ce 140.12	59 Pr 140.907	60 Nd 144.24	61 Pm (145)	62 Sm 150.35	63 Eu 151.96	64 Gd 157.25	65 Tb 158.924	66 Dy 162.50	67 Ho 164.930	68 Er 167.26	69 Tm 168.934	70 Yb 173.04	71 Lu 174.97
7	5f (Actinides)	90 Th 232.038	91 Pa (231)	92 U 238.03	93 Np (237)	94 Pu (244)	95 Am (243)	96 Cm (247)	97 Bk (247)	98 Cf (251)	99 Es (254)	100 Fm (253)	101 Md (256)	102 (254)	103 Lw (256)

Note: A value given in parentheses denotes the mass number of the longest-lived isotope.
*Electron populations are given to indicate only the general order of subshell filling, which is not completely regular for the "d" and "f" subshells. Chemical relationships require helium to be placed in the inert gas column even though it has no "p" electrons.

Fig. 14-1. A modern version of the periodic table. (See page 26 for explanation of the letters s, p, d, and f.) Which of the elements listed do not occur in nature? (From *The Merck Index*, courtesy Merck & Co., Inc.)

Hydrogen can be prepared in the laboratory by allowing an acid to react with zinc:

Zn	$+ H_2SO_4$	$\rightarrow$	$ZnSO_4$	$+ H_2\uparrow$
Zinc	Sulfuric acid		Zinc sulfate	Hydrogen

It can be prepared also by the electrolysis of water or electrolyte solutions (see page 81). It is dangerous to have flames in contact with hydrogen since when the element is heated, it combines with oxygen with explosive force, forming water.

$$2\,H_2 + O_2 \rightarrow 2\,H_2O$$

Hydrogen, which forms compounds with most of the elements, always has a valence of 1 when combined. A few examples follow:

NaH	MgH_2	CH_4	H_2S	HCl
Sodium hydride	Magnesium hydride	Methane	Hydrogen sulfide	Hydrogen chloride

ALKALI METALS

The remaining members of the first vertical column often are called the *elements of group I*, or the *alkali metals*. Lithium, sodium, and potassium are the most important of these. They are extremely active chemically and when free are soft, light, silvery white metals. The alkali metals react violently with water and should be stored under oil.

$2\,Na$	$+ 2\,H_2O$	$\rightarrow$	$2\,NaOH$	$+ H_2\uparrow$
Sodium	Water		Sodium hydroxide	Hydrogen

When these elements are heated, they impart characteristic colors to the flame: yellow for sodium, carmine (red) for lithium, and violet for potassium, rubidium, and cesium.

ALKALINE-EARTH METALS

These are the elements listed in the second vertical column of the modern periodic table. Magnesium, calcium, barium, and radium are the most important of them. They are all much less reactive and much harder than are the alkali metals. In combined form they usually have a valence of 2+.

Many nonmetals were called "earths" by the early chemists. Calcium and magnesium oxides were found to neutralize acids as did alkalies, and were called *alkaline earths*. This name was retained for the free elements.

Magnesium reacts with boiling water to form magnesium hydroxide. Suspensions of this alkali are used in medicine under the name of *milk of magnesia*.

Mg	$+ 2\,H_2O$	$\rightarrow$	$Mg(OH)_2$	$+ H_2\uparrow$
Magnesium	Water		Magnesium hydroxide	Hydrogen

The element burns with a very bright white flame to form magnesium oxide, or magnesia.

Mg	$+ O_2$	$\rightarrow$	$2\,MgO$
Magnesium	Oxygen		Magnesium oxide

Flashlight powder is a mixture of an oxidizing agent and powdered magnesium.

Calcium is a silvery metal that is harder than lead. Like magnesium, it burns in air and reacts with water. An important compound of calcium is calcium carbonate, $CaCO_3$. This compound exists naturally as *marble* and as *limestone*. Sea shells, coral, and pearls are chiefly calcium carbonate.

Barium is most useful in medicine in the form of the white, insoluble powder, barium sulfate (see page 71).

Radium is discussed in Chapter 15.

BORON AND ALUMINUM

Boron forms very dense transparent crystals that are almost as hard as diamond (see page 133). Boron carbide, B_4C, is, except for diamond, the hardest known substance and is used as an abrasive. The element exists in nature in the form of complex minerals, the best known of which is *borax*. Borax, or sodium borate ($Na_2B_4O_7 \cdot 10H_2O$), is used in soldering metals, in tanning, in the manufacture of glazes and enamels, to artificially age wood, as a component of cleaning compounds, and to make fabric and woods fireproof; used alone, or with other antiseptics, it prevents the growth of wood fungus. *Boric acid,* H_3BO_3, is a white crystalline powder used in medicine as a mild antiseptic. A mixed solution of boric acid and borax can be used for treating cloth in order to make it resistant to flames.*

Aluminum is a light yet strong metal. It can be worked readily into different shapes and is used in the construction of many devices and machines, particularly when lack of weight is important. The pure element burns in air when it is heated strongly. However, under ordinary conditions it becomes coated with a layer of aluminum oxide (Al_2O_3) by reaction with oxygen, and this layer protects the underlying metal against corrosion or noticeable reaction in air, even when moderate heat is applied, as in cooking.

Duraluminum is an alloy† containing aluminum (95 percent), copper (4 percent), manganese (0.5 percent), and magnesium (0.5 percent). It is stronger than aluminum but is more reactive. Devices made of it usually are protected from corrosion by a coating of pure aluminum.

The mineral known as *corundum* is principally aluminum oxide, Al_2O_3. Except for diamond, corundum is the hardest of the *naturally* occurring substances. Corundum and emery (an impure form of corundum) are used as abrasives. Rubies and sapphires are transparent crystalline forms of corundum.

Potassium alum, $Kal(SO_4)_2 \cdot 12\ H_2O$, and ammonium alum, $NH_4Al(SO_4)_2 \cdot 12\ H_2O$, have astringent properties (that is, cause tightening or shrinking of tissue) and sometimes are used in medicine.

Aluminum subacetate, $Al_2O(CH_3COO)_4 \cdot 4\ H_2O$, often is applied externally in the treatment of certain diseases of the skin.

*A pamphlet entitled *Making Household Fabrics Flame Resistant* can be obtained from The Superintendent of Documents, U. S. Government Printing Office, Washington, D. C. 20402, for five cents.

†An alloy is a metallic material containing two or more elements. Some are solid solutions, some are intermetallic compounds, and some are mixtures of two or more phases, each of which may be a solid solution or intermetallic compound. The simplest form of stainless steel is an alloy of iron and carbon.

SILICON, TIN, AND LEAD

Silicon is a steel-gray, brittle, metallike material in its elemental state. Most of the rocks and sands that cover the earth's surface are composed of compounds that contain this element.

Silicon dioxide or *silica*, SiO_2, occurs in several forms in nature—for example, as *quartz* and as white sand. When quartz is melted (at temperature approximating 1600° C) and allowed to cool, fused quartz, or silica glass, is formed. This type of glass withstands high temperatures without cracking and is used to make various types of chemical apparatus. It allows the passage of ultraviolet radiant energy and often is used to make ultraviolet lamps.

When silica is boiled with a solution of a strong alkali (such as KOH or NaOH) it slowly dissolves. The salts of several different silicic acids (such as H_4SiO_4, $H_6Si_2O_7$, and $H_4Si_3O_8$) are formed by this procedure. A concentrated solution of these salts is known commercially as *water glass*. Water glass is used in preserving eggs, as an adhesive, and in fireproofing wood and cloth.

Ordinary glass (soda-lime glass or soft glass) is made by heating a mixture of sodium carbonate or sulfate, limestone (mostly calcium carbonate), and sand, usually with a little added glass to catalyze the reaction. The clear, melted glass then can be molded or blown to the desired shape. *Pyrex glass* contains a small percentage of boron; it does not crack easily and is used to make glass vessels suitable for cooking or for heating liquids used in the chemical laboratory. The glazes used on kitchen utensils and bathtubs usually consist of a white pigment (titanium oxide or stannic oxide) mixed with an easily fusible glass.

Portland cement is a powder containing mainly calcium aluminate, $Ca_3Al_2O_6$, and calcium silicates, such as Ca_2SiO_4 and Ca_3SiO_5. When it is treated with water, complex crystalline compounds (calcium aluminosilicates) are produced. The crystals intermesh, forming hard cement.

Silicones are complex compounds of silicon, carbon, and oxygen. The most common structural unit is $—R_2Si—O—$, where R is a monovalent carbon-containing radical. Silicones have several physical forms, such as fluids (or oils), rubbers, resins, and powders. There are many industrial applications, including their use as lubricants, hydraulic oils, heat transfer media; as rubbers for electrical coatings, molding, and extruding; as ingredients of paints, varnishes, and enamels; as water repellents for textiles, paper, masonry, and concrete; and as lubricants for coating the edges of stainless steel razor blades.

Glass coated with a layer of silicone resembles the lining of the blood vessels in that it does not wet easily, and blood collected in silicone-coated glass vessels does not clot for long periods of time. Vials containing suspended drugs (such as procaine penicillin) often are siliconed in order to facilitate removal of the suspension from the vial.

Silicones are employed industrially as agents to break up foams (for example, in the beer industry), and this has led to an interesting medical application. Theoretically, one form of gastrointestinal distress is caused by the presence of foams (collections of small bubbles). When a silicone is administered by mouth, the tiny bubbles coalesce into one large bubble, which is expelled from the body by belching or by intestinal peristalsis.

"Bouncing putty" or "silly putty" is a silicone that can be stretched, shattered, molded, or caused to rebound like rubber when it is dropped on a hard surface. It has been used in physiotherapy to exercise the fingers.

Silicones have been incorporated in hand creams, lotions, and shaving creams to form a protective layer on the skin.

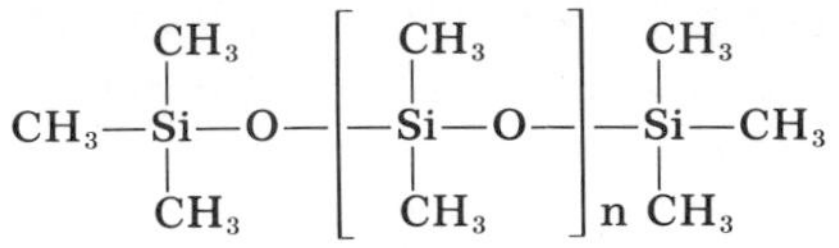

Polysiloxane
(a silicone polymer* used as a drug)

Well-known forms of minerals containing silicates are *zeolites* (used in softening water), *talc, mica,* and *asbestos. Lapis lazuli* is a silicate mineral with a rich blue color. The pigment known as *ultramarine* is prepared by grinding lapis lazuli to a fine power.

The principal *tin* mineral is *stannic oxide,* SnO_2, or *cassiterite.* The element is formed by heating this mineral with carbon.

SnO_2	+	C	→	Sn	+	$CO_2\uparrow$
Stannic oxide		Carbon		Tin		Carbon dioxide

Ordinary white tin is easily molded into various shapes and is used widely as tinfoil and as the familiar coating on tin cans. ("Tin" cans really are iron cans coated with a layer of tin in order to prevent corrosion.) At very low temperatures ($-40°$ C) white tin rapidly changes to so-called *gray tin,* which is a crumbly material. This same change occurs more slowly at any temperature below 18° C, and objects coated with tin should not be stored at temperatures lower than this for long periods of time. Tin sometimes has a valence of 2+, as illustrated by the compound *stannous oxide,* SnO.

Lead occurs principally as the ore known as *galena,* or lead sulfide (PbS). The free element is a soft, easily malleable (workable), bluish gray metal. It is widely used industrially in the manufacture of pipes, solder, foil, storage batteries, shot, plumbing, and many other products. Like tin it forms the two oxides, *plumbous oxide* (PbO) and *plumbic oxide* (PbO_2). PbO, an orange-yellow compound also known as *litharge,* is used in making glass and in glazing pottery. Another oxide of lead known as *red lead* (Pb_3O_4) is used as a red pigment and is an ingredient of flint glass. *Lead subcarbonate (basic lead carbonate),* $Pb_3(OH)_2(CO_2)_2$, is known commercially as *white lead.* White lead formerly was used in enormous quantities as a white pigment in the paint industry, but probably this use will be discontinued soon because of the danger of lead poisoning.

*A simple polymer is a large molecule made up of repeating chemical units. The n in the formula indicates that polymeric chains of different lengths can be produced, depending on the conditions under which the synthesis takes place. A mixed polymer is made up of more than one repeating unit. Usually two such units are involved.

The charged cell of an ordinary *storage battery* consists of a plate composed of spongy lead separated from a second plate impregnated with lead oxide (PbO_2) by a solution of sulfuric acid. The sulfuric acid is ionized and serves as a source of sulfate and hydrogen ions.

$$H_2SO_4 \rightleftarrows 2\,H^+ + SO_4^{--}$$

When the battery is discharged, the lead plate reacts with sulfate ions to form lead sulfate and electrons.

$$Pb + SO_4^{--} \rightarrow PbSO_4 + 2\,e^-$$

The PbO_2 of the second plate undergoes a reaction in which electrons are absorbed.

$$PbO_2 + 4\,H^+ + SO_4^{--} + 2\,e^- \rightarrow PbSO_4 + 2\,H_2O$$

Thus if the two plates are connected by means of a conductor, electrons flow into the conductor from the lead plate and out of it into the PbO_2. This passage of electrons through the conductor is the electric current (see page 81). When the battery is recharged, an electric current is passed through it in a reverse direction so that the above reactions are reversed.

NITROGEN, PHOSPHORUS, ARSENIC, ANTIMONY, AND BISMUTH

Free *nitrogen*, N_2, accounts for about four-fifths of the volume of air. It is a colorless, odorless, tasteless gas. In combined form it usually has a valence of 3−, 5+, or 3+ as illustrated by the following compounds:

NH_3	HNO_3	HNO_2
Ammonia	Nitric acid	Nitrous acid

Ammonia, NH_3, is a pungent, colorless gas. It readily dissolves in water to form ammonium hydroxide (ammonia water).

NH_3	$+ H_2O$	$\rightarrow$	NH_4OH
Ammonia	Water		Ammonia hydroxide

Many ammonium salts have been used as drugs.

Nitrogen combines with oxygen to form several oxides:

Nitrous oxide, N_2O, is an odorless, colorless gas. A mixture of this gas with oxygen is used as a general anesthetic for minor operations. Sometimes it is called "laughing gas."

Nitric oxide, NO, resembles nitrogen in its physical properties.

Nitrogen trioxide, N_2O_3, is unstable at room temperature. Mixtures of N_2O_3 and NO can be condensed to a dark blue liquid that boils at 3.5° C.

Nitrogen dioxide, NO_2, exists in equilibrium with *dinitrogen tetroxide*, N_2O_4. Both are gases.

NO_2	$\rightleftarrows$	N_2O_4
Red		Colorless

Nitrogen pentoxide, N_2O_5, an unstable white solid, reacts with water to form *nitric acid*, HNO_3.

$$N_2O_5 + H_2O \rightarrow 2\,HNO_3$$

The old-fashioned type of *gunpowder* was a mixture of potassium nitrate (KNO_3), 75 percent; charcoal, 15 percent; and sulfur, 10 percent.

Phosphorus exists in several crystalline forms, the most familiar of which are *white phosphorus* and *red phosphorus*. White phosphorus ignites spontaneously in air and should be stored under water. It is used in making rat poisons and smoke screens. Red phosphorus is used in the manufacture of safety matches, fertilizers, tracer bullets, and smoke screens. Phosphorus forms several oxides and exists widely in biology as the phosphate radical.

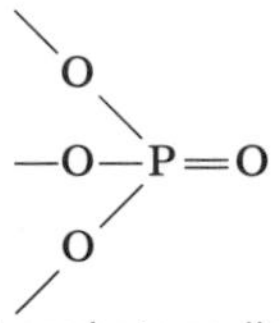

Phosphate radical

Arsenic in free form is a brittle, steel-gray crystalline mass or a heavy, grayish black powder. Some of its compounds, most of which are poisonous, are used as insecticides. Aresenic compounds formerly were used in the therapy of syphilis.

Antimony is a silvery, lustrous metal. One of its salts, antimony potassium tartrate, or *tartar emetic,* has been used in *small* doses in the treatment of certain tropical diseases.

Bismuth is a grayish white solid with a reddish tinge and a metallic luster. It is used in "silvering" mirrors. A suspension of *bismuth hydroxide,* $Bi(OH_3)$, known as *milk of bismuth* is used in the symptomatic treatment of diarrhea. *Bismuth subcarbonate* also is used for this purpose. Bismuth compounds formerly were used widely for the treatment of syphilis.

SULFUR

Sulfur exists in nature both combined and as the free element. It exists in several forms, but the usual stable type is a yellow, crystalline powder.

Hydrogen sulfide, H_2S, is a gas with an odor resembling that of rotten eggs.

Sulfuric acid, H_2SO_4, is one of the most important inorganic compounds used in industry. It is used in the manufacture of fertilizers, explosives, dyes, parchment paper, glue, and in the purification of petroleum.

HALOGENS

Fluorine, chlorine, bromine, and iodine are known collectively as the *halogens.* The word halogen is derived from the Greek and means "salt-producing"—the halogens combine with metals to form salts.

Fluorine is the most reactive of all the elements, and it forms compounds with all the other elements except the inert gases. *Hydrofluoric acid,* HF, attacks glass and is used to etch glass apparatus, the glass that is not to be etched being protected by a layer of paraffin. *Sodium fluoride,* NaF, is used as an ant poison. In recent years numerous organic compounds containing fluorine have become important commercially.

Chlorine was discovered by Karl Scheele (see page 42) in 1774. It is a greenish yellow gas with a choking odor. It combines with most of the elements to form chlorides. It has been used as a war gas. It is used in the manufacture of bleaching powders, as a disinfectant, and in the production of many important industrial chemicals. Chlorine forms several acids with hydrogen and oxygen:

HCl	$HClO_4$	$HClO_3$	$HClO_2$	$HClO$
Hydrochloric acid	Perchloric acid	Perchlorous acid	Chlorous acid	Hypochlorous acid

Sodium hypochlorite, NaClO, is the agent present in many household bleaching agents. *Sodium chlorate,* $NaClO_3$, and *sodium perchlorate,* $NaClO_4$, are used to kill weeds.

Bromine is a fuming, volatile, reddish brown liquid. Its fumes are highly irritating to the lungs and to the eyes. It attacks tissues and all metals. Some of its salts, such as sodium bromide, NaBr, and potassium bromide, KBr, are useful as sedatives. *Silver bromide,* AgBr (and also silver chloride and silver iodide), is used in making photographic emulsions.

Iodine exists in the form of bluish black scales with a metallic luster, a characteristic odor, and a sharp taste. *Tincture of iodine,* used in medicine as an antiseptic, contains iodine, potassium iodide (KI), water, and alcohol. Iodine is required for the formation of the hormone of the thyroid gland and is used in treating diseases of this gland (see pages 342 and 390).

NOBLE GASES

The *noble gases* also are known as the *rare gases* or *inert gases.* All of the elements in this group—*helium, neon, argon, krypton, xenon,* and *radon*—are chemically almost inert and hence rarely exist in combination with other elements. All of them except radon are present in trace amounts in ordinary samples of air. Helium is used for filling balloons. A mixture of helium and oxygen is more diffusible than is air, and sometimes is administered to patients with diseases of the lungs. Neon is used in the familiar neon lights. Argon is the gas used in most incandescent light bulbs. The use of radon in medicine is discussed in Chapter 15.

COPPER, SILVER, AND GOLD

Copper occurs naturally both as the free element and in numerous minerals. It is a lustrous, reddish, malleable metal. In moist air it gradually becomes coated with a layer of green basic carbonate (subcarbonate). It is used in the manufacture of brass, bronze, and other alloys and as copper wire. *Copper sulfate,* $CuSO_4$, known also as *blue vitriol* and as *bluestone,* is used in copper plating, in dyeing wool and silk, in tanning leather, in destroying algae in swimming pools, in insecticide mixtures, and for many other purposes. Formerly it was used as a mild astringent and antiseptic in medicine.

Silver is found in ores and in the free state in nature. It is a white metal and is more malleable than any other metal except gold. It blackens readily in the presence of sulfur compounds as a result of the formation of *silver sulfide,* Ag_2S. It is used in coinage, for electroplating, and in the manufacture of tableware, ornaments, and jewelry. *Silver nitrate,* $AgNO_3$, is used in medicine as a caustic *(lunar caustic).* Dilute solutions of this salt were formerly dropped in the eyes of newborn babies in order to ensure against gonorrheal infection.

Photographic film is prepared by coating a transparent material with a suspension of silver iodide (AgI) or silver chloride (AgCl) in a gelatin solution (in the dark or under a dull red light). The film is exposed by a brief projection on it of an illuminated image. The exposed film is "developed" by immersing it in a bath containing a reducing agent. Some of the silver salt present is reduced to finely divided metallic silver (which is black). The rapidity of this reduction is proportional to the intensity of the illumination that exposed it; hence the resulting image on the film is the "negative" of the original image (originally light areas are dark and vice versa). The action of the reducing agent is stopped at the desired point, and the film is immersed in a second bath containing sodium thiosulfate ($Na_2S_2O_3$ or "hypo"). This chemical dissolves out the unreduced silver salt. A "positive" print is made by exposing a second sensitized film to illumination allowed to pass through the negative, so that a second reversal of image intensity occurs. The positive print is developed and "fixed" as described for the negative.

Gold is widely distributed in nature. It is the most malleable of the metals. It is a soft yellow metal that is extremely inactive chemically. It can be dissolved by *aqua regia* (a mixture of nitric and hydrochloric acids):

Au +	4 HCl	+ 3 HNO_3	→	$HAuCl_4$	+ 3 NO_2↑	+ 3 H_2O
Gold	Hydrochloric acid	Nitric acid		Tetrachloroauric acid	Nitrogen dioxide	Water

Its primary use is in the manufacture of jewelry. It is the standard of currency in many areas of the world. Because of its softness, gold usually is alloyed with other metals in the jewelry industry. Pure gold is said to be 24 *carats*. Hence, the alloy in an object made of 18 carat gold would be 18/24 or 75 percent gold.

ZINC AND MERCURY

Zinc is a lustrous, bluish white metal. On exposure to air it becomes coated with a white coating of zinc subcarbonate. It is slowly soluble in mineral acids and reacts readily with concentrated metallic hydroxides, with the evolution of hydrogen gas:

Zn +	NaOH	+ H_2O	→	$NaHZnO_2$ + H_2↑
Zinc	Sodium hydroxide	Water		Sodium zincate

The metal has many industrial uses, such as in the manufacture of galvanized iron, dry cell batteries, bronze, brass, German silver, and dyes.

Zinc acetate, $Zn(C_2H_3O_2)_2 \cdot 2H_2O$, *zinc chloride,* $ZnCl_2$, *zinc oxide,* ZnO, and *zinc peroxide,* ZnO_2, are used topically as astringents and mild antiseptics. Zinc is present in preparations of insulin (see page 401). *Zinc undecylenate,* $Zn(C_{11}H_{20}O_2)_2$, is used topically in the treatment of fungous infections such as "athlete's foot."

Mercury, or *quicksilver,* is the only element that exists as a liquid at ordinary room temperature. (Cesium liquefies at 28.5° C and gallium, at 29.8° C.) It is heavy, silvery white, and extremely mobile. Mercury fumes are poisonous if inhaled over a long period of time. The element should not be poured into laboratory sinks, since it may form alloys with metals in plumbing, thus causing leaks, or may create reservoirs of mercury that serve as an unsuspected source of mercury vapor. It is used industrially in many ways: in thermometers and similar instruments, in ultraviolet lamps, and in dental amalgams.

Mercurous chloride, HgCl, also known as *calomel,* is a laxative. *Mercuric chloride (bichloride of mercury, corrosive sublimate),* $HgCl_2$, is extremely toxic, but in dilute solution is useful as an antiseptic. *Mercuric oxide (yellow oxide of mercury),* HgO, is used topically in the treatment of diseases of the eyes. *Ammoniated mercury,* $HgNH_2Cl$, is useful in the therapy of some diseases of the skin. Some organic salts of mercury are useful diuretics (agents that increase the loss of fluid from the body by way of the urinary tract). An organic form of mercury, methyl mercury, is present in some fish. If the level is higher than governmental standards permit, such fish cannot be sold.

IRON Metallic iron is a silvery white or gray, malleable, hard, magnetic solid. Iron containing from 0.05 percent to 2.0 percent of carbon is ordinary *steel*. *Stainless steel* contains about 14 percent of the element chromium. The rusting of iron has been discussed elsewhere (see page 46). Numerous iron compounds (ferric sulfate, ferrous carbonate, ferrous gluconate, saccharated iron oxide, iron and ammonium citrate) are used in the treatment of iron deficiency anemia (see page 341).

PRECIOUS STONES Most precious stones are complex minerals. In many cases only approximate formulas can be written for them. Their beautiful colors usually result from the presence of metallic impurities.

The hardness of precious stones is measured in terms of Mohs' scale, in which the diamond, the hardest natural substance, has been given a value of 10. Each stone will scratch all other stones below it in this scale. The most valuable stones are the diamond, ruby, sapphire, and emerald. The other stones sometimes are classified as semiprecious.

STUDY QUESTIONS

1. Who first developed a workable periodic table?
2. In your own words explain what is meant by the phrase "periodicity of the elements."
3. How does the modern periodic table differ from the Mendeléeff periodic table?
4. What type of element indicates the ending of each period of the modern table?
5. List some properties of hydrogen.
6. What is the most abundant element in nature?
7. Why is it dangerous to expose hydrogen to an open flame?
8. What valence has combined hydrogen? Hydrogen gas?
9. Name three important alkali metals.
10. Why should the alkali metals be stored under oil?
11. What colors are produced when the following metals, or compounds containing them, are heated in a flame: lithium, sodium, potassium?
12. Name four alkaline-earth metals.
13. What is the usual valence of the alkaline-earth metals in combined form?
14. What is milk of magnesia?
15. What is flashlight powder?
16. What is marble? Limestone?
17. For what purpose is barium sulfate used in medicine?
18. What synthetic compound is, except for diamond, the hardest known substance?
19. What is boric acid?
20. Why is aluminum particularly useful in the construction of airplanes?
21. What is duraluminum?
22. For what purpose are corundum and emery used in industry?
23. Name two salts of aluminum that are useful in medicine.
24. What is quartz? Glass? Water glass? Pyrex glass? Portland cement?
25. What are silicones? Why are they of interest in medicine?
26. Name several well-known minerals that contain silicon.
27. Why should materials coated with tin not be stored at very low temperatures?
28. Name some industrial uses of lead.
29. Explain how a storage battery works.
30. What percentage of the air is nitrogen?
31. What are the usual valences of nitrogen?
32. What is laughing gas? For what purpose is it used in medicine?
33. What is ordinary gunpowder?
34. What radical containing phosphorus is particularly important in biology?
35. Name some industrial uses of phosphorus compounds.
36. For what purposes have compounds containing arsenic, antimony, and bismuth been used in medicine?
37. Describe sulfur.
38. What gas is responsible for an odor resembling that of rotten eggs?
39. Name some uses for sulfuric acid.
40. Name the halogens. From what is their family name derived?
41. What is the most reactive element?
42. Why are hydrofluoric acid solutions stored in paraffin or plastic containers?
43. Who discovered chlorine? Oxygen?

44. What is the appearance of chlorine gas? What are some of its uses? Why do swimming pools often have a "chlorine odor"?
45. What is a household use for sodium hypochlorite?
46. For what purpose are bromides used in medicine?
47. What is tincture of iodine?
48. Name the noble gases. What other names are used to refer to them?
49. How do the noble gases differ from other elements?
50. Name a use for each of the following elements: helium, argon, neon.
51. Name some uses of copper and its compounds.
52. What is the cause of the darkening of ordinary silverware used in the home?
53. How is silver nitrate used in medicine?
54. Explain how it is possible to take a picture with photographic film.
55. What is meant by "malleable"? Name the most malleable element.
56. What is aqua regia?
57. What is the percentage of gold in an ornament labeled "14 carat gold"?
58. What gas is formed when zinc reacts with acids and alkalies?
59. Name two zinc compounds and state their use in medicine.
60. What is quicksilver?
61. What element is a liquid at room temperature?
62. Name five elements that are gases at room temperature.
63. Why should waste mercury not be poured into a laboratory sink?
64. What is calomel? Corrosive sublimate?
65. What is steel? Stainless steel?
66. Name three iron compounds that are used in medicine.
67. Name the four most valuable precious stones.

CHAPTER 15

Nuclear chemistry and atomic energy

INTRODUCTION

The startling developments in the fields of nuclear chemistry and atomic energy, brought forcibly to the attention of the world when the first atomic bomb exploded in World War II, make it mandatory that students of nursing and medicine acquaint themselves with the elementary principles involved. Otherwise it will not be possible for medical science to cope with the new types of bodily injury that could be encountered in modern warfare. Indeed, the modern nursing curriculum includes a unit in which this problem is discussed, and a knowledge of the facts given in this chapter should make this unit more interesting and comprehensible to the student.

Radioactive isotopes are being used extensively as tracers for studying the normal and pathological reactions that take place in living tissues, and some of them are becoming increasingly useful in the diagnosis and treatment of disease.

NATURAL RADIOACTIVITY

In 1896 Henri Becquerel accidentally discovered that salts of the element uranium could darken a photographic plate in the complete absence of visible light. Later, Marie Curie, working with her husband, Pierre Curie, found two other elements, polonium and radium, that had this same interesting property. Still later, another naturally occurring radioactive element, thorium, was discovered. Further work indicated that these elements emit three types of "rays" capable of affecting the photographic plate: alpha particles, beta particles, and gamma rays.

Alpha particles are identical with the nucleus of the helium atom. They contain 2 neutrons and 2 protons and thus have a charge of 2+ and an atomic weight of approximately 4.

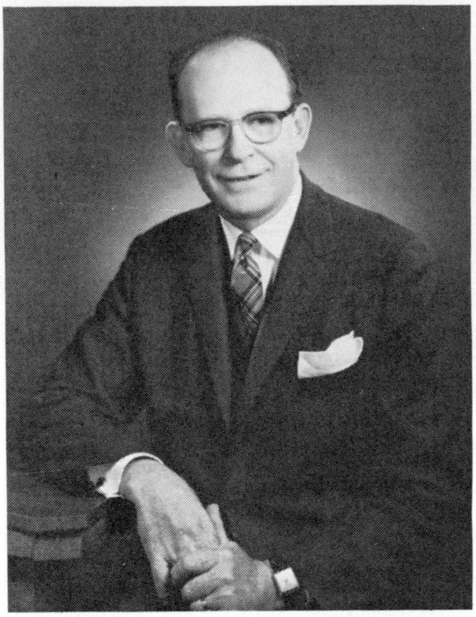

Fig. 15-1. Dr. Willard F. Libby, Professor of Chemistry and Director of the Institute of Geophysics and Planetary Physics of the University of California at Los Angeles, received the Nobel Prize in chemistry in 1960 for the carbon-14 method of age determination. Using this method, the age of many ancient objects has been estimated. For what purpose is radium used in medicine?

Beta particles are electrons traveling at very high speed.

Gamma rays are very similar to x-rays except that they are more penetrating than are the latter.

It is known now that the emission of these subatomic particles indicates the spontaneous change of one element into another. When an alpha particle is emitted from an atomic nucleus, two positive charges are lost, and the remaining nucleus thus belongs to an element having an atomic number lower by 2 than that of the original element. For example, radium (atomic number 88 and atomic weight 226) spontaneously loses an alpha particle to form the element radon (atomic number 86 and atomic weight 222). We may write an equation describing this nuclear reaction as follows:

$$^{226}\mathrm{Ra} \rightarrow \mathrm{He}^{++} + {}^{222}\mathrm{Rn}$$

The small numbers indicate the atomic weight, and the symbol He^{++} is the shorthand expression for an alpha particle (that is, a helium atom that has lost 2 electrons).

If we use the small letter e to indicate a beta particle (that is, an electron moving at high speed), some of the reactions that occur when radium disintegrates are described in the following equations:

$$^{226}\mathrm{Ra} \rightarrow \mathrm{He}^{++} + {}^{222}\mathrm{Rn}$$
$$^{222}\mathrm{Rn} \rightarrow \mathrm{He}^{++} + {}^{218}\mathrm{Po}$$
$$^{218}\mathrm{Po} \rightarrow \mathrm{He}^{++} + {}^{214}\mathrm{Pb}$$
$$^{214}\mathrm{Pb} \rightarrow \mathrm{e} - {}^{214}\mathrm{Bi}$$
$$^{214}\mathrm{Bi} \rightarrow \mathrm{e} + {}^{214}\mathrm{Po}$$
$$^{214}\mathrm{Po} \rightarrow \mathrm{He}^{++} + {}^{210}\mathrm{Pb}$$
$$^{210}\mathrm{Pb} \rightarrow \mathrm{e} + {}^{210}\mathrm{Bi}$$
$$^{210}\mathrm{Bi} \rightarrow \mathrm{e} + {}^{210}\mathrm{Po}$$
$$^{210}\mathrm{Po} \rightarrow \mathrm{He}^{++} + {}^{206}\mathrm{Pb}$$

The isotope of lead (Pb) of atomic weight 206 is stable and does not disintegrate further. The overall result of the above reactions is that radium has been converted to lead, and that alpha particles, beta particles, and gamma rays (not shown in the above equations) have been emitted.

The rates of the above reactions are known, so it is possible to make estimates of the age of the earth (or more exactly, of a given sample of naturally occurring radium) by determining the amount of lead and the amount of radium present in pitchblende, an ore containing radium. Radium has a *half-life* of 1,590 years. This means that a sample of radium weighing 100 mg today will weight 50 mg 1,590 years from now. Since the other elements in the above equation disintegrate rapidly (half-lives of 0.0001 second to 3.82 days), practically all of the 50 mg that disappeared will have been converted to lead. When another 1,590 years shall have passed, only 25 mg (half of the 50 mg) of the radium will remain, and so on. Estimates of the age of the earth, based on this type of evidence, vary from 3.3 billion to 4.5 billion years.

Radium and radon are used in the treatment of cancer. Since radium has a very long half-life, it must be placed in the vicinity of the cancer in a suitable container so that it can be removed after the patient has received as much irradiation as his healthy tissues can stand without injury. Radon is a gas, and ordinarily is placed in short, sealed pieces of gold tubing for use in medicine. These radon seeds, or implants as they are called, are inserted into the cancer itself or around its periphery. It is unnecessary to remove them, since radon has a half-life of 3.82 days. A simple calculation will prove that practically all of the radioactive radon will have disappeared within a month.

BOMBARDMENT WITH CHARGED PARTICLES

In many cases atoms existing in nature can be converted to artificially created atoms by bombardment with particles traveling at high velocity. In 1919 Lord Rutherford and his collaborators in Cambridge, England, converted nitrogen to an isotope of oxygen by bombarding the nitrogen atoms with alpha particles.

$$^{14}N + He^{++} \rightarrow {}^{17}O + H^{+}$$

Table 15-1. The transuranium elements

Name	Atomic symbol	Atomic number
Neptunium	Np	93
Plutonium	Pu	94
Americium	Am	95
Curium	Cm	96
Berkelium	Bk	97
Californium	Cf	98
Einsteinium	E	99
Fermium	Fm	100
Mendelevium	Md	101
Nobelium	No	102
Lawrencium	Lr	103
*		104
*		105

*Rutherfordium and hahnium have been proposed as names for elements 104 and 105, respectively, by scientists at the University of California who believe they are the discoverers. But Russian scientists also claim their discovery and names have not been adopted by the International Union of Pure and Applied Chemistry.

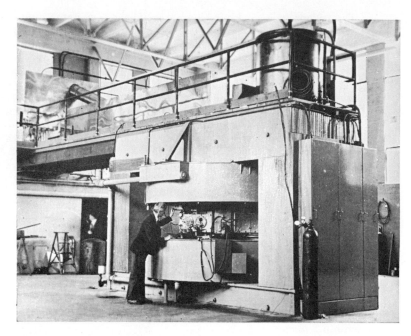

Fig. 15-2. Five of the 13 transuranium elements were first made in this 60-inch cyclotron at the University of California. Shielding used when in operation is not shown. Why are these elements spoken of as "transuranium elements"? (Courtesy Dr. Glenn T. Seaborg.)

As the equation indicates, the other product of the reaction was a proton (that is, a hydrogen ion).

In the early experiments an isotope of the element bismuth (^{83}Bi), which emits alpha particles, was used as a source of particles with which to bombard atoms. In more recent years several methods of accelerating particles have been devised. One type of device, known as the *Van der Graaff generator,* can accelerate electrically charged particles under a potential of from 2 million to 5 million volts. The *cyclotron* was invented by E. O. Lawrence at the University of California in 1929. Dr. Lawrence received the Nobel Prize for this achievement. In principle, positively charged particles are caused to move in a powerful electric field. A magnetic field is applied in such a way that the particles are forced to follow a large spiral pathway. As the particles spin around this spiral pathway, they move at faster and faster speeds so that eventually they contain the energy that would be imparted by a voltage of 7 million to 200 million volts in the Van der Graaff machine. The positively charged particles usually employed in the cyclotron are the deuteron (which consists of a proton and a neutron and is the nucleus of an atom of "heavy hydrogen," or deuterium) and the proton. Many elements have been bombarded with these two particles with the result that many new isotopes, both radioactive and stable, have been discovered.

More recent devices for accelerating particles are the *synchrotron,* the *betatron,* and the *linear accelerator.*

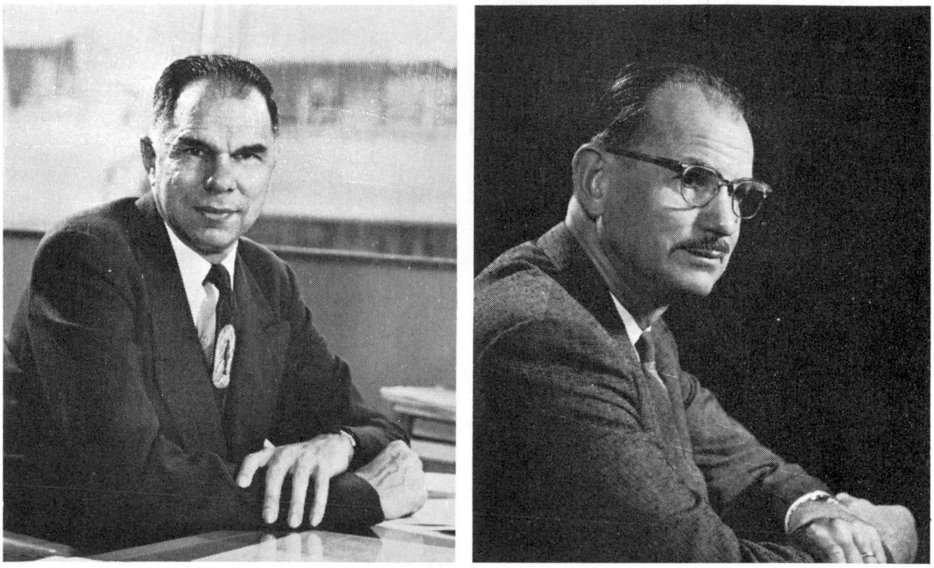

Fig. 15-3. Dr. Glenn T. Seaborg (left), formerly Chairman of the Atomic Energy Commission, and Dr. Edwin M. McMillan (right) were awarded the Nobel Prize in chemistry in 1951 for their work with transuranium elements and the discovery of plutonium. How were the transuranium elements discovered?

Uranium, a metal, has the highest atomic number (92) of the elements that we presently know to occur normally in nature. However, in recent years it has been possible to produce thirteen elements of higher atomic number in the laboratory by experiments in which naturally occurring elements have been bombarded by subatomic particles. These newly discovered elements are known as the transuranium elements. Dr. Edwin M. McMillan and Dr. Glenn T. Seaborg of the University of California were awarded the Nobel Prize in 1951 for their part in these discoveries.

BOMBARDMENT WITH NEUTRONS

It will be recalled that neutrons are subatomic particles that do not possess an electric charge. Hence it is not possible to accelerate them by electric or magnetic fields. However, many radioactive elements spontaneously emit neutrons. In most of the early experiments a mixture of the elements radon and beryllium was used to produce neutrons. The alpha particles from the radon reacted with the beryllium in two ways. Using ^{1}n to represent neutron, the reactions were as follows:

$$^{9}Be + He^{++} \rightarrow {}^{12}C + {}^{1}n$$
$$^{9}Be + He^{++} \rightarrow 3\,{}^{4}He + {}^{1}n$$

More recently the *uranium reactor* or *uranium pile* has been used as a device for bombardment with neutrons. Each sample of naturally occurring uranium (^{238}U) contains 0.71 percent of ^{235}U. When atoms of this isotope of uranium are struck by neutrons, they break into two or more smaller atoms, liberating additional neutrons in the process. If the sample of uranium is small, these newly created neutrons escape and the reaction ceases. However, if the sample is large enough, the newly formed neutrons will strike other atoms of ^{235}U and the reaction continues as a *chain reaction.* The uranium pile consists of a large number of lumps of uranium piled together with bricks of graphite (see page 133). The graphite slows down the neutrons formed from the fission of ^{235}U and increases the probability that they will strike other ^{235}U atoms rather than escape from the pile. The pile also contains a number of cylindrical holes into which rods made of the metal cadmium can be inserted if it is desired to stop or slow down the reactions going on in the pile. The nuclei of cadmium atoms readily capture neutrons and thus prevent their reaction with ^{235}U.

One important use of the uranium pile is to manufacture plutonium (^{239}Pu), which is one of the elements best suited as a source of energy for the manufacture of the atomic bomb and other devices for utilizing atomic energy. Neutrons liberated by the breakdown of ^{235}U atoms react with the ^{238}U atoms to form ^{239}U. This isotope emits a beta particle to form an unstable isotope of neptunium (^{239}Np). ^{239}Np is spontaneously converted to plutonium.

$$^{238}U + {}^{1}n \rightarrow {}^{239}U$$
$$^{239}U \rightarrow {}^{239}Np + e$$
$$^{239}Np \rightarrow {}^{239}Pu + e$$

ATOMIC ENERGY

The nucleus of the atom under ordinary circumstances probably contains only protons and neutrons (see page 20). Since the protons are positively charged and since like electrical charges repel each other, it will be apparent that an enormous amount of energy would be required to bring protons as close to each other as they must be in an atomic nucleus. Because energy cannot be destroyed (although it can be converted to matter and vice versa), this vast store of energy would be released if the protons were separated from each other; that is, if the nucleus of the atom were broken up into the individual subatomic particles of which it is made. It can be calculated that 1 g of helium, one of the lightest elements, contains sufficient nuclear energy to run an ordinary 100-watt light bulb for about 30,000 years. It is evident, then, that tremendous amounts of energy are released under controlled conditions in the atomic pile, or more suddenly when an atomic bomb explodes. Probably the atomic bombs used in World War II contained two or more pieces of relatively pure ^{235}U of insufficient mass to allow a chain reaction to occur. At the time of explosion these masses presumably were brought together to make one large mass, which then exploded as a result of the chain reaction.

It has been calculated that the complete fission of one pound of ^{235}U would produce energy equivalent to 1,000,000,000,000 calories. This is about 2.5 million times the energy that results from the complete combustion of a pound of coal. Undoubtedly we are entering an era in which many of the machines so valuable to mankind will be powered by atomic energy. Dr. Linus Pauling has expressed the view that the discovery of atomic fission and its control is the greatest discovery made since primitive man learned to control fire.

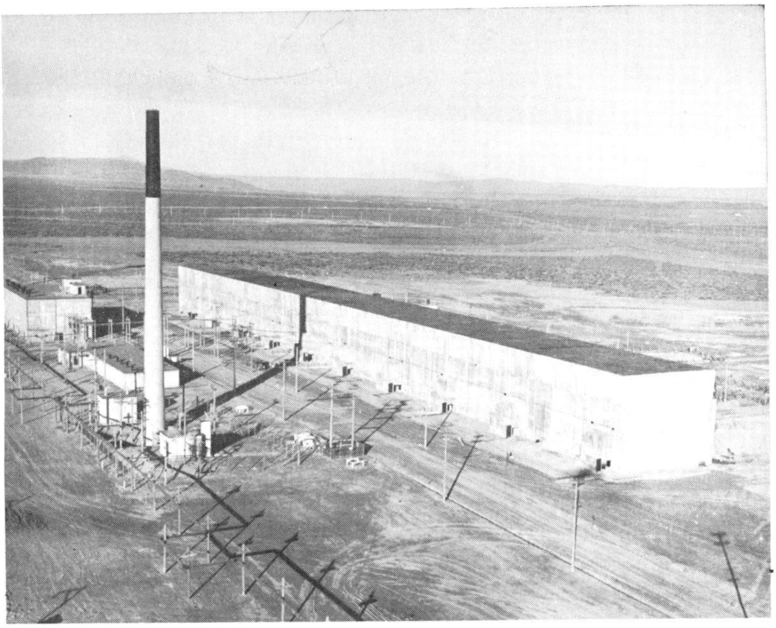

Fig. 15-4. This separation plant at the Hanford project of the Atomic Energy Commission is 800 feet long and has thick concrete walls. Called a canyon building, it is used to separate plutonium from uranium and other process materials. Why is plutonium important? (Courtesy Atomic Energy Commission.)

The nucleus of an atom of uranium (^{235}U) contains 92 protons and 143 neutrons. They are packed into a sphere that is about 1^{-12} cm in diameter. When an atom of ^{235}U absorbs an extra neutron, the spherical shape is distorted. The deformed nucleus then becomes 2 spherical balls connected by a stretched, ropelike mass. Usually the larger sphere contains 50 protons plus some neutrons and the smaller sphere, 50 neutrons plus some protons. The ropelike mass has about 20 particles—both protons and neutrons. When fission occurs, the split usually occurs at the midpoint of the ropelike mass, and thus each sphere receives an equal amount of this connecting mass. Occasionally the ropelike portion splits close to one of the spheres. If this occurs, one of the resulting fragments has much more internal energy (much of which has been in the stretched, ropelike material) than does the other. Of course, large amounts of energy are released.

NUCLEAR FUSION

It should be apparent from what has just been read that the matter present in atomic nuclei can be converted to energy and vice versa. A vivid natural illustration of this phenomenon is the conversion of hydrogen atoms to helium atoms—the principal reaction responsible for the energy of the sun.

$$4\,^{1}H \rightarrow\ ^{4}He + \text{Energy}$$

Since the atomic weight of hydrogen is 1.008 and that of helium is 4.003, it is evident that some loss of weight occurs when the above reaction takes place (since $4 \times 1.008 = 4.032$). Although this weight loss is small, it is very large indeed when measured as energy. Enormous temperatures would be required to cause the fusion of hydrogen atoms to form helium atoms. Many scientists believe that, using the temperature generated by an atomic explosion, it might be possible to convert certain isotopes of hydrogen to helium. These isotopes are *deuterium* (hydrogen of atomic weight 2; its nuclei contain 1 proton and 1 neutron) and *tritium* (hydrogen of atomic weight 3; its nuclei contain 1 proton and 2 neutrons). These isotopes occur in trace amounts in natural samples of hydrogen. The postulated reaction is as follows:

$$^{2}H + {}^{3}H \rightarrow {}^{4}He + {}^{1}n + \text{Energy}$$

One theoretical way to make a "hydrogen bomb" would be to surround an atomic bomb with a mixture of deuterium and tritium. When the atomic bomb exploded, the deuterium and tritium might fuse to form helium, with the release of an enormous amount of energy. Probably the resulting explosion could be several thousand times as violent as that of the ordinary atomic bomb. So-called hydrogen bombs have been made and tested experimentally.

USE OF RADIOACTIVE ELEMENTS AS TRACERS

Scientists working in the Atomic Energy Commission's establishment at Oak Ridge, Tennessee, have discovered many radioactive isotopes of elements important in biology and medicine and have made them available to scientists for study. For example, a very useful isotope is ^{14}C, a radioactive isotope of carbon. It is prepared in the uranium pile, using nitrogen (^{14}N) as a starting material:

$$^{14}N + {}^{1}n \rightarrow {}^{14}C + {}^{1}H$$

Table 15-2. Some radioactive isotopes of medical interest

Element	Isotope	Half-life	Energy emitted as	Form used
Hydrogen (tritium)	^{3}H	12.3 years	β-rays	H_2O
Carbon	^{14}C	5600 years	β-rays	Carbonates, CO_2, and organic compounds
Sodium	^{24}Na	14.9 hours	β-rays; γ-rays	NaCl
Phosphorus	^{32}P	14.3 days	β-rays	Na_2HPO_4
Potassium	^{42}K	12.5 hours	β-rays; γ-rays	K_2CO_3
Chromium	^{51}Cr	26 days	γ-rays	$CrCl_3$
Iron	^{59}Fe	46 days	β-rays; γ-rays	Ferric ammonium citrate
Cobalt	^{60}Co	5.2 years	β-rays; γ-rays	Metallic Co
Gallium	^{72}Ga	14.1 hours	β-rays; γ-rays	Gallium citrate
Strontium	^{90}Sr	24 years	β-rays	Beta ray applicator
Iodine	^{131}I	8 days	β-rays; γ-rays	NaI
Gold	^{198}Au	2.69 days	β-rays; γ-rays	Colloidal Au
Lead	^{210}Pb	22 years	β-rays; γ-rays	Beta ray applicator
Radon	^{222}Rn	3.825 days	β-rays; γ-rays; α-particles	Rn gas
Radium	^{226}Ra	1590–1690 years	β-rays; γ-rays; α-particles	$RaBr_2$

Most of the compounds in foods and in biological materials contain natural carbon (^{12}C), which is not radioactive. However, the chemist can prepare these same compounds in the laboratory in such a way that some of the carbon atoms are ^{14}C. This makes it possible to locate this compound or products formed from it later by using an instrument that detects radioactivity. For example, if an animal is allowed to breathe CO_2 labeled with ^{14}C, many important substances later isolated from the animal's tissues can be shown to contain radioactive ^{14}C. This experiment proves beyond doubt that CO_2, until recent years thought to be a waste product incapable of undergoing reactions in animal tissues, can be converted in the body into compounds of value to the animal. As another example of an experiment that can be done very simply with radioactive isotopes: suppose it is desired to find out how long a time elapses between the eating of some common table salt (NaCl) and its first appearance in the bloodstream. This problem can be solved by using table salt labeled with radioactive sodium atoms. The subject places his hand in front of an instrument that detects radioactivity, and then swallows the salt. As soon as the salt enters the blood and passes to his hand, the instrument registers, indicating that passage of the salt into the blood has taken place.

THERAPEUTIC AND DIAGNOSTIC USES OF RADIOACTIVE ISOTOPES.* Several of the many radioactive isotopes now available are used in the treatment and diagnosis of human diseases, and undoubtedly many more will prove to be useful for these purposes in the future.

Compounds labeled with radioactive *phosphorus* are used in the treatment of chronic myelogenous leukemia. This disease is characterized by a rapid production of white blood cells. Probably because these cells are multiplying more rapidly than are most other cells in the body, and perhaps also because white blood cells contain a high percentage of phosphorus, the radioactive phosphorus isotope tends to concentrate in these cells and destroys some of them by emission of radiant energy. This treatment will not bring about cure (nor, indeed, will any other), but the patient appears clinically to have fewer disabling signs and symptoms during his illness than would be the case without therapy.

In the form of a colloidal dispersion of chromic phosphate ^{32}P has been given intravenously in the therapy of diseases of the spleen and liver. When this colloidal dispersion is adsorbed on blotting paper, it can be applied topically in the treatment of superficial skin diseases.

Erythremia (polycythemia vera), a disease in which there is an overproduction of red blood cells, also frequently can be controlled by the administration of radioactive *phosphorus*. Some slight benefit has been reported following the treatment of multiple myeloma, a malignant disease of the bones. Radioactive *strontium* also has been used for this purpose. Certain compounds labeled with various radioactive elements (phosphrous, potassium, copper, iodine) appear to concentrate preferentially in brain tumors, and are used both in making a diagnosis and in locating the exact site of the tumor.

Iodine concentrates preferentially in the cells of the thyroid gland, probably because that gland converts it to thyroglobulin, a protein having hormonal activity (see page 390). Radioactive iodine compounds have been used with some success

***CRC Handbook of Radioactive Nuclides* (1968) is a useful reference book. It is edited by Yen Wang, MD, DSc (Medicine) and is published by the Chemical Rubber Company, 18901 Cranwood Parkway, Cleveland, Ohio 44128 ($15.00).

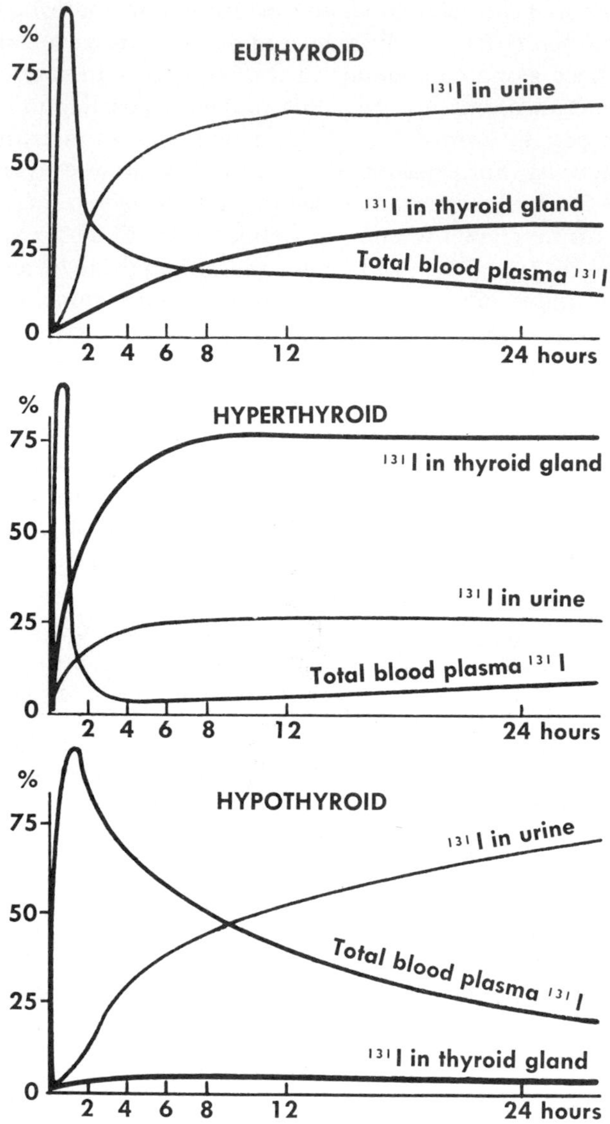

Fig. 15-5. Graphs illustrating the distribution of radioactive iodine after patients have swallowed a solution containing it. What percentage of the ingested iodine usually is taken up in 24 hours by the thyroid of a normal individual? (From Therapeutic Notes; courtesy Parke, Davis & Co.)

in treating hyperthyroidism (overactivity of the thyroid gland) and cancer of the thyroid. Cancers frequently metastasize—that is, cells break away from the parent tumor and locate at some distant site in the body. This makes radioactive iodine a particularly intriguing agent for therapy, since it should localize in the cancerous thyroid cells no matter where they may be located in the patient's body. Compounds containing radioactive iodine also have been placed in the chest cavity in the treatment of patients with cancer of the lungs. This procedure does not eradicate the cancer, but it may abolish the troublesome pleural effusion (accumulation of fluid in the chest cavity) that sometimes is present.

Studies of the function of the pancreas (see page 325) and the degree of absorption of fat from the intestinal tract can be made by administering a fat (usually triolein) labeled with radioactive iodine (^{131}I).

Methyl iodide tagged with radioactive iodine (^{131}I) has been injected into the bloodstream in order to measure circulation time, to determine the presence of abnormal passages between the chambers of the heart, and to locate aneurysms (abnormal dilated areas in blood vessels, or abnormal connections between arteries and veins).

One test of thyroid function (see page 390) is the *iodine uptake test*. The patient swallows ^{131}I (usually as NaI) in distilled water. A standard is prepared by placing an identical amount of the same solution ingested by the patient in a volumetric flask. Twenty-four hours later the standard is placed 10 inches from a scintillation probe (radiant energy counter) and a 3-minute count is taken. Then the probe is placed 10 inches from the region of the patient's thyroid and another 3-minute count is taken. From these two measurements it is possible to calculate the percentage of ingested iodine that is in (that is, has been taken up by) the patient's thyroid. In hypothyroidism the figure usually ranges from 0 to 15 percent; in normal function, from 15 to 45 percent; in hyperthyroidism, more than 45 percent.

An isotope of *gold* that has a relatively short half-life has been used in the form of a colloidal dispersion of the metal. It is injected into or in the vicinity of the cancer in much the same way as radon seeds are implanted (see page 119). Colloidal radioactive gold also has been injected into the chest cavity in the attempt to prevent pleural effusion in patients with cancer of the lungs. Radiogold colloid can be injected intravenously, and has been used in this way to treat patients with chronic leukemia.

Gallium is a metal whose salts tend to concentrate in the bones when it is injected into a patient. Radioactive gallium is used in the treatment of cancers of the bones. The cells of the cancer are multiplying much more rapidly than are the normal bone cells and preferentially take up the gallium.

Radioactive *cobalt* has a long half-life and is a powerful gamma ray emitter. It is being used increasingly as a substitute for radium. Indeed, it has been possible to make machines containing a sufficient amount of this radioactive metal so that large areas of the body can be irradiated at one time. These machines may some day replace the standard x-ray machines now used for therapy.

Radioactive *iron* salts can be used to determine the total circulating red cell volume in patients. A suitable salt is injected into a donor and after a period of time some of it becomes incorporated in the hemoglobin (see page 227) present in the donor's red blood cells. A sample of blood now is taken from the donor and is injected into the bloodstream of the patient. After this injected blood has become thoroughly mixed with that of the patient, a sample of the patient's blood is removed and the radioactivity of the red blood cells present is measured. Suppose, as an example, that 30 ml of labeled red blood cells were injected into the patient, and that subsequent study of the patient's blood indicated that these cells had been diluted 100 times by admixture with the patient's red blood cells (that is, the cells removed had $1/100$ the amount of radioactivity present before injection). Then the volume of circulating red blood cells in the patient would be calculated to be 3,000 ml (30 ml $\times$ 100). Human serum albumin (see page 353) labeled with radioactive iodine also is used to measure blood volume.

After the injection of small amounts of a radioactive iron salt intravenously it is possible to measure with a suitable detection device the rate at which iron is entering and leaving the plasma (liquid portion of the blood) of the patient. The information thus obtained sometimes is useful in establishing a diagnosis in certain blood diseases.

As a rule, substances injected into the bloodstream do not easily diffuse from the blood into the fluid present in and around the brain (cerebrospinal fluid). When a brain tumor is present, however, diffusion at its site takes place more readily. If a compound containing a radioactive element is injected into the blood, frequently the location and approximate size of brain tumors can be ascertained with the aid of a suitable external detection device (Geiger-Mueller counter or scintillation counter). Diiodofluorescein, an organic dye, and iodinated human serum albumin (see page 353), a protein – each containing radioactive iodine – have been used for this purpose. The use of an external counter is possible because the radioactive iodine emits gamma rays that pass through the patient's tissues and so reach the measuring device.

Compounds containing radioactive phosphorus (^{32}P) have been injected into the blood during operations for brain tumors. They also localize in the tumors. Since ^{32}P emits beta rays, which penetrate only a few millimeters in tissue, it is necessary to place the detector in close contact with the source of beta rays. A so-called probe counter that can be introduced directly into the brain tissue during the operation has been used for this purpose.

The amount of body water in man has been determined by injecting small amounts of tritium oxide. (Tritium is radioactive hydrogen of atomic weight 3, ^{3}H.) A sample of body fluid then is taken, and its content of tritium oxide is measured. A simple calculation indicates how many fold the injected tritium oxide has been diluted by H_2O (water), thus making it possible to calculate the content of body water. By this method normal adults of average build are found to be about 51 to 55 percent water. This is somewhat lower than the figure obtained by older methods (see page 51).

The absorption of vitamin B_{12} is impaired in pernicious anemia (see page 324). The *Schilling test,* in which vitamin B_{12} labeled with radioactive cobalt is used, is one test for this disease. This test can be used also in persons without pernicious anemia as a measure of the efficiency of absorption of vitamin B_{12} from the intestinal tract. Briefly, a small dose (a few micrograms) of labeled vitamin B_{12} is given by mouth to a patient with an empty urinary bladder. Two hours later a much larger dose (usually 1 mg or 1000 micrograms) of unlabeled vitamin B_{12} is injected subcutaneously. Any labeled vitamin B_{12} that has been absorbed becomes mixed in the body with this large amount of injected vitamin B_{12}. Because the body cannot store all of the large amount injected, some of the vitamin is eliminated in the urine. The urine is collected over a 24-hour period, and the amount of radioaotivity present is measured. In normal persons about 13 to 15 percent of the dose administered by mouth is excreted in the urine in the first 24 hours. Patients with pernicious anemia excrete less than 3 percent in 24 hours.

Scanning and photographic techniques. When appropriate compounds containing radioactive isotopes are injected into the body they tend to concentrate in certain organs. In some cases they are most concentrated in a pathological area (in a brain tumor, for example) and in other cases they concentrate in the normal tissue rather than in the lesion (in normal liver tissue rather than in a cancerous region of the liver, for example). In either case, detection of the radiation coming from the organ by an appropriate device makes it possible to obtain a rough "picture" of the extent of the pathological area.

One device is a mobile scanner. When this instrument is used, a scanner containing a sensitive crystal moves back and forth across the region until the entire area has been scanned. Radiation from the tissue strikes the crystal and causes the emission of gamma rays. These rays strike a photographic film inside the instrument and are translated into a series of dots. The intensity of the dots is correlated with the intensity of the radiation emitted by the tissue (Fig. 15-6, *A*).

One disadvantage of the scanner is that an appreciable time is required for the complete scanning process. If changes in the content of radioactive isotope occur quickly, the final dot pattern may be distorted. In order to overcome this, the scintillation camera has been developed. It uses a single large, stationary crystal and

A 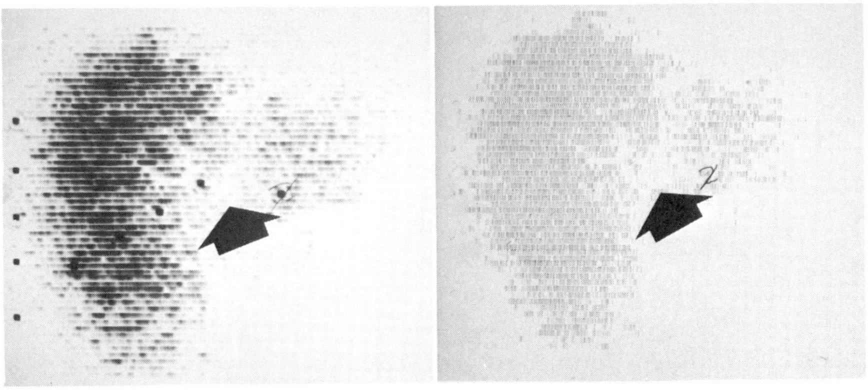 B

Fig. 15-6. Photoscan, **A,** and scintillation photograph, **B,** of the region of the liver of a patient who had received an injection of ^{198}Au colloid. The clear areas indicated by the arrows suggest the presence of a lesion (probably cancer) in which the gold isotope did not concentrate. What is the theoretical advantage of the scintillation photographic technic? (Courtesy Dr. Stanley M. Becker and Dr. Hugo C. Pribor, Institute of Laboratory Medicine, Perth Amboy General Hospital, Perth Amboy, N. J.)

Table 15-3. Some radioisotopes in the environment*

Radioisotope	Physical half-life	Metabolic behavior	Removal rate from body	Samples of importance for testing and monitoring
Iodine 131	8 days	Collects in thyroid gland	Fast	Air, water, plants, milk, thyroid
Barium 140	13 days		Fast (physical decay)	Plants, milk
Strontium 89	51 days	Like calcium, collect in bone	Relatively fast (physical decay)	Soil, plants, dairy products, aquatic foods, bone
Strontium 90	28 years		Slow	
Cesium 137	30 years	Like potassium, collects in bone	Relatively fast (biological halflife of 140 days)	Soil, plants, meats, dairy products, aquatic foods, whole body

*From Dairy Council Digest, a publication of the National Dairy Council.

takes an instantaneous photograph. Again, gamma rays emitted by the irradiated crystal appear on the developed film as a series of dots (Fig. 15-6, *B*).

Use of heavy particles in therapy. As used for therapy, high energy, heavy, charged particles (usually protons or alpha particles) differ from gamma rays or x-rays. They do not scatter very much in tissues and will not penetrate too deeply. It is possible to use a pencil-like beam with equal intensity along its path, or several external beams can be caused to come together at a point in the tissue. This latter method results in greatly decreased intensity in tissues away from the point of convergence. Such beams have been used to suppress the activity of the pituitary gland (useful in some cases of metastatic breast cancer; acromegaly, page 405; diabetic retinal disease; and Cushing's disease, page 406). Tumors of the brain and soft tissues have been treated also with high energy, heavy particles.

In some cases charged pions (pi-mesons, Table 4-1, page 21) have been used. This particle has a mass 276 times as great as that of an electron. It is unstable and spontaneously changes to a muon (mu-meson) within 20 billionths of a second. When the negatively charged pion comes to rest in the tissue, it is captured by an atom of oxygen, carbon, or nitrogen, causing its nucleus to explode into alpha particles, protons, and neutrons. These secondary particles attack the tumor or other lesion. Thus pions can traverse healthy tissue without causing much damage and can, if properly used, deliver a high therapeutic dose to a tumor.

RADIOACTIVE FALLOUT Natural radioactivity always has been a part of man's environment. The occurrence of nuclear explosions has caused an increase in the amount of this environmental radioactivity. Some scientists have been concerned about the amounts of radioactive chemicals that find their way into foods, and hence into the bodies of humans. Table 15-3 lists some of the more important of these radioactive isotopes.

STUDY QUESTIONS

1. Why is it important for students of nursing to learn something about nuclear reactions?
2. Define: alpha particles, beta particles, gamma rays.
3. Who discovered radioactivity?
4. Who discovered radium?
5. What is meant by the term "halflife"?
6. How can radioactivity be used to estimate the age of the earth?
7. Write the equation describing the conversion of radium to radon.
8. What stable element is the end result of the nuclear disintegration of the elements in the radium series?
9. How are radium and radon used in medicine?
10. Name several machines used to accelerate charged particles of atomic and subatomic size.
11. What is meant by the term "transuranium elements"?
12. Why cannot neutrons be accelerated by an electric field?
13. In your own words describe the uranium pile and how it works.
14. What do you think is meant by the term "chain reaction"?
15. How is plutonium manufactured? Why is this element important?
16. Explain why energy is released when uranium undergoes fission.
17. What reaction is responsible for most of the sun's energy?
18. What is deuterium? Tritium?
19. How might a "hydrogen bomb" be manufactured?
20. Give several possible uses not mentioned in the text for radioactive tracers.
21. Name one medical use for radioactive isotopes of each of the following elements: phosphorus, iodine, gold, gallium, cobalt, iron.
22. Explain how tritium can be used to estimate body water.
23. How can the absorption of vitamin B_{12} be measured?
24. Name several ways in which radioactive iodine is used in medicine.
25. Name several radioactive elements that contribute to radioactive fallout.
26. What is meant by "scanning the liver to detect a lesion"?
27. When radioactive compounds are injected into the body, do they tend to concentrate in healthy tissues or in diseased tissues? Explain your answer.
28. Describe how heavy, high energy, charged particles are used in therapy.
29. Explain why charged pions sometimes are useful in destroying tumors.

CHAPTER 16

Introduction to organic chemistry

Organic chemistry was first used as a term to designate those chemical compounds produced by living cells. This seemed logical to the chemists of a former day because they supposed that some "vital force" that man could never hope to master was required to make such substances. Fortunately for the present state of chemistry and medicine, Friedrich Wöhler, a German chemist, proved this conception was wrong in 1828 when he prepared urea (found in blood and urine) from ammonium isocyanate, a compound not present in living cells; it thus became unnecessary to assume that some unknown "vital force" was responsible for the synthesis of the compounds of the tissues. A vast number of compounds found in plants and animals have been made in the laboratory since Wöhler's time.

Most compounds made by cells contain the element carbon. Today we define organic chemistry as that branch of chemistry that deals with the carbon compounds, even though many such compounds have no relation to life. Inorganic chemistry includes all those substances that do not contain carbon (see page 67).

At first it may seem strange that we should divide chemical substances into two groups and, perhaps, stranger still that we should place in one of these groups the compounds of only one of the elements. There are, however, excellent reasons for such a division. Organic compounds far outnumber inorganic ones. Moreover, carbon compounds have certain properties not found in other compounds. For example, all organic compounds turn dark and decompose when they are heated. Also, many organic substances exhibit the phenomenon of *isomerism* (see page 160). This means that organic molecules may contain the same number and kinds of atoms and yet represent entirely different substances. Sixteen different compounds, including glucose, the sugar found in blood, have the formula $C_6H_{12}O_6$. This is explained by assuming that the carbon, hydrogen, and oxygen atoms are connected in different ways. That is, all 16 of these compounds have the same *empirical* formula, but each one has a different *structural* formula. Such compounds are called *isomers*.

SOURCES OF ORGANIC COMPOUNDS

Plant and animal tissues are an ever present source of organic substances. The fats, sugars, starches, and proteins that we use as foods are examples of compounds from these sources. Many of the hormones and vitamins used in treating human and animal diseases can be extracted from the tissues of animals or plants, although most of these substances are now made more economically in the laboratory. Alcohol, dyes, perfumes, flavoring agents, drugs, and a multitude of other useful products are made by chemists from plant and animal substances.

Decomposition products of animals and plants that lived centuries ago furnish another rich source of carbon compounds. Coal, coke, petroleum, and natural gas belong in this group. Gasoline, kerosene, paraffin, and lubricating oils are prepared from petroleum. Coal and wood yield valuable substances when they are heated in closed containers, and the vapors thus formed are condensed, a process known as *destructive distillation*.

IMPORTANCE OF ORGANIC SUBSTANCES

Chemical reactions involving carbon compounds make up a large majority of the reactions that take place in living tissues. To understand how our bodies function, therefore, we must know something about such compounds. The foods we eat, the tissues we build from them, the waste products we excrete, the vitamins and hormones that spell the difference between normal and abnormal body function, and, in some cases, between life and death—all these are organic substances.

The list of products the organic chemist has given us seems almost endless. Drugs, dyes, perfumes, fuels, solvents, varnishes, household cement, plastics, synthetic fibers, and a host of other useful things were made in his laboratory. Some cynic has remarked that even the beauty of a modern woman's face is a tribute to his skill!

COMPARISON OF ORGANIC AND INORGANIC REACTIONS

The fundamental laws of chemistry discussed in preceding chapters apply to inorganic and organic reactions alike. Organic reactions, however, are very much slower than inorganic ones. This is explained by the fact that reactions between inorganic substances usually represent reactions between ions in solution; carbon compounds ionize only slightly or not at all. This means that catalysts are particularly important in organic chemistry. Enzymes catalyze the organic reactions occurring in the body; without their aid life, if it existed at all, would indeed be a sluggish affair.

CARBON AS AN ELEMENT

Carbon exists in three elementary forms: amorphous carbon, diamond, and graphite. Amorphous means "without structure," and such forms of carbon as lampblack, charcoal, coal, and coke are said to be amorphous because they do not show crystalline structure even if examined with a microscope. We know now, however, as a result of x-ray studies, that these substances probably do exist as exceedingly small crystals. Charcoal has the property of adsorbing many gases and colored compounds. Brown impurities present in natural products such as sugar are removed by it.

The adsorbing material in one type of gas mask is largely charcoal. This substance is sometimes administered to patients in an attempt to adsorb gases in the intestinal tract.

Diamond is a crystalline form of carbon and is the hardest substance found in nature. Rich natural deposits of diamonds are found in southern areas of South America, Africa, and Asia. Diamonds that have flaws and cannot be used for jewelry are used to make instruments for cutting glass, drilling through rock formations, and for cutting and shaping ornamental diamonds. Artificial diamonds have been made, but they are too small and imperfect to be of commercial value.

Natural deposits of graphite are located in Asia, southern Europe, and New York. Artificial graphite is made by heating coal to high temperatures. Crystals of graphite are minute, flat plates that slide readily on each other. This explains the use of this substance as a lubricating material. The "lead" of lead pencils is a mixture of graphite and clay. Vessels that must withstand high temperatures are often made of graphite.

IMPORTANT PROPERTIES OF THE CARBON ATOM

The carbon atom has 4 electrons in its outer electron shell. This means that carbon has a valence of 4. Carbon does not ionize, and when it unites with other elements it does so by means of covalent linkages. Elements having either negative or positive valence can unite with carbon by sharing electrons. This fact, together with the fact that *carbon atoms readily unite with each other*, explains why so many organic compounds exist.

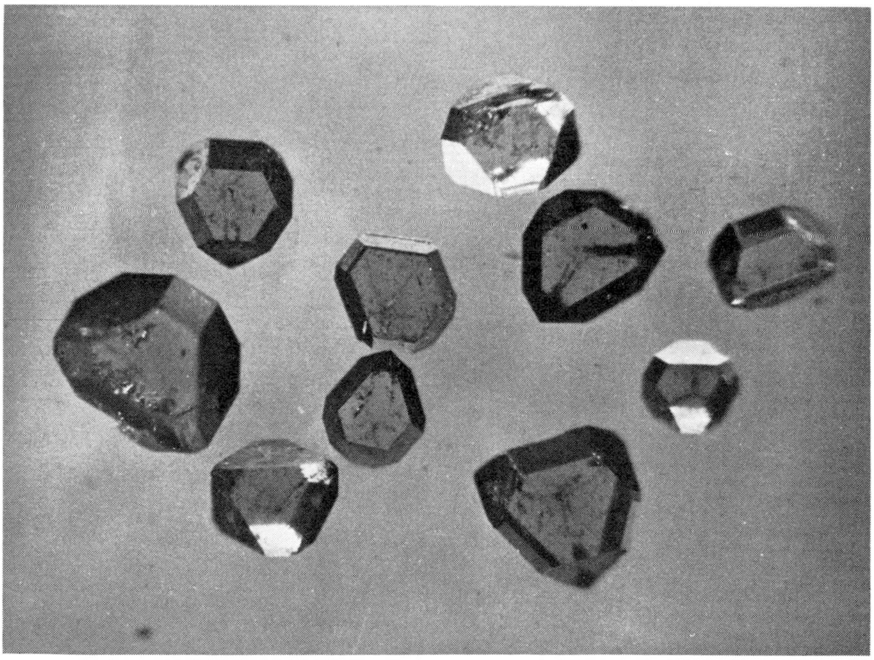

Fig. 16-1. Photomicrograph of artificial diamonds made in the General Electric Research Laboratory. Why are they not valuable commercially? (Courtesy General Electric Research Laboratory.)

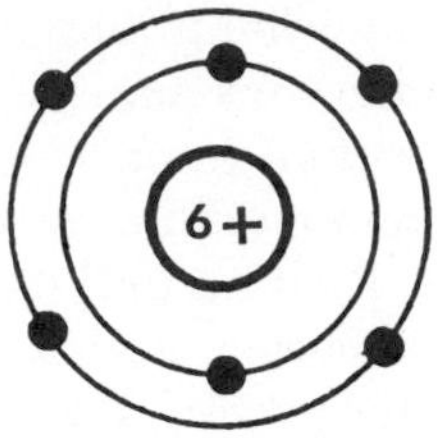

Fig. 16-2. Diagram of the carbon atom. What is the most probable valence of carbon, as indicated by this diagram?

USE OF STRUCTURAL FORMULAS IN ORGANIC CHEMISTRY

It will be recalled (see page 35) that structural formulas represent "maps" of molecules in the sense that they indicate how the atoms that compose the molecule are linked. Carbon atoms in structural formulas have 4 bonds, —C—, because the valence of carbon is 4 (remember that chemical bonds represent valence; each bond represents 1 valence). A carbon atom is thus capable of uniting with 4 univalent atoms or radicals. In the following compounds chlorine and hydrogen atoms each have only one bond, since the valence of these elements is 1.

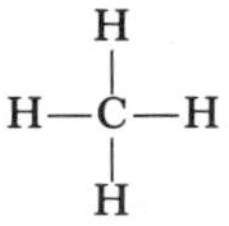
CH_4
Methane

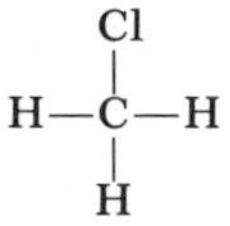
CH_3Cl
Methyl chloride

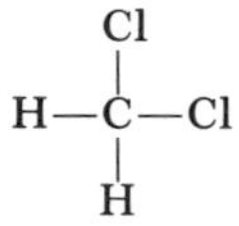
CH_2Cl_2
Methylene chloride

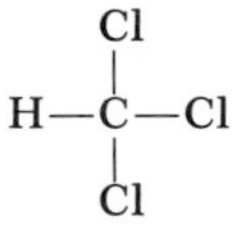
$CHCl_3$
Chloroform

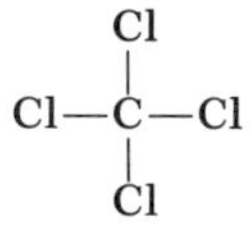
CCl_4
Carbon tetrachloride

Notice that carbon unites with elements having either positive or negative valence (chlorine has a valence of 1− and hydrogen has a valence of 1+) because the linkage is of the covalent type. The Cl and H atoms in the above formulas are not present as ions—as they frequently are in inorganic compounds. Electrons have not been exchanged; they are merely shared. Figs. 16-3 and 16-4 may assist in making this point clear. The diagrams also show that the bonds used in writing organic formulas represent *pairs* of shared electrons. This is the same as saying that such bonds represent valence.

Carbon can combine also with divalent and trivalent elements, as the compounds that follow illustrate:

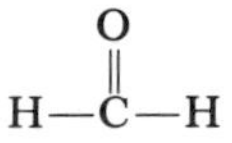
HCHO
Formaldehyde

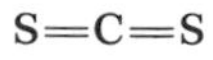
CS_2
Carbon disulfide

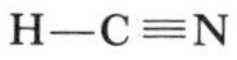
HCN
Hydrocyanic acid

Notice that O and S are each connected to C by 2 bonds, since the valence of these elements is 2. N is connected by 3 bonds; its valence here is 3. Each C atom has 4 bonds.

Carbon atoms have an important property not commonly found in other

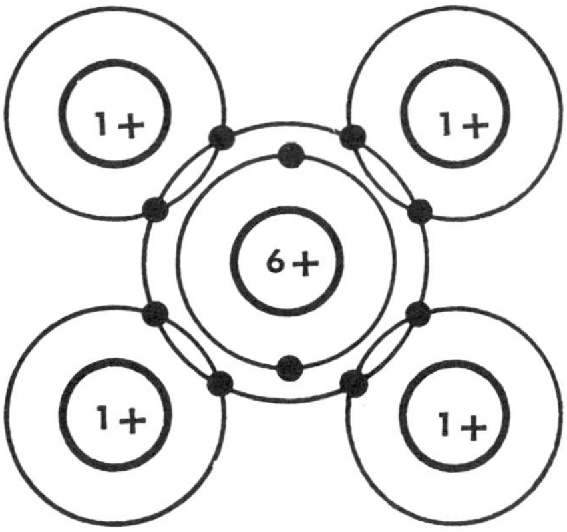

Fig. 16-3. Diagram of the methane molecule, CH_4. Here carbon has combined with an element (hydrogen) that ordinarily has positive valence. Is the linkage covalent or electrovalent?

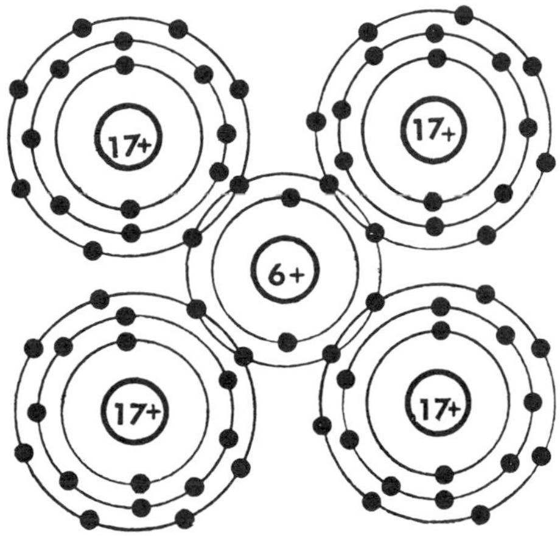

Fig. 16-4. Diagram of the carbon tetrachloride molecule, CCl_4. Here carbon has combined with an element (chlorine) that ordinarily has negative valence. Why is carbon tetrachloride a nonelectrolyte?

elements, the property of uniting with other carbon atoms to produce chains or rings of such atoms.

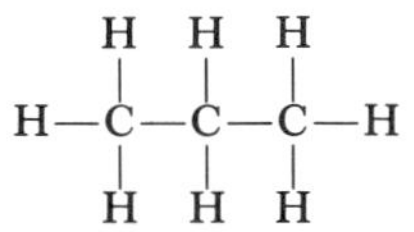

C_3H_8

Propane
(A chain of C atoms)

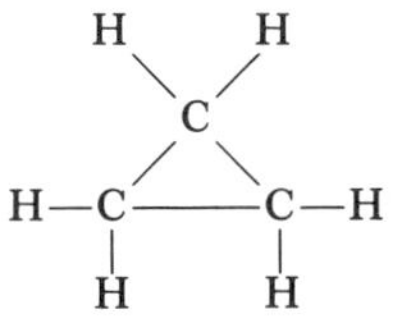

C_3H_6

Cyclopropane
(A ring of C atoms)

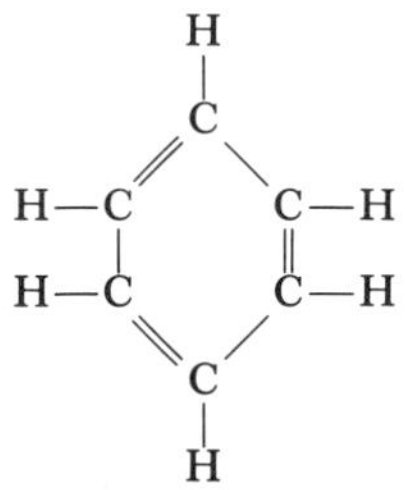

C_6H_6

Benzene
(A ring of C atoms)

The organic chemist is able to obtain either a ring of carbon atoms or an open chain of them by appropriate treatment of the reacting substances.

SATURATED AND UNSATURATED COMPOUNDS

Compounds containing only single bonds *between carbon atoms* are said to be *saturated. Unsaturated* compounds contain double or triple bonds *between carbon atoms.*

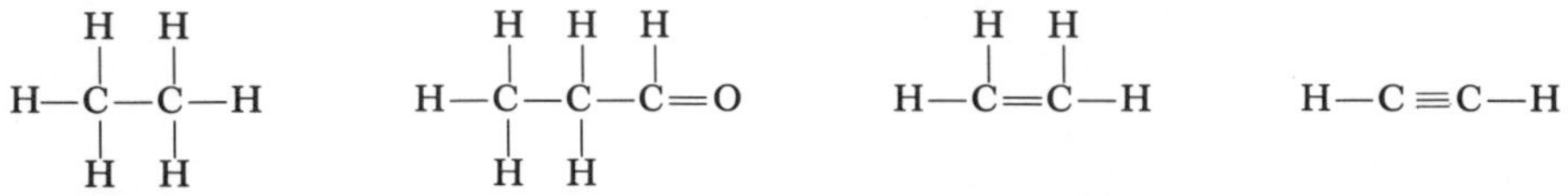

C_2H_6 Ethane (Saturated) | C_2H_5CHO Propionaldehyde (Saturated) | C_2H_4 Ethylene (Unsaturated) | C_2H_2 Acetylene (Unsaturated)

Notice that propionaldehyde is a saturated compound because the double bond present is *not between carbon atoms*. Ethylene contains 2 and acetylene 3 bonds between carbon atoms. These compounds are therefore unsaturated. The word unsaturated implies that more atoms could be made to unite with the carbon atoms in the molecule. By causing 2 hydrogen atoms to unite with 1 molecule of ethylene, for example, or by causing 4 atoms of hydrogen to unite with 1 molecule of acetylene, a molecule of ethane is formed. Verify this by studying the foregoing structural formulas. On the other hand, it is not possible to add any more hydrogen to ethane because no more bonds are available to unite with other atoms.

It is clear that unsaturated compounds are more *active* chemically than saturated ones; that is, they unite more readily with other atoms or radicals.

CHARACTERISTIC GROUPS

Organic chemistry is made somewhat simpler by the fact that reactions between organic substances seldom involve whole molecules. Usually only one small portion of the molecule is involved. This small reactive portion of the molecule is called the *characteristic group*, or *functional group*. This group may be regarded as an atom or radical that has taken the place of one of the hydrogen atoms attached to carbon in hydrocarbons (see page 138). The characteristic group in the following compounds is enclosed in a square:

C_2H_5OH Ethyl alcohol | CH_3COOH Acetic acid

Notice that the *empirical* formulas for the above compounds are written in such a way as to indicate the characteristic group. Thus, ethyl alcohol is written C_2H_5OH, or CH_3CH_2OH; acetic acid is written CH_3COOH. Ethyl alcohol may be thought of as a derivative of ethane, CH_3CH_3, in which 1 of the hydrogen atoms has been replaced by OH. Acetic acid is a derivative of methane, CH_4, in which COOH has substituted for 1 of the H atoms.

DIVISIONS OF ORGANIC COMPOUNDS

Organic compounds whose molecules are composed of open chains of carbon atoms to which atoms or radicals are attached are called *aliphatic compounds*. Compounds whose molecules contain rings of carbon atoms are *carbocyclic compounds*. In some cases ring compounds have elements in addition to carbon in the ring; such compounds are *heterocyclic*.

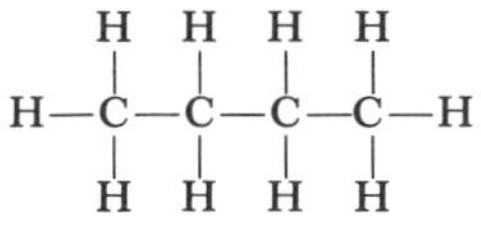

C_4H_{10} or $CH_3CH_2CH_2CH_3$

Butane
(Aliphatic)

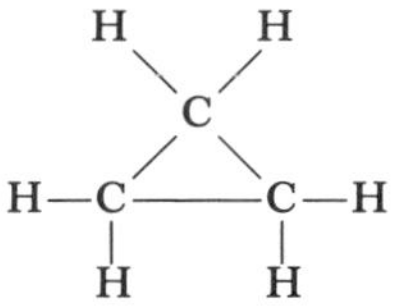

C_3H_6 or
$CH_2CH_2CH_2$
Cyclopropane
(Carbocyclic)

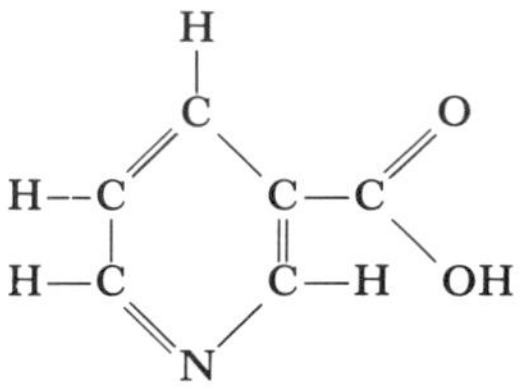

C_5H_4NCOOH

Nicotinic acid
(Heterocyclic)

Derivatives of the carbocyclic compound benzene are extremely important. Many of these compounds have an aromatic odor, and members of this series are often called the *aromatic compounds*. They are discussed in Chapter 19.

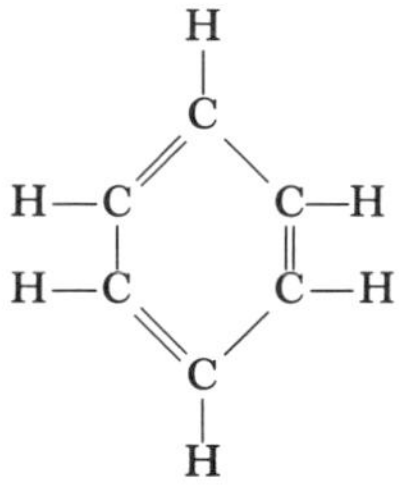

C_6H_6
Benzene
(Aromatic)

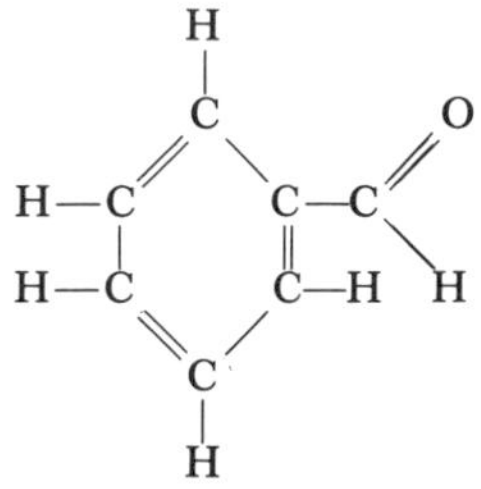

C_6H_5CHO
Benzaldehyde
(Aromatic)

STUDY QUESTIONS

1. Who first prepared an organic compound from a substance not found in living tissues? What compound did he make?
2. What is an organic compound? An inorganic compound?
3. Why are there so many more known organic compounds than inorganic compounds?
4. What is meant by isomerism? What is an isomer?
5. Name some of the sources from which organic compounds are obtained.
6. Do you believe that organic compounds are of sufficient importance to justify separate chapters in this book? Why?
7. How do organic and inorganic reactions differ?
8. What are the three elementary forms of carbon? What do you think would happen if a diamond were scraped with a steel file?
9. Draw a diagram showing the structure of the carbon atom. What is the valence of carbon? Is this valence positive? Negative?
10. Draw a diagram showing the structure of carbon dioxide, CO_2.
11. What is an unsaturated compound? Is CH_2CHCH_3 a saturated or unsaturated compound? How do you know?
12. Why are unsaturated compounds more active chemically than saturated ones?
13. What is a characteristic group?

Aliphatic organic compounds

HYDROCARBONS

SATURATED
ALIPHATIC
HYDRO-
CARBONS

Compounds containing only hydrogen and carbon are known as *hydro-carbons*. Aliphatic hydrocarbons may be considered as derivatives of methane, the simplest member of the group.

$$
\begin{array}{cccc}
& \overset{\displaystyle H}{\underset{\displaystyle H}{H-\overset{|}{\underset{|}{C}}-H}} & \overset{\displaystyle H\ \ H}{\underset{\displaystyle H\ \ H}{H-\overset{|}{\underset{|}{C}}-\overset{|}{\underset{|}{C}}-H}} & \overset{\displaystyle H\ \ H\ \ H}{\underset{\displaystyle H\ \ H\ \ H}{H-\overset{|}{\underset{|}{C}}-\overset{|}{\underset{|}{C}}-\overset{|}{\underset{|}{C}}-H}} & \overset{\displaystyle H\ \ H\ \ H\ \ H}{\underset{\displaystyle H\ \ H\ \ H\ \ H}{H-\overset{|}{\underset{|}{C}}-\overset{|}{\underset{|}{C}}-\overset{|}{\underset{|}{C}}-\overset{|}{\underset{|}{C}}-H}}
\end{array}
$$

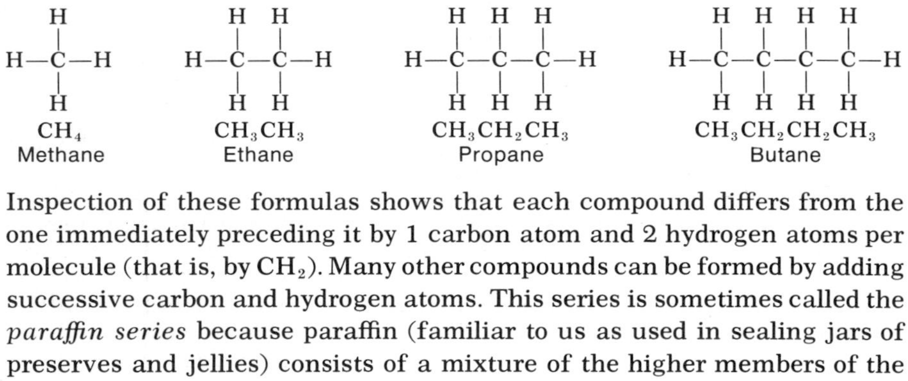

CH_4	CH_3CH_3	$CH_3CH_2CH_3$	$CH_3CH_2CH_2CH_3$
Methane	Ethane	Propane	Butane

Inspection of these formulas shows that each compound differs from the one immediately preceding it by 1 carbon atom and 2 hydrogen atoms per molecule (that is, by CH_2). Many other compounds can be formed by adding successive carbon and hydrogen atoms. This series is sometimes called the *paraffin series* because paraffin (familiar to us as used in sealing jars of preserves and jellies) consists of a mixture of the higher members of the series. Large quantities of the paraffins are found in nature. *Petroleum* consists of a mixture of them, and distillation of petroleum yields many useful products.

The lower members of the series are gases and are found in *natural gas*, which many communities burn for cooking and heating purposes. As the carbon chains become progressively longer, liquid compounds are found. *Gasoline* boils between 40° C and 150° C and consists chiefly of a mixture of paraffins containing 6, 7, and 8 carbon atoms per molecule. *Kerosene, mineral oil* (liquid petrolatum), and *lubricating oils* are mixtures of hydrocarbons with somewhat higher boiling points. Higher hydrocarbons are found in *solid petrolatum* and in *paraffin*. Highly volatile gasoline, called *petroleum ether*, is useful as a solvent for fats.

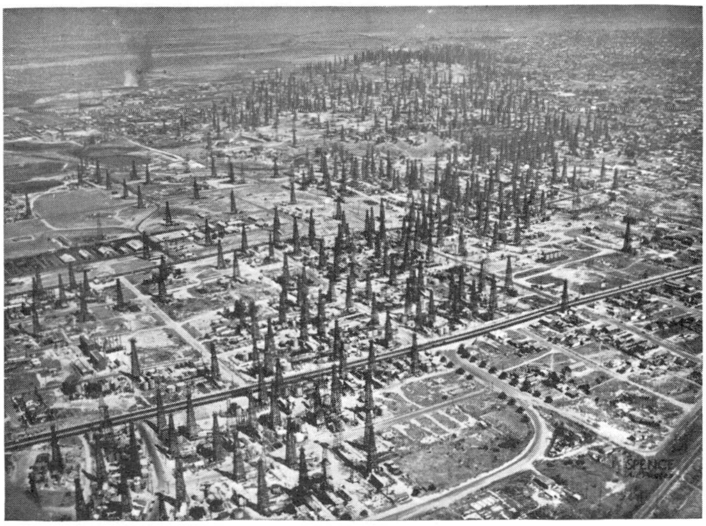

Fig. 17-1. Signal Hill oil field in southern California. The location of the derricks indicates the size of the field; the number of derricks indicates the enormous quantity of oil that must have collected in the underground pool, although a few wells uniformly distributed over the field would help conserve the nation's oil supply by producing a much larger yield at lower production costs. What is petroleum? (Courtesy Spence Air Photos.)

Methane is called *firedamp* by coal miners because it is sometimes liberated during the process of mining coal. It is formed by the decomposition of plants that occurs in marshes and is also called *marsh gas*. The "ghost fires" of such marshes are usually burning methane. The bacteria of the lower intestinal tract form it (as well as hydrogen and small amounts of carbon dioxide) from undigested carbohydrate. Some years ago a group of scientists found that methane and hydrogen in sufficient quantity to keep a small flame burning day and night was thus formed in the intestinal tract of a single cow!

NOMENCLATURE. A meeting of organic chemists was held in Geneva, Switzerland, in 1892 for the purpose of devising a uniform system of naming organic compounds. The system devised was modified and simplified somewhat by the International Union of Chemistry, which met at Liège, Belgium, in 1930. According to this latter system (the IUC system) a compound is named as a derivative of the hydrocarbon corresponding to the *longest continuous carbon chain*. Where there is branching of the carbon chain, the name is modified according to the kind and position of the groups attached to the longest continuous carbon chain. The chain is numbered from the end nearest the branching, and the positions of the alkyl (aliphatic) or other groups attached are indicated by numbers. Just as a house number indicates the relative location of the house in the block, so the numbers in the IUC system indicate the positions of the groups attached to the carbon chain. To illustrate how the system works the formulas and names of the isomers of hexane, C_6H_{14}, are given on page 141. The small n- stands for normal; that is, the form of hexane that exists as a straight, unbranched chain of carbon atoms. Note the names of organic radicals given in Table 17-1.

The student should avoid the error of placing a carbon below the end carbon in

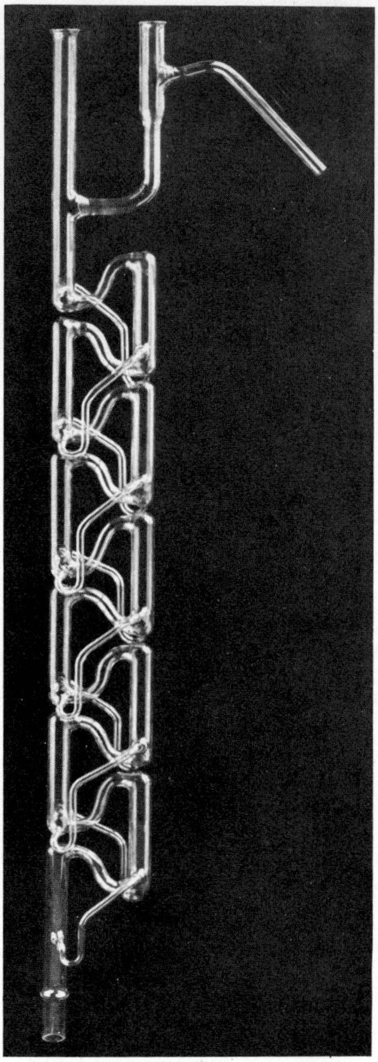

Fig. 17-2. A distilling column. Columns of this type are used in separating volatile compounds that have different boiling points, such as the components of paraffin hydrocarbon mixtures. The mixture is heated, and the vapors are allowed to pass up the distilling column. The less volatile components collect near the bottom of the column, and the most volatile, near the top. Could such a column be used to separate gasoline from kerosene? (Courtesy Eastman Kodak Company Research Laboratories.)

a horizontal chain in the belief that this represents a branch. It should be borne in mind that the representation of a compound on a flat surface such as a sheet of paper is inadequate, since molecules actually possess three dimensions in space. Even though the carbon atoms usually are written in a straight line, it must not be thought that the bonds between the atoms are like rigid steel wires. Rather, they should be thought of as similar to rubber bands that may be bent in various directions at will, still leaving the carbon atoms in a continuous chain.

Table 17-1. Physical constants of paraffin hydrocarbons

Molecular formula	**Name**	**Melting point °C**	**Boiling point °C**	**Name of alkyl radical**	**Formula of alkyl radical**
CH_4	Methane	−184.0	−161.5	Methyl	CH_3—
C_2H_6	Ethane	−172.0	− 88.3	Ethyl	C_2H_5—
C_3H_8	Propane	−189.9	− 44.5	Propyl	C_3H_7—
C_4H_{10}	Butane	−135.0	0.6	Butyl	C_4H_9—
C_5H_{12}	Pentane	−131.5	36.2	Pentyl (Amyl)	C_5H_{11}—
C_6H_{14}	Hexane	− 94.2	69.0	Hexyl	C_6H_{13}—
C_7H_{16}	Heptane	− 90.0	98.4	Heptyl	C_6H_{13}—
C_8H_{18}	Octane	− 56.5	124.6	Octyl	C_8H_{17}—
C_9H_{20}	Nonane	− 51.0	150.6	Nonyl	C_9H_{19}—
$C_{10}H_{22}$	Decane	− 32.0	174.0	Decyl	$C_{10}H_{21}$—
$C_{11}H_{24}$	Undecane	− 26.5	19.5	Undecyl	$C_{11}H_{23}$—
$C_{12}H_{26}$	Dodecane	− 12.0	214.5	Dodecyl	$C_{12}H_{25}$—
$C_{13}H_{28}$	Tridecane	− 6.2	234.0	Tridecyl	$C_{13}H_{27}$—
$C_{14}H_{30}$	Tetradecane	5.5	252.5	Tetradecyl	$C_{14}H_{29}$—
$C_{15}H_{32}$	Pentadecane	10.0	270.5	Pentadecyl	$C_{15}H_{31}$—
$C_{16}H_{34}$	Hexadecane	20.0	287.5	Hexadecyl	$C_{16}H_{33}$—
$C_{17}H_{36}$	Heptadecane	22.5	303.0	Heptadecyl	$C_{17}H_{35}$—
$C_{18}H_{38}$	Octadecane	28.0	317.0	Octadecyl	$C_{18}H_{37}$—
$C_{19}H_{40}$	Nonadecane	32.0	330.0	Nonadecyl	$C_{19}H_{39}$—
$C_{20}H_{42}$	Eicosane	38.0	—	Eicosyl	$C_{20}H_{41}$—

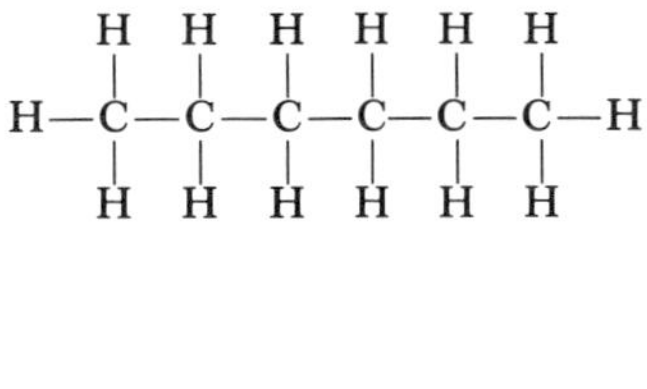

n-Hexane

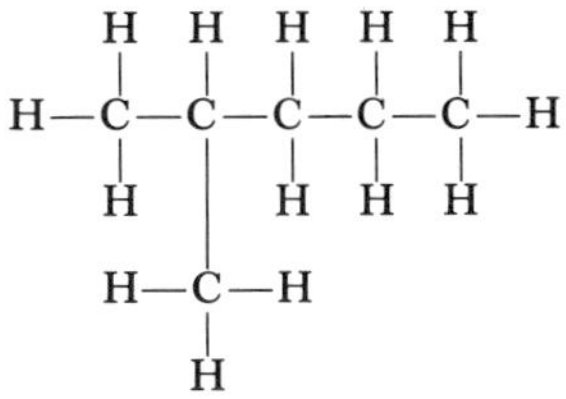

2-Methylpentane

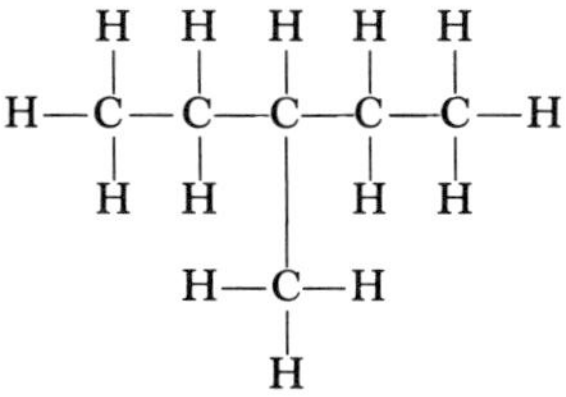

3-Methylpentane

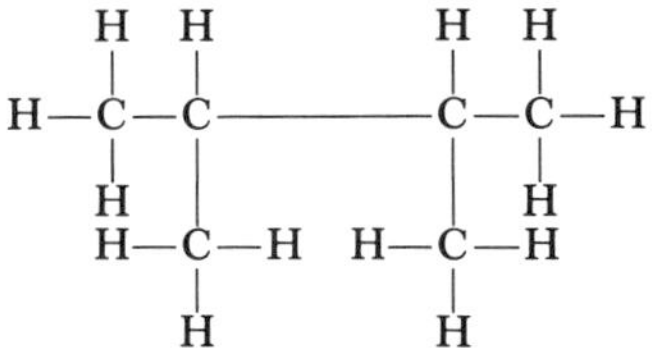

2,3-Dimethylbutane

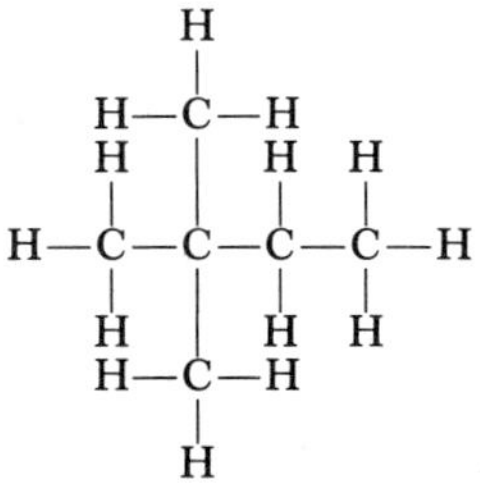

2,2′-Dimethylbutane

Another error often made by the unintiated is in assuming that the following formulas represent two isomers:

These really are formulas of the same compound; the one-carbon side chain is attached to the first carbon from the end of the longest continuous chain in both cases; they are only two ways of representing the same thing.

UNSATURATED ALIPHATIC HYDROCARBONS

Unsaturated aliphatic hydrocarbons contain double or triple bonds between carbon atoms and are more active chemically than the saturated compounds. The two members of this series that are of most interest in medicine are the gases ethylene and acetylene. *Ethylene* has been used, particularly in the United States, as an anesthetic. *Acetylene* also has anesthetic properties and is preferred by some European surgeons. When acetylene is burned in the presence of oxygen, intense heat is produced. Oxyacetylene torches are used in cutting and welding metals. Even sheet steel can be cut this way.

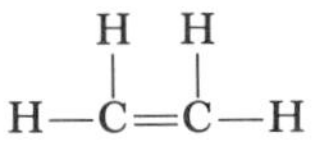

C_2H_4
Ethylene

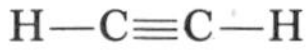

C_2H_2
Acetylene

Natural rubber apparently consists of huge molecules formed by the union of many molecules of the unsaturated hydrocarbon *isoprene*.

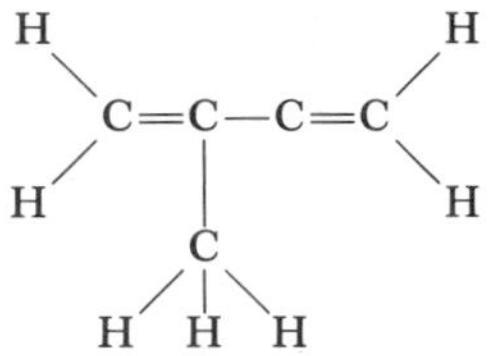

Isoprene

Chemical substances related to isoprene are used widely in the manufacture of rubberlike materials often incorrectly referred to as synthetic rubber.

REACTION OF HYDROCARBONS WITH OXYGEN

All hydrocarbons readily combine with oxygen, carbon dioxide and water being formed by the reaction. Methane burns so readily that a mixture of this substance with oxygen is explosive in the presence of an open flame.

$$CH_4 + 2\,O_2 \rightarrow CO_2 + 2\,H_2O$$

Gasoline also explodes when mixed with air, and the force of this explosion is used as a source of power in gasoline motors. If the reaction is incomplete, carbon monoxide (CO) is formed. This gas combines with hemoglobin, the red protein of the blood that carries oxygen from the lungs to the tissues. In carbon monoxide poisoning, then, the tissues cannot obtain a sufficient supply of oxygen, and abnormal reactions often leading to death or injury to the nervous system take place. Automobile exhaust gas and many illuminating gases are poisonous because they contain carbon monoxide.

$$2\,CH_3CH_2CH_2CH_2CH_2CH_3 + 13\,O_2 \rightarrow 12\,CO + 14\,H_2O$$

Hexane, found in gasoline

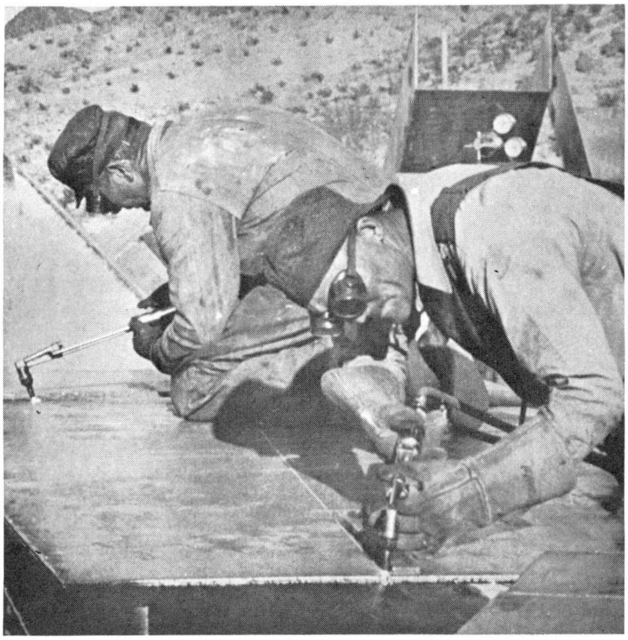

Fig. 17-3. Heavy steel plates being cut with the oxyacetylene cutting torch at the site where they are to be used. The heat liberated by the combustion of the acetylene melts the steel, and a jet of oxygen rapidly converts the molten iron to iron oxide that flies away as sparks. Write an equation illustrating the burning of acetylene. (Courtesy Linde Air Products Co.)

The reaction of organic compounds with oxygen is of special interest, inasmuch as many such compounds combine with oxygen in the tissues with the production of caron dioxide, water, and energy.

REACTION OF HYDROCARBONS WITH HALOGENS

The word halogen means "salt former." The four elements fluorine, chlorine, bromine, and iodine have similar chemical properties, and all combine with hydrogen to form salts. These elements are called *halogens*.

Halogen derivatives of the hydrocarbons are formed when one or more of the hydrogen atoms of hydrocarbon molecules is replaced by halogen atoms.

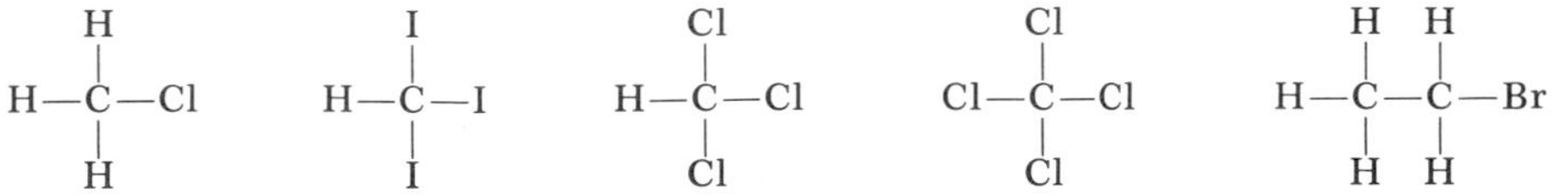

CH_3Cl	CHI_3	$CHCl_3$	CCl_4	CH_3CH_2Br
Methyl chloride	Iodoform	Chloroform	Carbon tetrachloride	Ethyl bromide

Methyl chloride, CH_3Cl, and *ethyl chloride*, CH_3CH_2Cl, are gases at room temperature. When placed in glass containers under pressure they liquefy. By releasing this pressure a spray of methyl chloride or ethyl chloride gas can be directed against the skin. This spray evaporates rapidly and freezes the area of skin. Since the nerves in the skin are not sensitive at freezing temperatures, this is a method of producing local anesthesia for minor surgical procedures, such as lancing boils.

Iodoform, CHI_3, is a yellow solid having a characteristic odor. It is slightly antiseptic and is often used in treating wounds and ulcers. Its antiseptic properties appear to be from the slow liberation of iodine as iodoform decomposes in the tissues. When ethyl alcohol (grain alcohol) is mixed with iodine in the presence of an alkali, iodoform is formed. This is a common test for grain alcohol.

Chloroform, $CHCl_3$, is an oily liquid. It is colorless and volatile and has a characteristic odor. Chloroform is used as a general anesthetic in surgery and obstetrics. It sometimes poisons the heart muscle and the liver and is not used as much now as it was formerly. It has the decided advantage, however, of being *noninflammable* and so can be used in the presence of an open flame. Chloroform is also used as a solvent for fats and fatlike substances.

Carbon tetrachloride, CCl_4, is a colorless, heavy liquid that does not burn. It is an excellent solvent for fats and grease and is used extensively in dry cleaning. It is given internally to stupefy hookworms, which can then be washed out of the intestinal tract by means of a saline cathartic such as magnesium sulfate (Epsom salt). Carbon tetrachloride is also used in some types of the fire extinguishers (see page 45).

Halothane (trademark: Fluothane) is a colorless, heavy, volatile liquid general anesthetic. It has a sweet odor. One to 3 percent in air is effective. It will not burn and is nonexplosive.

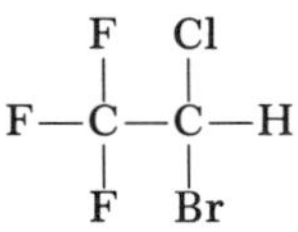

Halothane

HYDROCARBON RADICALS

Hydrocarbon radicals may be thought of as hydrocarbons that have lost 1 or more hydrogen atoms. It will be recalled that inorganic radicals do not exist in a free state but only in chemical union with other radicals or atoms. Organic radicals do not differ in this respect from inorganic ones.

The *methyl radical,* CH_3, occurs in methyl chloride, CH_3Cl, and in methyl alcohol (wood alcohol), CH_3OH. Ethyl alcohol (grain alcohol), CH_3CH_2OH, and ethyl chloride, CH_3CH_2Cl, contain the *ethyl radical,* CH_3CH_2 (also written C_2H_5). *Lead tetraethyl* has the property of making gasoline explode more slowly and completely and is a component of "ethyl gasoline." This type of gasoline should not be used for dry cleaning or solvent purposes, since breathing its vapor over a long period of time may result in lead poisoning.

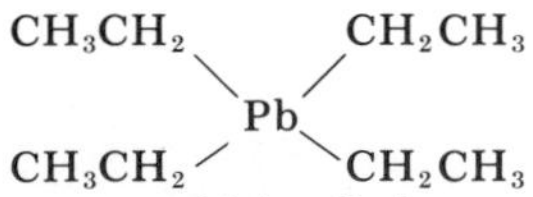

Lead tetraethyl

ALCOHOLS

DEFINITION *Alcohols* are hydrocarbon derivatives in which 1 or more of the hydrogen atoms of the hydrocarbon have been replaced by the OH radical. In other words, they consist of hydrocarbon radicals in combination with OH radicals.

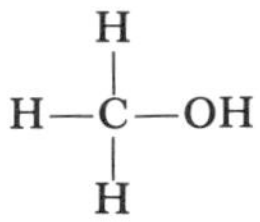

CH_3OH
Methyl alcohol

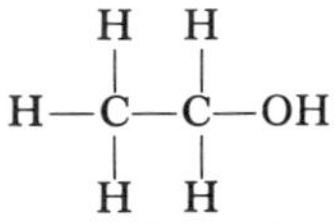

CH_3CH_2OH
Ethyl alcohol

TYPES OF ALCOHOL Alcohols that contain only 1 OH radical per molecule are called *monohydric alcohols*. *Dihydric alcohols* contain 2, and *trihydric alcohols* 3, OH groups in each molecule.

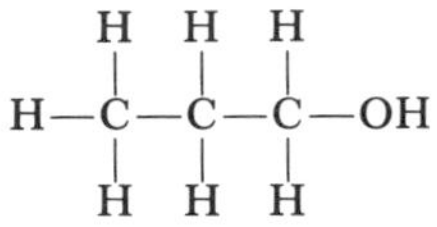

$CH_3CH_2CH_2OH$
Propyl alcohol
(Monohydric)

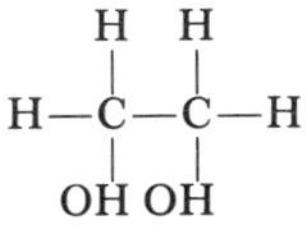

CH_2OHCH_2OH
Glycol
(Dihydric)

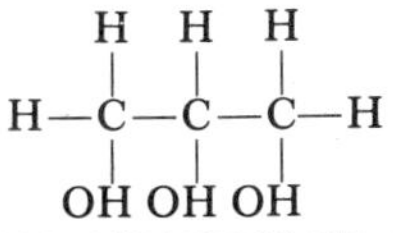

$CH_2OHCHOHCH_2OH$
Glycerol (glycerin)
(Trihydric)

Monohydric alcohols may be further classified as primary, secondary, or tertiary. If the OH is attached to a C atom at the end of a hydrocarbon chain, the compound is a *primary alcohol*. When the C atom to which the OH is attached is connected to 2 other C atoms and to 1 H atom, the compound is a *secondary alcohol*. *Tertiary alcohols* contain OH groups attached to a C atom that is connected to 3 other C atoms.

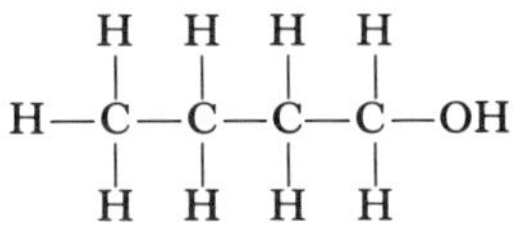

$CH_3CH_2CH_2CH_2OH$
Butyl alcohol
(Primary)

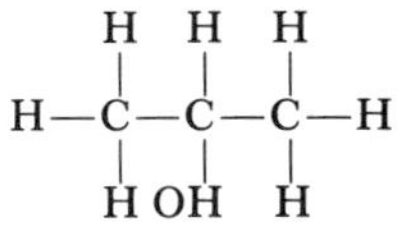

$CH_3CHOHCH_3$
Isopropyl alcohol
(Secondary)

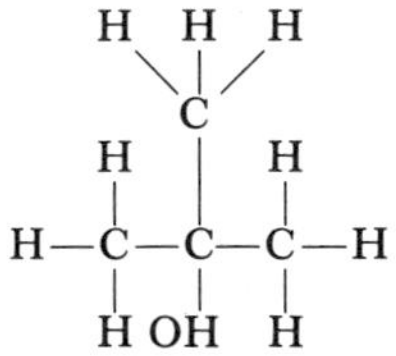

$(CH_3)_3COH$
Trimethylcarbinol
(Tertiary)

COMPARISON OF ALCOHOLS AND INORGANIC HYDROXIDES In general, the reactions that alcohols undergo are similar to those of the inorganic hydroxides. Alcohols do not ionize, however, and their reactions are much slower than inorganic reactions. We can verify the statement that solutions of alcohols do not contain OH^- ions by testing such solutions with litmus paper. No color change of the paper will be observed, in contrast to the blue color produced by solutions of inorganic hydroxides. Alcohols, like inorganic hydroxides, react with acids to form a new compound and water. This new compound is called an *ester*.

NaOH	+	HCl	→	NaCl	+ H_2O
Sodium hydroxide (Inorganic hydroxide)		Hydrochloric acid (Acid)		Sodium chloride (Salt)	Water

$$\underset{\substack{\text{Methyl alcohol}\\ \text{(Alcohol)}}}{CH_3OH} + \underset{\substack{\text{Hydrochloric acid}\\ \text{(Acid)}}}{HCl} \rightarrow \underset{\substack{\text{Methyl chloride}\\ \text{(Ester)}}}{CH_3Cl} + \underset{\text{Water}}{H_2O}$$

REACTIONS WITH OXYGEN

Alcohols burn, with the formation of carbon dioxide and water. This reaction yields a great deal of heat. When 1 g of ethyl alcohol oxidizes completely in the tissues, about 7 large calories (7,000 small calories) of heat are produced.

$$CH_3CH_2OH + 3\ O_2 \rightarrow 2\ CO_2 + 3\ H_2O$$

Many oxidizing agents readily break down to yield oxygen atoms. In the presence of easily oxidized compounds these atoms of oxygen may react before they have time to combine with each other to form oxygen gas (O_2). This kind of oxygen, which is extremely reactive, is called *nascent* oxygen. Primary alcohols react with nascent oxygen (that is, with oxidizing agents) to form *aldehydes*. *Ketones* are formed by the mild oxidation of secondary alcohols.

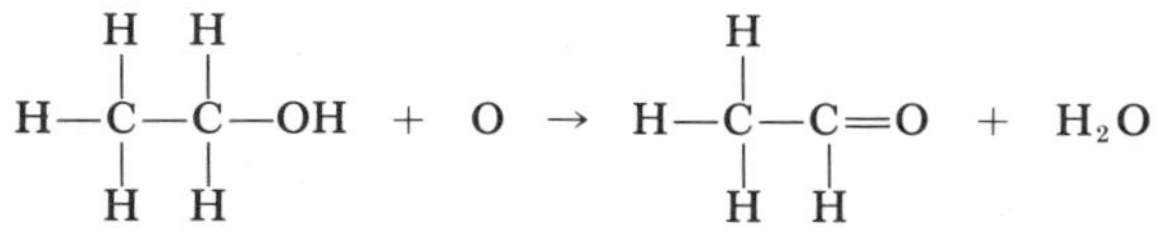

CH_3CH_2OH — Ethyl alcohol (Primary alcohol) → CH_3CHO — Acetaldehyde (Aldehyde)

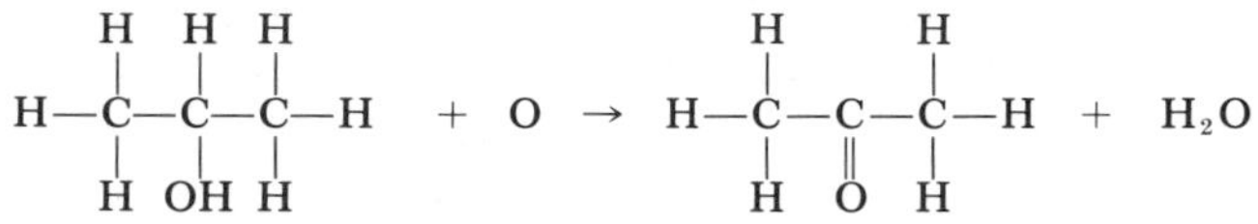

$CH_3CHOHCH_3$ — Isopropyl alcohol (Secondary alcohol) → CH_3COCH_3 — Acetone (Ketone)

Aldehydes and ketones are converted to organic acids by further oxidation, and organic acids can be oxidized to carbon dioxide and water.

SOME IMPORTANT ALCOHOLS

Methyl alcohol, CH_3OH, is also known as *methanol* or wood alcohol. It is a colorless, volatile liquid that mixes with water in all proportions and that burns with a pale blue flame. This substance can be made by the dry distillation of wood. *Methyl alcohol is poisonous when taken internally.* Even mild poisoning may result in blindness, and more profound poisoning causes death. Wright's stain, used to stain blood smears intended for microscopic examination, consists of a dye dissolved in methyl alcohol.

Ethyl alcohol, CH_3CH_2OH, is the ordinary grain alcohol (ethanol) in wines and liquors. (Usually the alcoholic content is designated as "proof" and can be converted to percentage by dividing by 2. Thus "100 proof" would mean 50 percent alcohol by volume.) It is volatile and mixes in all proportions with water. It burns with a yellow flame. Yeast has a mixture of enzymes, *zymase,* that catalyzes the conversion of some sugars to alcohol and carbon dioxide.

$$\underset{\text{Glucose, a sugar}}{C_6H_{12}O_6} \xrightarrow{\text{(Zymase)}} \underset{\text{Ethyl alcohol}}{2\ CH_3CH_2OH} + 2\ CO_2$$

This reaction, known as *fermentation,* is used to manufacture alcohol. A 70 percent solution of ethyl alcohol is used to sterilize the skin for minor procedures, such as the insertion of a needle into a vein. *Rubbing alcohol* contains ethyl alcohol mixed with water and mild poisons that prevent its use as an intoxicating beverage. Alcohol is an excellent solvent for many organic compounds. Much of the alcohol used commercially has been *denatured* by the addition of some poison, such as methyl alcohol or formaldehyde.

Alcohol taken internally in small doses causes an increased secretion of gastric juice and has a mild stimulating action on the intestinal musculature. Weak solutions are sometimes given to patients when samples of gastric juice are to be taken for chemical and microscopic analysis. In larger amounts alcohol is irritating to mucous membranes and produces a gastritis (inflammation of the lining of the stomach). The higher nervous centers are depressed by alcohol, and the so-called "mental stimulation" produced by it is really caused by the depression of some of the normal inhibitions. That is, people under the influence of alcohol often do things

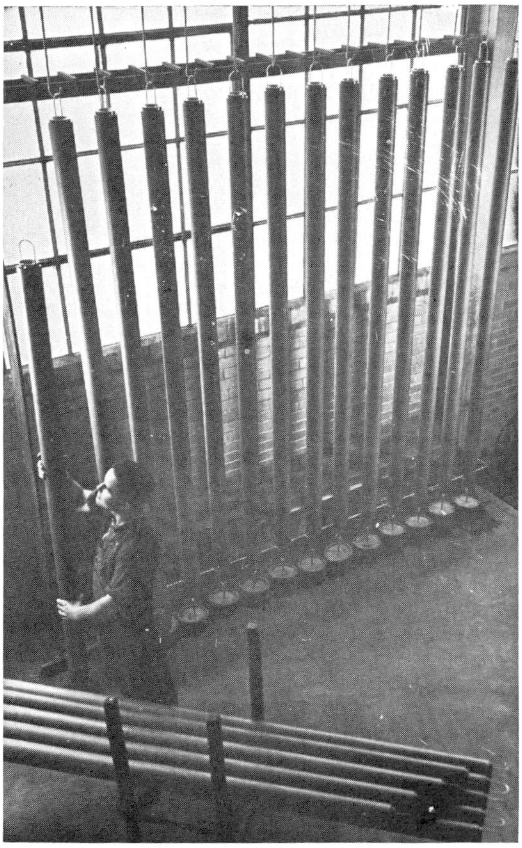

Fig. 17-4. Nitroglycerin in long, laminated Bakelite shells used for shooting oil wells. The force of the explosion breaks the oil-retaining sandstone, thus releasing the oil. The shells made of Bakelite shatter into small particles, thereby minimizing danger to workers and drilling equipment. For what purpose is nitroglycerin used in medicine? (Courtesy Bakelite Corporation.)

and say things that social and psychological inhibitions normally would prevent. Mental processes are slowed so that reactions to situations requiring rapid thought and decision cannot be carried out as quickly as usual. This effect of alcohol explains why intoxication is responsible for many automobile accidents.

The dihydric alcohol *glycol* (CH_2OHCH_2OH) is used industrially as a solvent. It is thought to be toxic when taken internally.

Glycerol, $CH_2OHCHOHCH_2OH$, also known as *glycerin,* is found in chemical combination in all fats and is made commercially by the hydrolysis of fats. This trihydric alcohol was discovered by Scheele, who also discovered oxygen, in 1779. Glycerol is an oily, slippery, colorless liquid, soluble in all proportions in water and alcohol. Some preparations used as drugs contain it as a solvent and preservative. The derivative of it prepared by replacing the OH groups with the nitrate (NO_3) radical is called *nitroglycerin.* Nitroglycerin is an explosive. It is used in medicine in doses of 0.5 to 1 mg as a heart stimulant. It causes a dilation of the coronary arteries and hence an increased supply of blood to the heart muscle. Glycerol is not intoxicating.

ALDEHYDES AND KETONES

DEFINITIONS   Compounds containing the characteristic group $-C\begin{subarray}{l}\diagup O \\ \diagdown H\end{subarray}$ 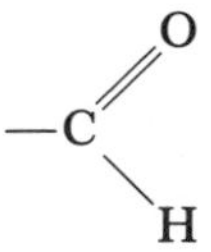 are called *aldehydes;* they may be regarded as hydrocarbon derivatives in which 2 of the H atoms attached to a C at the end of a hydrocarbon chain have been replaced by an O atom. The characteristic group of ketones is $-\underset{\underset{O}{\parallel}}{C}-$ 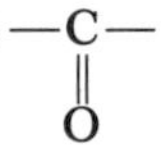; they are formed when the 2 H atoms attached to a C that is *not* at the end of a chain are replaced by O.

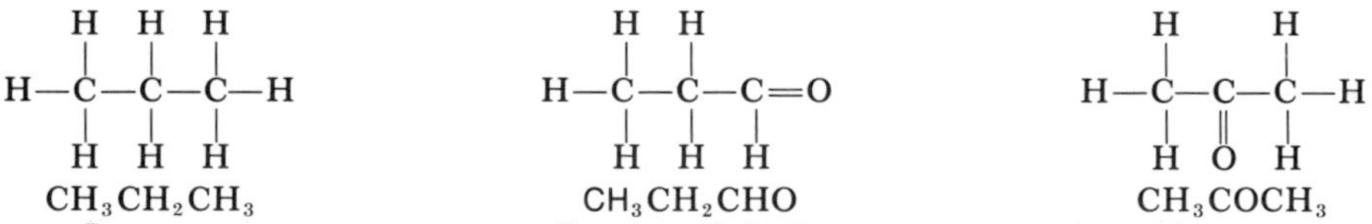

H H H	H H	H H
H—C—C—C—H	H—C—C—C=O	H—C—C—C—H
H H H	H H H	H O H
$CH_3CH_2CH_3$	CH_3CH_2CHO	CH_3COCH_3
Propane	Propionaldehyde	Acetone
(Hydrocarbon)	(Aldehyde)	(Ketone)

REACTIONS   We have already seen that aldehydes are produced by the oxidation of primary alcohols and that ketones result when secondary alcohols are oxidized. Organic acids are formed by the oxidation of aldehydes and ketones.

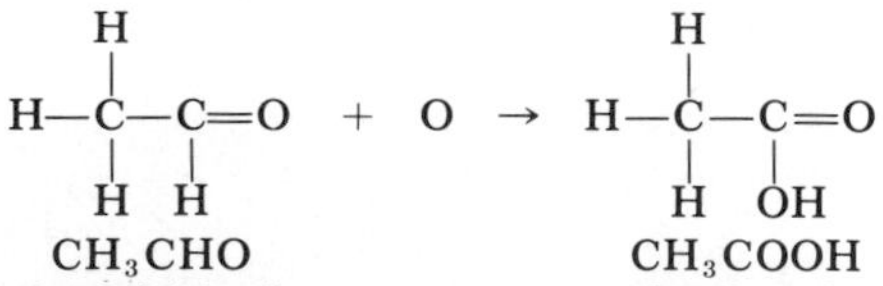

$$\begin{array}{ccc} H & & H \\ | & & | \\ H-C-C=O & +\ O\ \rightarrow & H-C-C=O \\ |\ \ | & & |\ \ \ | \\ H\ \ H & & H\ \ OH \end{array}$$

CH_3CHO CH_3COOH
Acetaldehyde   Acetic acid
(Aldehyde)   (Acid)

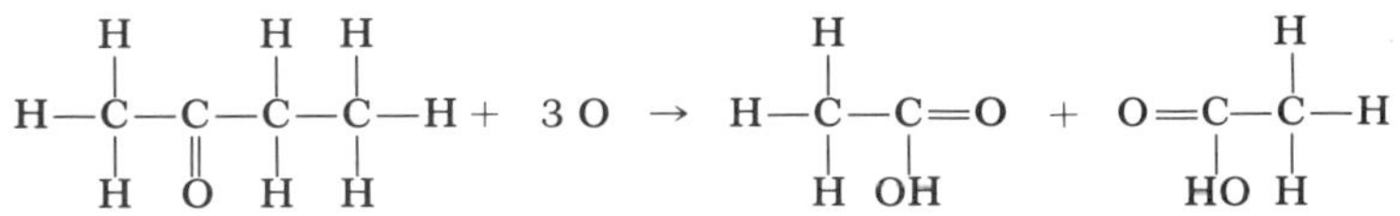

$CH_3COCH_2CH_3$ Methyl ethyl ketone (Ketone) → CH_3COOH Acetic acid (Acid) + CH_3COOH Acetic acid (Acid)

Since aldehydes and ketones are readily oxidized, it follows that they are good *reducing agents*. This property is important in physiologic chemistry because the simple sugars contain either aldehyde or ketone groups. *Benedict's reagent,* which contains cupric ions (Cu^{++}) in solution, is used in testing urine for the presence of sugar (glucose). If sugar is present, the Cu^{++} is reduced to Cu^{+} and insoluble cuprous oxide, Cu_2O, is deposited in the test tube as a brick-red or yellow precipitate.

IMPORTANT ALDEHYDES

Formaldehyde, HCHO, can be prepared by the oxidation of methyl alcohol, CH_3OH.

$$CH_3OH + O \rightarrow HCHO + H_2O$$

Formaldehyde is a gas having a characteristic pungent odor. A 40 percent solution of the gas in water, known as *formalin,* is used as a preservative for tissues and as a disinfectant. Formaldehyde, in common with other aldehydes, exhibits the phenomenon of *polymerization*. That is, molecules of formaldehyde tend to unite with each other to form new molecules, each containing 3 formaldehyde molecules. The substance thus formed, known as *paraformaldehyde* $(HCHO)_3$, is said to be a *polymer* of formaldehyde. Paraformaldehyde yields formaldehyde gas when heated and is used in the form of candles for disinfecting purposes. Some people are sensitive to formaldehyde and should wear rubber gloves when handling formalin in order to prevent a troublesome skin rash. Formalin is poisonous if taken internally.

Acetaldehyde, CH_3CHO, polymerizes to form *paraldehyde,* $(CH_3CHO)_3$, used in medicine as a hypnotic (sleep-producing drug) and sedative (drug that depresses the nervous system). Paraldehyde is colorless; it has a pungent odor and unpleasant taste. It is usually administered by rectum. Its chief disadvantage lies in the fact that it is partly eliminated in the lungs and imparts an unpleasant odor to the breath for some hours after its administration. Another hypnotic made from acetaldehyde is *chloral,* CCl_3CHO. This compound combines with water to form a crystalline solid known as chloral hydrate.

Glucose, the sugar normally found in blood, contains both alcohol and aldehyde groups. Its chemistry and metabolism will be discussed in subsequent chapters.

IMPORTANT KETONES

Acetone, CH_3COCH_3, is widely used as a solvent in industry. This substance is found in traces in normal blood and urine. In certain pathological conditions, such as diabetes mellitus, large amounts of it may be present in the blood, urine, and expired air. *Acetoacetic acid,* CH_3COCH_2COOH, which contains both a ketone (CO) and an acid (COOH) group, also occurs in blood and urine in diabetes mellitus. *Fructose,* a sugar, contains a ketone group in addition to alcohol groups.

ORGANIC ACIDS AND SALTS

DEFINITIONS AND PROPERTIES

Organic acids are compounds formed by replacing one of the hydrogen atoms of a hydrocarbon by the characteristic group 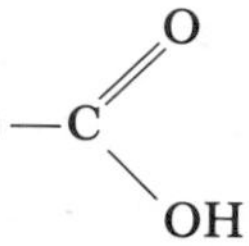 or by forming this group by the oxidation of the terminal carbon atom of an organic compound. This group, often written COOH, is called the *carboxyl group.* The simplest organic acid, formic acid, does not exactly conform to this definition, since it consists merely of a hydrogen atom combined with the carboxyl group (HCOOH).

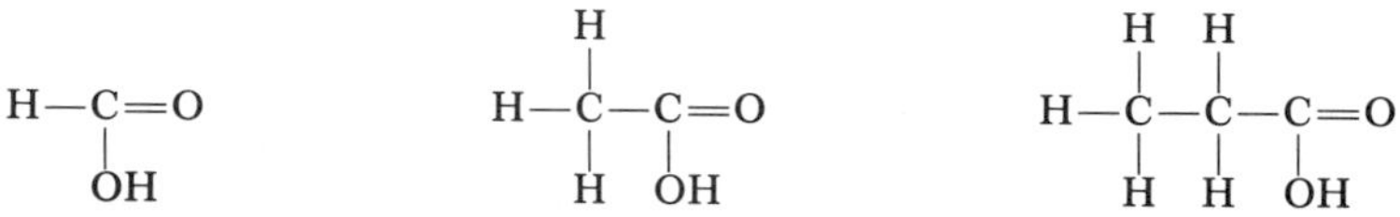

$HCOOH$ Formic acid — CH_3COOH Acetic acid — CH_3CH_2COOH Propionic acid

Organic acids ionize slightly in solution to form hydrogen ions.

$$\underset{\text{Acetic acid}}{CH_3COOH} \rightleftarrows \underset{\text{Acetate ion}}{CH_3COO^-} + \underset{\text{Hydrogen ion}}{H^+}$$

Organic acids are much weaker than inorganic acids, however, and reac-

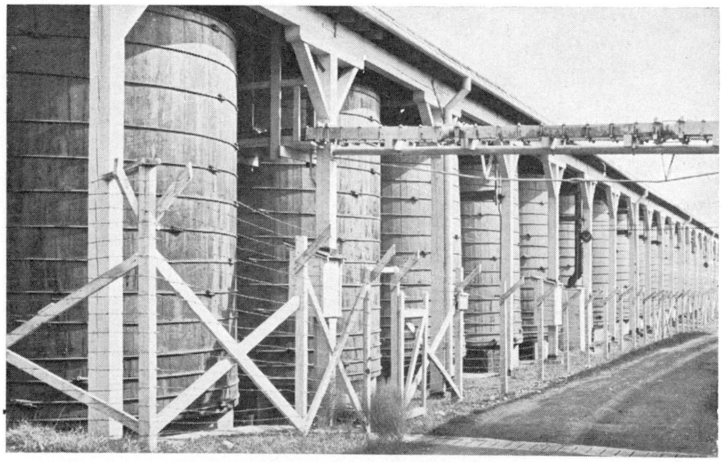

Fig. 17-5. Tanks in which cider vinegar is aged. The apple juice imparts to this type of vinegar characteristic flavors and odors that are not found in vinegars made from ethyl alcohol by the "quick vinegar process." Good cider vinegar is as carefully produced as fine old wine. Why does wine sometimes turn sour when exposed to air? (Courtesy H. J. Heinz Co.)

tions in which they are involved are slower. Only about 1 molecule out of 250 is ionized in a 6-percent solution of acetic acid.

Organic acids react with inorganic bases to produce salts and water; in this respect they resemble inorganic acids.

HCl	+	$NaOH$	→	$NaCl$	+	H_2O
Hydrochloric acid (Inorganic acid)		Sodium hydroxide (Inorganic base)		Sodium chloride (Inorganic salt)		

CH_3COOH	+	$NaOH$	→	CH_3COONa	+	H_2O
Acetic acid (Organic acid)		Sodium hydroxide (Inorganic base)		Sodium acetate (Organic salt)		

Organic acids derived from the aliphatic hydrocarbons are often called *fatty acids* because many of them can be obtained by the hydrolysis of fats. The fatty acids with short carbon chains are liquids that are soluble in water. As the chain becomes longer, the acids become less soluble and possess a rancid odor. When the number of carbon atoms in the chain becomes 10 or more, the acids become solid and odorless. Fatty acids are readily reduced with the formation of aldehydes.

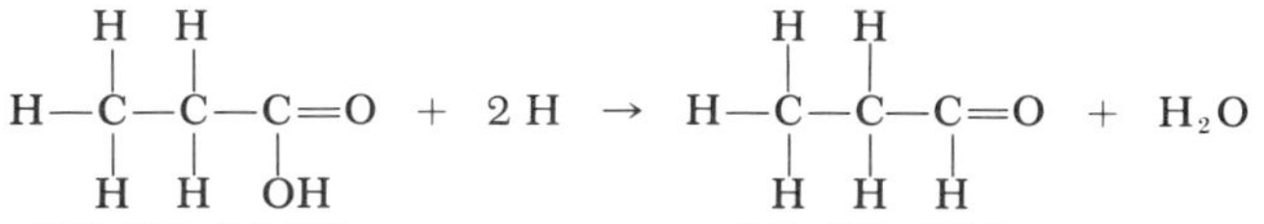

CH_3CH_2COOH Propionic acid → CH_3CH_2CHO Propionaldehyde

In the above equation 2 H, instead of H_2, is written to indicate that the propionic acid has reacted with a reducing agent that furnishes active hydrogen atoms (nascent hydrogen) and not with hydrogen gas.

TYPICAL ORGANIC ACIDS

Formic acid, HCOOH, is said to have been prepared originally by distilling ants (the Latin word for ant is *formica*). It is responsible for the sting accompanying the bite of many insects. It is a colorless liquid and has an irritating odor.

Acetic acid, CH_3COOH, can be prepared by the oxidation of ethyl alcohol (CH_3CH_2OH) or acetaldehyde (CH_3CHO). Wine exposed to air may turn sour as the result of its formation. Vinegar contains 3 to 5 percent acetic acid. The acid is prepared commercially by the distillation of wood. One hundred percent acetic acid is called *glacial acetic acid. Lead acetate,* often called *sugar of lead,* is a poisonous salt used in making white lead paint and is applied externally in the treatment of skin diseases and poison ivy. Dilute *aluminum acetate* solution (Burow's solution) is also used to treat skin diseases.

Lactic acid, $CH_3CHOHCOOH$, is a hydroxy acid; that is, it contains both an alcohol group (OH) and an acid group (COOH). It is formed by the action of certain bacteria on lactose (milk sugar) and is responsible for the taste of sour milk. (The Latin word for milk is *lac.*) This acid is produced in the tissues when muscles contract and is a normal component of the blood.

ESTERS

DEFINITION AND PROPERTIES *Esters* are compounds formed by the reaction between alcohols and acids. They are similar in some ways to salts but, unlike salts, they do not furnish ions in solution.*

$$\underset{\text{(Inorganic hydroxide)}}{NaOH} + \underset{\text{(Inorganic acid)}}{HCl} \rightarrow \underset{\text{(Inorganic salt)}}{NaCl} + H_2O$$

$$\underset{\text{(Inorganic hydroxide)}}{NaOH} + \underset{\text{(Organic acid)}}{CH_3COOH} \rightarrow \underset{\text{(Organic salt)}}{CH_3COONa} + H_2O$$

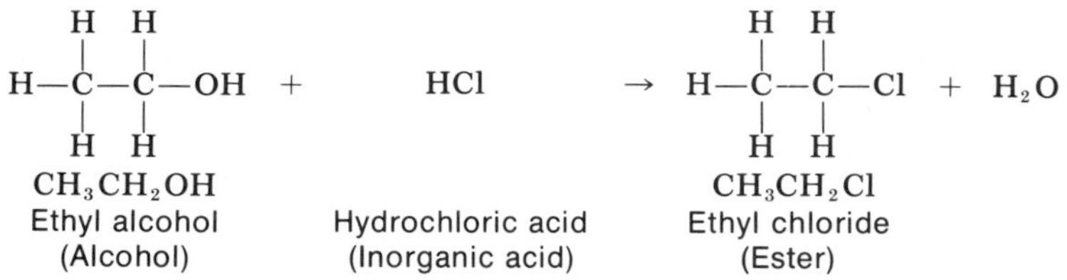

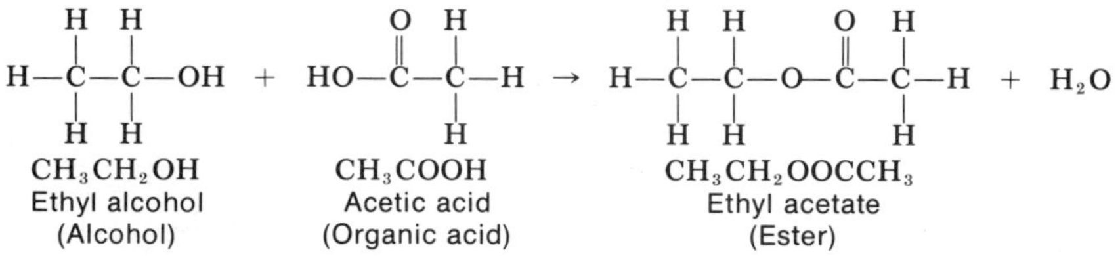

Most esters are colorless liquids that are only slightly soluble in water. Many of them have pleasant, fruity odors and are used in manufacturing synthetic (artificial) flavors. Isoamyl isovalerate has the flavor of apples; ethyl butyrate, of pineapples; isoamyl acetate, of pears; octyl acetate, of oranges; amyl acetate, of bananas; and amyl butyrate, of apricots.

IMPORTANT ESTERS *Ethyl acetate* is used externally in the treatment of parasitic skin diseases. *Methyl salicylate* is responsible for the odor of oil of wintergreen and is an ingredient of many liniments and of analgesic (pain-relieving) balms. *Phenyl salicylate,* also known as *salol,* occasionally is used as an enteric coating for pills, that is, as a coating that will not dissolve in the acid gastric juice and that, therefore, does not dissolve until the pill reaches the intestinal tract. *Benzyl benzoate* depresses the activity of smooth muscle and formerly was used to relieve the smooth muscle spasms that cause dysmenorrhea (painful menstruation) and asthma. It is used also for the treatment of scabies. *Acetylsalicylic acid* (aspirin) is an ester also containing a COOH group. It is used to relieve pain. *Glyceryl trinitrate* (nitroglycerin) dilates the coronary arteries supplying the heart muscle and lowers blood pressure. It is used in treating coronary heart disease. An alcoholic solution of *ethyl nitrite,* also known as spirit of ethyl nitrite and as sweet

*When one molecule of an alcohol reacts with a molecule of an organic acid, one of the hydrogen atoms in the molecule of water that is formed by the reaction comes from the alcohol and the OH radical in the water molecule comes from the acid.

spirit of niter, is a diuretic (increases the flow of urine). We have already learned that *ethyl chloride* and *methyl chloride* are anesthetics. *Procaine* is an ester that is used as a local anesthetic.

We shall see later that *fats* are esters. They yield glycerol (an alcohol) and fatty acids on hydrolysis.

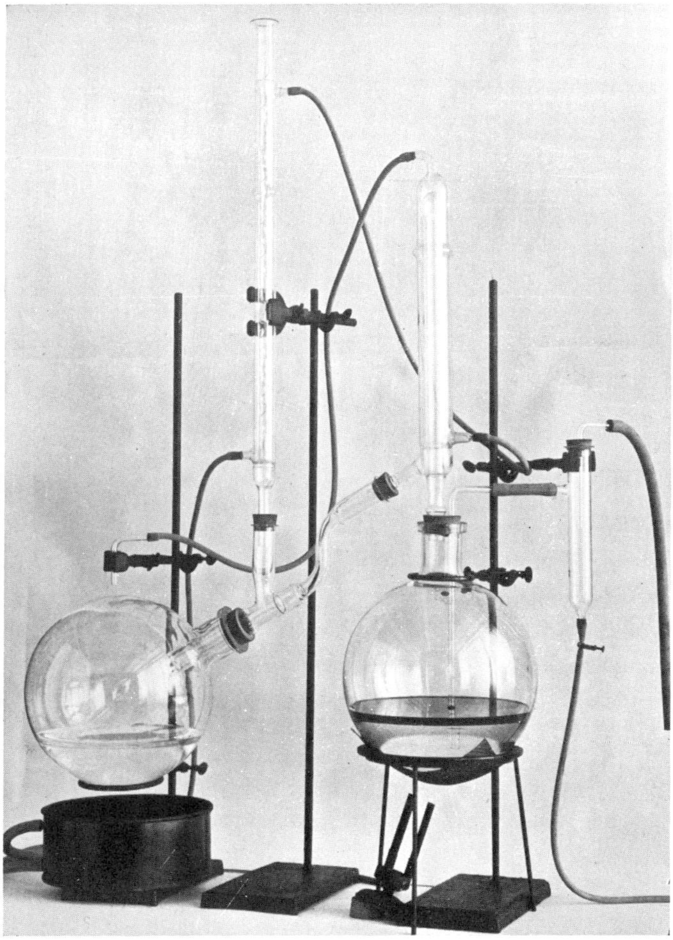

Fig. 17-6. Compact apparatus for steam distillation. Volatile compounds with boiling points higher than that of water can often be separated from impurities by allowing steam to pass through a mixture of the organic compounds and boiling water. The steam carries the volatile compound along with it and thus separates it from the impurities. In the apparatus shown above steam enters through the rubber tube at the far right. The flask on the right contains the impure organic compound; the two upright condensers cause the hot vapors to cool and condense; the flask at the left collects the distillate. Notice that the impure organic mixture floating on the water in the flask on the right is dark in color; the purified organic liquid floating on the surface of the water in the flask on the left has a much lighter color. Esters often can be purified in this way. How do you know that many esters are volatile? (Courtesy Eastman Kodak Company Research Laboratories.)

ETHERS

Ethers may be compared in structure to the inorganic oxides. They are compounds in which 2 hydrocarbon radicals are linked together by means of an oxygen atom.

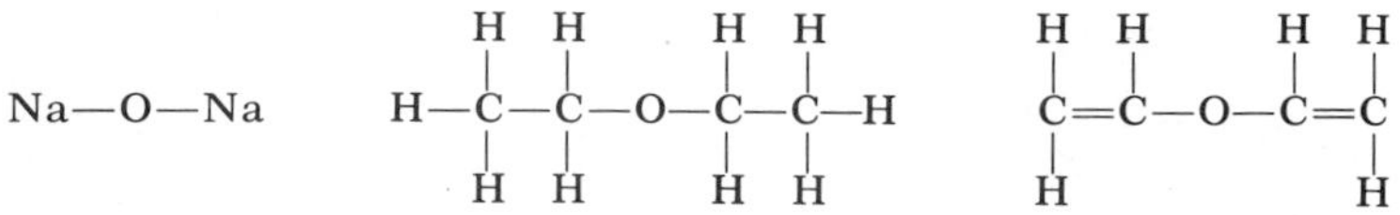

Na_2O — Sodium oxide (Oxide)

$CH_3CH_2OCH_2CH_3$ or $(C_2H_5)_2O$ — Diethyl ether (Ether)

$CH_2CHOCHCH_2$ or $(CH_2CH)_2O$ — Divinyl ether (Ether)

Diethyl ether is the common "ether" used as an anesthetic. It is prepared by the reaction between ethyl alcohol and sulfuric acid. Ethylsulfuric acid, an ester, is formed by this reaction. The addition of excess ethyl alcohol then converts ethylsulfuric acid to diethyl ether and sulfuric acid.

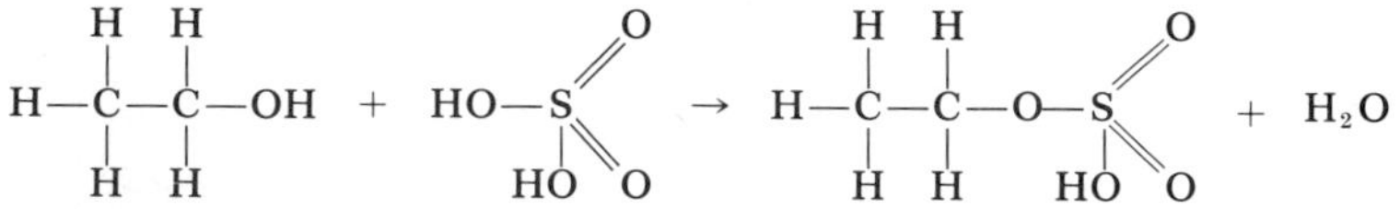

CH_3CH_2OH Ethyl alcohol + H_2SO_4 Sulfuric acid → $CH_3CH_2OSO_3H$ Ethylsulfuric acid + H_2O

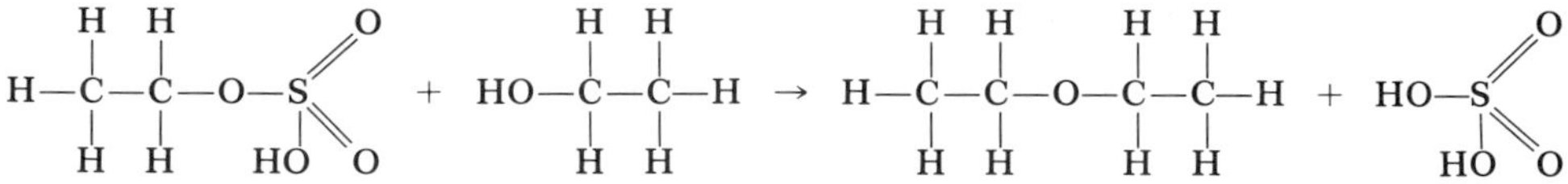

$CH_3CH_2OSO_3H$ Ethylsulfuric acid + CH_3CH_2OH Ethyl alcohol → $CH_3CH_2OCH_2CH_3$ Diethyl ether + H_2SO_4 Sulfuric acid

Since the sulfuric acid required to initiate the reaction is released again at the end, only a relatively small amount of this substance is required.

Diethyl ether is, in some respects at least, the most satisfactory anesthetic. It is easy to administer; it causes excellent muscular relaxation; there is less danger of an overdose than with most other anesthetics; and it does not alter the pulse rate, the rate of respiration, or the blood pressure very much. It has certain disadvantages, however, which explains its gradual decline in popularity in recent years. These disadvantages are: (1) it is irritating to the mucous membrane of the respiratory passage; (2) there is some danger of postoperative pneumonia; (3) nausea is a usual postoperative symptom; (4) it causes the accumulation of harmful acids in the blood if administered over a long period of time; and (5) there is some slight damage to the liver and kidneys.

Divinyl ether is another anesthetic that, like diethyl ether, can be administered by dropping it on a gauze cone or piece of gauze held over the patient's nose and mouth. Both diethyl ether and divinyl ether are highly volatile liquids. Ethers form explosive mixtures with air, and flames or sparks must be carefully avoided in the operating room.

Methoxyflurane (trademark: Penthrane) is used as an inhalant general anesthetic. It is not flammable or explosive at room temperature. It is a liquid with a boiling point of 105° C. A concentration of 0.5 to 1.5 percent in air is used.

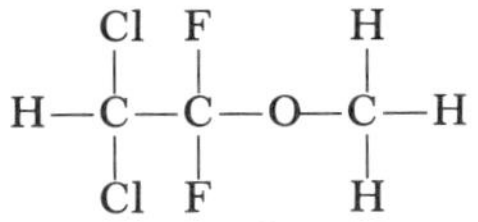

Methoxyflurane

Fluroxene (trademark: Fluomar) is an inhalant general anesthetic. It is a clear, colorless, volatile liquid with a mild ethereal odor. It is flammable.

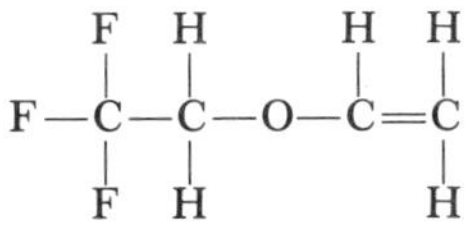

Fluroxene

AMINES

Amines are organic compounds containing the characteristic *amino* 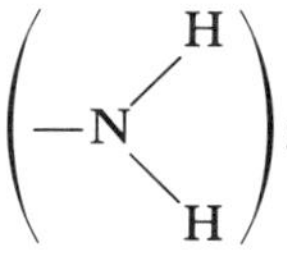 group. They may equally well be regarded as derivatives of ammonia, NH_3, in which 1 or more of the hydrogen atoms of ammonia has been replaced by an organic radical.

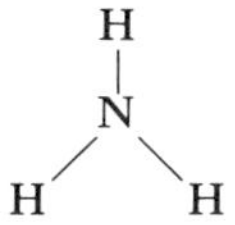

NH_3
Ammonia

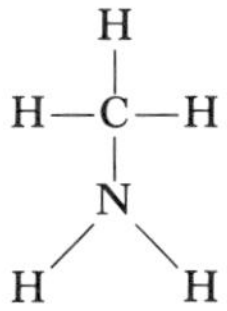

CH_3NH_2
Methyl amine

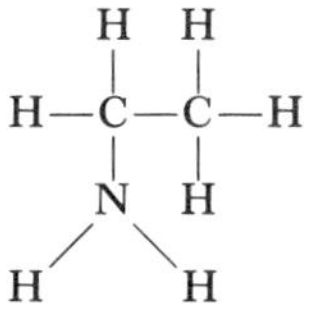

$CH_3CH_2NH_2$
Ethyl amine

Amines, like ammonia, react with inorganic acids and, in this respect, act like bases.*

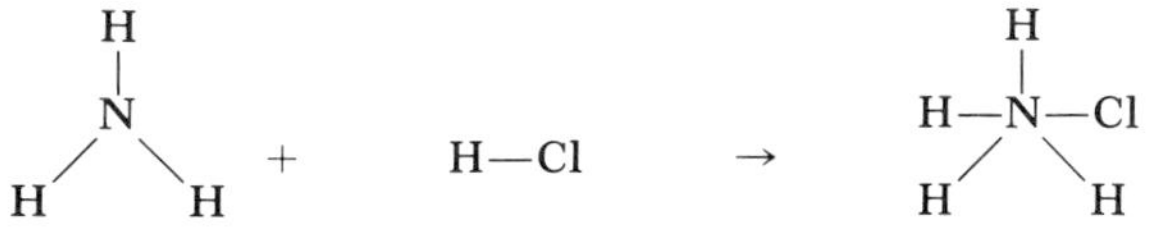

NH_3	HCl	NH_4Cl
Ammonia	Hydrochloric acid	Ammonium chloride

*See discussion of coordinate covalence, page 91.

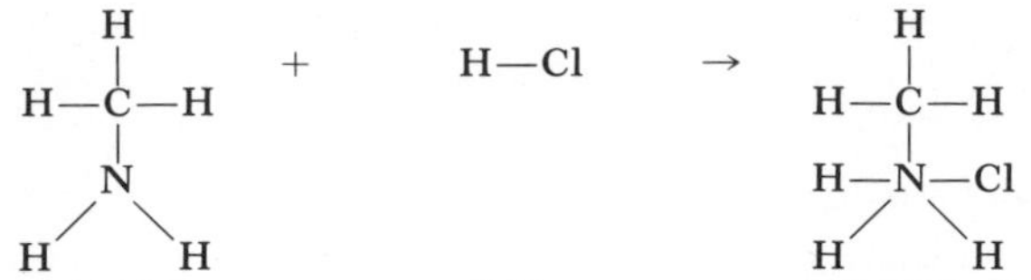

CH_3NH_2 Methyl amine | HCl Hydrochloric acid | CH_3NH_3Cl Methyl amine hydrochloride

When 2 of the 3 hydrogen atoms of ammonia are replaced by organic radicals, the compound is called a *secondary amine*. *Tertiary amines* contain 3 organic radicals attached to nitrogen.

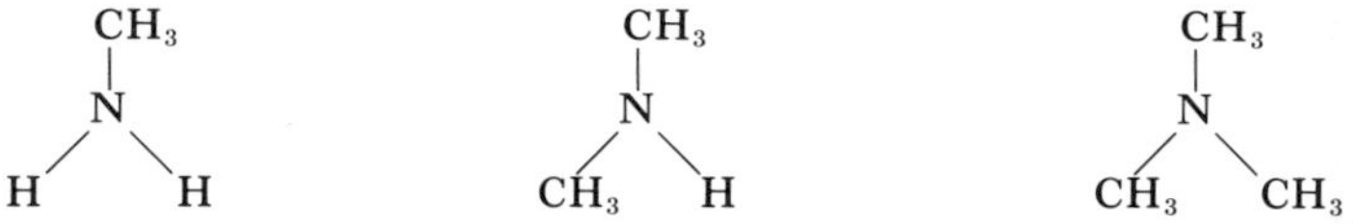

Methyl amine (Primary) | Dimethyl amine (Secondary) | Trimethyl amine (Tertiary)

Amino acids are compounds containing both an amino (NH_2) group and an acid (COOH) group. The proteins are composed of such compounds linked chemically together to form huge molecules. The COOH group of amino acids can react with bases, and the NH_2 group will react with acids. Compounds that can thus act either as acids or as bases are called *amphoteric* compounds.

Amines formed by the bacterial decomposition of protein-containing foods are called *ptomaines*. Spoiled foods contain such substances; they may be formed sometimes in the intestinal tract. Ptomaines cause a marked fall in blood pressure and death if they are injected directly into the bloodstream, but when they are placed in the intestinal tract, they enter the bloodstream, are taken directly to the liver, which causes them to be so changed chemically that they become relatively harmless, and are then eliminated from the body in the urine. In view of these facts it appears probable that true *ptomaine poisoning* does not exist. So-called "ptomaine poisoning" is usually caused by eating foods contaminated with pathogenic (harmful) bacteria or with toxic substances produced in the cells of such bacteria.

Quaternary ammonium compounds are formed by the reaction of an excess of alkyl (aliphatic) halide with a tertiary amine.

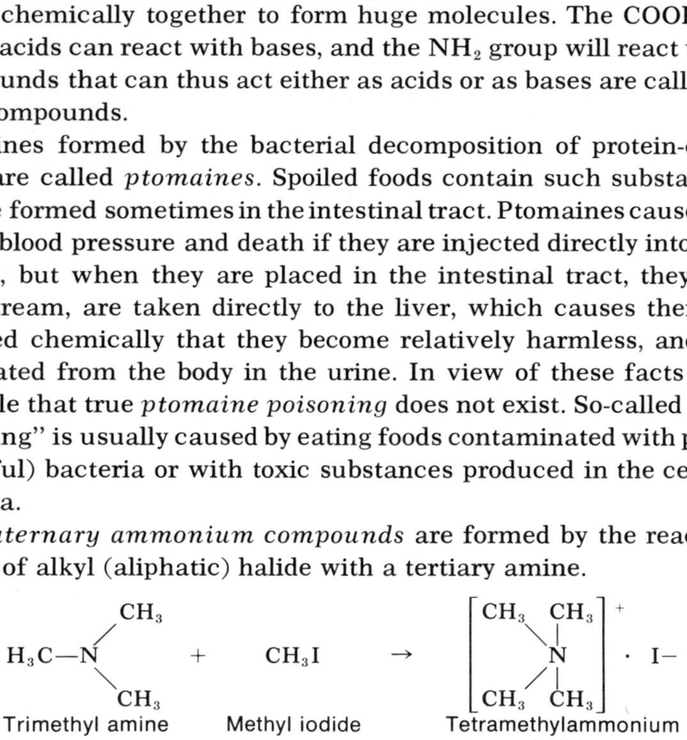

Trimethyl amine | Methyl iodide | Tetramethylammonium iodide

As the method of writing the formula illustrates, quaternary compounds exist as electrically charged ions held together by electrostatic forces. It will be helpful in understanding this structure if the discussion of coordinate covalence on page 91 is reviewed.

Many drugs used in medicine are quaternary ammonium compounds. They include antiseptics, antispasmodics, agents to lower blood pressure, local anesthetics, and agents useful in liquefying thick, ropy fluids in body cavities and in wounds.

CHELATES

A chelate* is a complex formed by the binding of a metal ion by an organic molecule to form a heterocyclic ring structure. The metal is bound by 2 or more ions within the organic molecule, which is called a *ligand*. Some of the atoms of the ligand "donate" electrons to the metal atom and "share" electron pairs with the metal ion (see covalence, page 90).

The properties of a chelate differ from those of the metal and the ligand. Optical activity (see Chapter 18), stability, color, chemical reactivity, catalytic properties, and solubility are some of the properties that change as a result of chelation.

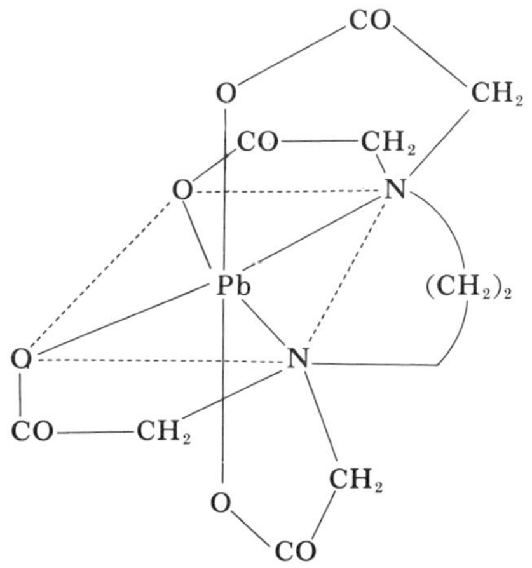

Three-dimensional formula of the lead chelate of EDTA

Ethylenediaminetetraacetic acid (EDTA) is a chelating agent that has been used widely in medicine. In most cases its sodium salt, or a salt of both sodium and calcium, has been employed.

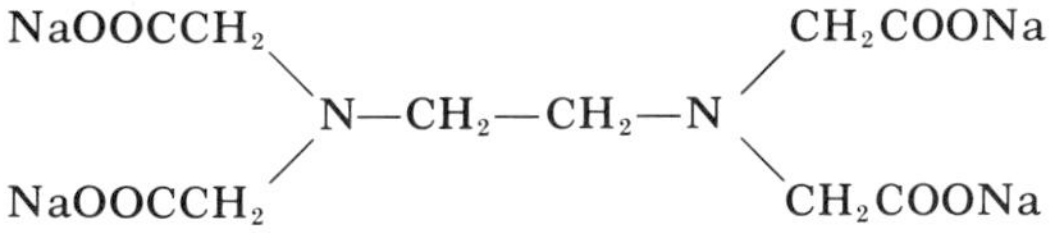

EDTA tetra sodium salt

This agent forms chelates with several metals that make it useful as a therapeutic agent.

When EDTA is injected into the body, it forms a chelate with calcium and is excreted as the calcium chelate, thus removing calcium from the body. This is desirable in emergency situations such as hyperparathyroid-

*The word chelate is derived from the Greek word *chele*, which refers to the claw of a lobster. The term describes the pincerlike binding of metal ions by a ligand (the "lobster").

ism (see page 397), bone metastases (cancer), and hypervitaminosis D (see page 441).

When EDTA is used to rid the body of undesirable metals, it is injected as the calcium disodium salt in order to avoid depleting the body of calcium. It is used in the treatment of poisoning by lead, arsenic, chromium, manganese, nickel, and radioactive metals such as plutonium.

Another chelating agent that is used in the treatment of poisoning by arsenic and mercury is British anti-lewisite* (BAL).

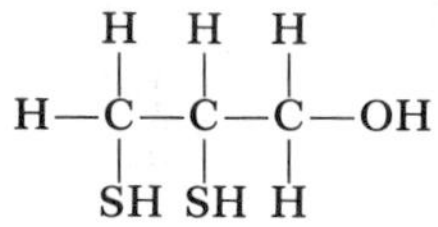

BAL (2,3-Dimercapto-1-propanol)

Penicillamine is a chelating agent that is employed to remove excess copper from the body. It is used principally to treat patients with the rare disorders known as Wilson's disease (see pages 289–342) and cystinuria.

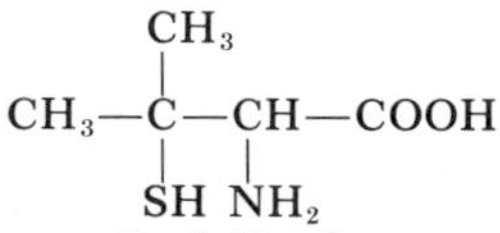

Penicillamine

*This compound derives its name from the fact that it was synthesized by British chemists during World War II to counter the effects (irritation of the skin and lungs) of a war gas known as lewisite.

STUDY QUESTIONS

1. What is the characteristic group of each of the following types of organic compound: alcohol, aldehyde, ketone, acid, ether, amine?
2. Draw structural formulas for each of the following compounds and state what type of compound each is: $CH_3CHOHCH_3$; CH_3CHO; $CH_3CH_2CH_3$; CH_3COOH; CH_3COCH_3; CH_3OOCCH_3; CH_3OCH_3; CH_3OH; $CH_2OHCHOHCH_3$; $CH_3CH_2NH_2$; CH_3CH_2Br.
3. Define chelate. Name one used in medicine. For what is it used?
4. What are paraffins? Name some products obtained from petroleum.
5. Give two other names for methane. From what type of food do bacteria make methane in the intestinal tract?
6. Name two unsaturated aliphatic hydrocarbon gases used as anesthetics. Is there any other use for either of them?
7. What are the products formed by burning hydrocarbons?
8. Why is carbon monoxide a poisonous gas?
9. What is a halogen? Name the four halogens. Name two halogen hydrocarbon derivatives used as local anesthetics.
10. What is iodoform? Why is it antiseptic?
11. Describe a common test for grain alcohol.
12. Discuss the advantages and disadvantages of chloroform and diethyl ether as anesthetics.
13. What are the uses of carbon tetrachloride?
14. What are hydrocarbon radicals? Name two of them.
15. Why is it dangerous to use "ethyl gasoline" for dry cleaning?
16. List the different types of alcohol. What characteristic group is common to all of them?
17. What is nascent oxygen? Nascent hydrogen?
18. How could you distinguish between methyl alcohol and ethyl alcohol if you had no apparatus except two beakers and a match?
19. How much heat is liberated when a gram of alcohol is burned in the tissues?
20. Give two other names for methyl alcohol. Why is it dangerous to drink methyl alcohol?

21. How is ethyl alcohol manufactured? What is zymase? Give some of the uses for alcohol.
22. Is alcohol a stimulating substance when taken by mouth? Discuss your answer.
23. What is glycerol? Nitroglycerin?
24. What is produced by the oxidation of a primary alcohol? Of a secondary alcohol? Of an aldehyde? Of a ketone? Of an organic acid?
25. What is produced by the reduction of an organic acid? Of an aldehyde?
26. Are aldehydes oxidizing or reducing agents? What test is sometimes used in testing urine for the presence of sugar?
27. Name some aldehydes and ketones and state why they are important in medicine.
28. Write an equation illustrating the formation of an organic salt.
29. Do organic acids ionize in solution? Are they weaker or stronger than inorganic acids?
30. What are fatty acids? What is glacial acetic acid?
31. Name some organic acids and salts and state why they are important in medicine.
32. Name some esters used in medicine and describe their uses.
33. What two ethers are used as anesthetics? Why is it a rule in many operating rooms that electric switches cannot be turned on or off while an anesthetic is being administered?
34. How is diethyl ether made? Why is it not a perfect anesthetic?
35. Amines are said to be basic even though they do not contain OH ions in combination. How do you explain this?
36. Define and give an example for each of the 3 types of amine.
37. What are ptomaines? What is "ptomaine poisoning"?
38. Define quaternary ammonium compound.

CHAPTER **18**

Isomerism of organic compounds

The hydrocarbon known as butane has the molecular formula C_4H_{10}. If we attempt to draw the structural formula for C_4H_{10}, we discover that two different arrangements of the atoms are possible.

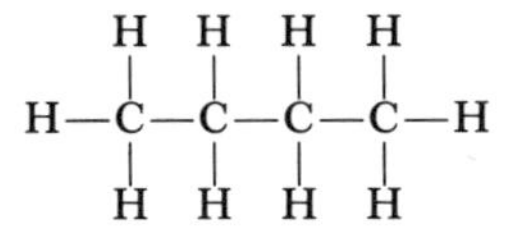

Normal butane (or Butane)

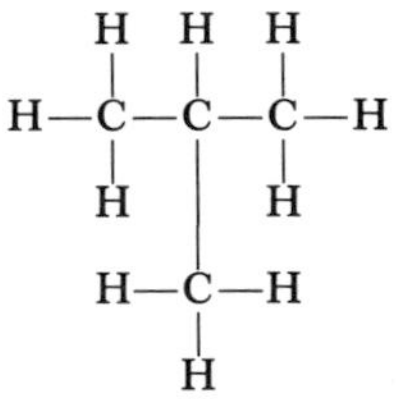

Isobutane

This phenomenon of two or more compounds having the same molecular formula but possessing different physical and chemical properties is known as isomerism (see page 131). The compounds themselves are known as *isomers*. The necessity for having available some means of distinguishing between isomers emphasizes the importance of the structural formulas, which show the spatial relationship of the carbon atoms as well as the mode of linkage of the various atoms in the molecule. The existence of isomers is somewhat analogous to the fact that with a given amount of mortar and a given number of bricks many different types of house can be built.

CHAIN OR NUCLEAR ISOMERISM

The type of isomerism illustrated by butane is known as *chain* or *nuclear* isomerism because the differences occur in the linkages in the carbon chain. As the number of carbon atoms in a compound increases, the number of isomers increases at a rapid rate. For example, the aliphatic hydrocarbon having 6 carbon atoms has 5 isomers, and there are 75 compounds having the molecular formula $C_{10}H_{22}$.

GEOMETRIC OR CIS-TRANS ISOMERISM

This type of isomerism can be illustrated by the acids, maleic and fumaric.

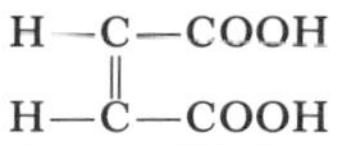

Maleic acid (Cis isomer)

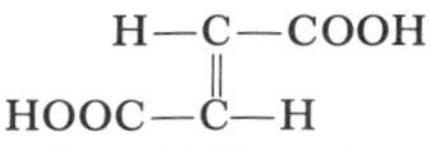

Fumaric acid (Trans isomer)

In order to understand more fully the reason for geometric isomerism let us suppose that we represent the carbon atom as a tetrahedron. Each of the 4 points of the tetrahedron represents one of the 4 valences of carbon. Two carbon atoms united by a single bond can be represented by tetrahedra joined through 1 corner of each tetrahedron. In this arrangement free rotation can be assumed to take place around an axis through the point of attachment of the 2 tetrahedra. This arrangement for ethane, C_2H_6, is illustrated in Fig. 18-1.

In order to represent the union of 2 carbon atoms by a double bond it is necessary to join the tetrahedra at 2 corners, that is, join them along an edge. When the carbon atoms are combined in this manner, the possibility of free rotation or spin is lost.

Fig. 18-1, *II* and *III*, shows that the carboxyl (—COOH) groups of maleic acid are closer to each other in space than are the carboxyl groups of fumaric acid. Since there is no possibility of free rotation, the positions of the carboxyl groups are fixed; this explains the existence of isomeric compounds with different chemical and physical characteristics.

In geometric isomerism the isomer having the 2 groups under considera-

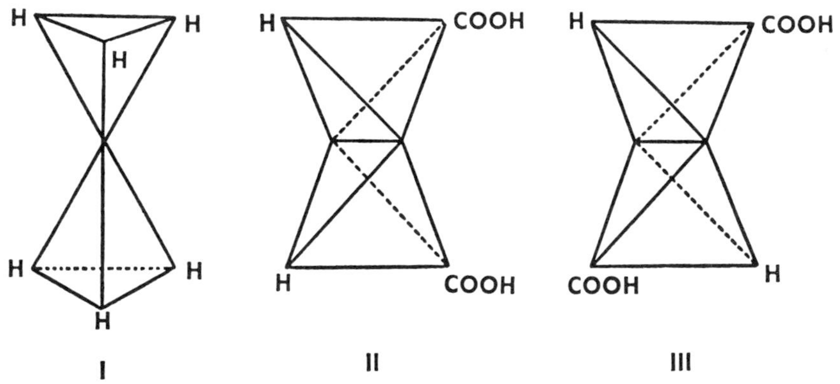

Fig. 18-1. I, Tetrahedral formula for ethane, showing possibility of free rotation of the carbon atoms. **II,** Maleic acid. The presence of the double bond, indicated by the union of tetrahedrons along an edge, prevents free rotation of the carbon atoms and gives rise to geometric isomerism. Maleic acid is the isomer that forms an anhydride because the carboxyl groups are nearer to each other in space than they are in fumaric acid. **III,** Fumaric acid, the trans isomer, does not form an anhydride because the carboxyl groups are too far removed from each other in space. How does geometric isomerism differ from chain isomerism?

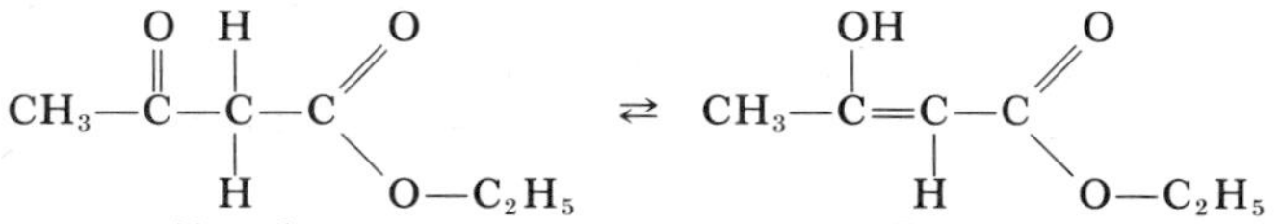

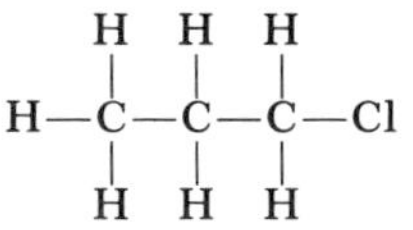

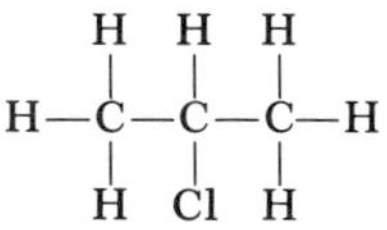

tion (the carboxyl groups in this instance) on the same side of the plane established by the double bond is known as the *cis* form. In the *trans* isomer these groups are on opposite sides, or across the plane of the double bond from each other.

A convenient aid in recalling the relative positions of the groups in the 2 isomers is to remember that the Latin prefix *trans* means *across*. This prefix occurs in such common words as transcontinental (across the continent) and transport (carry across).

This type of isomerism can be illustrated by the compound known as acetoacetic ester or, more properly, ethyl acetoacetate, $CH_3COCH_2COOC_2H_5$. The chemical properties of this compound puzzled chemists for years and were the subject of many investigations. As would be expected from the formula given above, the compound undergoes reactions indicating the presence of a ketone ($-CO$) group. In addition, however, it gives reactions characteristic of a hydroxyl ($-OH$) group.

No one formula that would explain satisfactorily these 2 types of reaction could be written, and the explanation that ethyl acetoacetate existed simultaneously in 2 forms was proposed. Later researches proved this to be true. One of the hydrogen atoms of the methylene group ($-CH_2-$) can shift to the carbonyl group, giving a hydroxyl group, and at the same time forming a double bond.

$$CH_3-\overset{\overset{\displaystyle O}{\|}}{C}-\overset{\overset{\displaystyle H}{|}}{\underset{\underset{\displaystyle H}{|}}{C}}-C\overset{\displaystyle O}{\underset{\displaystyle O-C_2H_5}{\diagup}} \quad \rightleftarrows \quad CH_3-\overset{\overset{\displaystyle OH}{|}}{C}=\overset{}{\underset{\underset{\displaystyle H}{|}}{C}}-C\overset{\displaystyle O}{\underset{\displaystyle O-C_2H_5}{\diagup}}$$

Keto form   Enol form

Careful experimental work has demonstrated that at room temperature ethyl acetoacetate consists of an equilibrium mixture containing about 8 percent of the hydroxyl (enol) form and 92 percent of the keto form. If a reagent that reacts with one form is added, more of this form will be regenerated by intramolecular rearrangement, which maintains the equilibrium condition.

This type of isomerism in which a compound passes back and forth from one structural form to another is known as *tautomerism* or *dynamic isomerism*.

In this type of isomerism the difference between the isomers is solely due to a difference in the position of an atom or group in the molecule.

$$H-\overset{\overset{\displaystyle H}{|}}{\underset{\underset{\displaystyle H}{|}}{C}}-\overset{\overset{\displaystyle H}{|}}{\underset{\underset{\displaystyle H}{|}}{C}}-\overset{\overset{\displaystyle H}{|}}{\underset{\underset{\displaystyle H}{|}}{C}}-Cl \qquad\qquad H-\overset{\overset{\displaystyle H}{|}}{\underset{\underset{\displaystyle H}{|}}{C}}-\overset{\overset{\displaystyle H}{|}}{\underset{\underset{\displaystyle Cl}{|}}{C}}-\overset{\overset{\displaystyle H}{|}}{\underset{\underset{\displaystyle H}{|}}{C}}-H$$

Normal propyl chloride   Isopropyl chloride
(n-Propyl chloride)   or
or   2-Chloropropane
1-Chloropropane

The only difference between the 2 propyl chlorides is the position of the chlorine atom in the molecule. These 2 compounds have different physical properties even though they have the same molecular formula.

OPTICAL ISOMERISM

This type of isomerism is well illustrated by lactic acid, a hydroxy acid.

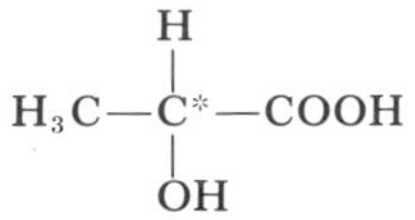

Lactic acid

The carbon atom marked with an asterisk will be seen to have 4 *different* groups or atoms attached to it. This type of carbon atom is designated as an asymmetric carbon atom. In other words, *an asymmetric carbon atom is defined as one whose valences are satisfied by 4 different kinds of atoms or groups.*

We can appreciate best the significance of an asymmetric carbon atom in a molecule if we return to the concept of the carbon atom situated at the center of a regular tetrahedron with the valences directed toward the corners. From purely geometric considerations if we represent the 4 differ-

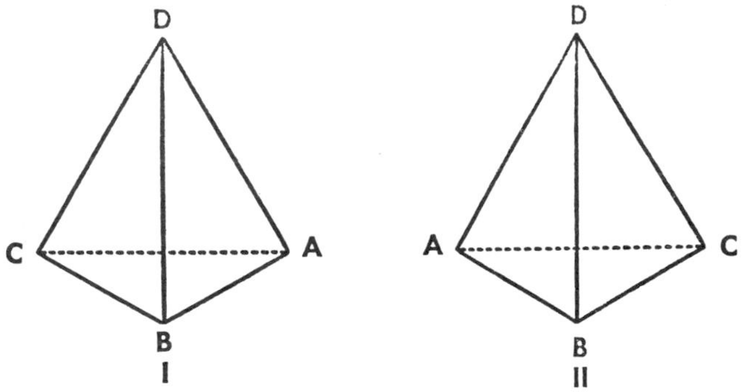

Fig. 18-2. Spatial arrangement of groups in optical isomers. Models **I** and **II** are mirror images of each other, and if 3-dimensional models are constructed, it is easily demonstrated that they cannot be superimposed. What is an asymmetric carbon atom?

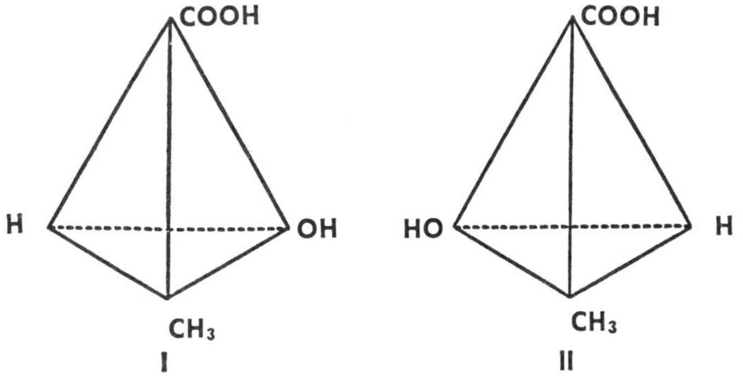

Fig. 18-3. Optical isomers of lactic acid. How would examination of the formula for lactic acid allow you to predict that it is an optically active compound?

ent groups by A, B, C, and D, then there are 2, and only 2, possible spatial arrangements that cannot be superimposed. These arrangements are represented by *I* and *II* in Fig. 18-2.

The 2 arrangements, or forms (if actual compounds are being considered), bear the same relationship to each other as a right hand to a left hand. If models are used, it will be seen that the 2 forms cannot be superimposed. Right and left hands can be placed together palm to palm and they will coincide, but one cannot be superimposed on the other and made to coincide. A similar situation exists in the case of the 2 compounds. The 2 forms are said to be *mirror images* of each other, since the image in a mirror of either form has the structure of the other one. The spatial relationship of the groups in the 2 forms of lactic acid are represented by *I* and *II* in Fig. 18-3.

The formulas for the optical isomers of lactic acid that are commonly encountered really are modifications of the projections of the three-dimensional figures on a flat surface. The conventional formulas of the 2 forms of lactic acid are:

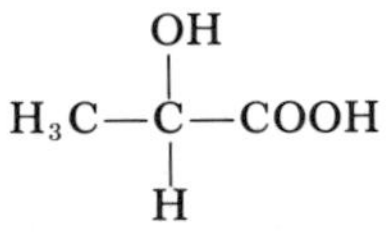

(I)

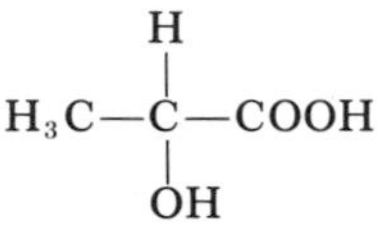

(II)

At this point it is necessary to explain what is meant by polarized light. Ordinary light is a form of energy propagated in the form of waves that are vibrating in all planes at right angles to the direction of propagation. If ordinary light is passed through a crystal of calcium carbonate ($CaCO_3$), only 2 beams are transmitted. Each of these is vibrating in a plane perpendicular to the plane of vibration of the other. A Nicol prism is composed of 2 sections of crystalline calcium carbonate (calcite) so cut and cemented together that one of the beams is refracted to the side. Consequently *the light that passes through it is vibrating in only one plane*. Such light is said to be polarized or, since all of its vibrations are in one plane, often it is termed *plane polarized light*.

The polarizing action of a Nicol prism can be demonstrated easily by holding 2 such prisms between a source of light and the eye. When the axes of the prisms are in line, or parallel, the source of light is visible, but when the axes of the prisms are at right angles the intersection of the 2 prisms is opaque. This is represented diagrammatically in Fig. 18-4.

The magnitude of rotation of plane polarized light by an optically active substance is measured in an instrument known as a polarimeter (Fig. 18-5). The essential parts of the polarimeter are shown in Fig. 18-6.

L is a source of light. Monochromatic light (light of one wavelength), is required for accurate polarimetric measurements and can be obtained by passing light through a filter made of a special kind of glass that transmits light of only one wavelength. The source of light also can be an asbestos gauze saturated with sodium chloride and heated with a Bunsen burner. The sodium flame thus obtained gives practically monochromatic light.

F is a glass light filter such as is used in the polarimeter illustrated in Fig. 18-5.

C is a condensing lens to concentrate the light on the polarizing prism.

P is a fixed Nicol prism for polarizing the light.

T is the sample tube in which the solution of optically active material is placed.

A is a movable Nicol prism known as the analyzer.

S is the scale that indicates the amount of rotation of the analyzer.

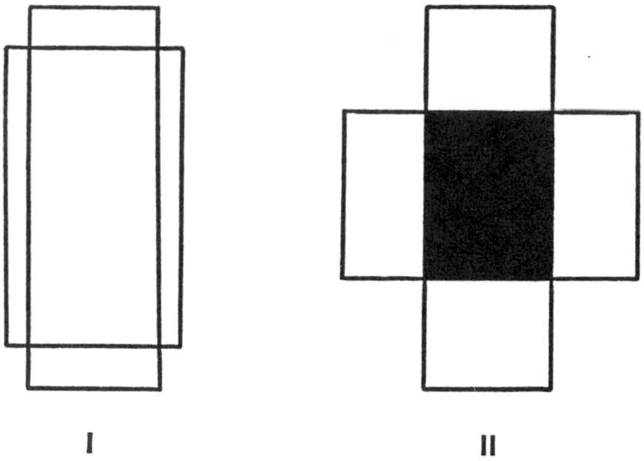

Fig. 18-4. Polarizing action on light of Nicol prisms. In position I the prisms are parallel, and light passes through both prisms. In position **II** the prisms are at right angles, and light polarized by the first prism is screened out by the second. What is the chemical composition of a nicol prism?

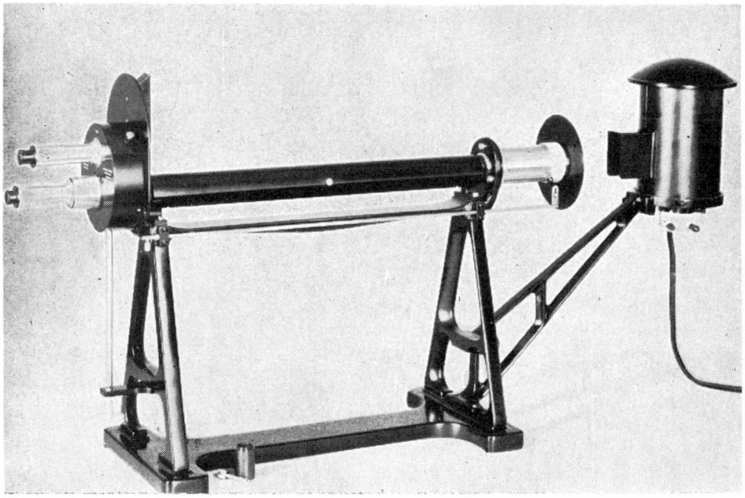

Fig. 18-5. Polarimeter used for the accurate measurement of the rotation of polarized light by optically active substances. For what purpose is this instrument used? (Courtesy Bausch & Lomb Optical Co.)

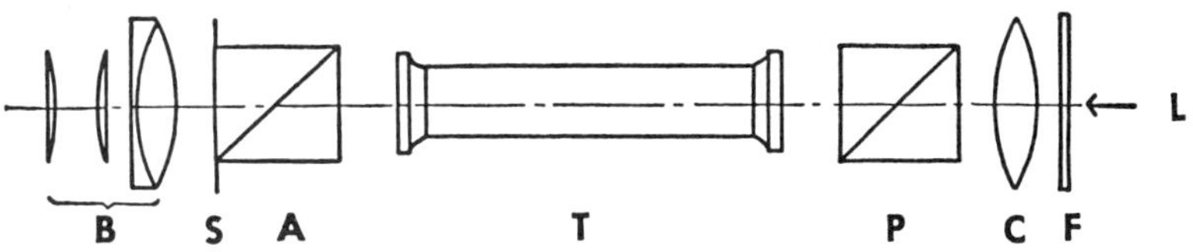

Fig. 18-6. Diagram of the essential parts of a polarimeter. Explain how the polarimeter works.

B represents a system of condensing lenses in the eyepiece for focusing on the field produced by the light passing through the analyzer. In addition there is a similar set of lenses (not shown) in the upper telescope (Fig. 18-5) to magnify the small divisions of the scale, thus enabling an accurate reading of the degrees of rotation.

To increase the accuracy of the instrument a small auxiliary Nicol prism often is placed at a slight angle to the polarizer. In this case the field of view in the eyepiece is divided into two halves. If the analyzer is set at an angle of 90 degrees to the plane of vibration, one-half of the field will be dark. When a solution of optically active substance is placed in the sample tube the dark half will become lighter, and the division between the two halves will be indistinct. The analyzer is turned then until the original condition, obtained with only water in the sample tube, is restored. The amount of this rotation is read from the scale.

The amount of rotation is dependent on several factors: (1) temperature, (2) wavelength of light used, (3) concentration of the optically active substance in solution, and (4) length of the tube containing the solution. The formula for expressing the specific optical rotation of a compound (at some constant temperature) is as follows:

$$[\alpha]_D = \frac{100\ a}{1\ c}$$

$[\alpha]$ = specific optical rotation
D = the bright yellow line of the sodium spectrum
a = observed rotation in angular degrees
1 = length of tube in decimeters (1 decimeter = 10 cm)
c = concentration in g per 100 ml of solution

One form of lactic acid is found to rotate plane polarized light to the right and is known as the dextro (sometimes abbreviated D or +) form. The other form of lactic acid rotates the plane of polarized light exactly the same amount to the left and is known as the levo (sometimes abbreviated L or −) form. Compounds such as these 2 forms of lactic acid, which differ from each other only in their effect on plane polarized light, are known as *optical isomers, optical antipodes*, or *enantiomorphic forms*. Substances that rotate the plane of polarized light are said to be optically active, or to possess optical activity.

Dextrolactic acid, also called sarcolactic acid, occurs naturally in the muscles and other tissues. The levorotatory form is obtained when sugar is fermented by certain bacteria.

A mixture of equal parts of the dextro and levo isomers has no effect on polarized light. The tendency of the levo form to rotate the light to the left is neutralized by the effect of the dextro form to rotate the light to the right. Such a mixture is known as a *racemic mixture*.

Lactic acid synthesized in the laboratory by the usual chemical procedures is a racemic mixture (optically inactive). This is a result of the operation of the law of probability. Billions of molecules are involved, and the probability of forming the levo form is just as great as is the probability of forming the dextro form.

Optically active compounds related spatially to L-lactic acid are designated by the prefix L-, even though in some cases they rotate polarized light to the right. In this case the actual direction of rotation is indicated by a + (right) or − (left) sign. For example, the form of the amino acid glutamic acid (see page 364) that occurs in the body is L + glutamic acid. This means that this form of glutamic acid is related spatially to L-lactic acid, although it rotates plane polarized light to the right.

SUMMARY

The various types of isomerism discussed thus far can be summarized as follows:

1. *Chain or nuclear isomerism.* Involves branching of the carbon chain, as in the isomeric butanes.

2. *Position isomerism.* Due to the position of a particular group in the molecule, as in 1-chloropropane and 2-chloropropane.

3. *Tautomerism or dynamic isomerism.* Due to the simultaneous existence of more than one structural form of a compound.

4. *Stereoisomerism.* Due to differences in spatial relationships.
   (a) *Geometric or cis-trans isomerism*—cis and trans isomers, which differ in chemical and physical properties, as illustrated by fumaric and maleic acids.
   (b) *Optical isomerism*—isomers named dextro and levo; same properties except effect on plane polarized light.

ISOMERISM OF COMPOUNDS RELATED TO COPROSTANE

A number of biologically active compounds (bile acids, sterols, steroids, cardiac glycosides—such as digitalis and ouabain—and toadstool poisons) contain the four-ring system found in the substance coprostane. The various forms of vitamin D also are related chemically to this system.

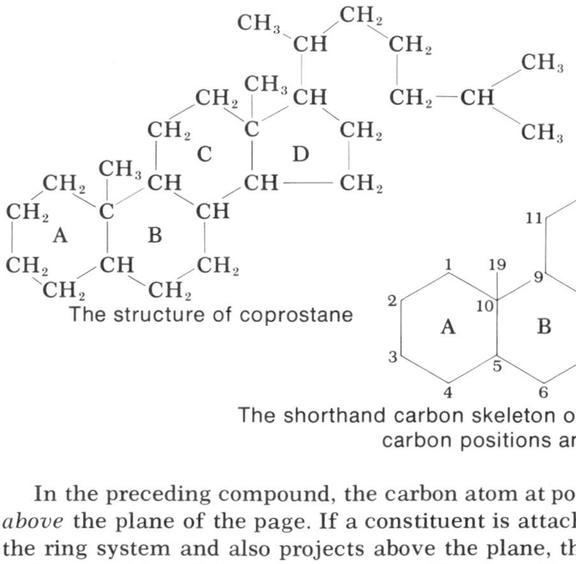

The structure of coprostane

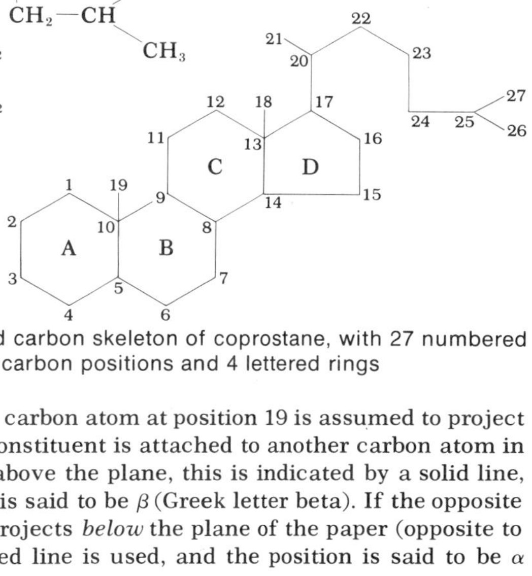

The shorthand carbon skeleton of coprostane, with 27 numbered carbon positions and 4 lettered rings

In the preceding compound, the carbon atom at position 19 is assumed to project *above* the plane of the page. If a constituent is attached to another carbon atom in the ring system and also projects above the plane, this is indicated by a solid line, and the position of the constituent is said to be β (Greek letter beta). If the opposite is true, that is, if the constituent projects *below* the plane of the paper (opposite to the direction of carbon 19), a dotted line is used, and the position is said to be α (Greek letter alpha).

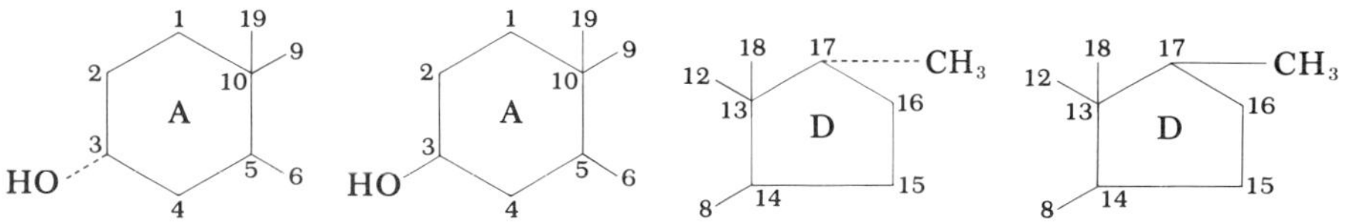

3 α-hydroxy- 3 β-hydroxy- 17 α-methyl- 17 β-methyl-

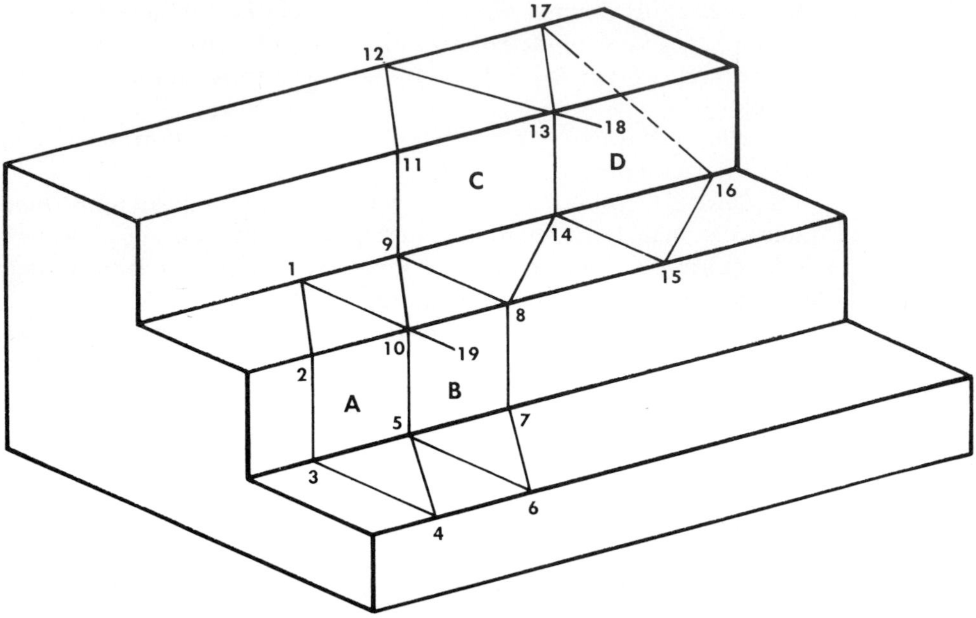

Trans (chair) form of rings A,B,C, and D

Fig. 18-7. Trans (chair) form of the ring system of compounds such as coprostane. What type of hormone has this trans ring system? (Drawing by James Skillman.)

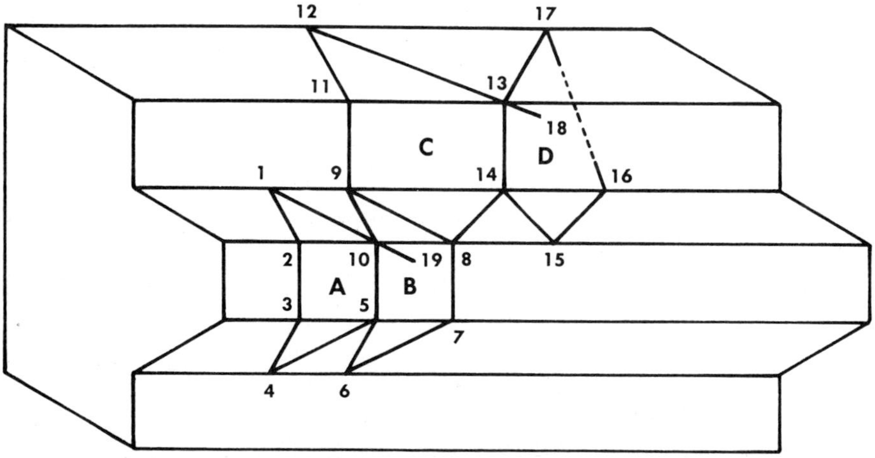

Cis (boat) form of rings A and B; trans form of rings C and D

Fig. 18-8. Cis (boat) form of the ring system of compounds such as coprostane. Why does the ring system in the estrogens not exhibit cis-trans isomerism? (Drawing by James Skillman.)

The four rings (*A, B, C,* and *D*) also exhibit isomerism. Rings *A* and *B*, for example, exist in a trans (chair*) form and in a cis (boat†) form (see Figs. 18-7 and 18-8). In many compounds of medical interest (hormones, bile acids, and sterols) rings *C* and *D* are trans, as illustrated in Figures 18-7 and 18-8. In the cardiac glycosides and toadstool poisons, the *C* and *D* rings are cis.

In the steroid hormones of the corpus luteum (page 385) and the adrenal cortex (page 399), the *A* and *B* rings are cis. In the male sex hormones (page 389), they are trans.

In the group of ovarian hormones known as estrogens (page 385) the *A* ring contains double bonds, and the carbon at position 19 is missing. In these compounds the *A* and *B* rings do not exhibit cis-trans isomerism, although the *C* and *D* rings are trans.

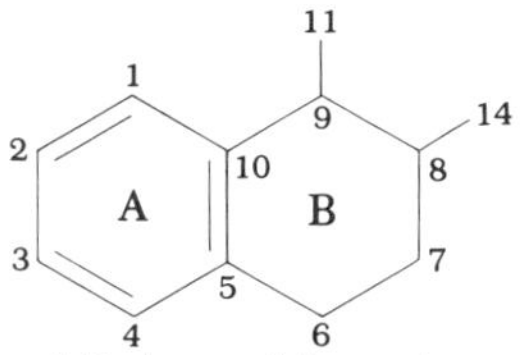

A and B rings of the estrogens

A shorthand way of indicating the cis position of the *A* and *B* rings is to indicate that the hydrogen attached to carbon 5 projects *above* the plane of the page.

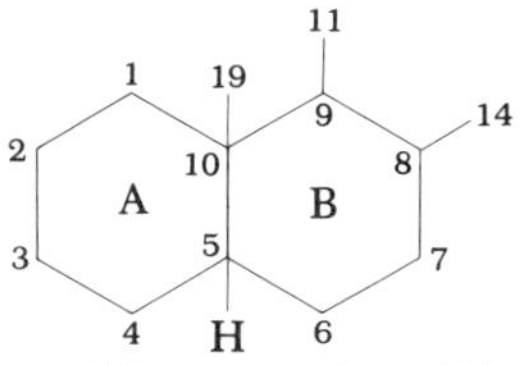

Rings A and B in coprostane (cis isomer)

In the isomer of coprostane known as cholestane, rings *A* and *B* are trans, and the H at carbon 5 is connected with a dotted line.

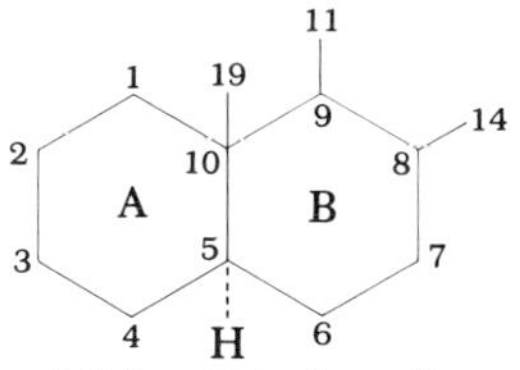

Rings A and B in cholestane (trans isomer)

*A conformation of a 6-membered ring in which 2 atoms directly opposite each other in the ring are outside the plane containing the other 4 atoms, one of the 2 atoms being above the plane, and the other, below the plane.

†A conformation of a 6-membered ring in which 2 atoms directly opposite each other in the ring are both either above or below the plane containing the other 4 atoms.

STUDY QUESTIONS

1. Make up a definition of isomerism.
2. What are isomers?
3. Give a definition of chain isomerisms; of nuclear isomerism.
4. How many isomers are represented by the formula C_6H_{14}?
5. Define geometric isomerism; cis-trans isomerism.
6. The 2 —COOH groups of maleic acid can react with each other, splitting out H_2O to form an anhydride. Fumaric acid does not form an anhydride. Explain.

7. How does a trans isomer differ spatially from a cis isomer?
8. Define tautomerism; dynamic isomerism.
9. Define position isomerism. Give several examples.
10. What is meant by optical isomerism?
11. What is an asymmetric carbon atom? What is its significance?
12. What is plane polarized light?
13. What is a polarimeter? What are its essential parts?
14. Name several factors affecting the magnitude of rotation of plane polarized light by a solution of an optically active compound.
15. What is the significance of the prefixes L- and D-? Of + and −?
16. Define: optical antipode; enantiomorphic form.
17. What is a racemic compound?
18. In what direction does a solution of L+ glumatic acid rotate plane polarized light?
19. What is meant by stereoisomerism?
20. What types of isomerism are found in compounds related to coprostane?

CHAPTER 19

Cyclic organic compounds

CYCLOPARAFFINS OR NAPHTHENES

Hydrocarbons known as *cycloparaffins* or *naphthenes* are present in some samples of petroleum. These compounds are similar to those of the paraffin series in their properties except that the carbon atoms are united in a closed cycle, from which the name is derived.

The simplest member of the cycloparaffin homologous* series is cyclopropane.

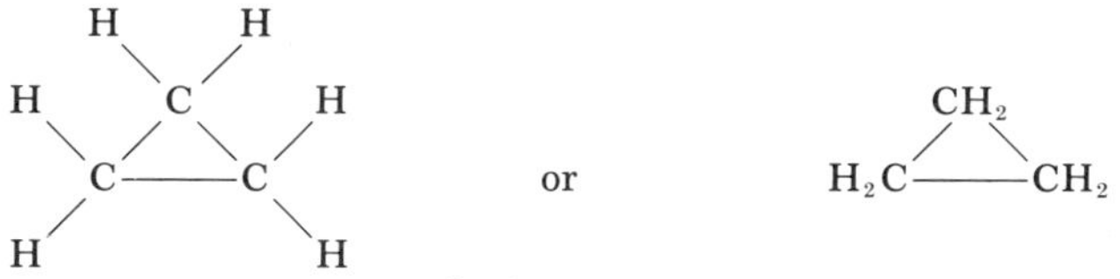

Cyclopropane

This compound does not occur in petroleum. It is made synthetically and is used in medicine as a general anesthetic. Some physicians believe it to be superior to other anesthetics since with cyclopropane muscular relaxation usually is good, induction and recovery times are short, and there is little postoperative vomiting.

The outstanding disadvantage of cyclopropane is the danger of explosion. The usual anesthetic mixture contains about 15 percent cyclopropane and 85 percent oxygen, which is well within the explosive range. Since a spark of static electricity may ignite the mixture, attendants at operations where cyclopropane is used often are requested not to wear silk garments or rubber-soled shoes, which may generate static electricity by friction.

Some of the cycloparaffins that have been identified in petroleum are: cyclobutane, cyclopentane, methyl cyclopentane, cyclohexane, methylcyclohexane,

*A homologous series is a group of similar compounds whose formulas differ by a constant amount, usually CH_2.

dimethylcyclohexane, trimethylcyclohexane, cycloheptane, and cyclooctane. These products are of special significance in gasoline because of their high antiknock properties.

The cyclohexane ring is found in a number of synthetic drugs.

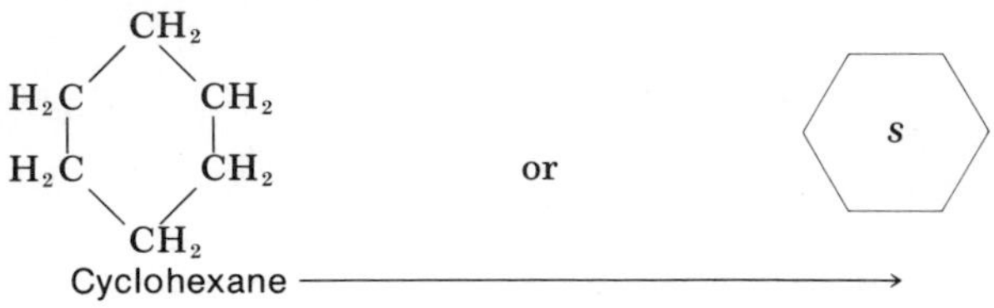

Cyclohexane

The small *s* in the hexagon formula for cyclohexane means "saturated"; that is, there are no double bonds present.

AROMATIC COMPOUNDS

The section of organic chemistry that we are to consider now is designated *aromatic* chemistry. The word "aromatic" originated from the observations of pioneer organic chemists that certain substances with similar chemical and physical properties all possess a pleasant aroma. Examples of such substances are those present in oil of wintergreen, oil of bitter almonds, and vanilla. Much later it was found that these substances contained some of their carbon atoms united in closed rings. The name "aromatic" was retained and is applied to the class of organic compounds that characteristically contain six carbon atoms in a closed ring or cycle. In a typical aromatic compound the ring of 6 carbon atoms contains 3 double bonds. It is known now that the property of possessing a pleasant aroma is not a characteristic property of aromatic compounds alone, for aliphatic esters as a rule also have agreeable odors. Moreover, there are certain compounds possessing a closed-ring type of structure that are odorless.

AROMATIC HYDROCARBONS

BENZENE

Benzene* occupies a more important place in aromatic chemistry than does methane in the aliphatic series of hydrocarbons. Many cyclic compounds are derivatives of benzene and many others are related structurally to it.

STRUCTURE OF BENZENE. An analysis for the elements and a molecular weight determination have shown that benzene has the molecular formula, C_6H_6. The graphic formula for benzene, however, can be proved only on the basis of chemical reactions. If benzene were an aliphatic compound, it would belong to the series having the general formula C_nH_{2n-6}. This would mean that benzene would be highly unsaturated. If we examine some of the properties of benzene, however, we find that it does not react like an unsaturated aliphatic hydrocarbon:

*Do not confuse *benzene* with *benzine*. Benzine is the name applied to a mixture of volatile compounds obtained during the distillation of petroleums. Benzine is more volatile than is gasoline.

1. Benzene does not react with hydrobromic acid (HBr) under ordinary conditions.

2. Benzene does not decolorize potassium permanganate ($KMnO_4$), a test for the type of double bond found in ethylene.

3. Benzene does not react when mixed with bromine.

4. Benzene does not react with nascent hydrogen.

Hence, judged by the criteria for aliphatic compounds, we must conclude that benzene behaves like a saturated compound. On the other hand, if we examine the reactions that benzene undergoes, we find that in the presence of finely divided nickel as a catalyst benzene adds 6 hydrogens to yield a compound with the formula C_6H_{12}. *This reaction indicates the presence of 3 double bonds in benzene.*

$$\underset{\text{Benzene}}{C_6H_6} + 3H_2 \xrightarrow{\text{Ni}} \underset{\text{Hexahydrobenzene}}{C_6H_{12}}$$

Although benzene does not react when mixed with bromine, substitution of bromine for hydrogen takes place if a catalyst such as iron filings is present.

$$\underset{\text{Benzene}}{C_6H_6} + Br_2 \xrightarrow{\text{Fe}} \underset{\text{Bromobenzene}}{C_6H_5Br} + \underset{\text{Hydrobromic acid}}{HBr}$$

Regardless of the conditions or the halogen used, *one and only one* monosubstituted derivative of benzene can be obtained. This reaction shows that all the hydrogens in benzene are equivalent; otherwise more than one monosubstitution product could result from the reaction. A structural formula for benzene that explains its reactions must take into account the presence of 3 double bonds and the equivalence of the 6 hydrogens.

The proposal of a formula for benzene that would meet these requirements satisfactorily was one of the most perplexing problems that confronted organic chemists in the middle of the nineteenth century. The formula that has stood most satisfactorily the test of time is the one proposed by Friedrich Kekulé in 1865. Kekulé, a German chemist, was teaching in London at the time. The story goes that he was sitting in front of his fireplace one night, dozing and dreaming. In one of his dreams, it is said, he saw a snake bite its tail. This gave him the idea of a ring structure for benzene. Whether or not inbibitions of a fermented beverage had an effect on the zoological nature of his dream is not reported.

The structural formula for benzene proposed by Kekulé is as follows:

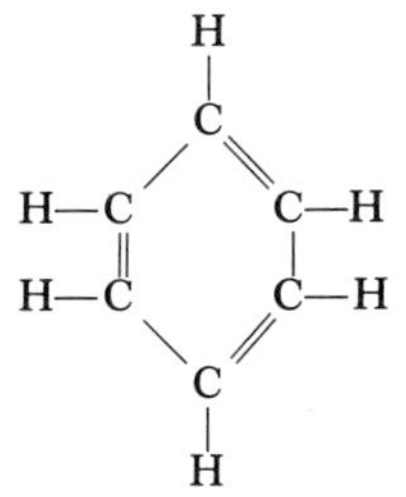

Benzene

The alternate double bonds account for the unsatisfied valences of carbon and explain the possibility of the addition of 6 hydrogen atoms. The relationship of each of the carbon atoms to the molecule is the same so that the hydrogen atoms attached to the carbon atoms are equivalent. This equivalence is reflected in the formation of only one monosubstitution product.

For convenience in writing formulas and in printing, the formula of benzene is represented frequently by a hexagon. Sometimes the double bonds are indicated and sometimes not. Probably it is best to include them in order to prevent confusing benzene with cyclohexane (see page 172). The hydrogen atoms are not shown, but the student should remember that a hydrogen atom is attached to each carbon atom unless some other group is indicated, signifying that one of the hydrogens has been replaced.

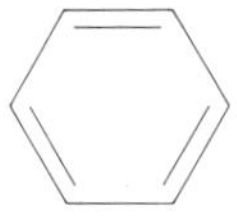

Benzene

From an examination of the Kekulé formula for benzene it could be predicted that there would be three disubstitution products of benzene. This has been found to be true. Assuming X to represent a group that has substituted for a hydrogen atom, the structures of the three isomers are:

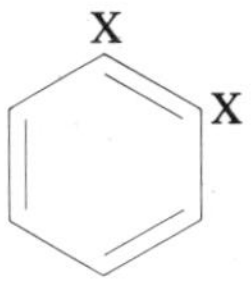

Ortho (o)

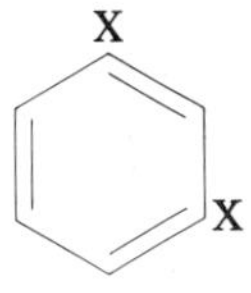

Meta (m)

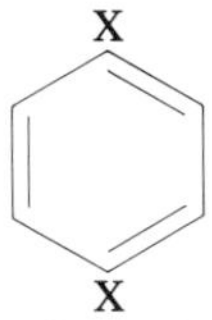

Para (p)

The isomer in which the substituted groups are on adjacent carbon atoms is termed *ortho,* abbreviated o-. The isomer having one carbon atom between the two substituted groups is known as *meta* (m-). The third isomer, in which the groups are on the carbon atoms across the ring from each other or in which there are 2 carbon atoms intervening, is called the *para* isomer (p-).

One objection that soon was raised to the formula for benzene proposed by Kekulé centers about its possession of double bonds. From the formula it would seem that there should be 2 compounds instead of only one when the substituted groups are adjacent to each other. It was pointed out that this necessarily would follow because in one instance the carbons carrying the 2 substituted groups would be connected by a double bond while in the other instance the carbons would be linked by a single bond. This objection to the Kekulé formula was met by the hypothesis that the double bonds in the proposed formula are not static but are shifting continually between 2 adjacent positions, as the following diagrams illustrate:

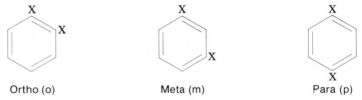

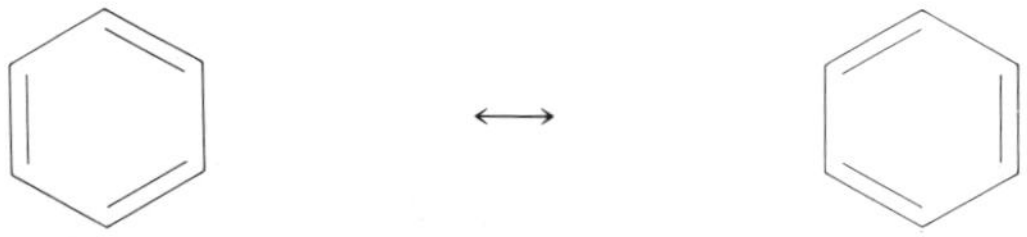

The 2 forms are equivalent and indistinguishable from each other; their interconversion requires only a redistribution of the valence electrons. Such a phenomenon is known as *resonance* (see page 94). It accounts for the relative stability and the lowered reactivity of benzene. X-ray data of crystalline derivatives of benzene show that all the C—C bonds in benzene are of the same length. They are slightly longer than an aliphatic C—C bond, but are slightly shorter than an aliphatic C=C bond. This supports the idea that benzene is a *resonating hybrid* (see page 95).

Another shorthand symbol for the benzene ring that is used frequently by organic chemists is:

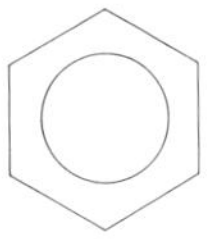

Benzene

PROPERTIES OF BENZENE. Benzene is a colorless liquid boiling at 80.4° C. It is insoluble in water but is soluble in alcohol and ether. Benzene is toxic to man. Taken internally it can cause death. If low concentrations of the vapor are inhaled over a long period of time, there is a decrease in the production of both the red and white blood cells, which may result in death. Contact with the skin also is harmful.

Chlorine and bromine can be introduced into the benzene ring by the direct action of the halogens on benzene in the presence of a catalyst. At high temperatures and with a high concentration of a halogen the dihalogen derivatives can be prepared. One of these compounds, p-dichlorobenzene, is used widely as an insecticide to protect woolens from moths and to protect peach trees from the peach tree borer.

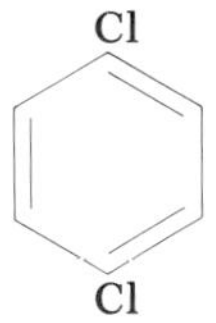

p-Dichlorobenzene

Benzene and other aromatic compounds react directly with concentrated nitric acid to form nitro compounds. Nitrobenzene, or oil of mirbane, is a pale yellow liquid with an odor resembling that of bitter almonds. It is poisonous. Because of its odor, it is used to replace oil of bitter almonds in perfumes, particularly those used in soaps. Its chief use, however, is in the preparation of aniline (see page 186).

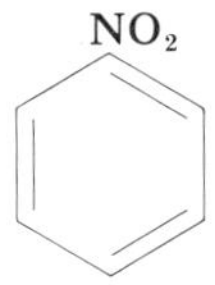

Nitrobenzene

In general, aliphatic saturated hydrocarbons are not affected by the action of sulfuric acid. Concentrated sulfuric acid containing dissolved sulfur trioxide (SO_3) reacts with the aromatic hydrocarbons to form *sulfonic acids*.

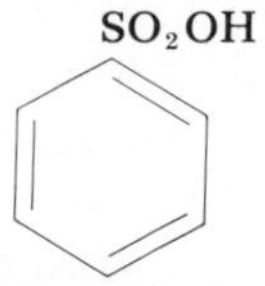

Benzenesulfonic acid

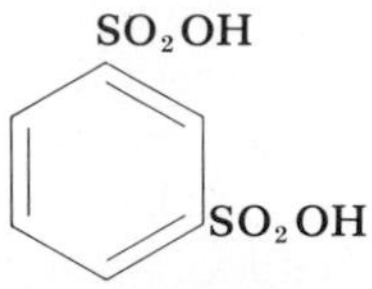

m-Benzenedisulfonic acid

USES OF BENZENE. Large quantities of benzene are used in motor fuels to increase the antiknock value. The so-called benzol blends are such mixtures. Benzene is used as a solvent for rubber, fats, and resins, and in the preparation of rubber cement. It is the starting material for the manufacture of a large number of other aromatic compounds such as synthetic phenol, nitrobenzene, aniline, chlorobenzene, and others.

OTHER IMPORTANT AROMATIC HYDROCARBONS

TOLUENE. This compound is the first higher homologue of benzene, in which 1 hydrogen atom has been replaced by a methyl group.

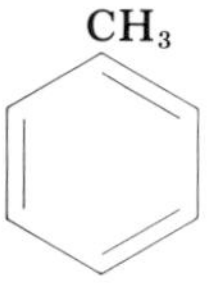

Toluene

Its chemical properties are similar to those of benzene. *Trinitrotoluene*, or TNT, is used as an explosive.

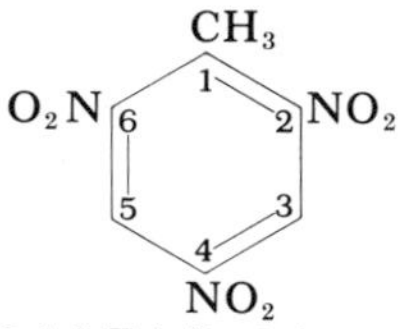

2,4,6-Trinitrotoluene

XYLENE. The second higher homologue of benzene contains 2 methyl groups and is known as xylene. As is true for all disubstitution products of benzene, there are 3 isomers:

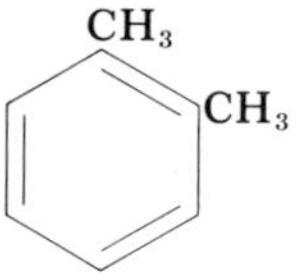

o-Xylene

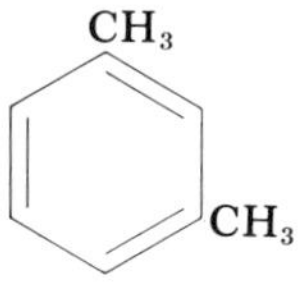

m-Xylene

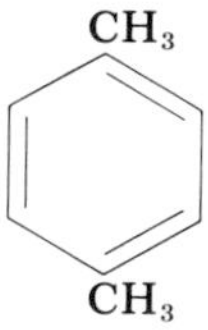

p-Xylene

NAPHTHALENE. Naphthalene is an aromatic compound containing 2 benzene rings. The rings are attached to each other at the points of 2 carbon atoms. Naphthalene is the simplest aromatic hydrocarbon with *condensed* or "fused" benzene rings, 2 carbon atoms being common to each benzene ring.

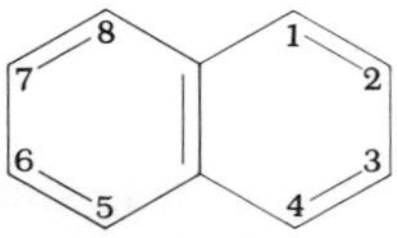

Naphthalene

As the small numbers indicate there are 8 replaceable hydrogens in the naphthalene molecule. The molecule is symmetrical in its structure so that positions 1, 4, 5, and 8 are identical (α), as are positions 2, 3, 6, and 7 (β). Thus there are 2 possible monosubstitution products of naphthalene; they are known as the *alpha* and *beta* forms.

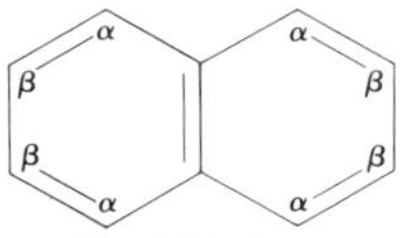

Naphthalene

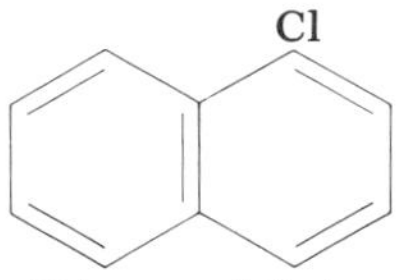

α-Chloronaphthalene

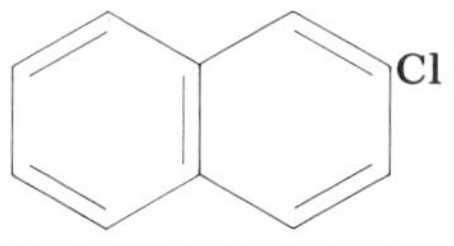

β-Chloronaphthalene

Purified naphthalene is the white solid familiar to everyone in the form of mothballs.

ANTHRACENE. Anthracene is present in the coal tar fraction that boils above 270° C. It forms colorless plates that exhibit a blue fluorescence. The anthracene structure is numbered as shown in order to facilitate the naming of derivatives.

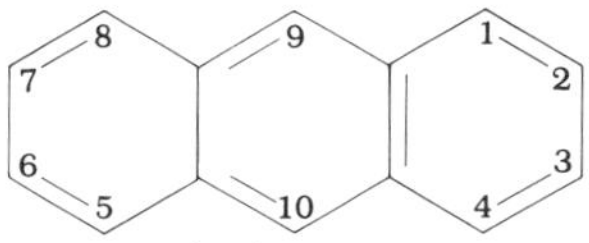

Anthracene

When nitric acid reacts with anthracene, it does not give rise to nitro derivatives; instead, anthraquinone is formed. Anthracene and anthraquinone are important products in the manufacture of dyes and dye intermediates.

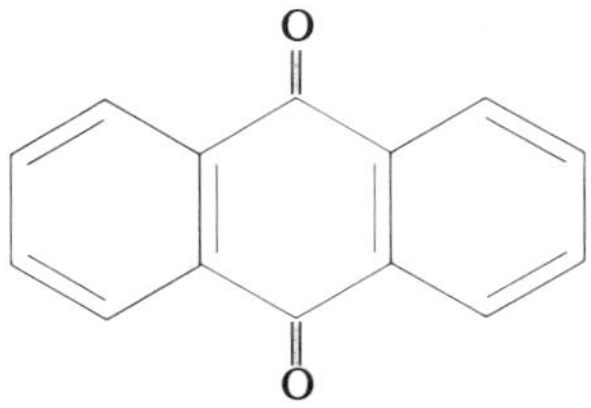

Anthraquinone

PHENANTHRENE. This compound has great theoretical importance in biology and medicine. Some compounds that can be considered to be derivatives of it are the male sex hormones, the female sex hormones, hormones of the adrenal cortex, bile acids, vitamin D, cholesterol, and the digitalis glycosides. It occurs also in a number of carcinogenic compounds (compounds that produce cancer in animals).

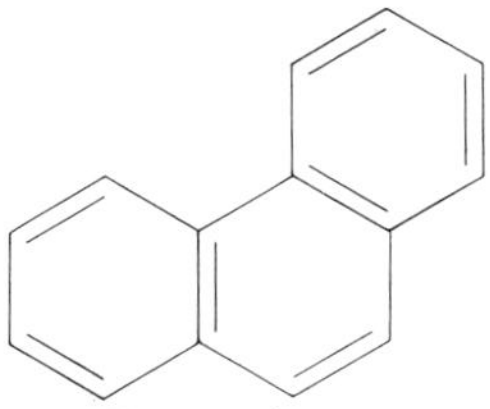
Phenanthrene

Oxygen derivatives of the aromatic hydrocarbons

Aromatic compounds have oxygen derivatives corresponding to the aliphatic oxygen compounds. Thus, there are aromatic alcohols, aldehydes, ketones, and acids. When the functional group of these derivatives is present in the side chain attached to the benzene ring, the compound behaves very much as does the corresponding aliphatic compound. This comparison also holds for other substitution groups present in side chains. For example, the chlorine atom in benzyl chloride, $C_6H_5CH_2Cl$, reacts in a manner similar to that of the chlorine atom in the aliphatic halide CH_3CH_2Cl.

AROMATIC ALCOHOLS

BENZYL ALCOHOL. The simplest aromatic alcohol, benzyl alcohol, occurs in the free state in balsams of Peru and Tolu and as an ester in jasmine, hyacinth, and other essential oils. It is a liquid and is useful in perfumes because of its pleasant odor.

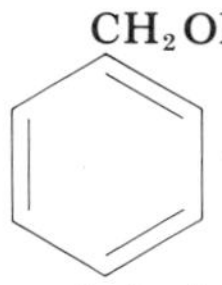

Benzyl alcohol

The chemical properties of benzyl alcohol are similar to those of the aliphatic alcohols. For example, on oxidation the aldehyde is found first; further oxidation yields the acid.

$$\underset{\text{Benzyl alcohol}}{C_6H_5CH_2OH} \xrightarrow{\text{oxidation}} \underset{\text{Benzaldehyde}}{C_6G_5CHO} \xrightarrow{\text{oxidation}} \underset{\text{Benzoic acid}}{C_6H_5COOH}$$

PHENETHYL ALCOHOL. This compound occurs in attar of roses and is used in making perfumes.

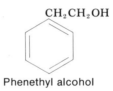

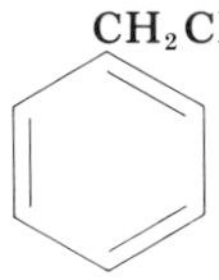

Phenethyl alcohol

PHENOLS

The aromatic derivatives in which the hydroxyl group is attached directly to the benzene ring are termed *phenols*. The properties of the phenols differ greatly from those of the aliphatic alcohols. The hydroxyl group in phenols is much more acidic than is the hydroxyl group in aliphatic alcohols. The phenols dissolve in dilute sodium hydroxide, whereas the aliphatic alcohols are no more soluble in alkaline solutions than they are in water.

PHENOL. Phenol is obtained from the middle oil fraction of coal tar.

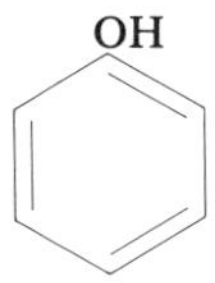

Phenol

Pure phenol is a white solid, melting at 41° C. On exposure to air and light it develops a red color. The presence of a small amount of water causes phenol to liquefy. The liquid form often is termed *carbolic acid*. Phenol is a poison when taken internally, and if it comes in contact with the skin in undiluted form it causes blisters and blanching of the skin. The solubility of phenol in water depends on the temperature. At room temperature it is soluble only to the extent of about 8 percent, but above 68° C (154° F) it is soluble in all proportions. It is soluble also in ether and in alcohol. If phenol is spilled on the skin, it is best to wash it off with an organic solvent such as rubbing alcohol rather than with water. If only water is available, large amounts should be used.

Chemical properties. Phenol reacts with an alkali to form a phenolate and H_2O.

$$\underset{\text{Phenol}}{C_6H_5OH} + NaOH \rightarrow \underset{\text{Sodium phenolate}}{C_6H_5ONa} + H_2O$$

Halogens readily react with phenol. Pentachlorophenol is used to protect wood against degrading agents such as termites and decay.

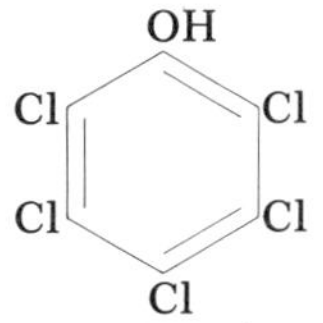

Pentachlorophenol

Phenol is reduced to the corresponding hydrocarbon when it is distilled at high temperature with zinc dust.

$$\underset{\text{Phenol}}{C_6H_5OH} + Zn \xrightarrow{\Delta} \underset{\text{Benzene}}{C_6H_6} + ZnO$$

Sodium phenolate reacts with aliphatic (alkyl) halides to give mixed aromatic-aliphatic ethers. The ether formed with methyl iodide is known as *anisole*. It is a solid with a pleasant odor and is used in the manufacture of perfumes.

$$\underset{\text{Sodium phenolate}}{C_6H_5ONa} + \underset{\text{Methyl iodide}}{CH_3I} \rightarrow \underset{\text{Methylphenyl ether (anisole)}}{C_6H_5OCH_3} + NaI$$

If phenol is heated to 100° C with nitric acid, 2,4,6-trinitrophenol is formed. This compound is known commonly as picric acid.

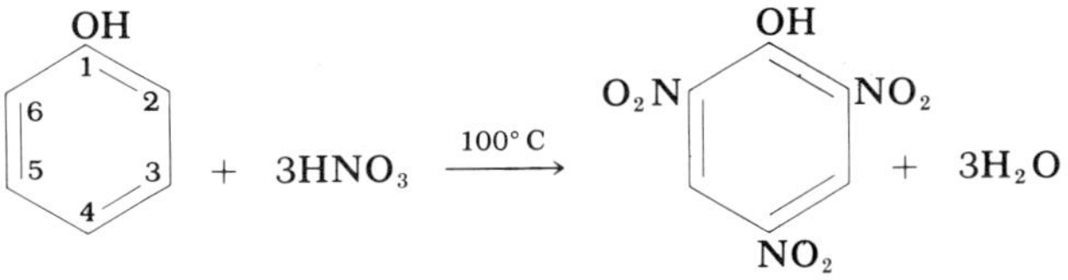

Phenol   Picric acid

Picric acid formerly was used in the treatment of burns. It is not used for this purpose today since there is danger of toxicity if too much of the compound is absorbed into the body through the burned skin.

When phenol is heated with formaldehyde, either in the presence of a base such as ammonium hydroxide or of an acid such as sulfuric acid, the first products formed are hydroxybenzyl alcohols.

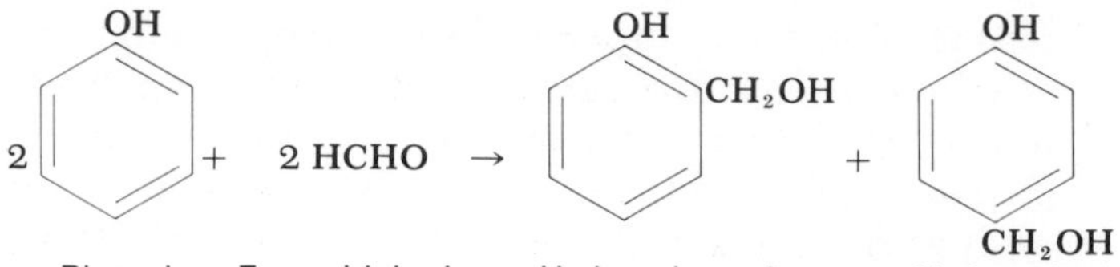

Phenol Formaldehyde o-Hydroxybenzyl alcohol p-Hydroxybenzyl alcohol

Upon further heating, with the elimination of water, these alcohols condense to form long chain molecules or linear polymers, a portion of which can be represented as having the following probable structure:

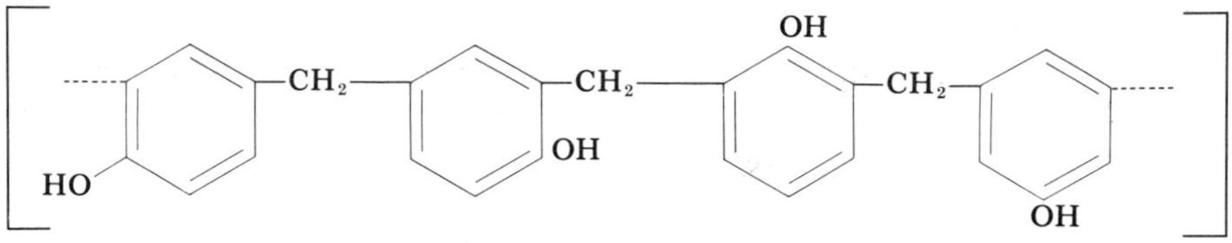

By varying conditions such as temperature, time, and the amount of formaldehyde, the resulting polymers are suitable for preparing quick-drying enamels and varnishes, or for preparing solid phenolic plastics. Bakelite is one such plastic.

Uses of phenol. Large quantities of phenol are used in the manufacture of dyes, drugs (such as aspirin), photographic developers, and plastics. A 3 percent solution of phenol is an effective disinfectant for inanimate objects such as surgeons' instruments, containers, and the like. It is not a satisfactory disinfectant for substances containing high percentages of protein materials since the protein reacts with the phenol and removes it from solution.

Phenol is used in the refining of lubricating oils since the undesirable aromatic and naphthenic compounds are selectively dissolved, leaving the paraffinic components, which have better lubricating properties.

DIHYDROXYPHENOLS. The ortho-, meta-, and para-dihydroxyphenols have specific names.

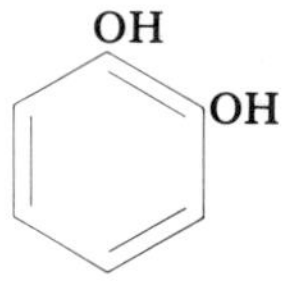

Pyrocatechol

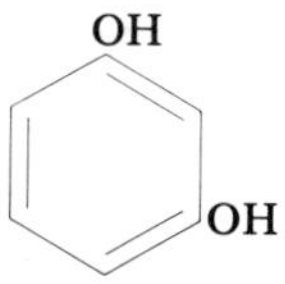

Resorcinol

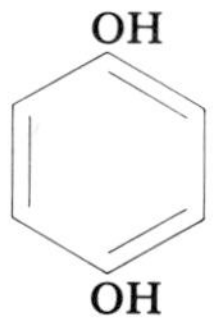

Hydroquinol

Pyrocatechol can reduce silver compounds and is used as a photographic developer (see page 113). The monomethyl ether of pyrocatechol, guaiacol, is obtained by distilling gum guaiac. Guaiacol has been used in cough syrups. Gum guaiac is used for detecting traces of blood in the stool (see page 332).

The major use of *resorcinol* is in the manufacture of dyes. If alcohol, sulfuric acid, and a solution of resorcinol are added to a sugar solution containing a ketose (see page 242), an intense red color develops (Selivanoff's test). *Hexylresorcinol* is used as an antiseptic and as a drug effective against hookworms.

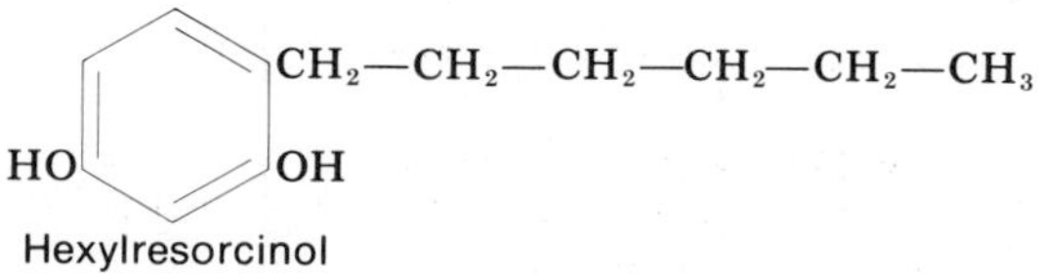

Hexylresorcinol

Hydroquinol is also known as hydroquinone. It is used widely in photographic developers.

TRIHYDROXYPHENOLS. There are two important trihydroxyphenols, pyrogallol and phlorglucinol.

Pyrogallol is obtained by heating gallic acid that has been secured from the tannins that occur in Chinese nutgalls.

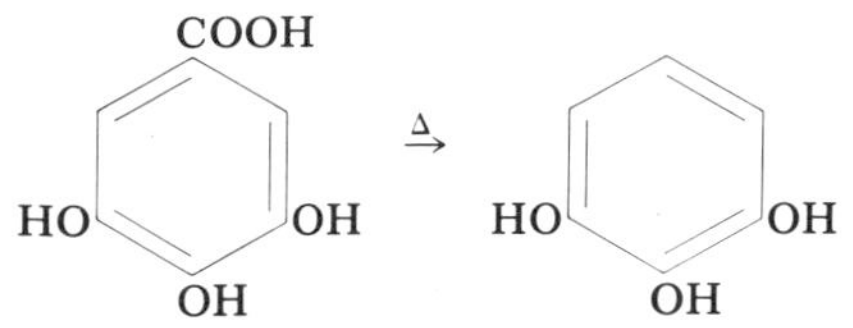

Gallic acid Pyrogallol

An alkaline solution of pyrogallol rapidly absorbs oxygen. Pyrogallol often is utilized in the quantitative absorption of oxygen from gaseous mixtures.

Phlorglucinol is a constituent of the glycoside phlorhizin (see page 266). It exists in two forms that are in equilibrium with each other.

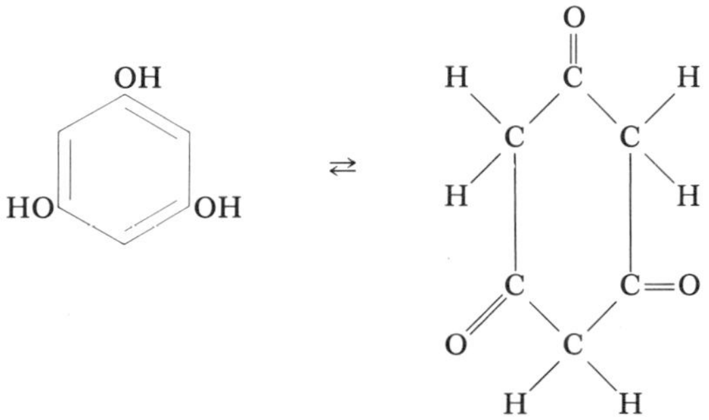

Phlorglucinol (Enol form) Phlorglucinol (Keto form)

Phlorglucinol is a component of some photographic developers and is used in testing for the presence of pentoses (see page 242).

NAPHTHOLS The monohydroxy derivatives of naphthalene are known as naphthols. There are two isomeric naphthols; they differ in the position of the hydroxyl group (see page 177).

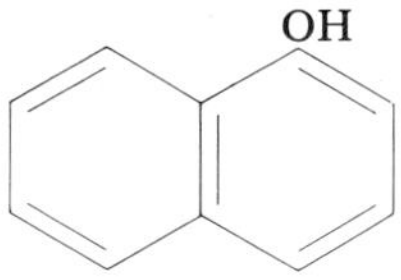

α-Naphthol

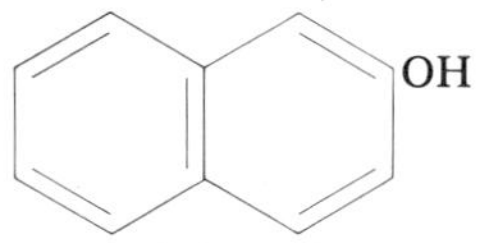

β-Naphthol

A test (Molisch) for the presence of carbohydrate in protein material involves the use of α-naphthol. β-Naphthol is used in the manufacture of dyes. It is used in the synthesis of β-phenylnaphthylamine, a compound used as an antioxidant for natural and synthetic rubbers.

ALKYLATED PHENOLS* The *cresols* are methyl derivatives of phenol. There are three isomers—ortho, meta, and para.

*Phenols containing an aliphatic side chain.

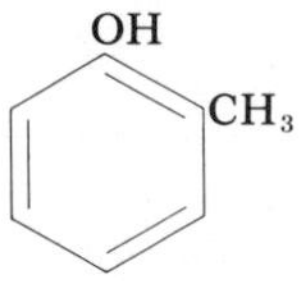

o-Cresol

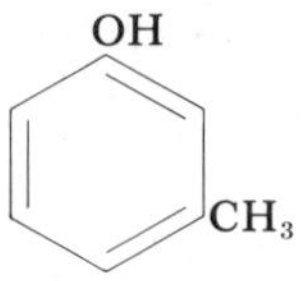

m-Cresol

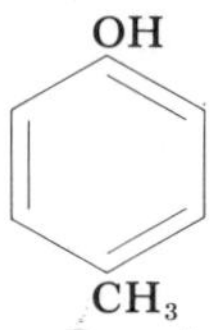

p-Cresol

A mixture of the three isomers is known as "cresylic acid." The crude mixture separated from coal tar is known as creosote oil and is employed as a wood preservative. The cresols are stronger disinfectants than is phenol and they are less toxic to man. They are only slightly soluble in water, but the addition of soap makes them water soluble. Lysol is a disinfectant that contains cresols and soap. Cresols are used in the manufacture of synthetic resins.

Thymol, or 3-hydroxy-1-methyl-4-isopropylbenzene, is a pleasant-smelling, crystalline compound obtained from the oils of thyme and mint.

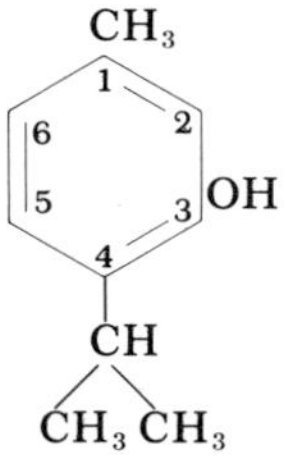

Thymol

It is used as an antiseptic in toothpastes and mouthwashes. It has been used to remove hookworms from the intestinal tract.

AROMATIC ALDEHYDES

The aromatic aldehydes contain the same functional group, 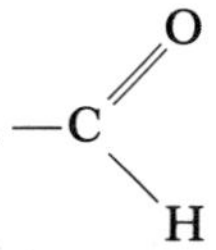 as do the aliphatic aldehydes. Many of their reactions are similar to those of the aliphatic aldehydes. The aromatic aldehydes can contain the functional group —CHO attached to one of the carbons in the benzene ring or attached to a carbon in a side chain. The class of aldehydes in which the aldehyde group is separated from the benzene ring by one or more carbon atoms undergoes reactions so similar to those of the aliphatic aldehydes that further consideration of this group will be omitted.

BENZALDEHYDE. The simplest purely aromatic aldehyde is benzaldehyde. It is a constituent of amygdalin, a naturally occuring glycoside (see page 249) found in bitter almonds and in the kernels of many fruits such as cherries, peaches, and plums. The characteristic odor of oil of bitter almonds is due to benzaldehyde.

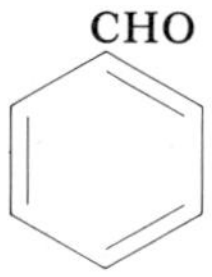

Benzaldehyde

Benzaldehyde is a liquid that is soluble in water to the extent of 0.5 percent; it is soluble in ether in all proportions. The compound readily undergoes oxidation in the presence of oxygen to form benzoic acid.

$$\underset{\text{Benzaldehyde}}{C_6H_5CHO} + O_2 \rightarrow \underset{\text{Benzoyl hydrogen peroxide}}{C_6H_5C(=O)\text{—}O\text{—}O\text{—}H}$$

$$\underset{\text{Benzoyl hydrogen peroxide}}{C_6H_5C(=O)\text{—}O\text{—}O\text{—}H} + \underset{\text{Benzaldehyde}}{C_6H_5CHO} \rightarrow \underset{\text{Benzoic acid}}{2\ C_6H_5COOH}$$

Vanillin is a compound that can be considered to be a derivative of benzaldehyde. It is the active component of vanilla extract and is present in vanilla beans to the extent of about 2 percent.

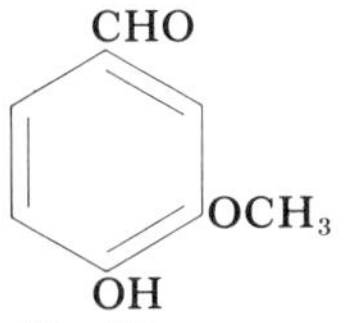

Vanillin

Cinnamic aldehyde. This unsaturated aldehyde is present in oil of cinnamon.

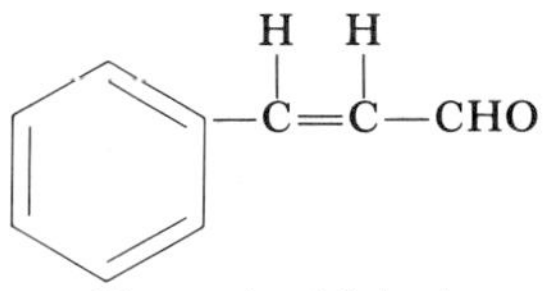

Cinnamic aldehyde

AROMATIC KETONES

It will be recalled that ketones can be thought of as compounds containing a carbonyl group ($\text{—}\overset{O}{\overset{\|}{C}}\text{—}$) to which 2 radicals are attached ($R\text{—}\overset{O}{\overset{\|}{C}}\text{—}R'$). Aromatic ketones of 2 types occur. In one type both R and R′ are aromatic; in the other R is aromatic and R′ is aliphatic.

BENZOPHENONE. Benzophenone is an example of a simple aromatic ketone; that is, both R and R′ are aromatic.

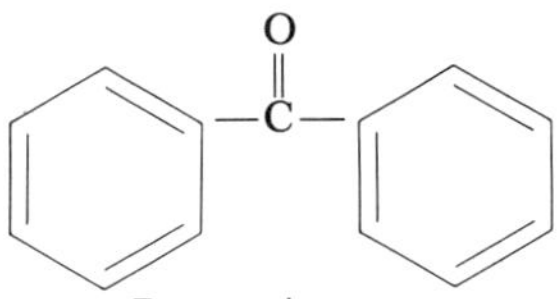

Benzophenone

Benzophenone is a colorless solid with an agreeable odor. In general, its reactions are similar to those of the aliphatic ketones.

ACETOPHENONE. This is the simplest mixed (aromatic-aliphatic) ketone.

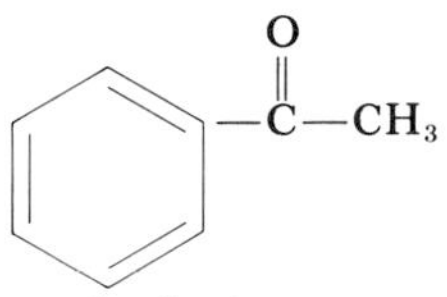

Acetophenone

This compound is a colorless oil with a fragrant odor. Formerly, under the name *hypnose*, it was used as a hypnotic (drug to induce sleep). Its reactions also are similar to those of the aliphatic ketones.

CHLORACETOPHENONE. This compound is one type of "tear gas."

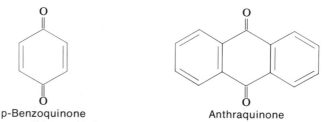

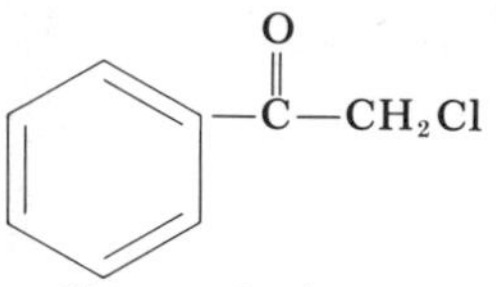

Chloracetophenone

QUINONES As we have seen, aromatic ketones contain a carbonyl group attached to one of the carbons in the benzene ring. Compounds known as *quinones* contain a carbonyl group as a part of the benzene ring itself.

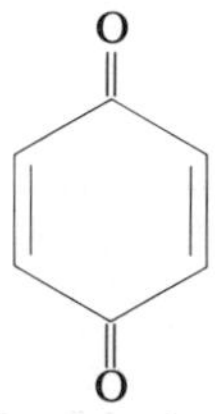

p-Benzoquinone

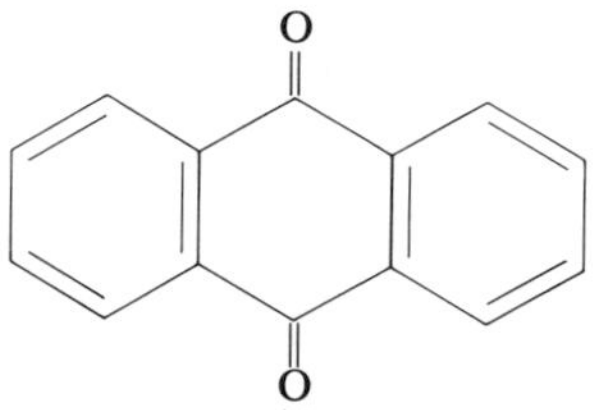

Anthraquinone

Compounds having the quinoid structure (2 double bonds in the 6-carbon ring and 2 double bonds connecting oxygen atoms to the ring) are colored. Quinones are used in the manufacture of dyes.

AROMATIC ACIDS There are 2 types of aromatic acid. In one type the carboxyl group is attached directly to the benzene ring; in the other type it is attached to a side chain. The aromatic acids form salts and neutralize alkalies just as do aliphatic acids.

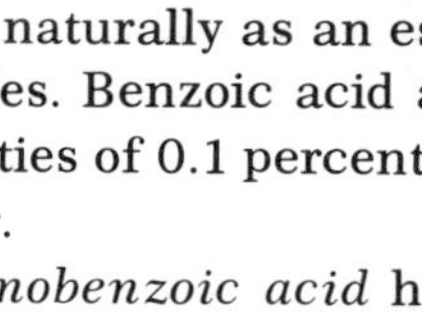

Benzoic acid

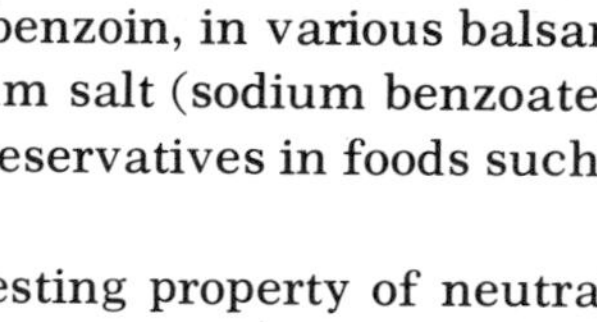

Phenylpropionic acid

BENZOIC ACID. Benzoic acid is a white crystalline solid that melts at 122° C. It is sparingly soluble in cold water but is more soluble in hot water. It occurs naturally as an ester in gum benzoin, in various balsams, and in cranberries. Benzoic acid and its sodium salt (sodium benzoate) are used in quantities of 0.1 percent or less as preservatives in foods such as catsup and cider.

p-*Aminobenzoic acid* has the interesting property of neutralizing the bacteriostatic action of sulfonamide drugs (page 187).

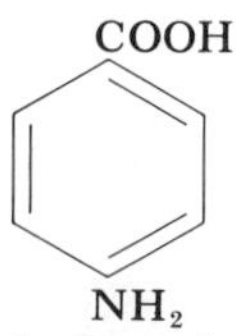

p-Aminobenzoic acid

Salicylic acid. Salicylic acid occurs as the methyl ester (methyl salicylate) in fairly large amounts in oil of wintergreen. It is a white crystalline solid and, like benzoic acid, is sparingly soluble in cold water but more soluble in hot water. It is used in the form of ointments and lotions to treat fungous infections of the skin. Its sodium salt is used as an analgesic. Salicylic acid and some of its most useful derivatives have the following structural formulas:

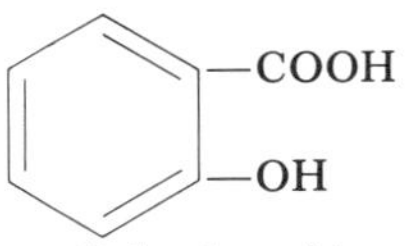

Salicylic acid

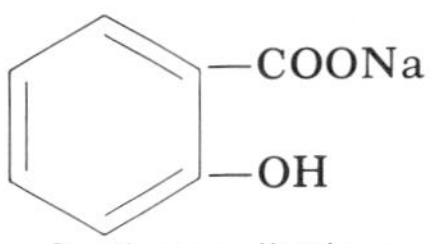

Sodium salicylate

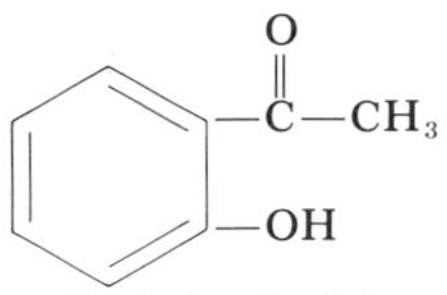

Methyl salicylate

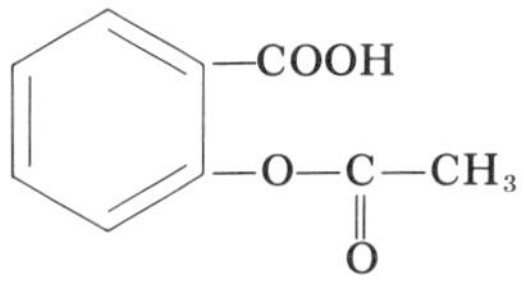

Acetylsalicylic acid (aspirin)

Methyl salicylate is a liquid that has the pleasant odor of wintergreen. It is used as a flavoring agent in toothpastes and in candies. It is used topically to relieve muscular and joint pain.

Aspirin is familiar to almost everyone. It is used as an analgesic and antipyretic (drug that reduces fever). Millions of pounds of it are manufactured annually in the United States.

Gallac acid. Gallic acid is not obtained from coal tar. It is produced by the hydrolysis of tannins that are found in tea, coffee, walnuts, and many other plants. The propyl ester of gallic acid is used in small quantities in foods as a preservative and antioxidant.

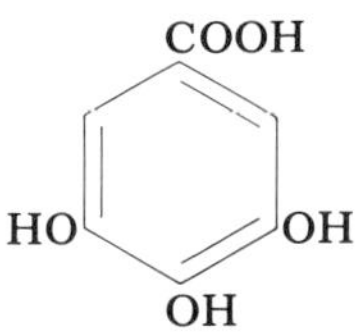

Gallic acid

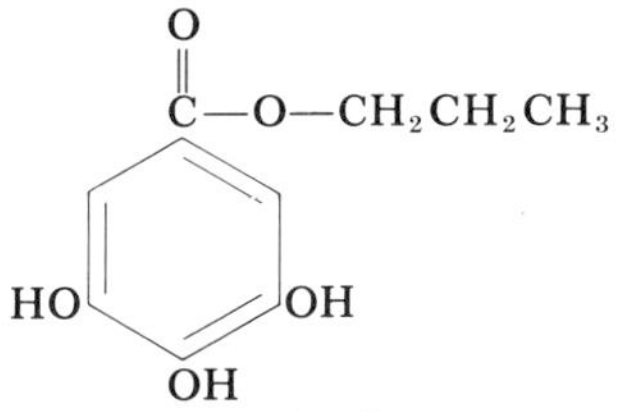

Propyl gallate

Tannins are glycosides (see page 249). They contain not only gallic acid but other hydroxy aromatic acids as well. They are responsible for the bitter flavor when tea and coffee are brewed improperly. They react with ferric salts to form a dark bluish black solution. This property has led to their use in inks. They react with ferrous salts to form ferrous tannate, a soluble, colorless compound. This compound is present in the familiar blue-black inks. On exposure in thin layers to air, the ferrous tannate is oxidized rapidly to the black insoluble ferric tannate. An organic dye used in the ink gives the original color to the ink so that the writing is not invisible before the oxidation reaction takes place.

Tannins react with proteins (see page 276). The reaction is used in the tanning of leather.

Phthalic acid. There are 3 dicarboxylic acid derivatives of benzene, but the o-form, known as o-phthalic acid, or simply as phthalic acid, is of most importance. It forms a stable anhydride when it is heated.

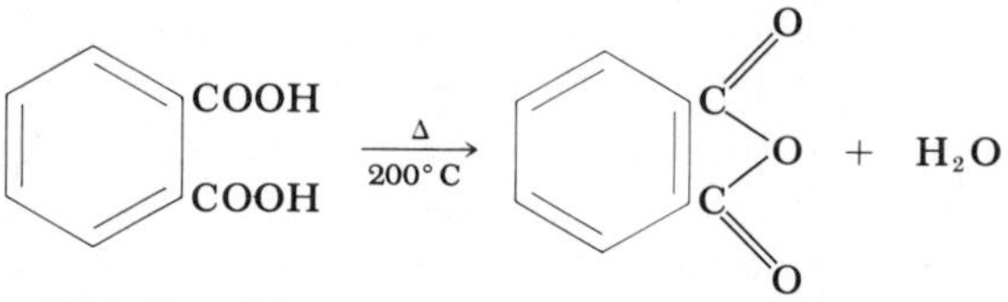

Phthalic acid Phthalic anhydride

Phthalic acid is used in the manufacture of dyes. Both phthalic acid and phthalic anhydride are used to manufacture complex polymers known as alkyd resins. These resins are used in surface coatings such as enamels and lacquers.

Aromatic amines

There are three classes of aromatic amines—primary, secondary, and tertiary. As in the case of aliphatic amines the basis of classification is the number of hydrogens in ammonia that are replaced by organic radicals, at least one of which must be aromatic.

PRIMARY AROMATIC AMINES

ANILINE. Aniline is by far the most important primary aromatic amine.

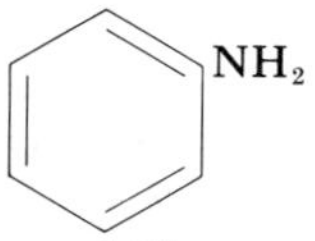

Aniline

Aniline readily dissolves in benzene, alcohols, and ether, but it is almost insoluble in water. It is a colorless oil when it is pure, but on contact with air it quickly turns brown. It is toxic to man. Contact with the liquid or inhalation of the vapors should be avoided.

In common with the aliphatic amines, aniline possesses basic properties and combines with inorganic acids to produce salts. Many compounds used in medicine contain primary amino groups. As a rule, such compounds are insoluble in water. In order to obtain a water-soluble substance the primary amino groups are converted to salts.

When aniline reacts with organic acids, *anilides* are formed.

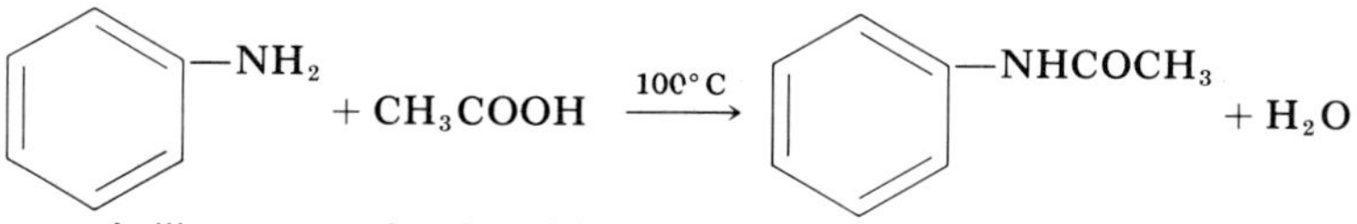

Aniline Acetic acid Acetanilide

Acetanilide is used in medicine as an analgesic and as an agent to reduce fever.

When aniline is heated with concentrated sulfuric acid, p-sulfanilic acid is formed.

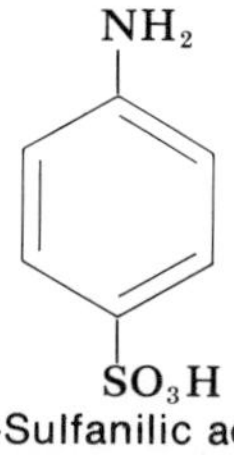

p-Sulfanilic acid

This compound is used in preparing the sulfonamide drugs.

In 1935 the German scientist Gerhard Domagk reported that a red dye, Prontosil Rubrum, given by mouth protected mice against otherwise fatal infection with hemolytic streptococci. In 1936 the French workers E. Fourneau, J. Trefouel, F. Nitti, and D. Bouvet announced that the action of Prontosil on microorganisms resulted from the fact that the dye was broken down in the body to yield sulfanilamide, which

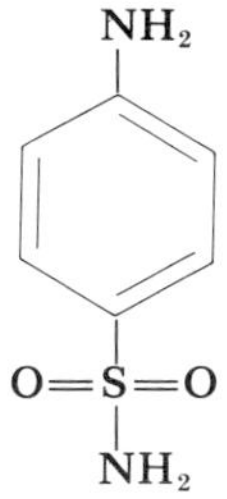

Sulfanilamide

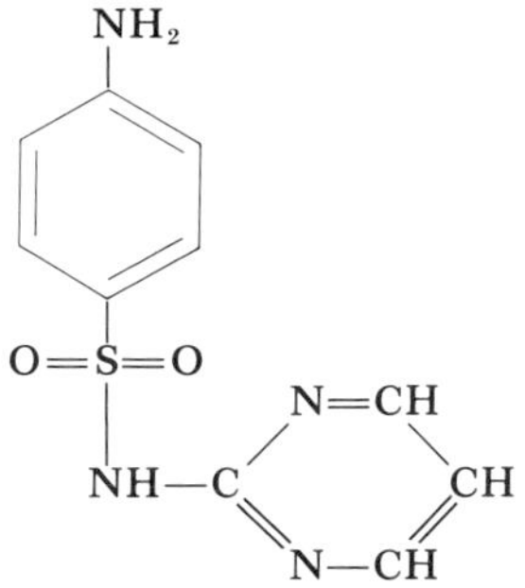

Sulfadiazine

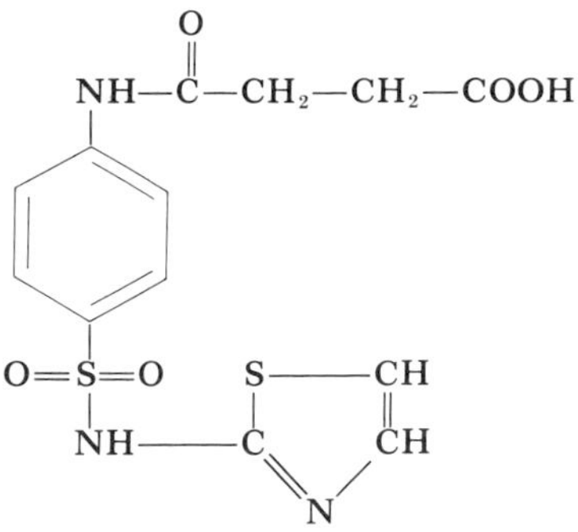

Succinylsulfathiazole

was the therapeutic agent. In 1937, Perrin H. Long and Eleanor A. Bliss and their co-workers at Johns Hopkins Medical School confirmed the findings of the French workers and used the new drug to treat streptococcal infections in human beings.

It soon became apparent, however, that sulfanilamide had numerous drawbacks. Its use often was accompanied by toxic signs and symptoms such as nausea, dizziness, cyanosis, psychoses, anemia, and methemoglobinemia (conversion of a portion of the hemoglobin of the blood to methemoglobin – see page 279). This has led to the development of a long list of sulfonamide derivatives now used in medicine. Some illustrative formulas are given directly above.

SECONDARY AROMATIC AMINES

The secondary aromatic amines may be of two types: (a) those in which there are alkyl (aliphatic) and aryl (aromatic) groups, and (b) those in which there are only aryl groups. Monomethylaniline (N-methylaniline*) is a representative of the first class.

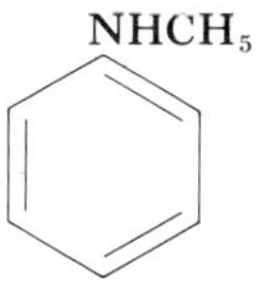

Monomethylaniline

Diphenylamine is an example of a purely aromatic secondary amine. It is used in smokeless gunpowder as a stabilizer to prevent spontaneous decomposition.

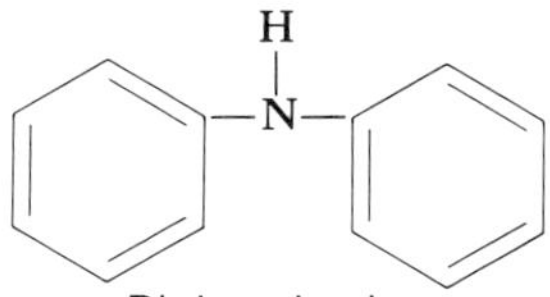

Diphenylamine

*This designation is used to indicate that the methyl group is combined with the nitrogen.

TERTIARY AROMATIC AMINES Tertiary aromatic amines contain a nitrogen to which are attached 3 organic radicals, at least one of which is aromatic. Two examples are:

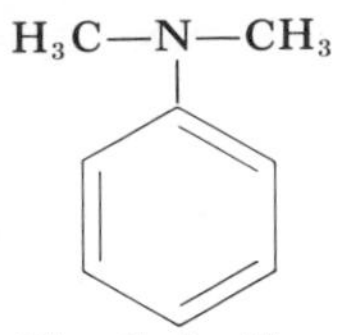

Dimethylaniline

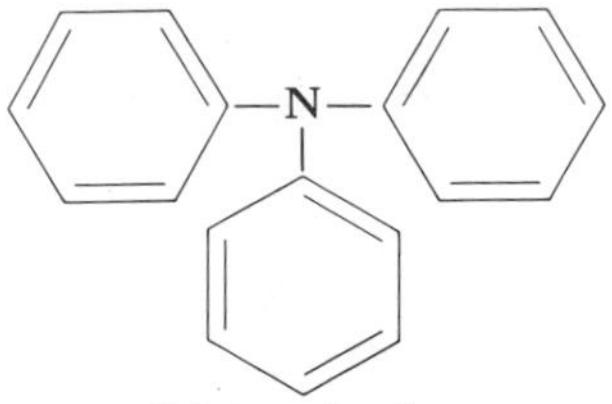

Triphenylamine

Dyes

Ordinary white light passed through a glass prism breaks up into its component colors, known as a spectrum. Substances are capable of absorbing or reflecting light. The color of a substance is dependent on the kind of light that it reflects or transmits—that is, on the kind of light that reaches our eyes. The absorption of light is dependent on the chemical structure of the substance absorbing the light. From a more fundamental standpoint this absorption of radiant energy is dependent on an unstable arrangement of electrons in the molecule.

Up to the middle of the last century all dyes were obtained from naturally occurring substances. The first dye to be synthesized, *mauve*, was prepared in 1856 in a private laboratory by the Englishman William Henry Perkin, then a lad only 18 years of age. The preparation, however, was quite unintentional. Perkin, working during his Easter vacation, was trying to prepare quinine by the oxidation of aniline. As sometimes happens to organic chemists he obtained a black tarry mass instead of the beautiful crystalline product he anticipated. He was washing out the tar with alcohol when he noted a violet color in the alcohol solution. It was an indication of his future greatness that the curiosity of this 18-year-old investigator led him to isolate the colored substance and to try it as a dye. He realized the commercial importance of his discovery and later he founded a profitable dye industry in England.

The discovery by Perkin that a dye could be made in the laboratory from substances that possess no color was the impetus for feverish attempts by organic chemists to synthesize other dyes. An important event in these attempts was Kekulé's announcement of the structural formula of benzene. Now there was some theoretical basis for aromatic chemistry. When Perkin discovered his dye, the structural formula for aniline was not even known. An indication of the influence of the development of the theoretical side of organic chemistry was the synthesis for the first time of a naturally occurring dye by Karl Graebe and Karl Liebermann in 1868. This dye, alizarin, had been obtained previously only from the madder root. Other chemists were working on a similar process. In fact, Graebe and Liebermann filed their patent application for a commercial method of manufacturing alizarin on June 25, 1869, one day before Perkin filed a patent application for the same process.

We have noted before that the development of color depends on the absorption of certain portions of visible light and the reflection of the remainder. It has been found that certain groupings must be present before compounds exhibit this phenomenon. These groups that cause the absorption of some light in the visible range and the reflection or transmission of that part which accordingly gives color to the compound are known as *chromophore groups*. Hence *a chromophore group can be defined as any group of atoms that gives color to a compound.* A few of the more important chromophore groups occurring in dyes are:

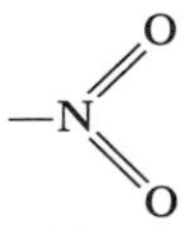

Nitro

—N=N—

Azo

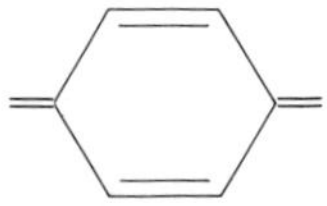
Quinoid

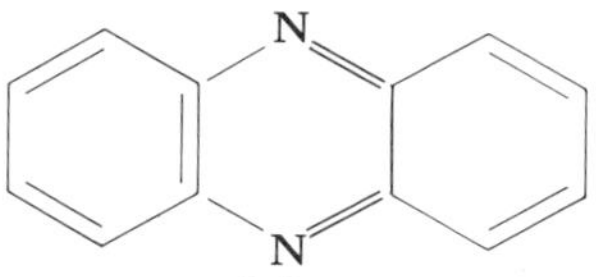

Azine

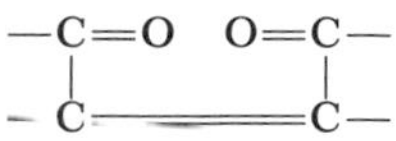

Indigoid

Not all colored compounds are dyes. The color must be capable of being permanently attached to the fiber, leather, or other solid material. In order for a substance to function as a dye it must contain *auxochrome* groups, which enable the dye to be fixed to the solid material. The auxochrome groups can be divided into two classes: the basic groups and the acidic groups. The basic groups are the primary amino group, —NH_2, the secondary amino group, —NHR, and the tertiary amino group, $-N\begin{matrix} R \\ R' \end{matrix}$. They deepen and intensify the color. The acidic groups, such as the carboxyl group, the sulfonic acid group, and the hydroxyl group, usually do not intensify the color. It will be noted that all the auxochrome groups are salt-forming groups and are important in rendering the dye soluble.

Representative formulas of dyes are:

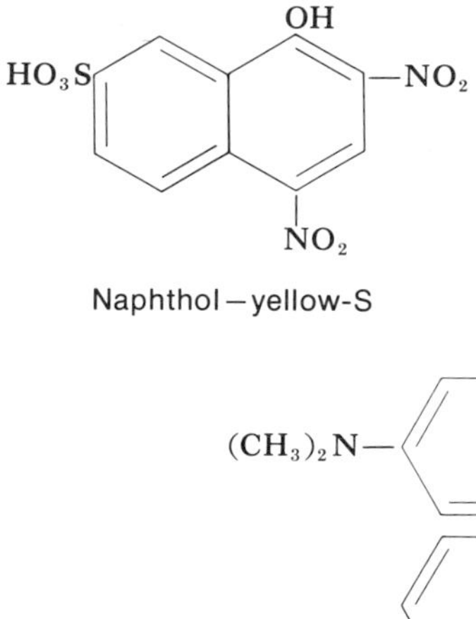

Naphthol–yellow-S

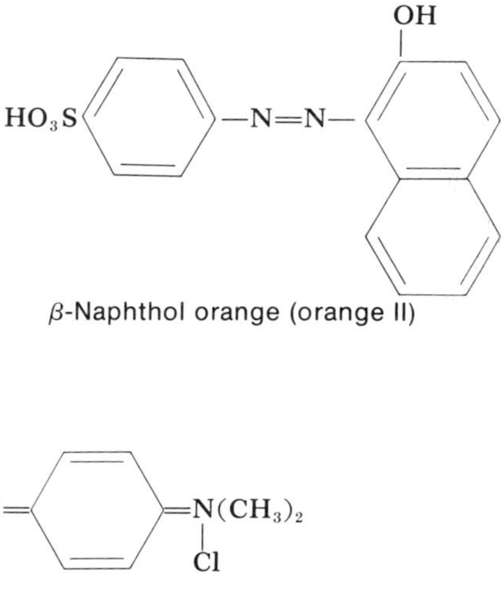

β-Naphthol orange (orange II)

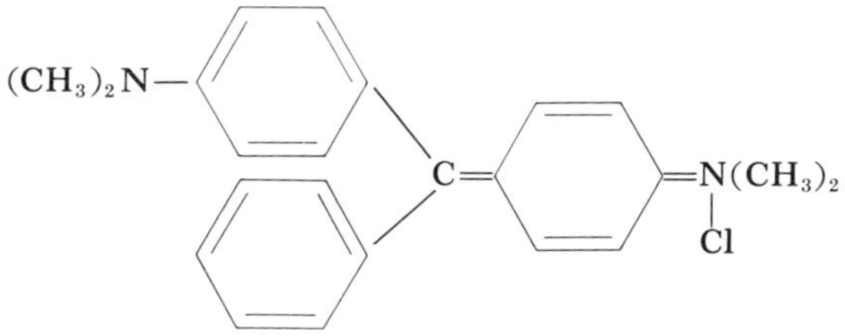

Malachite green

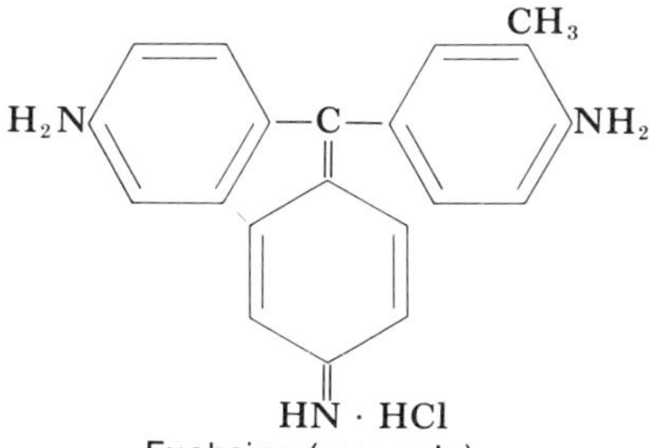

Fuchsine (magenta)

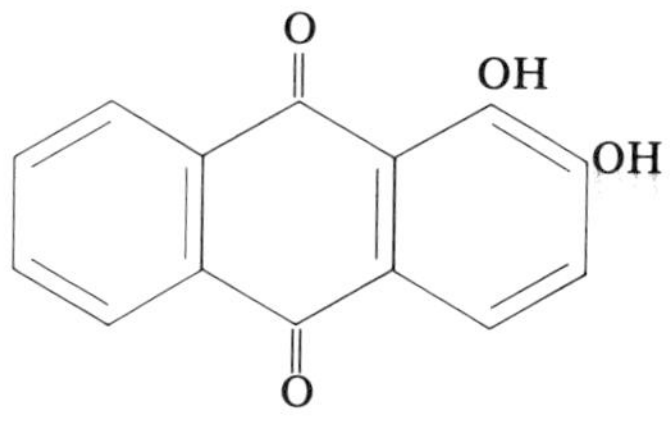

Alizarin

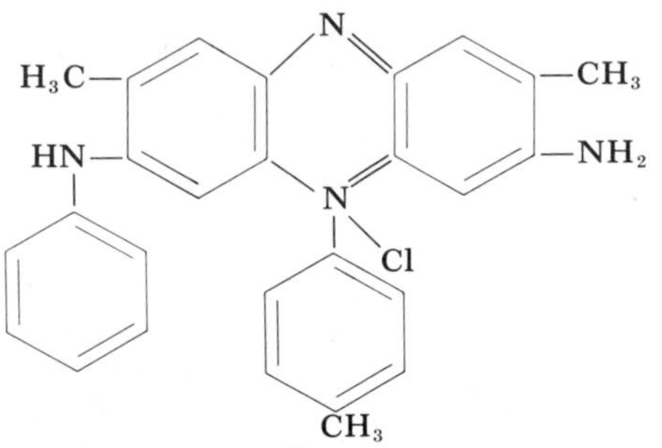

Mauve

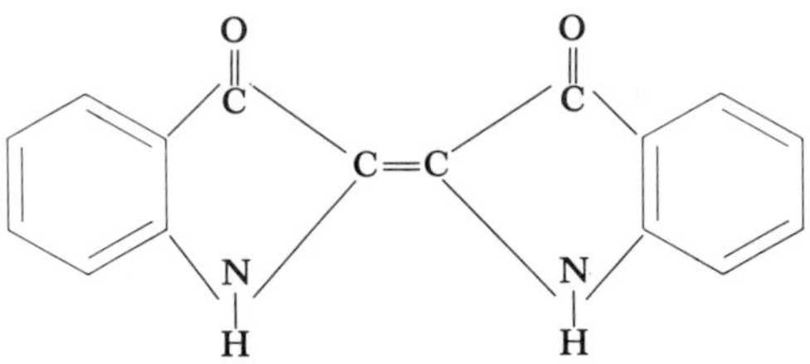

Indigo blue

HETEROCYCLIC COMPOUNDS

Most of the cyclic compounds studied thus far have contained only carbon atoms in the ring. These compounds often are called *homo*cyclic or *carbo*cyclic compounds. The class of compounds to be considered now contains atoms other than carbon in the ring structure; these compounds are termed *hetero*cyclic compounds. The prefix *hetero-* is derived from the Greek word meaning "other" or "different."

In the more common heterocyclic compounds the "hetero" atom is oxygen, sulfur, or nitrogen. In some cases phosphorus or selenium may act as the noncarbon atom in forming the ring. The more important heterocyclic compounds contain 5- or 6-membered rings, or contain these rings condensed with a benzene ring.

Heterocyclic compounds with five-membered rings

FURANE. The heterocyclic compound containing oxygen and 4 carbon atoms in the ring is known as furane.

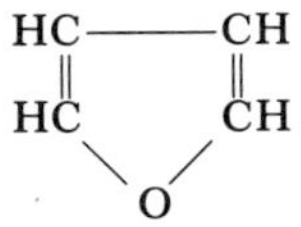

Furane

THIOPHENE. The sulfur analogue of furane is a compound called thiophene. It occurs along with benzene in coal tar.

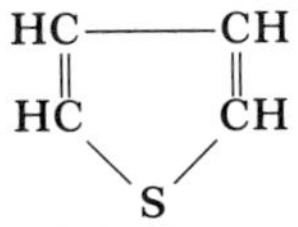

Thiophene

THIAZOLE. A heterocyclic compound containing both nitrogen and sulfur in a 5-membered ring is thiazole. One of the sulfonamide drugs (sulfathiazole) and vitamin B_1 (see page 422) contain the thiazole ring in their structures.

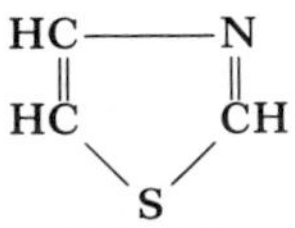

Thiazole

Penicillin is another compound containing a substituted thiazole ring. There are several useful forms of this compound. The first widely used penicillin was pencillin G.

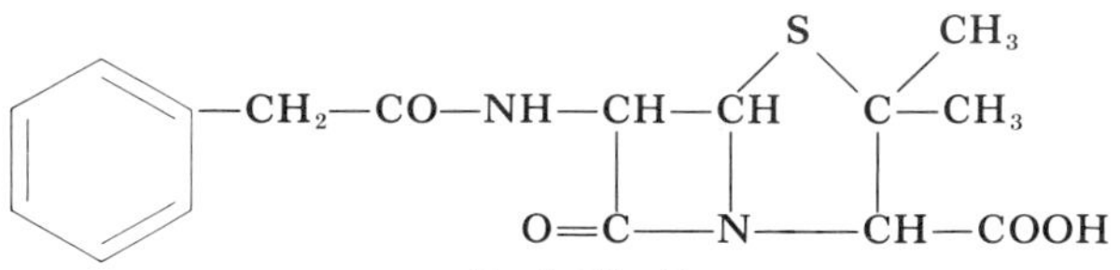

Penicillin G

PYRROLE. The 5-membered heterocyclic ring containing 1 nitrogen atom is known as pyrrole.

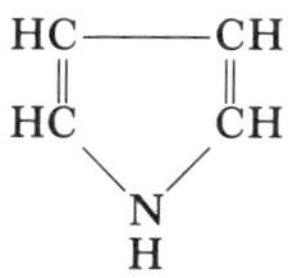

Pyrrole

Pyrrole is important since many natural products are complex derivatives of it. Important biological substances are hemoglobin, the red pigment of blood (see pages 277 and 288 for structure of heme); chlorophyll, the green pigment of plants; and bilirubin, a pigment of bile.

If a pinewood splint moistened in hydrochloric acid is held in the vapors of pyrrole, a fiery red color is produced. This is a characteristic reaction of pyrrole and is used for detecting the presence of the compound in unknown solutions. The word *pyrrole* is derived from Greek and Latin words meaning "fiery red."

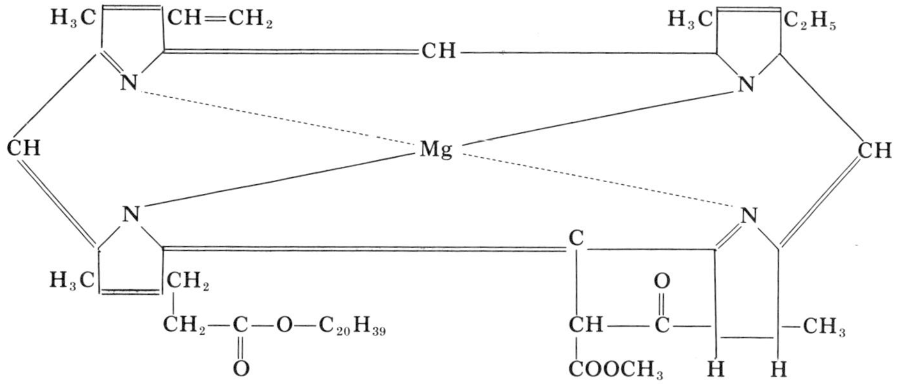

Chlorophyll a
(The dotted lines represent weak secondary chemical bonds.)

IMIDAZOLE. Another heterocyclic compound containing a 5-membered ring is imidazole. Histidine and histamine (page 292) contain this heterocyclic structure.

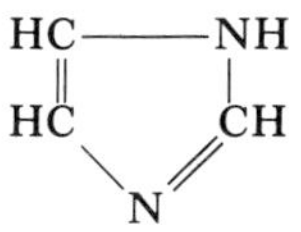

Imidazole

Heterocyclic compounds with six-membered rings

PYRIDINE. Pyridine can be thought of as benzene in which a CH group has been replaced by a nitrogen atom.

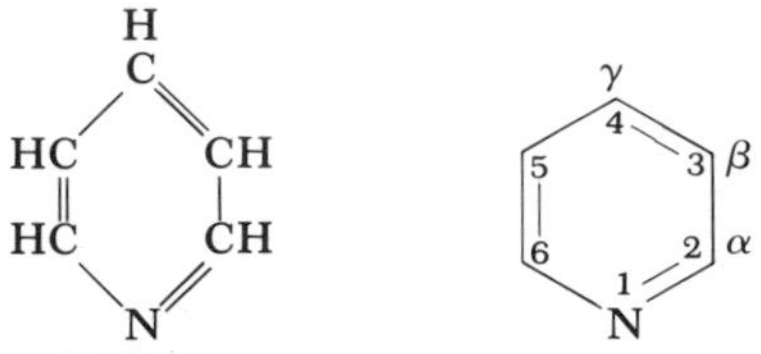

Pyridine

The numbering and positions in the ring are indicated by the numbers and Greek letters. This compound occurs in the middle oil fraction of coal tar.

Pyridine is very stable and for this reason often is used as a solvent in which other compounds react with each other. It is a tertiary amine and forms stable salts. It also reacts with alkyl halides to form quaternary compounds (see page 156) known as pyridinium derivatives. The higher alkylpyridinium salts, such as cetylpyridinium chloride,* are used as antiseptics.

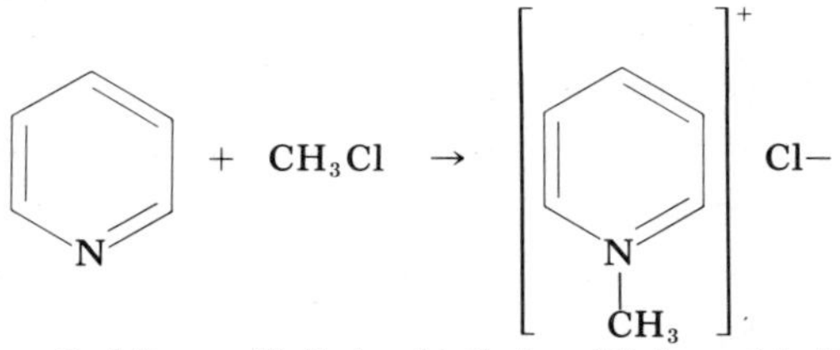

Pyridine Methyl chloride Methyl pyridinium chloride

On reduction with sodium and alcohol, pyridine combines with 6 atoms of hydrogen to form piperidine.

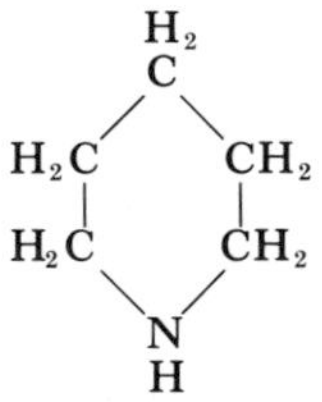

Piperidine

Piperidine was first obtained as a decomposition product of piperine, the alkaloid in pepper, from whence it obtained its name.

Heterocyclic compounds with condensed rings

INDOLE. The heterocyclic compound whose formula corresponds to a fusion of a benzene ring with pyrrole is known as *indole*.

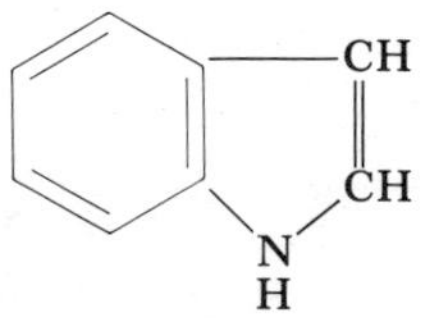

Indole

*The cetyl radical contains 16 carbon atoms.

Indole is formed in the intestinal tract as a result of bacterial putrefaction of undigested protein material, and is present in feces (see page 331). It also occurs in jasmine flower oil and in oil of orange blossoms. As ordinarily obtained it possesses an unpleasant fecal odor. Strangely enough, when it is purified and mixed in the desired dilution with other perfume ingredients, the odor of fresh flowers is imparted to the mixture.

Skatole, β-methylindole, is produced from the amino acid tryptophan in the intestinal tract (page 331). It has powerful repugnant odor.

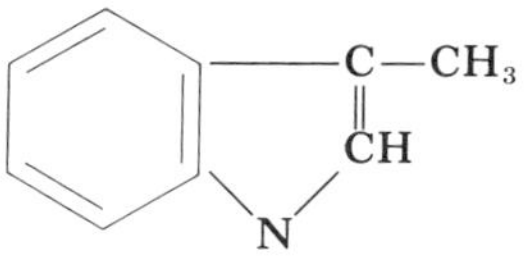

Skatole

QUINOLINE. From a structural viewpoint quinoline represents the fusion of pyridine with a benzene ring, the union being in the α-β-positions of the pyridine.

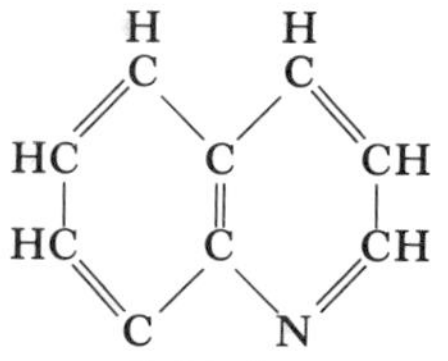

Quinoline

Quinoline is important because the antimalarial drugs quinine (see page 196) and plasmochin are derivatives of it.

Coumarin. Coumarin is a substance with the odor of new-mown hay. It is used in flavoring tobacco and in perfumery.

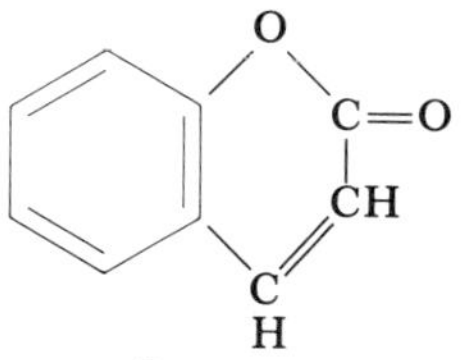

Coumarin

Other heterocyclic compounds

UREIDES. The reaction of urea with dicarboxylic acids (acids with 2 —COOH groups) leads to the formation of compounds known as ureides. As an example, the ureide of oxalic acid is formed by the reaction of urea and oxalyl chloride.

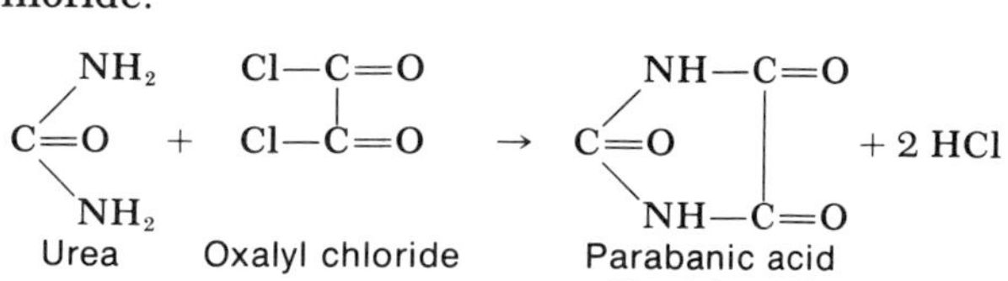

Urea Oxalyl chloride Parabanic acid (Oxalyl urea)

Of greater importance is the ureide of malonic acid, barbituric acid.

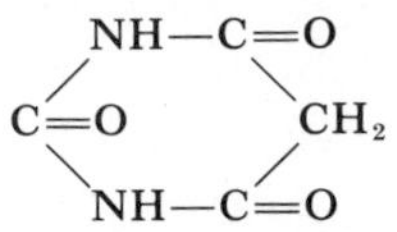

Barbituric acid
(Malonyl urea)

Barbituric acid is the parent substance for a number of important drugs used as sedatives and hypnotics. In 1903 Emil Fischer showed that diethylbarbituric acid, or barbital, was an excellent hypnotic. Since that time many other useful barbiturates (derivatives of barbital) have been made available as drugs.

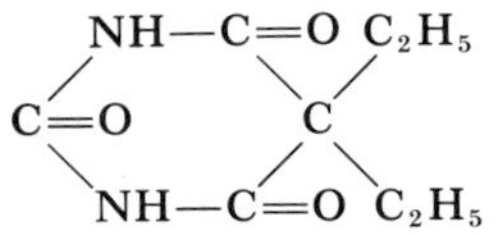

Barbital

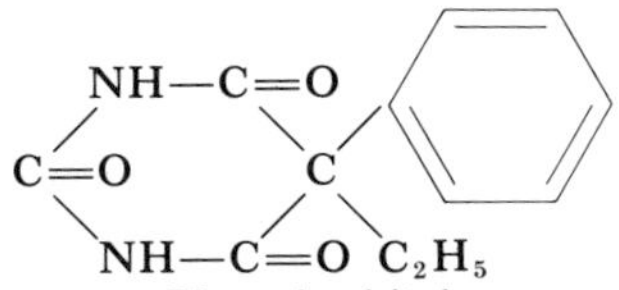

Phenobarbital

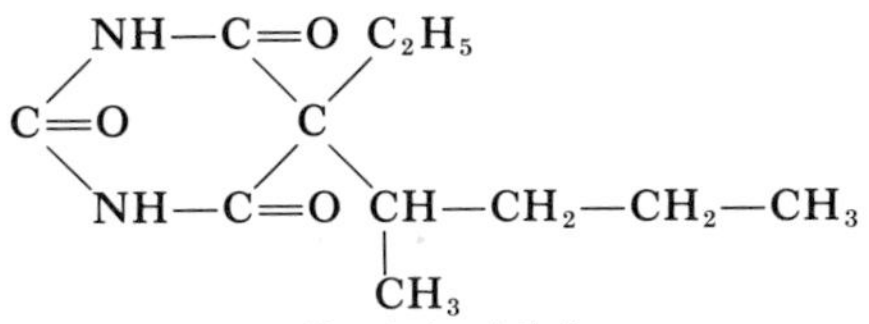

Pentobarbital

PYRIMIDINES. The cyclic structure present in barbituric acid and its derivatives is known as the pyrimidine nucleus. The simplest compound containing this nucleus is pyrimidine itself.

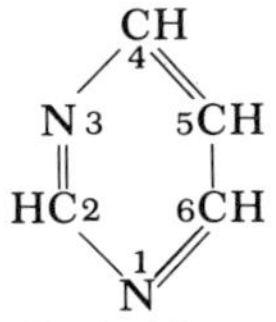

Pyrimidine

Derivatives of pyrimidine are of great importance since they occur in nucleic acids (see page 297). Those found in plants and animals are:

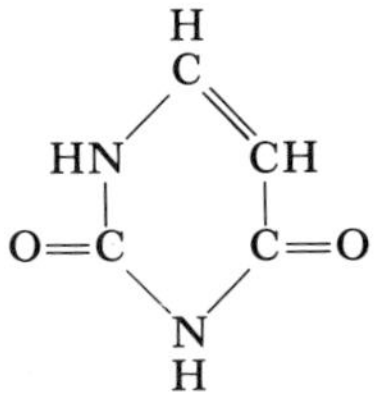

Uracil
(2,6-Dioxypyrimidine)

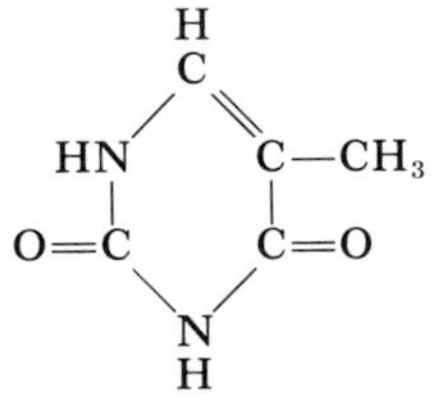

Thymine
(2,6-Dioxy-5-methylpyrimidine)

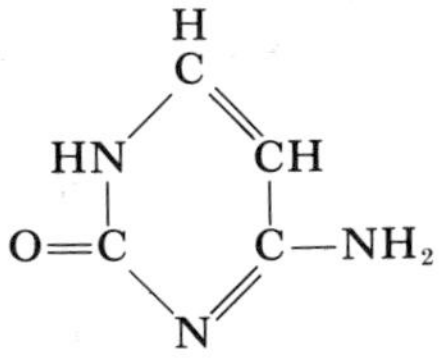

Cytosine
(2-Oxy-6-amino-pyrimidine)

Vitamine B_1, thiamine, contains a pyrimidine nucleus in its structure (see page 422).

PURINES. The purines also occur in nucleic acids. The parent substance is known simply as purine. It does not occur in nature.

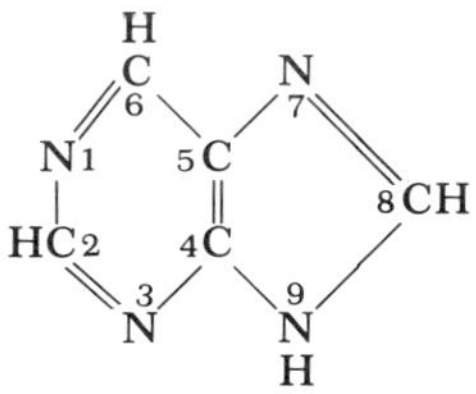

Purine

Guanine and adenine are the 2 purines that occur in nucleic acids. Xanthine, hypoxanthine, and uric acid are derived from these in the body (see page 313).

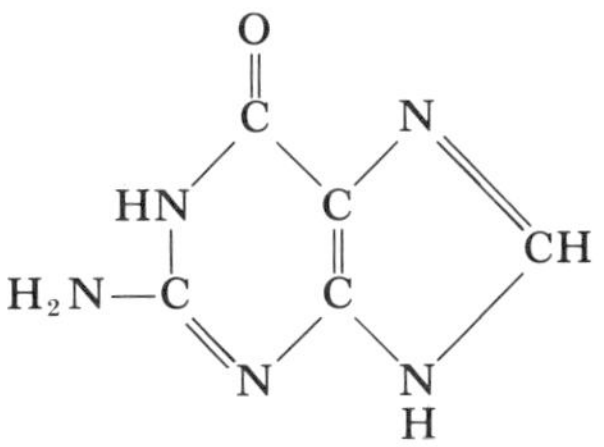

Guanine
(2-Amino-6-oxypurine)

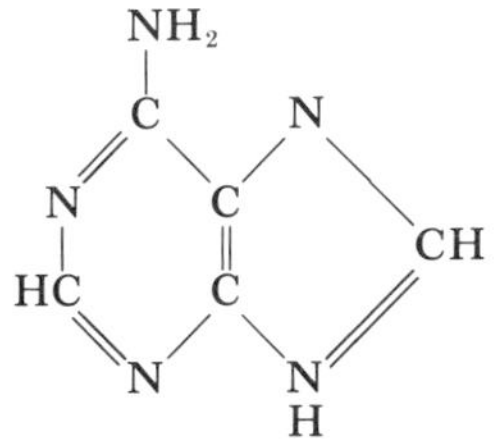

Adenine
(6-Aminopurine)

Three methyl purines are important in medicine. They are caffeine (1,3,7-trimethyl-2,6-oxypurine), theobromine (3,7-dimethyl-2,6-dioxypurine), and theophylline (1,3-dimethyl-2,6-dioxypurine). Caffeine occurs naturally in tea and in coffee. It stimulates the central nervous system and is a diuretic. Theobromine, theophylline, and their derivatives are used as mild diuretics, bronchodilators, and coronary vasodilators.

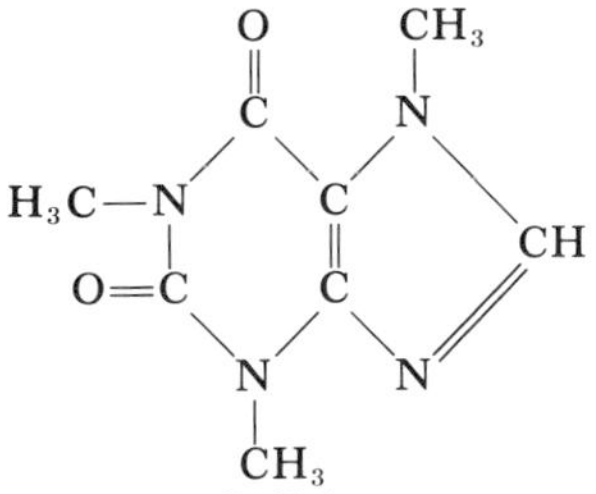

Caffeine

Alkaloids

Alkaloids are basic substances of plant origin that contain at least one nitrogen atom in a heterocyclic ring. Most of them are physiologically very active, and many of them are useful in medicine. As a rule alkaloids are present in plants as the salts of organic acids such as malic acid, tartaric acid, citric acid, oxalic acid, tannic acid, and succinic acid. A few of them are combined with a special acid. For example, quinine occurs as a salt of quinic acid, and morphine exists in the plant as a salt of meconic acid.

Most alkaloids are white crystalline solids that have bitter tastes, and most of them are insoluble in water. Nicotine is exceptional since it is a liquid and will dissolve in water. Berberine, formerly found in many proprietary brands of "eye drops," is yellow.

Nicotine is the principal alkaloid of tobacco. The pure compound is a colorless, oily liquid that dissolves in alcohol, ether, and water at room temperature. It is poisonous to man. Its principal use is in insect dusts and sprays used in orchards and gardens.

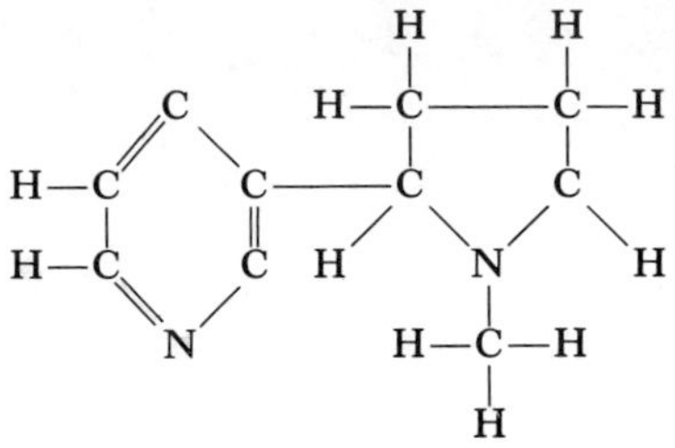

Nicotine

Cocaine is obtained from the leaves of the coca plant. It is a crystalline solid that is slightly soluble in cold water but is readily soluble in alcohol, ether, and benzene. It is used in medicine as a topical anesthetic. It has a stimulating effect when it is taken internally, but continued use of it leads to habit formation, mental deterioration, and insanity.

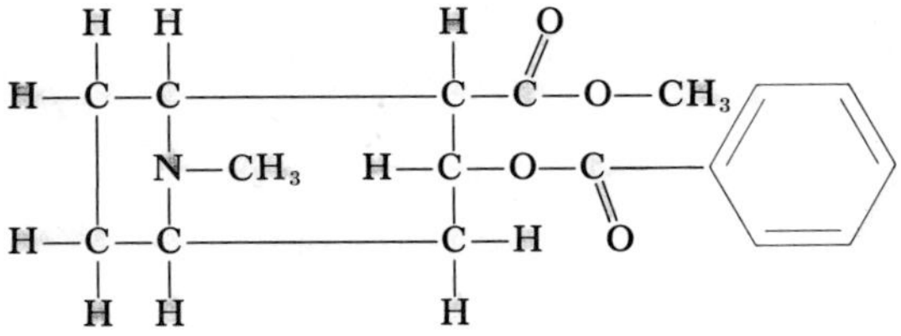

Cocaine

Atropine is found in the roots of the deadly nightshade. It is used as a mydriatic (drug that causes dilation of the pupil of the eye) and as an agent (antispasmodic) to combat cramping of the gastrointestinal tract. It also causes diminished secretion of saliva and mucus.

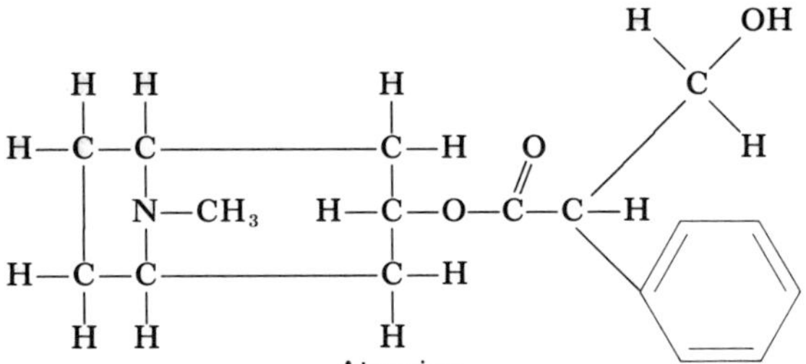

Atropine

Quinine is used in the treatment of malaria. It is obtained from the bark of the cinchona tree.

Morphine is the alkaloid that is responsible for much of the physiological activity of opium, which is obtained from the poppy plant. It was the first alkaloid to be isolated from plants. Morphine depresses the central nervous system and is used to abolish pain and to induce sleep. Continued use leads to addiction.

Codeine occurs also in opium. It can be prepared from morphine by the introduction of a methyl group into the morphine molecule.

Curare, an extract obtained from various plants used as arrow-tip poisons by

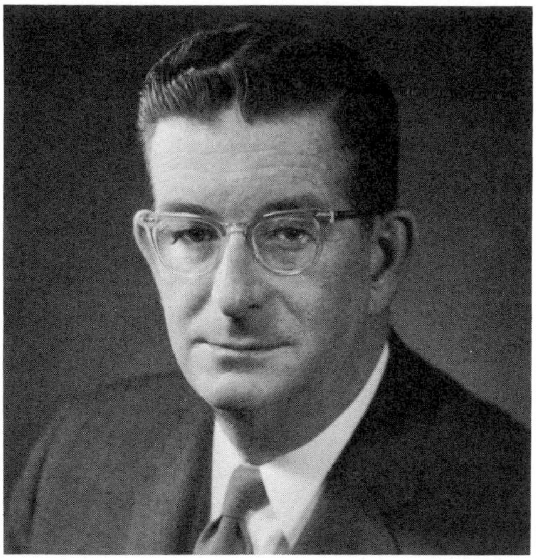

Fig. 19-1. Dr. Robert Burns Woodward of Harvard University received the Nobel Prize in Chemistry in 1965 for his "meritorious contributions to the art of chemical synthesis." He and his collaborators have synthesized a number of natural products, including quinine, patulin, cortisone, lysergic acid, cholesterol, strychnine, lanosterol, reserpine, colchicine, and chlorophyll. Also, they have worked out the molecular structures of strychnine, oxytetracycline, aureomycin, cevine, carbomycin, tetrodotoxin, and a number of other complex natural substances. What is an alkaloid?

certain South American Indians, contains several alkaloids, the most active of which is known as D-tubocurarine. A purified form of this extract now is employed in medicine. It causes muscular relaxation and is used along with the usual general anesthetics in surgery.

Strychnine is found in nux vomica seeds. It is highly toxic and in poisonous doses causes convulsions involving most of the muscles of the body. Larger doses cause paralysis. Sometimes it us used in very small dosage as a tonic.

STUDY QUESTIONS

1. Both propane and cyclopropane contain 3 carbon atoms; both are saturated hydrocarbons, yet the latter molecule contains 2 fewer hydrogen atoms than does the former molecule. How do you account for this seeming contradiction?
2. Define cycloparaffin. Naphthene.
3. What is the structure of cyclopropane? For what purpose is it used in medicine?
4. Explain what is meant by the term "homologous series."
5. What is the structure of cyclohexane?
6. Explain how an important branch of organic chemistry became known as "aromatic chemistry."
7. Write the structural formula for benzene. Give in your own words the evidence that this structure is correct.
8. Who first proposed the structural formula for benzene?
9. Is benzine the same as benzene?
10. Explain why only one monosubstituted derivative of benzene can be obtained with a given radical or element.
11. Name the three disubstituted products that can be formed by the reaction of chlorine and benzene.
12. What is meant by the statement that "benzene is a resonating hybrid"?
13. What are some uses of benzene?
14. Write formulas of compounds that could result from reactions of benzene with chlorine, nitric acid, or sulfuric acid.
15. What is the formula for toluene?
16. What is a use for trinitrotoluene?
17. Write formulas and names for the three isomers of xylene.

18. Write formulas for α-bromonaphthol and for β-bromonaphthol.
19. Explain why there are only two possible monochloro derivatives of naphthalene.
20. Write the chemical structure of mothballs.
21. Write chemical structures for anthracene and anthraquinone.
22. Why is phenanthrene important in physiological chemistry? What is its formula?
23. Name and write formulas for two aromatic alcohols.
24. What types of compound can be formed by the oxidation of aromatic alcohols?
25. How does a phenol differ structurally from an alcohol?
26. What is the structure of phenol?
27. What should be done if phenol is spilled on the skin?
28. What is carbolic acid?
29. Write an equation illustrating the reaction of phenol with an inorganic alkali.
30. What is the commercial use of pentachlorophenol?
31. What is meant by "mixed alkyl-aryl ether"? Write the structure for one of them.
32. Write the structural formula for picric acid.
33. Write equations and formulas illustrating the preparation of phenol-formaldehyde polymers. What are some uses of these polymers?
34. List a few uses of phenol.
35. Write structures and names for the three diphenols.
36. What is guaiacol? For what purpose has it been used in medicine?
37. What is hexylresorcinol? What is its use in medicine?
38. Write structures for pyrogallol and phlorglucinol. How does the enol form of phlorglucinol differ from the keto form?
39. How does the structure of α-naphthol differ from that of β-naphthol? Would it be possible to prepare a γ-naphthol? Explain.
40. Write names and formulas for the three isomers of cresol.
41. What is Lysol?
42. What is the structure of thymol? What are its uses?
43. Are the chemical reactions of the aromatic aldehydes similar to those of the aliphatic aldehydes?
44. Write the name and structure of the simplest aromatic aldehyde.
45. Write equations illustrating the conversion of benzaldehyde to benzoic acid.
46. What is vanillin? Cinnamic aldehyde?
47. Write formulas illustrating the two types of aromatic ketone.
48. Write the name and formula of a compound used as "tear gas."
49. How do quinones differ from aldehydes?
50. Write structures illustrating the two types of aromatic acid.
51. Write an equation illustrating the reaction between an aromatic acid and an inorganic base.
52. Name a use for sodium benzoate. What is its structure?
53. For what purpose is each of the following compounds used in medicine: salicylic acid; sodium salicylate; methyl salicylate; aspirin? Write structures for these compounds.
54. What is the source of gallic acid? What is its structure?
55. For what purpose is propyl gallate used?
56. What causes the change in color from blue to black when blue-black ink is applied to paper?
57. Write formulas for phthalic acid and phthalic anhydride.
58. For what purposes are alkyd resins used commercially?
59. Define the three types of aromatic amine.
60. What is the structure of aniline?
61. List a few physical and chemical properties of aniline.
62. What is an anilide? Write the structure of an anilide used as a drug.
63. Who should receive credit for the discovery of the sulfonamide drugs?
64. Write the formula for a sulfonamide drug. What is its name?
65. Write formulas illustrating the two types of secondary aromatic amine.
66. What is the meaning of the N in the name N-methylaniline?
67. Write formulas for the following tertiary aromatic amines: diethylaniline, phenylethylaniline, dibenzylaniline. (Clue: review structure of benzyl alcohol.)
68. Who first synthesized a dye? What was it?
69. How do you explain the production of color by a dye?
70. What is a chromophore group? List a few of them.
71. What is an auxochrome group? Name some of them.
72. How do heterocyclic compounds differ from carbocyclic compounds?
73. What does the prefix hetero- mean?
74. What elements other than carbon most commonly occur in heterocyclic rings?

75. How many atoms are present in most heterocyclic rings?
76. Write structures for the following compounds: furane, thiophene, thiazole.
77. What heterocyclic ring occurs in vitamin B_1?
78. Write the formula for penicillin G.
79. What is pyrrole? Why is it important?
80. Explain the derivation of the word pyrrole.
81. Name two substances of biological importance that contain the imidazole ring.
82. Write the structure for pyridine. List some of its properties.
83. Write a structure illustrating a pyridinium derivative.
84. What is piperidine?
85. Write formulas for indole and skatole. Where are they formed in the body?
86. What is a commercial use for indole? Why is this surprising?
87. Write formulas for quinoline and coumarin.
88. What is a ureide? Write the formula for a ureide not given in the text.
89. What is the structure for barbituric acid?
90. Why are barbiturates important in medicine?
91. Write formulas for the three pyrimidines found in nucleic acids. Name them.
92. What vitamin contains a pyrimidine nucleus in its structure?
93. Write names and formulas for the purines that occur in nucleic acid.
94. How does the purine structure differ from the pyrimidine structure?
95. Name three methyl purines that are used as drugs.
96. Define alkaloid. Name several alkaloids used in medicine.

part two
Physiological and pathological chemistry

CHAPTER **20**

Nature of enzymes

DEFINITIONS

Enzymes are the expert "chemists" that control and direct all the reactions that occur in the body. They may be defined as organic catalysts produced by living cells but independent of cells in their action. That is, an enzyme that has been isolated from the tissues will catalyze reactions in the test tube, even though no cells are present.

The substance undergoing chemical change in the presence of an enzyme is called the *substrate*, and the new substances present when the reaction reaches equilibrium are called *end products*. We have already observed that zymase, a mixture of enzymes present in yeast, catalyzes the change whereby glucose forms alcohol and carbon dioxide. Here glucose is the substrate and alcohol and carbon dioxide are the end products.

CHEMICAL NATURE OF ENZYMES

Enzymes are proteins (see page 268). Proteins are composed of a number of smaller molecules known as amino acids linked chemically together to form long (on the molecular scale) chains. Some proteins consist of a single chain. In others, there are 2 or more chains bound to each other by chemical cross linkages.

Each enzyme molecule is coiled in 3-dimensional space and has a characteristic surface. Some of the atoms on this surface are so arranged that a substrate or substrates readily combine loosely with a particular region of the surface. Thus, two molecules may so combine and be brought closely together. Under these circumstances they react with each other to form new substances. The new substances break away from the enzyme, and the enzyme can then attract more substrate molecules. This process can be repeated many times, because the enzyme itself is not changed; it is a true catalyst (see page 17).

Many enzymes have been isolated in pure crystalline form. A few of them are listed in Table 20-1.

SPEED OF ENZYME ACTION

Some factors that affect the speed of enzyme action are concentration of the enzyme, temperature, and pH.

CONCENTRATION OF THE ENZYME. The speed of chemical reactions catalyzed by enzymes varies with the concentration of enzyme present. That is, if we increase the amount of enzyme, the speed of the reaction that it catalyzes will also be increased even though the amount of substrate present has not been changed.

TEMPERATURE. It will be remembered that the speed of chemical reactions is increased two or three times for each 10° C rise in temperature. This is true also for reactions catalyzed by enzymes. However, we cannot raise the temperature too high because if we do, the enzyme will be made insoluble and its catalytic action will cease. The highest temperature at which an enzyme will act without danger of becoming inactive is called the *optimum temperature*. Many of the enzymes in the body have optimum temperatures ranging between 37° C and 50° C.

pH. For every enzyme there is a pH value at which the enzyme is most efficient as a catalyst. This pH value is called the *optimum pH* for the enzyme. If the pH value is too far removed from this optimum point, the enzyme will have no catalytic effect at all. For example, the optimum pH for pepsin, an enzyme found in the stomach, is about pH 2 when the substrate is food protein. If the pH is above 4 or below 0.1, pepsin has little or no activity.

ENZYME SPECIFICITY

Enzymes are said to be *specific*. This means that any given enzyme catalyzes chemical change for only one type of substrate. Catalase, which catalyzes the breakdown of hydrogen peroxide to form water and oxygen, will not catalyze the hydrolysis of fats. Pancreatic lipase, an enzyme that catalyzes the hydrolysis of fats, has no effect on the rate of breakdown of hydrogen peroxide.

PROENZYMES

Substances that are not enzymes when they are first made in the body cells but that become enzymes when they come in contact with some other substance are called *proenzymes*. The cells of the stomach secrete a proenzyme called pepsinogen. When pepsinogen comes in contact with the hydrochloric acid of the gastric juice, it is changed to the active enzyme pepsin. Trypsinogen is a proenzyme made in the pancreas. This proenzyme reacts with a substance secreted by the glands of the duodenum (first part of the small intestine) called enterokinase and is changed to trypsin, an enzyme. Substances that convert proenzymes to enzymes are often called *kinases*.

ACTIVATORS

Substances that are necessary for optimal activity of enzymes are known as *activators* or *accelerators*. *Metalloenzymes*, for example, contain a metal atom that is firmly bound chemically to the enzyme molecule. It cannot be removed by dialysis (see page 63). If it is removed chemically, the enzyme is not active.

Other enzymes are either not active at all, or are not maximally active, in the absence of specific metal ions. The most important of these ions are Na^+, K^+, Mg^{++}, Ca^{++}, Zn^{++}, Mn^{++}, Fe^{++}, Co^{++}, and Ni^{++}. In some cases, at least, the ion acts as a link between the surface of the enzyme and the sub-

Table 20-1. Some enzymes that have been crystallized from tissue

Crystalline enzymes	Substrates	End products
Urease	Urea	Ammonium carbonate
Pepsin	Proteins	Proteoses and peptones
Trypsin	Proteins, proteoses, and peptones	Peptides
Catalase	Hydrogen peroxide	Water and oxygen

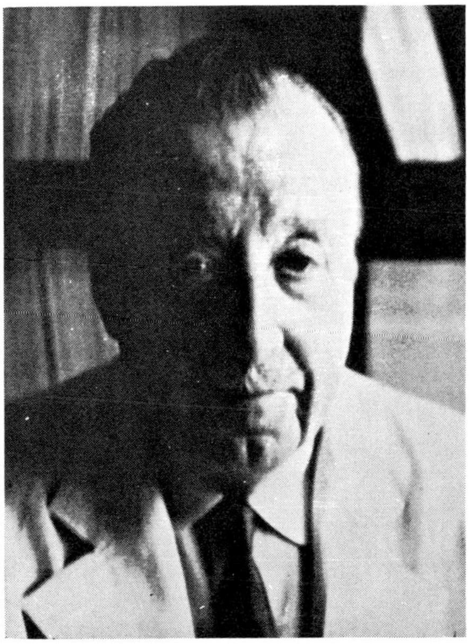

Fig. 20-1. Dr. John H. Northrop, Professor Emeritus of the Rockefeller Institute and now at the University of California, received the Nobel Prize in chemistry in 1946 in recognition of his pioneering work in the purification and crystallization of enzymes. Two other biochemists shared the award with Dr. Northrop. They were Dr. James B. Sumner (now deceased), who first crystallized an enzyme (urease), and Dr. Wendell M. Stanley, who first crystallized a virus. When the crystallization of urease was announced in 1926, many biochemists would not accept the hypothesis that enzymes were proteins. The careful, beautiful work of Dr. Northrop and his associates played a major role in establishing this concept. Today dozens, perhaps hundreds, of enzymes, all of which have been proteins, have been purified. Name two types of enzyme.

strate or substrates. Thus, the distinction between a true metalloenzyme and an enzyme that requires a metallic ion activator is only one of degree, depending on the firmness of the attachment of the ion to the enzyme.

Anions also may act as activators. It is believed that they may act by altering the degree of ionization of combined atoms in the protein surface. Amylase, an enzyme that catalyzes the hydrolysis of starch, is activated by Cl^-, Br^-, or NO_3^-. Fumarase, an enzyme that catalyzes the reaction between fumaric acid and water to form malic acid, is activated by citrate, phosphate, or arsenate ions.

Occasionally metallic ions may inhibit enzyme activity. Addition of a chemical that removes the inhibiting ion often will "activate" the enzyme.

COENZYMES

Some enzymes have a nonprotein organic group as a part of their molecules. If it is removed, the enzyme is inactivated. This group, in combined or noncombined state, is known as a *coenzyme*. In most cases, a part of the coenzyme molecule is one of the water-soluble vitamins (see Chapter 33). Indeed, these vitamins owe their biological activities to their roles as necessary constituents of enzymes.

The protein portion of enzymes that contain coenzymes or metals in their active structure is known as the *apoenzyme*. The active enzyme, containing the metal or coenzyme, is the *holoenzyme*.

INHIBITION OF ENZYMES

Since all enzymes are proteins, any substance or procedure that destroys proteins or modifies drastically their normal 3-dimensional structures will permanently inactivate them. Thus, exposure to heat, extremes of pH, x-rays, ultraviolet radiant energy, very high pressures, certain sound waves, and violent mechanical shaking will cause permanent inactivation.

Oxidizing agents, substances that precipitate proteins (see page 275), and some heavy metal ions react chemically with enzymes and inactivate them.

Obviously, chemical agents that react with substrates, activators, or coenzymes will inhibit enzymic activity. For example, cyanides, sodium azide (NaN_3), H_2S, and CO effectively inhibit metalloenzymes, especially those containing iron, copper, or zinc.

Many proteins, including enzymes, contain —SH groups, and agents that react with these groups often inhibit activity of enzymes.

In all of the cases mentioned above, the inactivation is permanent. This type of inactivation often is referred to as *noncompetitive inhibition*. In other cases, enzyme activity may be inhibited in such a way that activity can be restored by appropriate treatment. This type of inactivation is *competitive inhibition*.

For example, the enzyme creatine phosphokinase requires Mg^{++}, Mn^{++}, or Ca^{++} for maximal activity. Zn^{++} can combine with this enzyme and, if it does, will inhibit activity. This inhibition occurs because the sites where the activator ions can combine are occupied by the nonactive zinc ion. If, however, a high concentration of activator ion is provided, this ion will replace the Zn^{++}, and the enzyme will become active. In other words, Zn^{++} ions (which are *not* activators) compete with Mg^{++}, Mn^{++}, and Ca^{++} ions (which *are* activators).

Organic substances that are similar chemically to substrates may combine with an enzyme. Since this interferes with the combination of the true substrate with the enzyme, activity is inhibited. Increasing the concentration of the substrate often will displace the inhibiting compound, thus restoring activity. For example, the malonate ion will attach itself to the surface of the enzyme succinic dehydrogenase. The true substrate, succinic acid, thus cannot be activated by the enzyme unless enough of it is present to displace the malonate.

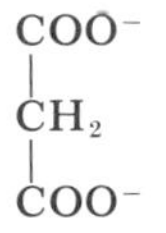

Malonate ion

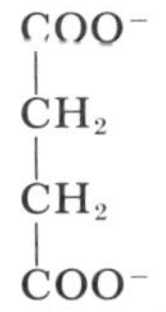

Succinate ion

One of two optical enantiomorphs (see page 166) often acts as a competitive inhibitor of the enzyme for which the other optically active substance is the substrate.

In some cases, compounds related chemically to the water-soluble vitamins will combine chemically with an apoenzyme (see page 206), thus preventing the union of the apoenzyme with its normal coenzyme to form the holoenzyme. A number of these *antivitamins* have been synthesized and tested biologically. It was hoped that they might inhibit an essential enzyme in pathogenic bacteria and thus act as chemotherapeutic agents. Unfortunately, although some of them did inhibit bacterial growth, they also inhibited essential enzyme activity in animals and humans and were highly toxic. Some of them are used in the desperate attempt to inhibit the growth of cancer. Cancer cells multiply more rapidly than do normal tissue cells, and the physician who uses antivitamins as therapeutic agents attempts to give just the right amount to cause some inhibition of cancer growth with minimal toxicity to the patient.

NOMENCLATURE

The word enzyme means "in leaven" or "in yeast." The name was coined by Kuhne in 1878. In 1898, Duclaux proposed that an enzyme be named by adding the last 3 letters of diastase (which had become a name for yeast enzymes) to a root indicating the substrate or the nature of the reaction catalyzed. Thus succinase is an enzyme for which succinate is the substrate. A dehydrogenase is an enzyme that catalyzes the removal of hydrogen (oxidation) from the substrate.

In 1961 the Commission on Enzymes of the International Union of Biochemists recommended nomenclature based both on the substrate and the type of reaction catalyzed. For example, succinic dehydrogenase is an enzyme that catalyzes the oxidation (removal of hydrogen from) the substrate, succinic acid.

CLASSIFICATION OF ENZYMES

The Commission on Enzymes of the International Union of Biochemists also adopted the following classification of enzymes:

1. *Oxidoreductases*, which catalyze oxidation-reduction reactions. Example: glucose-6-phosphate dehydrogenase catalyzes the oxidation of glucose-6-phosphate.

2. *Transferases*, which catalyze the transfer of a characteristic chemical group from one molecule to another. Example: glutamic oxalacetic aminopherase (transferase), which catalyzes the transfer of an amino group from glutamic acid to oxalacetic acid (see page 364).

3. *Hydrolases*, which catalyze reactions in which the substrate reacts with water (hydrolysis). Example: choline esterase, which catalyzes the

reaction of acetylcholine with water to yield acetic acid and choline. The digestive enzymes (see Chapter 28) are hydrolases.

4. *Isomerases,* most of which catalyze interconversions involving aldoses (sugars containing aldehyde groups, see page 242) and ketoses (sugars containing ketone groups).

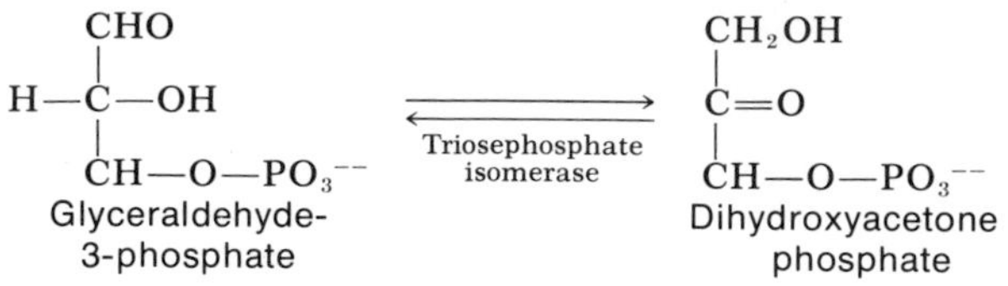

5. *Lyases,* which catalyze reactions in which a group is removed from the substrate in such a way that the substrate is converted to a compound having a double bond. (The reverse reaction also is catalyzed.)

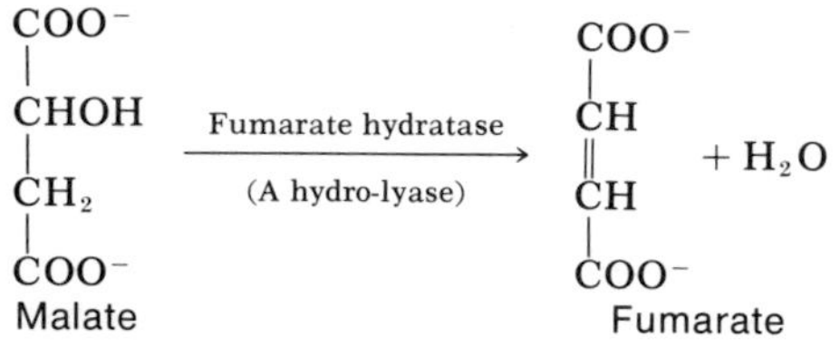

6. *Legases (synthetases),* which catalyze the coupling of 2 molecules of substrate with the simultaneous breakdown of adenosine triphosphate (see page 209) or a similar triphosphate.

OXYGENASES

These enzymes catalyze the direct interaction of gaseous oxygen with organic molecules. They participate in numerous catabolic and anabolic reactions (see page 228) in the body. They are involved also in the metabolic disposal of a number of drugs and foreign substances that gain entrance into the body. Iron is involved in most of these reactions, and iron-bound oxygen may represent an "activated" form of oxygen.

TEST FOR BLOOD. Hemoglobin, an important blood protein, can act as a peroxidase; and we often make use of this fact in testing for the presence of blood. Benzidine, an aromatic compound, forms a compound having a blue-green color when it is oxidized. Hydrogen peroxide, H_2O_2, is an oxidizing agent, but it is too weak to oxidize benzidine. If we mix a benzidine solution and a solution of hydrogen peroxide, we do not see any change. If, however, we add some blood (or a fluid containing blood) to the benzidine–hydrogen peroxide mixture a deep blue-green color appears. The peroxidase (hemoglobin or one of its derivatives) present in the blood has catalyzed the reaction between the benzidine and the hydrogen peroxide, and the benzidine has been oxidized. Less than one part of blood in 10,000 parts of water can be detected by this method.

THE ENERGY POWER PLANT OF ANIMAL CELLS

As we shall learn later, plant cells get their energy from sunlight, through a mechanism known as photosynthesis. Animal cells, however, must be provided with food (carbohydrates, fats, proteins) and derive the energy required to carry out the many functions of life by oxidizing these foods. This process, which requires molecular oxygen and produces carbon dioxide and water as end products, is referred to as *respiration.*

Most of the available energy in living cells is stored in the form of a compound known as adenosine triphosphate (ATP). This is a complex substance made up of adenine (see page 298), ribose (sec page 298), and three phosphate radicals. The terminal phosphate radical is attached by an energy-rich bond; when this bond is hydrolyzed, and the terminal phosphate radical is released from ATP (usually to be attached to a substrate molecule), large amounts of energy are released. Conversely, the same amount of energy is required to form ATP. The compound known as adenosine diphosphate (ADP) is formed when ATP loses its energy-rich phosphate radical.

$$ATP \rightleftarrows ADP + P + Energy$$

ATP, then, may be regarded as the cell's "charged" form of energy carrier, and ADP as the "discharged" form.

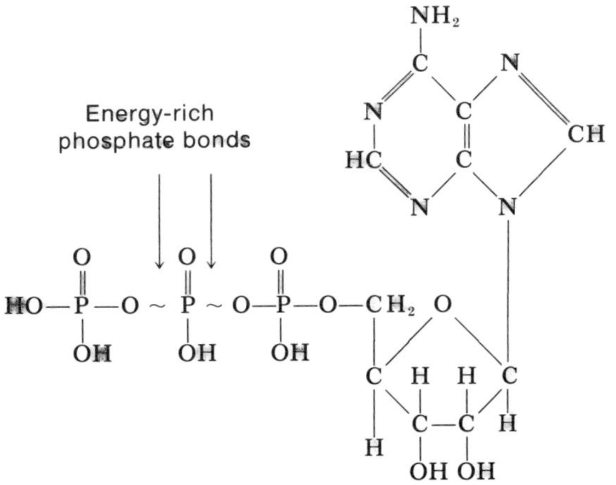

ATP
(ADP lacks the terminal phosphate radical.)

The generation of ATP in the cell involves the interaction of two important series of reactions. One series is known as the *Krebs cycle, citric acid cycle,* or *tricarboxylic acid cycle* (see page 259). Each of the reactions of this cycle is catalyzed by a specific enzyme. The other group of reactions involves the passage of electrons along a chain of complex molecules, at the end of which they, together with hydrogen ions, reduce molecular oxygen to water.

$$O_2 + 4H^+ + 4e \rightarrow 2H_2O$$

These two systems are located close to each other in a cellular structure known as a *mitochondrion*. Cells may contain from 50 to 50,000 mitochondria. They can be seen with the ordinary light microscope, but the fine structural details can be observed only with the electron microscope.

As illustrated in Fig. 20-2, the mitochondrion is sausage shaped. It has an outer and an inner membrane separated by a watery fluid. A number of

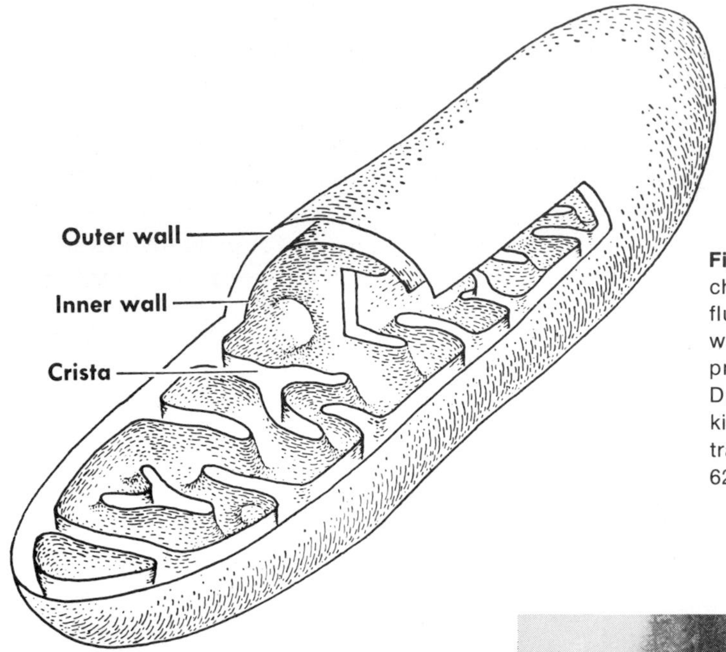

Fig. 20-2. The structure of a mitochondrion is basically that of a fluid-filled vessel with an involuted wall. How many mitochondria are present in a single cell? (Courtesy Dr. Albert L. Lehninger, Johns Hopkins University; from How cells transform energy, Sci. Amer. **205:** 62, Sept. 1961.)

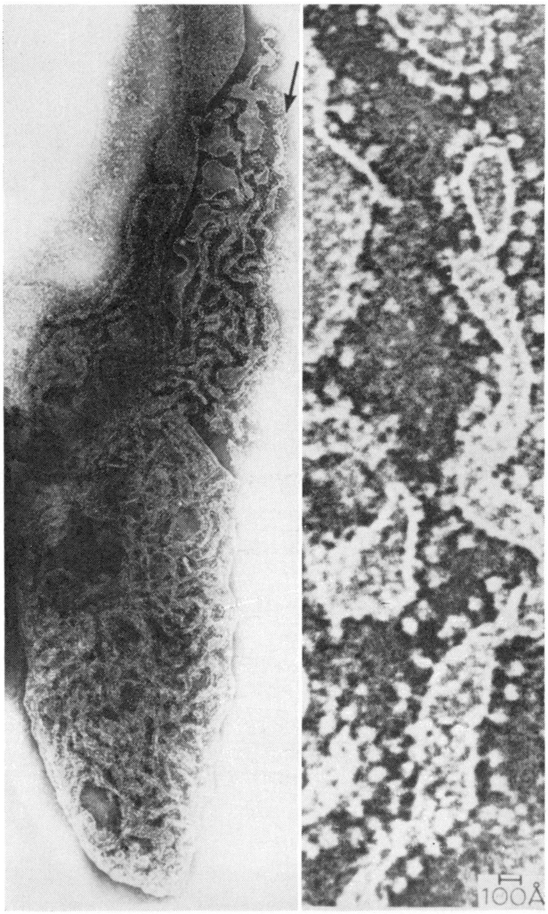

Fig. 20-3. Electron photomicrograph of a longitudinal cross section of a beef heart mitochondrion. What is the function of the mitochondrion? (Courtesy Dr. H. Fernandez-Moran, University of Chicago; from Green, D. E.: The mitochondrion, Sci. Amer. **210:**67, Jan. 1964.)

sacs called cristae extend from the inner membrane into the interior of the mitochondrion. Sprinkled over the surfaces of both membranes are thousands of small particles. Each of these particles is an elementary unit containing enzymes that carry out the chemical activities of the structure. Necessary coenzymes are present in the fluids between the membranes and serve to connect the two major oxidation-reduction enzyme systems already mentioned. The reactions that supply electrons (oxidation of glucose and the Krebs cycle reactions) occur in the particles located on the outer membrane. Particles attached to the inner membrane, and extending inward on short stalks, transfer the electrons along a chain of complexes, forming ATP in the process and finally reducing molecular oxygen to water.

The membranes of the mitochondrion are composed of protein, 80 percent, and of phospholipid, 20 percent. (See pages 268 and 220 for definitions of protein and phospholipid.)

The acetyl derivative of coenzyme A (CoA) is required as a link between the food to be oxidized and the Krebs cycle. On hydrolysis, CoA yields pantothenic acid (a vitamin; see page 435), adenine (see page 195), ribose (see page 298), phosphoric acid, and mercaptoethanolamine ($NH_2 \cdot CH_2 \cdot CH_2 \cdot SH$).

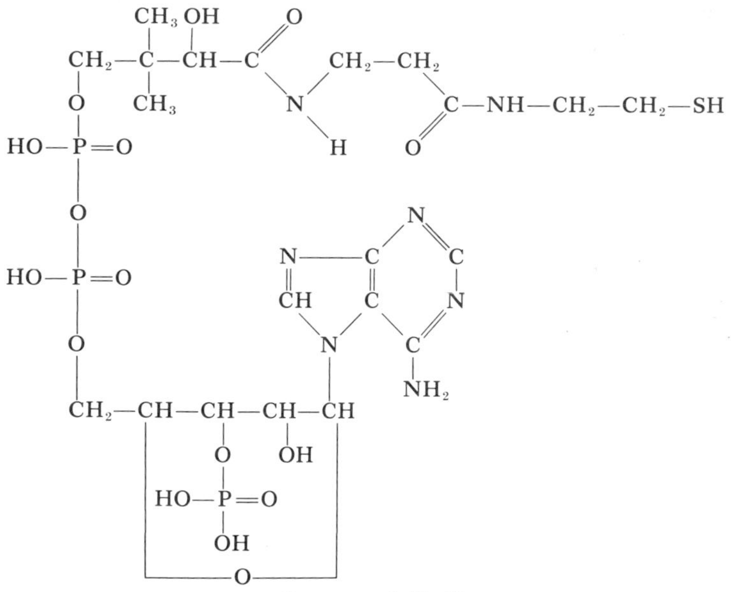

Coenzyme A (CoA)
(In acetyl CoA, the acetyl group is attached to the sulfur atom.)

The electrons formed on the outer membrane of the mitochondrion are carried across to the inner membrane by a coenzyme known as nicotinamide adenine dinucleotide phosphate (NAD^+). This coenzyme is alternatively reduced and oxidized as it transfers the electrons. (See page 425 for discussion of nicotinamide.)

$$NAD^+ + H^+ + 2e \rightleftharpoons NADH \text{ (reduced form)}$$

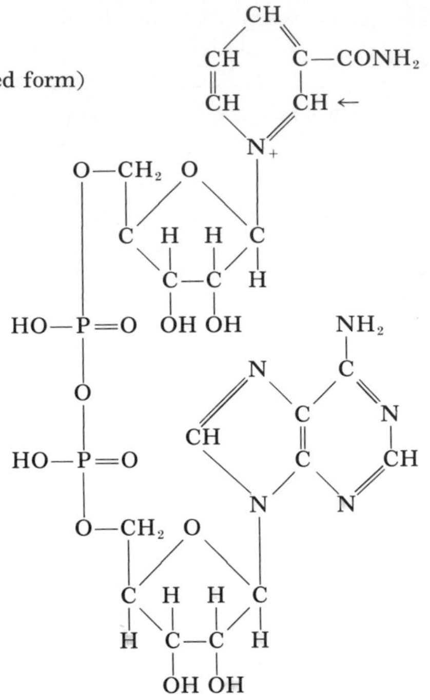

NAD+

(In NADH* the carbon atom indicated by the small arrow has one more H atom, with abolition of the double bond between this carbon and the nitrogen, and loss of the extra positive charge of the nitrogen.)

The chain of substances that conveys the electrons along (with the formation of ATP) is grouped into 4 complexes that contain 11 components, 10 of which are proteins. Another coenzyme (Q) serves to connect certain complexes (see Fig. 20-4). An iron-containing substance (a conjugated protein; see page 268) known as cytochrome C also exists in the chain. The

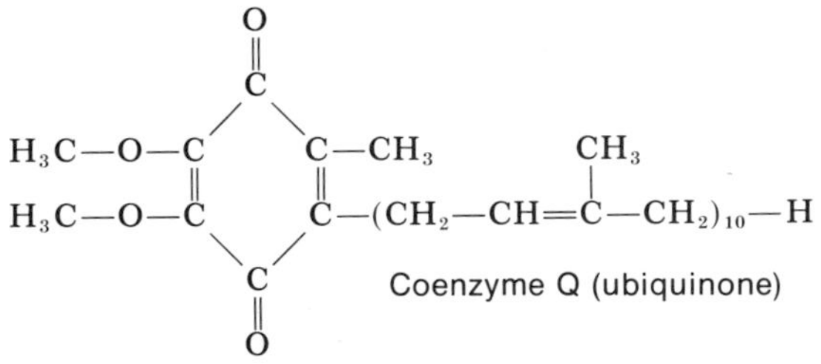

Coenzyme Q (ubiquinone)

(The number of $-(CH_2-CH=\underset{CH_3}{\underset{|}{C}}-CH_2)-$ groups (isoprenoid units) is 10 in mammalian coenzyme Q; it may be 6, 7, 8, or 9 in material isolated from bacterial sources.)

*2H are involved in the reduction of NAD^+. However, only one of these actually is added to the NAD^+ molecule; the other is used to combine with, or neutralize, the anion associated with the positively charged N. If, for example, this is OH^-, the reaction becomes: $H^+ + OH^- \rightarrow H_2O$. An older abbreviation for NAD^+ was DPN^+ (diphosphopyridine nucleotide).

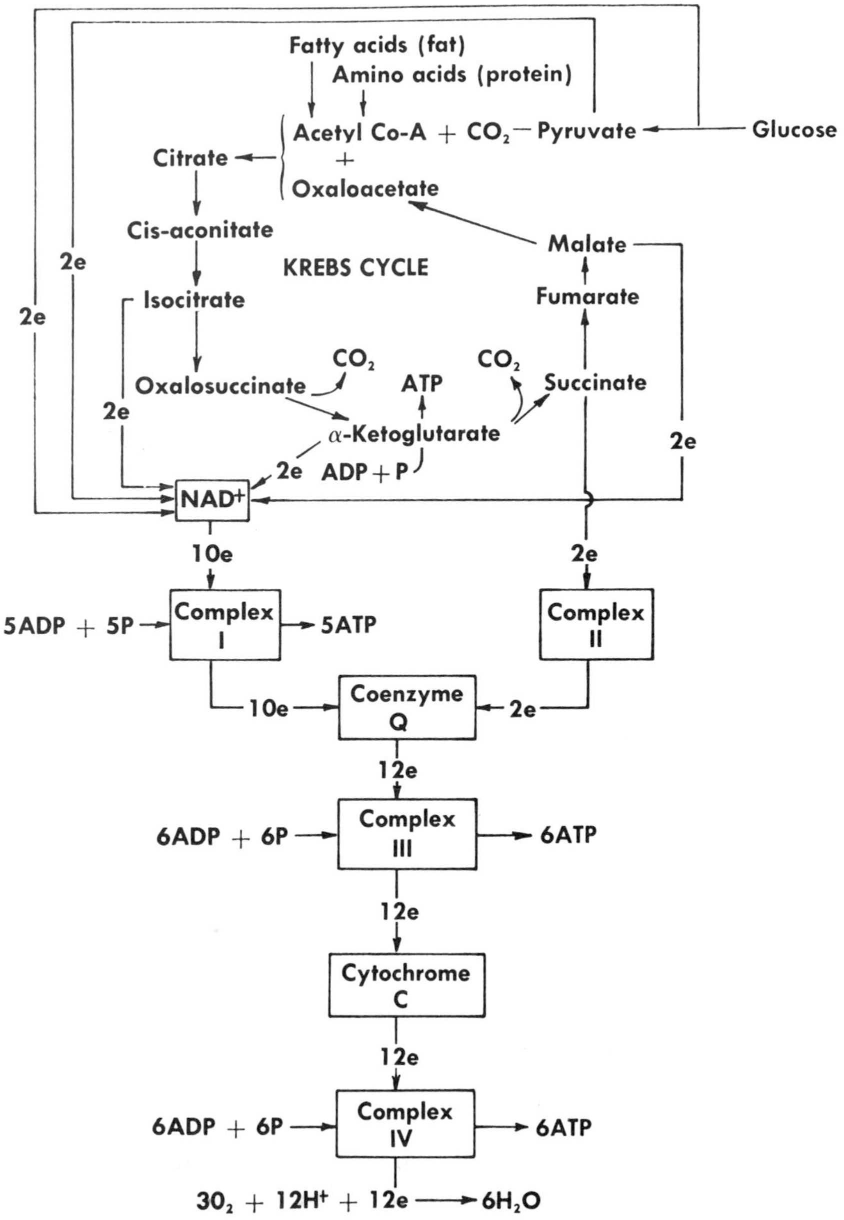

Fig. 20-4. Diagram illustrating the chain of reactions that takes place in the mitochondrion. How many ATP molecules are contributed by the Krebs cycle portion of the scheme? How many by the electron-transport system? (Drawing by James Skillman.)

scheme is illustrated in Fig. 20-4. Note that only one ATP molecule is contributed by the Krebs cycle portion of the scheme for each pyruvic acid molecule oxidized; the electron-transport system provides 17. Since 1 molecule of glucose yields 2 molecules of pyruvic acid, the oxidation of 1 molecule of this sugar yields 36 ATP molecules.

It will be observed that the end products produced are CO_2 (in the Krebs cycle) and H_2O (at the end of the electron-transport chain).

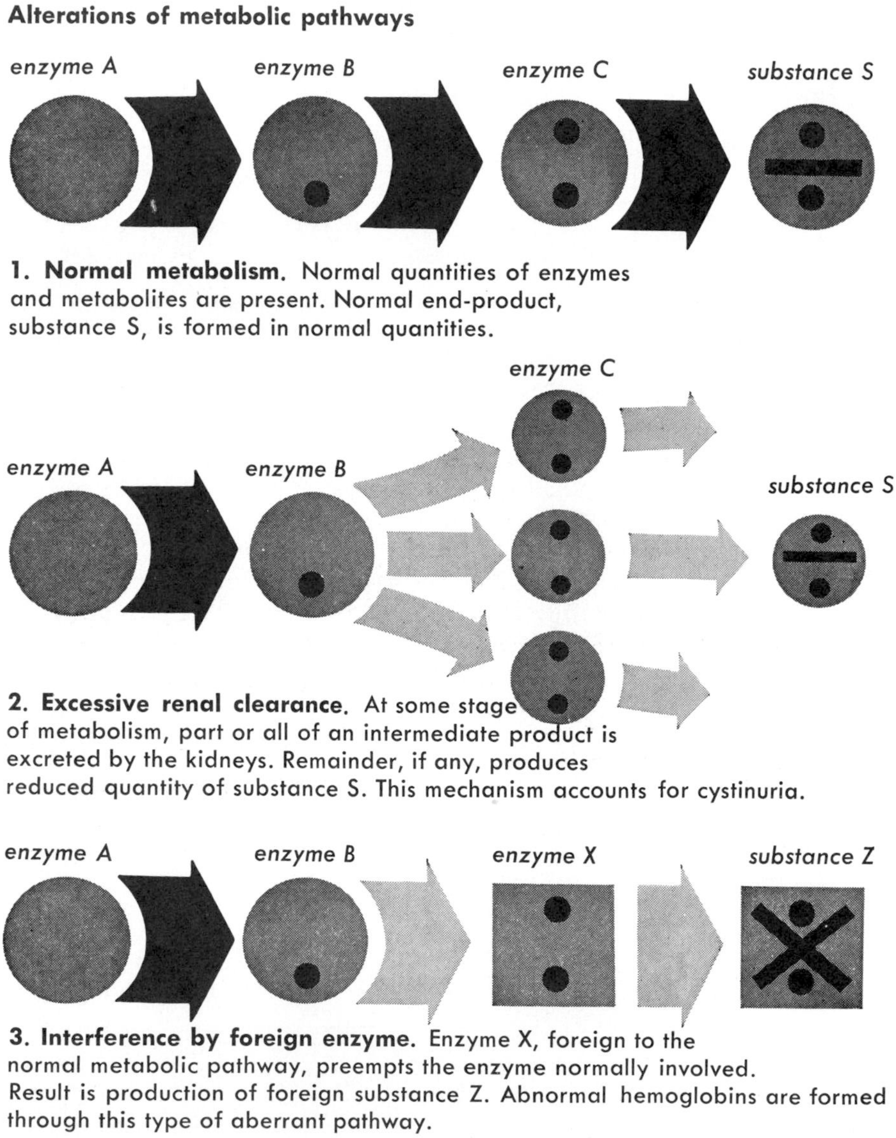

Alterations of metabolic pathways
enzyme A
enzyme B
enzyme C
substance S
1. Normal metabolism. Normal quantities of enzymes and metabolites are present. Normal end-product, substance S, is formed in normal quantities.
enzyme C
enzyme A
enzyme B
substance S
2. Excessive renal clearance. At some stage of metabolism, part or all of an intermediate product is excreted by the kidneys. Remainder, if any, produces reduced quantity of substance S. This mechanism accounts for cystinuria.
enzyme A
enzyme B
enzyme X
substance Z
3. Interference by foreign enzyme. Enzyme X, foreign to the normal metabolic pathway, preempts the enzyme normally involved. Result is production of foreign substance Z. Abnormal hemoglobins are formed through this type of aberrant pathway.

Fig. 20-5. What is meant by a disease of enzymic defect? (Courtesy Parke, Davis & Co.)

Molecular oxygen is utilized. The summarized reaction for glucose is: $C_6H_{12}O_6 + 6O_2 \rightarrow 6CO_2 + 6H_2O$.

MICROSOMES

Within the cytoplasm of most cells there is a fibrillar network that is known as *hyaloplasm*. Another term used to describe it is *cytoplasmic reticulum*.

When cells suspended in a sucrose solution are exposed to high-speed centrifugation, the cytoplasmic reticulum breaks down to form small structures known as *microsomes*. They vary in size and in composition. They contain many enzymes, and a number of drugs are metabolized (and thus inactivated) in the body by the microsomal enzymes. Oxygen and NADPH* are required for this activity.

AUTOLYSIS

When plant or animal tissue dies, it soon begins to liquefy even if bacteria are not present. The liquefaction, called *autolysis*, occurs mainly because of hydrolysis of the proteins in the cells and is catalyzed by a mixture of enzymes known as *cathepsin*. Sometimes autolysis occurs even before death. For example, in the disease known as acute yellow atrophy of the liver the liver tissue autolyzes. This disease is usually fatal. We have not yet learned what prevents autolysis in living, healthy tissue.

DISEASES OF ENZYMIC DEFECT

There are a number of *hereditary* diseases in which the causal factor appears to be a defective enzyme, lack of an enzyme, or the presence of a substance that interferes with the activity of an enzyme. These diseases often are referred to as *inborn errors of metabolism*.

In the disease known as *phenylketonuria* there is a deficiency of the enzyme phenylalanine hydroxylase, which normally is present in the liver. As a result, there is an interference with the conversion of the amino acid (see page 270) phenylalanine to another amino acid, tyrosine. This leads to high plasma and urinary levels of a metabolite of phenylalanine, phenylpyruvic acid. The disease is characterized clinically by mental retardation. Signs of the disease appear in early infancy. Diets low in phenylalanine are used in the treatment of these patients.

Certain compounds that are filtered from the blood in the kidneys are reabsorbed again in the kidney tubules (see page 372). In the disease known as *cystinuria* one or more of the enzymes in the kidney tubules is deficient or abnormal and there is an excessive excretion of some amino acids (cystine, arginine, lysine, and ornithine) in the urine. Cystine is not very soluble, and patients with cystinuria have recurrent formation of cystine kidney stones.

In the disease known as *congenital porphyria* an enzymic defect leads to a failure of the tissues to convert uroporphyrin 1 to coproporphyrin 1.† Clinical features of the disease include extreme sensitivity of the skin to light, excretion of a Burgundy red urine, excessive body hair, discoloration of bones and teeth, and an enlargement of the spleen.

One of the most interesting types of anemia (disease characterized by a deficiency of red blood cells) is *sickle-cell anemia*. In this disease the normal biconcave disc shape of the red blood cells changes to a crescent shape (sickle shape) when the oxyhemoglobin present in them is changed to reduce hemoglobin (see page 347) as a result of exposure to lowered oxygen pressure. About 8 percent of the Negro

*NADPH can be thought of as NADH (page 212) to which a third phosphate radical has been added. NADPH was formerly called TPN (triphosphopyridine nucleotide).

†These compounds are chemically related to heme, the prosthetic group of hemoglobin (see page 288).

Table 20-2. Some diseases of enzymic defect

Disorder	Organs chiefly involved	Metabolic defect	Page reference
Galactosemia	Liver, eyes	Absence of phosphogalactose uridyl transferase	256
Pentosuria	Not determined	Abnormal excretion of the pentose L-xylulose	266
von Gierke's disease	Liver, kidney	Deficiency of hepatic glucose-6-phosphatase	261
Cystinuria	Kidney	Defective renal reabsorption of cystine and other amino acids	215
Phenylketonuria	Liver, brain	Relative inability to hydroxylate phenylalanine to tyrosine	215
Albinism	Skin, hair, eyes	Inability to form the pigment melanin	290
Alkaptonuria	Connective tissue (adults)	Absence of hepatic homogentisic acid oxidase	291
Hemophilias A, B, and C	Blood	Lack of clotting factors	359, 361
Agammaglobulinemia	Lymphoid tissues	Inability to form γ-globulins (antibody proteins)	355
Gilbert's disease	Liver	Lack of uridine diphosphate glucuronide transferase	266
Porphyria	Liver	Increased excretion of uroporphyrins	288
Sickle-cell anemia	Blood	Abnormal hemoglobins	215
Thalassemia	Blood	Abnormal hemoglobins	279
Wilson's disease	Brain, liver, kidneys	Decreased ceruloplasmin; increased copper in liver and brain	342, 356
Hypophosphatasia	Bone	Deficiency of alkaline phosphatase	364
Gout	Joints	Excessive production of uric acid	313
Maple syrup urine disease	Brain	Absence of decarboxylation enzyme system for branched chain amino acids	292
Histidinemia	Brain (speech defect)	Histidase deficiency	292

population of the United States has red blood cells that can be made to sickle in the laboratory. Fortunately, only 1 in 40 of these has clinically significant anemia. The hemoglobin (hemoglobin S) present in these abnormal cells differs slightly from normal hemoglobin (hemoglobin A) in both chemical and physical properties. These individuals form the abnormal hemoglobin S because an enzyme in their tissues (bone marrow) concerned with the synthesis is abnormal. As blood passes through the capillaries, the oxygen tension of the blood decreases (see page 347), and about 85 percent of the hemoglobin S actually crystallizes in the red blood cells, thereby distorting them.

Some other diseases of enzymic defect are listed in Table 20-2.

ISOZYMES Certain enzymes exist in different chemical forms, and the proportion of the different forms may differ from tissue to tissue. For example, there are 5 known molecular forms of the enzyme lactic dehydrogenase. These 5 forms are said to be isozymes or isoenzymes: in this case, of lactic dehydrogenase. When tissues become diseased, some of the lactic dehydrogenase present is released into the blood. This is important clinically, because by studying the types present, often the tissue that has been damaged can be identified. For example, the increased blood enzymes resulting from a heart attack differ qualitatively from those resulting from acute liver disease.

Many proteins (and all known enzymes are proteins) consist of chains of substances known as amino acids joined together chemically (see page 273). When more than one chain is present in a molecule, cross chemical linkages bind them together. In the case of lactic dehydrogenase, there are 2 different kinds of chain present. One is designated the H (heart) type, and one, the M (muscle) type. The 5 forms of the enzyme have the following composition:

1. Pure H type = H_4 (four chains connected together)
2. Pure M type = M_4
3. M_3H
4. M_2H_2
5. MH_3

The so-called European numerical classification of the lactic dehydrogenase (LDH) isozymes is used in many American clinical laboratories. In this system, LDH_1 is H_4; LDH_2 is MH_3; LDH_3 is M_2H_2; LDH_4 is M_3H; and LDH_5 is M_4. (In the so-called American system, the subscript numbers are reversed; LDH_1 becomes LDH_5, LDH_5 becomes LDH_1, and so on.)

In normal subjects, LDH_1, LDH_2, and LDH_3 can be detected in the blood; LDH_4 and LDH_5 usually are absent (European system). In liver disease, LDH_5 is elevated. In myocardial infarction (coronary attack), LDH_1 and LDH_2 are increased.

LDH can be measured in red blood cells. LDH_5 is present mainly in young cells. If there is a high relative amount of LDH_1, it suggests that the cells are old. There is an elevation of LDH_1 and LDH_2 in hemolytic anemia (deficiency of red cells caused by hemolysis, or rupture, of red cells). In many cases of cancer there is an increase in LDH_3 and, to a lesser extent, in LDH_4 and LDH_5. A relative increase in LDH_5 usually means that cancerous (metastatic) lesions are present in the liver.

LYSOSOMES Certain structures located within the cytoplasm of all cells resemble small bags. They are filled with a mixture of powerful digestive enzymes. So long as their membranes remain intact, digestion is confined to substances that gain entrance into the lysosome. If, however, the membrane ruptures, and the enzymes leak out, the cytoplasm itself may be digested and the cell destroyed. It has been postulated that this occurs in certain types of disease.

Probably the lysosomes serve as the "digestive tract" of the cell. Their membranes can fold in, forming a pocket into which substrate (food) molecules can enter. The membrane then can completely surround this food, and by unfolding on the inner side, transfer it from the cytoplasm to the interior of the lysosome. Here it can be digested. The products of digestion then diffuse through the membrane into the cytoplasm.

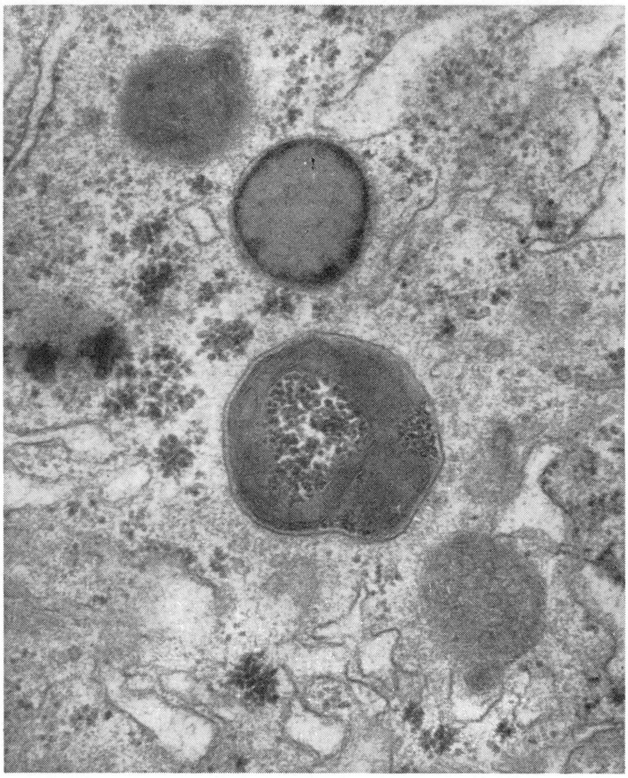

Fig. 20-6. The two prominent round structures in this electron photomicrograph are lysosomes present in the cell of a rat liver. The lower lysosome has ingested and largely digested a mitochondrion. What type of biologically active compound is present in lysosomes? (Courtesy Dr. Carl Bruni and Dr. Keith R. Porter, Harvard University; from The fine structure of the parenchymal cell of the normal rat liver. I. General observations, Amer. J. Path. **46:**691, May 1965.)

CYCLIC AMP

Investigations of the mechanism of action of epinephrine (page 262) and glucagon (page 265) in causing a rise of blood sugar led to the discovery that adenosine-3′,5′-monophosphate, better known as cyclic AMP, is important in metabolism.

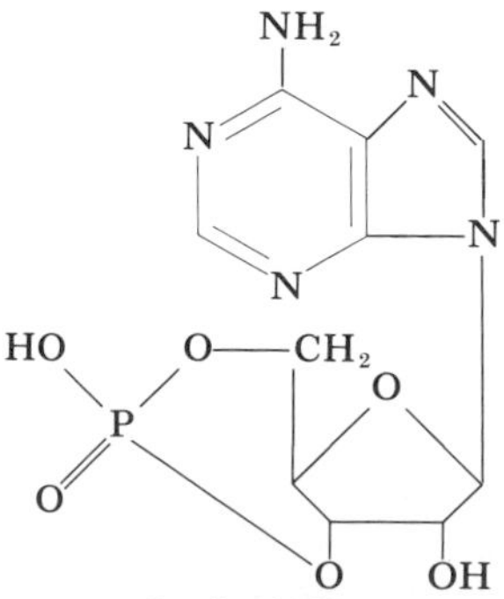

Cyclic AMP

These substances increase the rate of breakdown of liver glycogen (page 257) by increasing the rate of formation of cyclic AMP. This, in turn, causes an increased rate of formation of active phosphorylase, an enzyme required for glycogen breakdown.

The enzyme, adenyl cyclase, in the presence of magnesium ions, catalyzes the conversion of ATP (page 209) to cyclic AMP and inorganic pyrophosphate. Another enzyme, phosphodiesterase, catalyzes the conversion of cyclic AMP to adenosine-5′-monophosphate.

Several hormones (see Chapter 32, page 381) – epinephrine, norepinephrine, parathormone, glucagon, LH, ACTH, TSH, vasopressin – produce some of their effects by stimulating adenyl cyclase. This, in turn, leads to an increase in cyclic AMP. The effects of insulin in liver (page 262) can be attributed to its ability to *lower* the level of cyclic AMP. Some other active substances – histamine (page 292), serotonin (page 292), acetylcholine – probably are active because they alter the level of cyclic AMP in target organs.

All of these substances, then, probably act by increasing the activity of adenyl cyclase or, in some cases, by lowering it, or by an effect on phosphodiesterase.

STUDY QUESTIONS

1. What is an enzyme?
2. What is the substrate? What are the end products?
3. What is the chemical nature of enzymes?
4. Name some enzymes that have been obtained in crystalline form.
5. Name three factors that influence the rate of enzyme-catalyzed reactions.
6. What is meant by the optimum temperature? The optimum pH?
7. Why are enzymes said to be specific?
8. What is a proenzyme? Give two examples.
9. Explain the following terms: activator; inhibitor. Give an example of each.
10. What is a coenzyme? How are coenzymes related to vitamins?
11. Name several procedures that inactivate enzymes.
12. What types of chemicals will inactivate enzymes?
13. Define: competitive inhibition; noncompetitive inhibition. Give an example of each.
14. Define: apoenzyme; holoenzyme.
15. What is an antivitamin? Why are antivitamins toxic? Are they ever used as drugs?
16. What is the derivation of the word, enzyme?
17. What 3 letters form the terminal letters of the names of enzymes?
18. Name and define 6 classes of enzyme.
19. What type of reaction is catalyzed by an oxygenase? What metal usually takes part in reactions catalyzed by oxygenases?
20. Describe the mitochondrion.
21. What two systems of respiratory enzymes occur in the mitochondrion?
22. What is ATP? NAD^+?
23. Name an important function of the microsomal enzymes.
24. Describe the benzidine test for blood. Do you think this test would allow you to distinguish between human blood and dog blood?
25. What is meant by autolysis? What is cathepsin? Can autolysis occur during life?
26. Make up a definition for "diseases of enzymic defect." Why are they spoken of as "inborn errors of metabolism"?
27. Name a disease in which there is a deficiency of an enzyme. Name another in which an enzyme is abnormal.
28. Why do you suppose scientists believe that most drugs' activity consists in interacting in some way with an enzyme?
29. What is an isozyme?
30. How many isozymes of lactic dehydrogenase are known?
31. Why are isozymes of interest in diagnosis?
32. What is a lysosome?
33. What is the probable function of lysosomes?
34. Define: cyclic AMP; adenyl cyclase; phosphodiesterase.
35. Name several biologically active substances that owe their activity to changes in the concentration of cyclic AMP in target organs.

CHAPTER 21

Chemical nature of lipids

DEFINITION OF LIPID

The class of compounds known as *lipids* are soluble in many organic liquids but are nearly or completely insoluble in water. They are either compounds that yield fatty acids when they are hydrolyzed (combined with water) or they are complex alcohols capable of combining with fatty acids to form esters. All of the lipids found in nature are made in the tissues of plants and animals; that is, lipids take part in the normal chemical reactions of living things.

TYPES OF LIPID

For convenience of study we divide the lipids into three main groups: simple lipids, compound lipids, and derived lipids.

1. *Simple lipids* are esters. When they are hydrolyzed, alcohols and fatty acids are produced. Fatty acids, we remember, are acids that may be thought of as hydrocarbons in which one of the hydrogen atoms has been replaced by a carboxyl (COOH) group. The two important kinds of simple lipid are the *fats* and the *waxes*. Fats are lipids that break down into fatty acids and glycerol (an alcohol) when they are hydrolyzed. Simple lipids that break down to fatty acids and to some alcohol other than glycerol on hydrolysis are called *waxes*.

Fat + H_2O → Fatty acids + Glycerol
Wax + H_2O → Fatty acids + Alcohol (other than glycerol)

2. *Compound lipids* also yield alcohols and fatty acids when they are hydrolyzed. In addition, however, other compounds are formed by the reaction. For example, when *phospholipids* are hydrolyzed, the products formed are fatty acids, alcohol, phosphoric acid, and a nitrogen-containing compound.

Phospholipid + H_2O → Fatty acids + Alcohol
+ Phosphoric acid + Nitrogen-containing compound

Glycolipids (also called *cerebrosides* because they are found in high concentration in the cerebrum, a portion of the brain) form fatty acids, sphingosine (an alcohol), and a sugar when they are hydrolyzed. The sugar obtained from most glycolipids is *galactose*.

$$\text{Glycolipid} + H_2O \rightarrow \text{Fatty Acid} + \text{Sphingosine} + \text{Galactose}$$

3. *Derived lipids* are the water-insoluble substances obtained by the hydrolysis of simple or compound lipids. The *fatty acids* themselves are important derived lipids. *Sterols* are solid alcohols having a high molecular weight. Sterols are found both as a free alcohols and combined with fatty acids as esters. *Glycerol* is not regarded as a lipid because it is soluble in water.

TYPES OF FATTY ACID

Most of the fatty acid molecules found in nature contain an even number (2, 4, 6, 8, etc) of carbon atoms. Fatty acid molecules containing odd numbers (3, 5, 7, 9, etc) of carbon atoms, however, have been prepared in the laboratory. Both saturated and unsaturated fatty acids are known.

Linoleic acid, linolenic acid, and *arachidonic acid* are unsaturated fatty acids that have a special nutritional importance. Linoleic and linolenic acids occur in both plant and animal tissues. Arachidonic acid is synthesized from linoleic acid by animals and is found only in animal tissues. These acids sometimes are called the *essential fatty acids*. Linoleic acid has 18 carbon atoms per molecule and 2 double bonds between carbon atoms; linolenic acid, 18 carbon atoms and 3 double bonds; and arachidonic acid, 20 carbon atoms and 4 double bonds. If these acids are not present in the diet of rats, the animals lose weight, develop a scaly skin disease, show blood in the urine, and finally die with badly diseased kidneys. These conditions can be prevented by adding small amounts of linoleic or arachidonic acid to the diet. (Linolenic acid is active only in promoting growth.)

Table 21-1. Some fatty acids found in nature

Name	Formula	Number of carbon atoms
Acetic acid	CH_3COOH	2
Butyric acid	$CH_3CH_2CH_2CH_2COOH$	4
Caproic acid	$CH_3(CH_2)_4COOH$	6
Caprylic acid	$CH_3(CH_2)_6COOH$	8
Capric acid	$CH_3(CH_2)_8COOH$	10
Lauric acid	$CH_3(CH_2)_{10}COOH$	12
Myristic acid	$CH_3(CH_2)_{12}COOH$	14
Palmitic acid	$CH_3(CH_2)_{14}COOH$	16
Oleic acid	$CH_3(CH_2)_7CH{=}CH(CH_2)_7COOH$	18
Stearic acid	$CH_3(CH_2)_{16}COOH$	18
Chaulmoogric acid	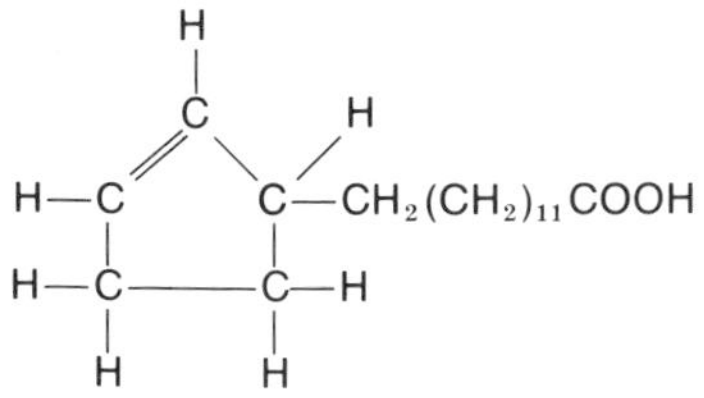	18

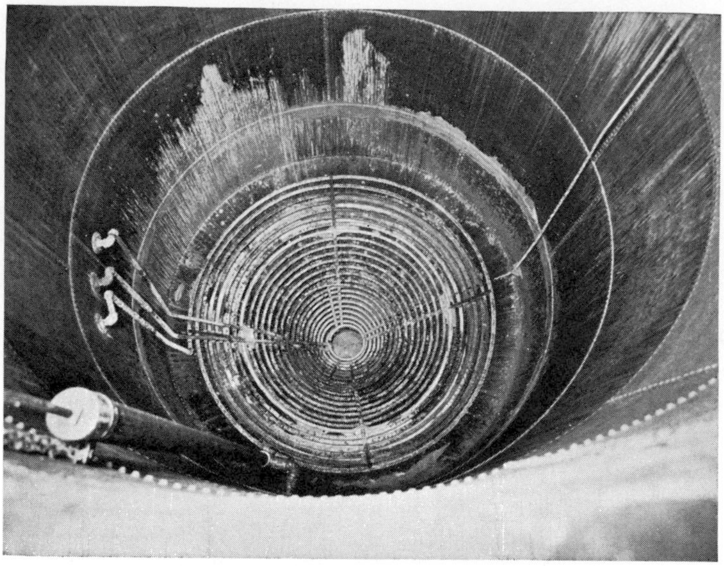

Fig. 21-1. Saponification on a large scale. An empty soap kettle that is three stories deep. Such a kettle is stocked for each batch with approximately 130,000 pounds of fat and 75,000 pounds of caustic solution, from which a yield of about 150,000 pounds of toilet soap and 14,000 pounds of glycerol are obtained. What is meant by the term saponification? (Courtesy Procter & Gamble Co.)

Chaulmoogric acid and *hydnocarpic acid* are cyclic fatty acids that occur in chaulmoogra oil. This oil has been used in the treatment of leprosy. *Ethyl chaulmoograte,* an ester of ethyl alcohol and chaulmoogric acid, also has been used to treat leprosy.

SOAPS

The salts of fatty acids are called *soaps*. Stearic acid, for example, reacts with sodium hydroxide to form sodium stearate, a soap. This type of reaction in which a soap is produced is called *saponification.**

$CH_3(CH_2)_{16}COOH$ +	$NaOH$	→	$CH_3(CH_2)_{16}COONa$ +	H_2O
Stearic acid (Fatty acid)	Sodium hydroxide (Inorganic base)		Sodium stearate (Soap)	Water

Since pure fatty acids are expensive, soaps are prepared commercially by boiling fats with inorganic bases. In this process the fat is hydrolyzed, yielding glycerol and a mixture of fatty acids. The fatty acids then react with the base to form soaps. Incidentally, this is also a commercial method of obtaining glycerol. *Castile soap* is made by boiling olive oil with sodium hydroxide.

Sodium and potassium soaps mix with water to form milky colloidal

*Organic chemists frequently use the term saponification to indicate the hydrolysis of esters (whether or not they are fats—see page 152) in alkaline solution. This reaction results in the formation of an alcohol and an organic salt, which will be a soap, of course, if the original ester was a fat.

solutions. Sodium soaps are solids; the ordinary cake soaps we use for cleansing purposes are sodium salts of fatty acids. Potassium soaps are liquids or semisolids at ordinary temperatures. The *tincture of green soap* used in hospitals is a solution of potassium soap in alcohol. Sodium and potassium soaps are *surface active substances* (see page 60) and lower surface tension. This means they are *emulsifying agents*. The cleansing action of soaps results from their ability to cause particles of grease and dirt to become suspended in water.

Calcium and magnesium soaps are not soluble in water, but they will dissolve in some organic liquids and are used in dry cleaning. Water containing calcium and magnesium salts is called *hard water* (see page 74). When a sodium or potassium soap is added to such water, calcium and magnesium soaps are formed and these precipitate. This explains why soap does not lather well in hard water.

$$2\,CH_3(CH_2)_{14}COONa + CaCl_2 \rightarrow (CH_3(CH_2)_{14}COO)_2Ca\downarrow + 2\,NaCl$$

2 $CH_3(CH_2)_{14}COONa$ +	$CaCl_2$	→	$(CH_3(CH_2)_{14}COO)_2Ca\downarrow$ +	2 NaCl
Sodium palmitate (Soluble soap)	Calcium chloride (Calcium salt)		Calcium palmitate (Insoluble soap)	Sodium chloride

Soaps are *emulsifying agents*. If a lipid, like olive oil, is shaken with water in the presence of a sodium or potassium soap, small drops of lipid will remain suspended in the water for some time. This type of emulsion in which small drops of lipid are suspended in water is called an oil-in-water or lipid-in-water emulsion. If olive oil is shaken with water in the presence of calcium or magnesium soap, on the other hand, water drops will be suspended in the oil and a water-in-oil or water-in-lipid type of emulsion will be formed.

Soaps have *antiseptic* properties. Surgeons and nurses who handle instruments in the operating room formerly scrubbed their hands and arms with soap and water for ten minutes. This procedure removes the majority of bacteria on the skin, but more effective antiseptic agents are used now.

CHEMICAL NATURE OF FATS

Fats are *esters* formed by the chemical union of glycerol and fatty acids. Glycerol is a trihydric alcohol (each molecule has 3 OH groups) and therefore combines with 3 molecules of fatty acid.

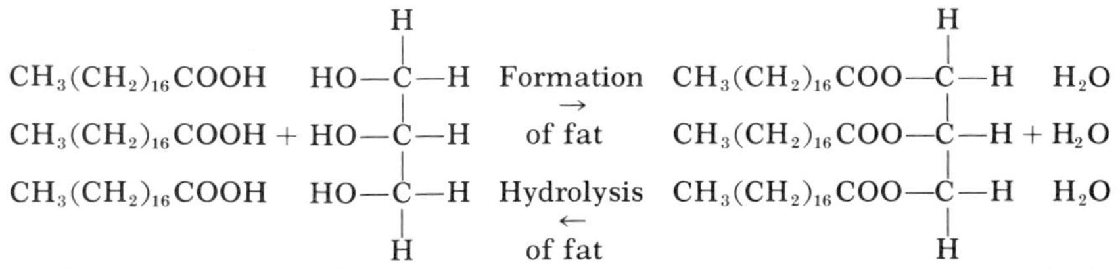

Stearic acid (3 Molecules of fatty acid)	+	Glycerol (1 Molecule of glycerol)	⇄	Stearin (1 Molecule of fat)	+	Water (3 Molecules of water)

This is the reaction living things use to make fats. If this reaction is reversed—that is, if the fat is *hydrolyzed*—we see that 1 molecule of fat will yield 1 molecule of glycerol and 3 molecules of fatty acid. Fats are hydrolyzed when they are digested in the intestinal tract.

Most fats found in nature form glycerol and a *mixture* of different fatty acids when they are hydrolyzed. That is, natural fats contain more than one kind of fatty acid in their molecules. Such a molecule, for example, may contain 1 molecule of glycerol combined with 1 molecule of stearic acid, 1 molecule of palmitic acid, and 1 molecule of oleic acid. Solid fats contain mainly *saturated* fatty acids; liquid fats contain a majority of *unsaturated* fatty acids in their molecules. Many animal fats are liquid at body temperature but become solid at ordinary room temperatures. They contain a mixture of saturated and unsaturated fatty acids.

Fats are not soluble in water, but they will dissolve in certain organic liquids, called *fat solvents*. Petroleum ether, alcohol, diethyl ether, chloroform, and carbon tetrachloride are examples of fat solvents. Fat droplets can be suspended in water with the aid of emulsifying agents to form emulsions. We have already learned that soaps owe their cleansing action to the fact that they are good emulsifying agents. Dry cleaning fluids are fat solvents; they remove fatty stains by dissolving them.

OILS Liquid fats are frequently called *oils*. We must remember, however, that not all oils are fats. Mineral oil and lubricating oils are mixtures of hydrocarbons—not fats. Many substances responsible for the odor and flavor of aromatic plants are oily liquids called *volatile oils*. Oil of peppermint, oil of clove, oil of rose, and oil of orange are examples of volatile oils used as flavors and perfumes. Liquid fats are not very volatile at ordinary temperatures and for this reason are sometimes called *fixed oils*.

HYDROGENATION OF FATS Unsaturated fatty acids are converted to saturated fatty acids when they unite with hydrogen.

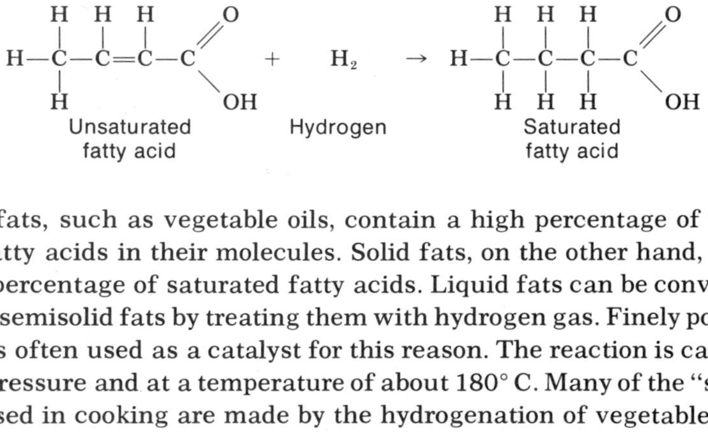

Liquid fats, such as vegetable oils, contain a high percentage of unsaturated fatty acids in their molecules. Solid fats, on the other hand, contain a high percentage of saturated fatty acids. Liquid fats can be converted to solid or semisolid fats by treating them with hydrogen gas. Finely powdered nickel is often used as a catalyst for this reason. The reaction is carried on under pressure and at a temperature of about 180° C. Many of the "shortenings" used in cooking are made by the hydrogenation of vegetable oils.

ACROLEIN TEST When fats are heated to high temperatures, some of the fat is hydrolyzed, and free glycerol (as well as free fatty acid) is formed. If heating is continued, a sharp, somewhat irritating odor will be noticed. This odor is from the formation of *acrolein*. The reaction occurs at a lower temperature in the presence of a dehydrating agent such as potassium bisulfate, $KHSO_4$.

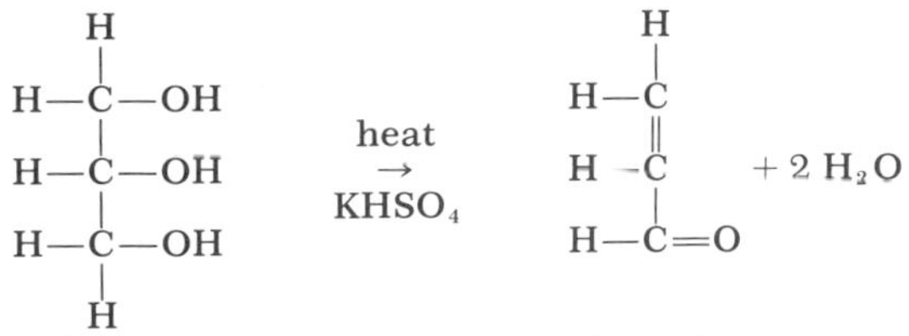

Glycerol Acrolein

Anyone who has done much cooking will have noticed this odor when cooking fat has been overheated. Acrolein is irritating to the mucous membranes lining the digestive tract. Some clinicians are of the opinion that the indigestion some people experience after eating fried foods may be caused by the presence of this substance.

The formation of acrolein is really a test for glycerol, but it is also used as a test for fats since all fats yield glycerol when they are heated.

RANCIDITY OF FATS

Fats allowed to stand in contact with the air frequently develop an unpleasant odor and taste; we say the fat has become *rancid*. Rancidity is caused by a combination of *hydrolysis* and *oxidation*. Hydrolysis causes the formation of free fatty acids, some of which have disagreeable odors and tastes. Most of the unsaturated fatty acids present in fats are slowly oxidized in contact with air, with the formation of products with "rancid" odors and tastes. The drying of linseed oil in paints can be compared with oxidative rancidity; the drying of the paint results from the oxidation of the linseed oil.

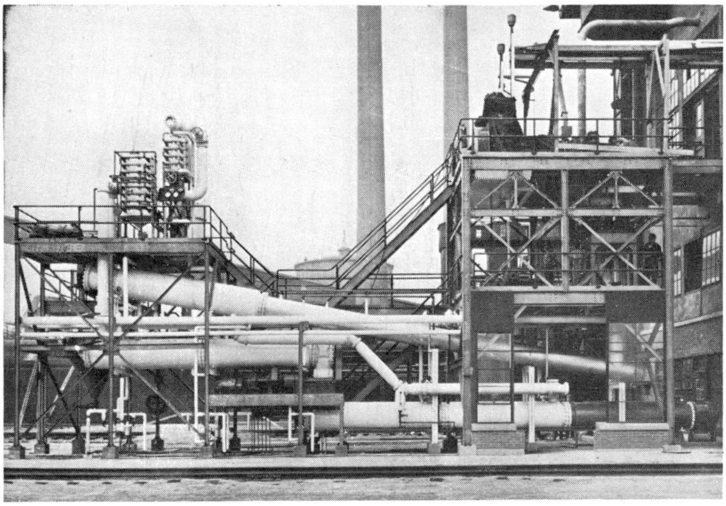

Fig. 21-2. Solvent extraction plant for soybeans. One of the principal solvents is *n*-hexane, which extracts lecithins as well as the oil. Lecithins are used in the candy industry, in gasolines to prevent corrosion, and in the formation of oil-in-water emulsions. Soybean oil is a component of many paints and varnishes. The protein obtained from the "cake" after the oil has been removed is being used in the manufacture of plastics, and a synthetic fiber has been made from this protein material. What are the products of hydrolysis of lecithin? (Courtesy Ford Motor Co.)

PHOSPHOLIPIDS Phospholipids are present in every tissue of the body. They are present in high concentrations in the nervous system, particularly in the sheath (myelin sheath) surrounding many nerve fibers.

Lecithins hydrolyze to form 1 molecule of glycerol, 2 molecules of fatty acid, 1 molecule of phosphoric acid, and 1 molecule of choline for each molecule of lecithin (see page 292). Choline is a nitrogen-containing substance that neutralizes acids. Lecithins are good emulsifying agents and form stable emulsions in water. It appears likely that fats are partly converted to lecithins in the body and are transported in this form from one tissue to another by the blood. Lecithins are important sources of the phosphoric acid used in building new cells in the body.

Some snake venoms contain an enzyme called lecithinase A. This enzyme catalyzes the loss of 1 fatty acid molecule from lecithin molecules. The substance that remains after the loss of fatty acid is called a *lysolecithin*.

$$\text{Lecithin} \xrightarrow{\text{(Lecithinase A)}} \text{Lysolecithin} + \text{1 molecule of fatty acid}$$

Lysolecithins cause hemolysis (disintegration of red blood cells).

Cephalins are the phospholipids that are important in blood clotting. The products of hydrolysis of cephalins are the same as those of lecithins except that aminoethyl alcohol, $CH_2NH_2CH_2OH$, is formed instead of choline.* It is believed that the disintegration of blood platelets (small pieces of tissue floating in the blood) with the formation of thromboplastin, a cephalin-protein complex, is the first step in blood coagulation. In certain diseases known as *purpuras,* where the blood platelets are greatly reduced in number, the patient literally may bleed to death. Cephalins, like lecithins, are a source of phosphoric acid.

Sphingomyelins form a fatty acid, sphingosine (an alcohol), phosphoric acid, and choline when they are hydrolyzed. They were originally isolated from the brain. Large quantities of phospholipids, chiefly sphingomyelins, accumulate in the liver and spleen of children suffering from Niemann-Pick's disease. This disease is rapidly fatal and occurs chiefly in the first two years of life. Fortunately, Niemann-Pick's disease is rare.

A variant of a phospholipid, in which a fatty acid is replaced by vinyl alcohol, is known as a *plasmalogen*. Plasmologens occur in traces in various tissues, including brain, bone marrow, and heart.

GLYCOLIPIDS *Glycolipids* or *cerebrosides* are similar chemically to the sphingomyelins. On hydrolysis, however, they yield galactose (a sugar) instead of phosphoric acid and choline. One of the glycolipids, known as *kerasin,* is found in large quantities in the spleen in cases of the rare disorder known as Gaucher's disease.

WAXES *Waxes* are of importance in medicine chiefly because they are used as ointment bases. Most natural waxes are mixtures of several substances.

*Some cephalin molecules contain serine (an amino acid, page 480) or inositol ($C_6H_{12}O_6$; hexahydroxy benzene) instead of aminoethyyyl alcohol.

Beeswax, made by the common honeybee; spermaceti, obtained from the sperm whale; and lanolin, obtained from wool, are examples. The shiny appearance of apple peel is duc to the presence of waxes. Paraffin wax is not a true wax since it is a mixture of hydrocarbons.

STEROLS Sterols are solid alcohols of high molecular weight. *Cholesterol* has been called the characteristic animal sterol because it is found in every cell in the body. It exists in the bloodstream partly as free sterol and partly in chemical combination with fatty acids (in other words, as an ester) and protein. It is found in largest amounts in the tissues of the nervous system and is excreted from the body in the bile. Some of the cholesterol that gains entrance into the intestinal tract by way of the bile is reduced to *coprosterol,* another sterol, by intestinal bacteria.

Several of the sterols form substances having high vitamin D activity when they are exposed to ultraviolet light. *Ergosterol,* a sterol found in certain lower plants (the fungi), is the most important of these. A series of compounds is formed by exposing ergosterol to ultraviolet light, and one of them, called *calciferol,* is an active vitamin. The mixture of compounds made by irradiating ergosterol has been called *viosterol.* A sterol, *7-dehydrocholesterol,* found in animal tissues also yields vitamin D when exposed to ultraviolet rays.

The *bile acids,* which are responsible for the low surface tension and emulsifying properties of bile, are chemically closely related to cholesterol. Other related substances include the sex hormones and the hormones of the cortex (outer portion) of the adrenal gland.

STUDY QUESTIONS

1. What is a lipid?
2. What are the three main types of lipid? Give a definition of each type.
3. What are fats? Waxes? Phospholipids? Glycolipids? Cerebrosides? Fatty acids? Sterols?
4. What is peculiar about the number of carbon atoms found in most natural fatty acids?
5. Name the essential fatty acids.
6. What diseases have been treated with ethyl chaulmoograte?
7. What is a soap? How are soaps made commercially? What is Castile soap?
8. How do you explain the cleansing action of soaps?
9. Why does soap not lather well in hard water?
10. What type of emulsion do sodium and potassium soaps form? What type do calcium and magnesium soaps form?
11. Why is the nurse who assists the surgeons in the operating room called a scrub nurse?
12. Why do surgeons and nurses scrub their hands and arms before an operation?
13. Name several substances that are chemically related to cholesterol.
14. What are the products of hydrolysis of fats? What are the products of digestion of fats?
15. What is the chemical difference between solid fats and liquid fats?
16. List some of the important properties of fats.
17. Make up a dcfinition for "oil."
18. What is meant by hydrogenation of fats? How is it used commercially?
19. Describe the acrolein test. For what is it a test?
20. What happens when fats become rancid? What happens when paint dries?
21. What are lecithins? What is lecithinase A?
22. Name an important function of cephalin.
23. Name a disease in which sphingomyelins accumulate in the liver and spleen.
24. What sugar is formed by the hydrolysis of most glycolipids? What glycolipid is important in Gaucher's disease?
25. Are waxes of any importance in medicine? Name several waxes.
26. What is the most important animal sterol? What is coprosterol?
27. Name two sterols that form substances with vitamin D activity when they are exposed to ultraviolet rays. What is viosterol?

CHAPTER 22

Metabolism of lipids

DEFINITION OF METABOLISM

From the point of view of physiological chemistry *metabolism* means all of the chemical changes that occur in the body. Those chemical reactions that build new tissue, replace old tissue, and prepare substances used as reserve food supplies or as catalysts make up *anabolism*. Reactions that result in the destruction of tissues or in the production of energy by the oxidation of foods are collectively called *catabolism*. Anabolic reactions, then, usually build complex molecules from simpler molecules; catabolic reactions usually change complex molecules to simpler molecules, often with the production of energy.

SUMMARY OF FAT DIGESTION

The fat molecule cannot be absorbed efficiently from the digestive tract until it has been hydrolyzed to glycerol and fatty acids—a process called *digestion*.* The gastric juice of the stomach contains an enzyme called *gastric lipase*, which begins fat digestion. We shall see later (see page 322), however, that only *emulsified fats* can be digested efficiently by the digestive enzymes. Gastric lipase, then, only catalyzes the hydrolysis (digestion) of fats that are already emulsified before they are eaten—for example, the emulsified fat of egg yolk. The majority of fat digestion occurs in the small intestine. Here fat is first emulsified by the bile. Its digestion is then catalyzed by *pancreatic lipase (steapsin)*, an enzyme made in the pancreas. (The pancreas is an organ that empties its digestive fluid into the first part of the small intestine.) The end products of fat digestion are *glycerol* and *fatty acids*. These substances enter the cells lining the intestinal tract where they recombine again to form fat. This fat enters the

*It has been demonstrated that fat (and also mineral oil) can be absorbed from the intestinal tract unhydrolyzed if it is very finely emulsified. Some scientists believe that this fine state of emulsification is produced normally in the intestine by the action of bile and partially hydrolyzed fats, and that, therefore, appreciable quantities of food fat may be absorbed without first undergoing digestion.

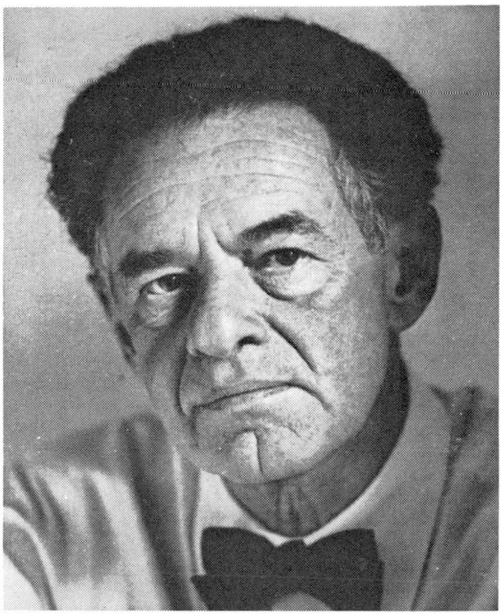

Fig. 22-1. Dr. Fritz Lipmann, now a member of the Rockefeller Institute, was awarded the Nobel Prize in medicine and physiology in 1953 for his work in cell metabolism and for his discovery of coenzyme A. What role does this coenzyme play in fatty acid metabolism?

lymph vessels (often called lacteals) that drain the intestinal tract and passes by means of these vessels to the bloodstream. The blood then distributes the fat to the various tissues of the body.

ANABOLIC PRODUCTS OF FATTY ACIDS

The two principal anabolic products formed from fatty acids are *stored,* or *depot, fat,* and the *lipids necessary for the formation of protoplasm,* the material of which cells are made. Depot fat is found beneath the skin and around many of the organs in the body. Fat deposits, for example, surround the heart and kidneys and line the bony orbit in which the eye rotates. These fat deposits are also spoken of as *adipose tissue.*

The tissues begin the formation of a fatty acid by adding 2 carbon atoms to acetic acid, thus forming butyric acid (4 carbon atoms). Two more carbon atoms then are added to butyric acid to form caproic acid (6 carbon atoms). This process continues until the proper chain length has been achieved. It will be obvious that the natural fatty acids, built by 2-carbon additions, have even numbers of carbons in their molecules.

An important coenzyme found in tissues is known as coenzyme A (or CoASH; see page 211). On hydrolysis coenzyme A yields pantothenic acid (a vitamin; see page 211), adenine (see page 195), ribose (see page 298), phosphoric acid, and mercaptoethanolamine ($NH_2 \cdot CH_2 \cdot CH_2 \cdot SH$).

The first step in the synthesis of a fatty acid in the tissues is the formation of acetyl coenzyme A (acetyl CoA).

$$\underset{\text{Acetic acid}}{CH_3 \cdot COOH} + \underset{\text{Coenzyme A}}{CoASH} \rightarrow \underset{\text{Acetyl CoA}}{CH_3 \cdot CO \cdot SCoA} + H_2O$$

Acetyl CoA then reacts with carbon dioxide to form malonyl CoA.

$$\underset{\text{Acetyl CoA}}{CH_3 \cdot CO \cdot SCoA + CO_2} \rightarrow \underset{\text{Malonyl CoA}}{CH_2\begin{cases} COOH \\ CO \cdot SCoA \end{cases}}$$

A second molecule of acetyl CoA then reacts with the malonyl CoA to form an intermediate compound.

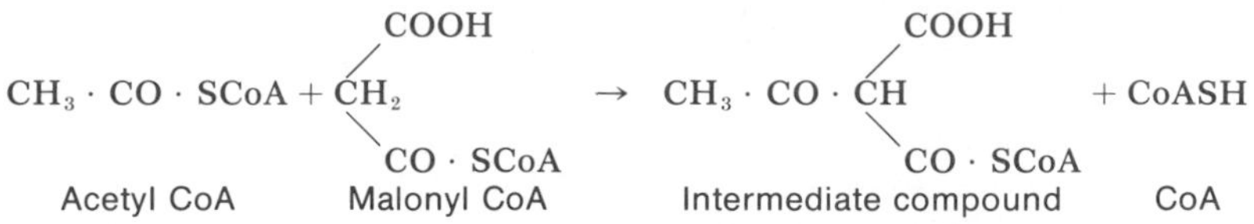

Further reactions result in reduction (addition of H atoms to the intermediate compound).

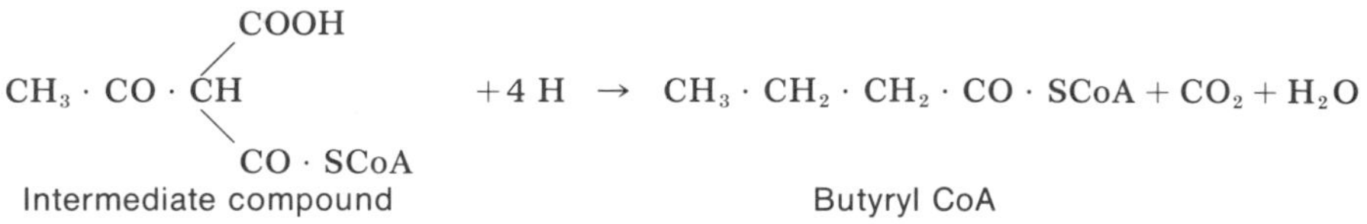

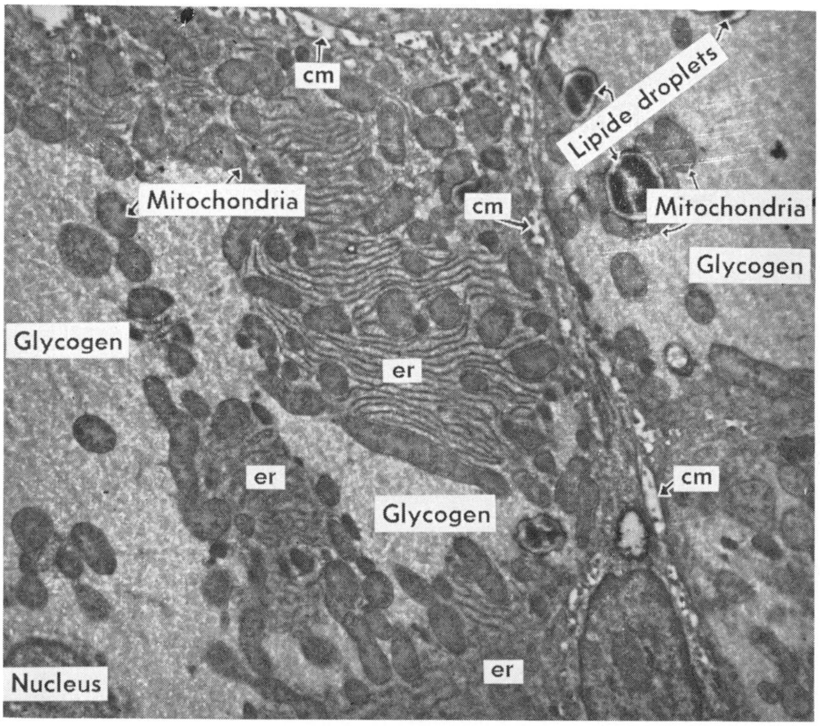

Fig. 22-2. Electron photomicrograph of liver cells. The microsomal particles (parallel strands) probably are the site of the synthesis of fatty acids. **cm,** Cell membrane; **er,** endoplasmic reticulum, or microsomes. The mitochondria (small oval structures) are the sites of fatty acid catabolism and also of the combining of glycerol and fatty acids to form fat. Lipid droplets can be seen lying adjacent to mitochondria at the upper right. Fats also are present as part of the membranes surrounding the mitochondria and cell walls (whitish boundaries at top and right center). The structures are magnified about 5700-fold. Can carbon dioxide undergo chemical reactions in the body? (Courtesy George E. Palade; from Green, D. E.: The synthesis of fat, Sci. Amer. **202:**46, 1960.)

The butyryl CoA, like the acetyl CoA, can condense with a molecule of malonyl CoA to form the coenzyme A ester of caproic acid (6 carbon atoms). This process is repeated until the final fatty acid is formed.

$$\underset{\text{Palmityl CoA}}{CH_3 \cdot (CH_2)_{14} \cdot CO \cdot SCoA} + H_2O \rightarrow \underset{\text{Palmitic acid}}{CH_3 \cdot (CH_2)_{14} \cdot COOH} + \underset{\text{CoA}}{CoASH}$$

FUNCTIONS OF DEPOT FAT

1. Depot fat is a reserve food supply. Most body cells ordinarily prefer to oxidize carbohydrate to furnish energy. (Heart muscle apparently prefers to oxidize fatty acids and to use carbohydrate as an alternative source of energy.) If the carbohydrate stores are used up, however, as they may be in starvation and in certain other conditions, depot fat is oxidized.

2. The adipose tissue beneath the skin is a poor conductor of heat and helps to protect the interior of the body against changes in outside temperature. In general, fat people suffer from cold less than do thin people. Thin people have the advantage in hot weather, however, because they are able to lose body heat more easily than are fat individuals.

CATABOLISM OF FATTY ACIDS

Fatty acids are oxidized in the body to form carbon dioxide and water. This reaction results in the production of a relatively large amount of energy—about 9 large calories of heat for each gram of fat oxidized. This is more than twice the energy obtained by the oxidation of the same amount of either carbohydrate or protein.

The physiological chemist F. Knoop was the first to explain the way in which fatty acids burn (see oxidized) in the tissues, and his explanation is often called *Knoop's theory of β-oxidation*. According to this theory, fatty acids are oxidized *2 carbon atoms at a time*.

$$CH_3 \cdot CH_2 \cdot CH_2 \cdot CH_2 \cdot CH_2 \cdot COOH + CoASH \rightleftarrows CH_3 \cdot CH_2 \cdot CH_2 \cdot CH_2 \cdot CH_2 \cdot CO \cdot SCoA + H_2O$$

$$CH_3 \cdot CH_2 \cdot CH_2 \cdot CH_2 \cdot CH_2 \cdot CO \cdot SCoA + FAD^* \rightleftarrows CH_3 \cdot CH_2 \cdot CH_2 \cdot CH{:}CH \cdot CO \cdot SCoA + FADH_2$$

$$CH_3 \cdot CH_2 \cdot CH_2 \cdot CH{:}CH \cdot CO \cdot SCoA + H_2O \rightleftarrows CH_3 \cdot CH_2 \cdot CH_2 \cdot CHOH \cdot CH_2 \cdot CO \cdot SCoA$$

$$CH_3 \cdot CH_2 \cdot CH_2 \cdot CHOH \cdot CH_2 \cdot CO \cdot SCoA + NAD^+ \rightleftarrows CH_3 \cdot CH_2 \cdot CH_2 \cdot CO \cdot CH_2 \cdot CO \cdot SCoA + NADH$$

$$CH_3 \cdot CH_2 \cdot CH_2 \cdot CO \cdot CH_2 \cdot CO \cdot SCoA + CoASH \rightleftarrows CH_2 \cdot CO \cdot SCoA + CH_3 \cdot CH_2 \cdot CH_2 \cdot CO \cdot SCoA$$

$$CH_3 \cdot CH_2 \cdot CH_2 \cdot CO \cdot SCoA + H_2O \rightleftarrows CH_3 \cdot CH_2 \cdot CH_2 \cdot COOH + CoASH$$

It will be seen that the acid with 6 carbon atoms (caproic acid) loses 2 carbon atoms during one reaction cycle (fatty acid cycle).

KETONE BODIES

Acetoacetic acid (diacetic acid or β-ketobutyric acid), β-hydroxybutyric acid, and acetone are called the *ketone* or *acetone bodies*.

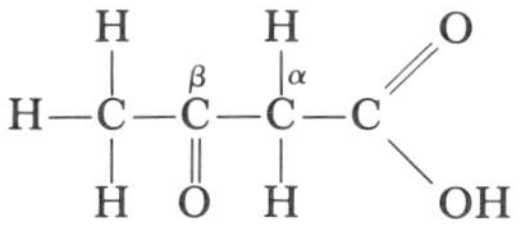

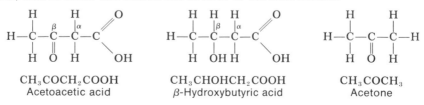

CH_3COCH_2COOH
Acetoacetic acid

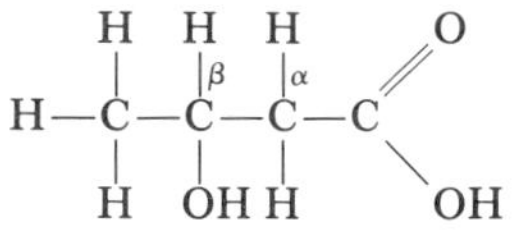

$CH_3CHOHCH_2COOH$
β-Hydroxybutyric acid

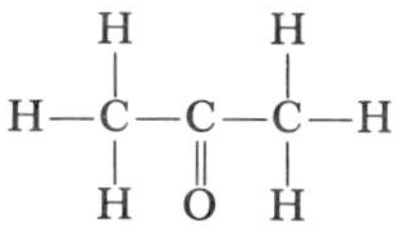

CH_3COCH_3
Acetone

*FAD (flavin adenine dinucleotide) is a coenzyme found in tissues.

Probably small amounts of the ketone bodies are present normally in the blood and urine. They are formed during the catabolism of fatty acids. Hydroxy acids and keto acids are formed during the oxidation of fatty acids. The third ketone body, acetone, is formed from acetoacetic acid.

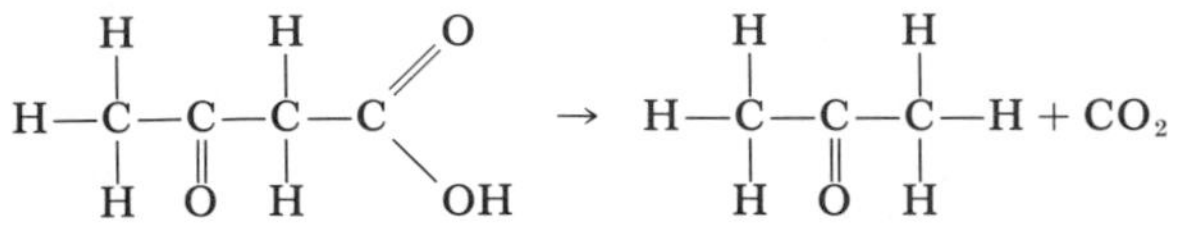

CH_3COCH_2COOH Acetoacetic acid → CH_3COCH_3 Acetone + Carbon dioxide

In any condition in which carbohydrate cannot be burned or converted to fat at a normal rate in the body, *the amount of ketone bodies in the blood and urine greatly increases.* This increase of ketone bodies in blood and urine is called *ketosis.*

The substances in the blood capable of neutralizing acids make up the *alkali reserve* of the blood. When the alkali reserve is lower than normal, the condition is called *acidosis.* This name is misleading to some extent because the blood is never actually acid during life; that is, the pH of the blood never falls below 7, even with very low values for the alkali reserve. One of the important substances constituting the alkali reserve is sodium bicarbonate, $NaHCO_3$. Acetoacetic acid and β-hydroxybutyric acid combine with sodium bicarbonate, forming sodium salts, carbon dioxide, and water.

$$\underset{\text{Acetoacetic acid}}{CH_3COCH_2COOH} + \underset{\text{Sodium bicarbonate}}{NaHCO_3} \rightarrow \underset{\text{Sodium acetoacetate}}{CH_3COCH_2COONa} + \underset{\text{Carbon dioxide}}{CO_2} + \underset{\text{Water}}{H_2O}$$

$$\underset{\beta\text{-Hydroxybutyric acid}}{CH_3CHOHCH_2COOH} + \underset{\text{Sodium bicarbonate}}{NaHCO_3} \rightarrow \underset{\text{Sodium }\beta\text{-hydroxybutyrate}}{CH_3CHOHCH_2COONa} + \underset{\text{Carbon dioxide}}{CO_2} + \underset{\text{Water}}{H_2O}$$

These sodium salts are then excreted in the urine. Of course, this causes a decrease in the amount of sodium bicarbonate and, therefore, of alkali reserve in the blood. *Ketosis, then, is a cause of acidosis.* If acidosis is severe and if it lasts for a sufficient length of time, the patient becomes drowsy and dull, then unconscious, and finally dies. This state of unconsciousness is similar to that produced by anesthetics. It is often called coma.

CAUSES OF KETOSIS

Some causes of ketosis are starvation, diabetes mellitus, severe liver damage, and ketogenic diets.

STARVATION. Only a small amount of carbohydrate is stored in the body at any one time. This is soon used up in starvation, and the body cells are then compelled to burn an increased amount of fat for energy purposes. Ketosis results as it always does when carbohydrate metabolism is impaired.

DIABETES MELLITUS. This is a disease that appears to result, in most cases, either from a failure of the pancreas to manufacture *insulin* or from ineffective use of the insulin produced. Carbohydrate cannot be burned efficiently in the absence of this substance, and again the body is forced to burn an increased amount of fat. Moreover, apparently the liver is unable to form fat at a normal rate from carbohydrate (perhaps by way of the ketone bodies) in this disease (see page 263). The resulting ketosis often causes *diabetic acidosis,* and untreated patients develop *diabetic coma.* Diabetic coma is serious, and prompt treatment is necessary to save the patient's life.

Examination of the reactions of the tricarboxylic acid cycle, given on page 259, shows that acetyl CoA (see page 229) is oxidized by means of these reactions. In the diabetic patient carbohydrate metabolism is impaired and one or more of the compounds required for operation of the cycle is not formed in large enough amounts. Because of this, large amounts of acetyl CoA (which is generated during fatty acid catabolism – see page 231) are shunted into the formation of acetoacetyl CoA, which is a precursor of the ketone bodies. This may be one reason, if not the only one, for the ketosis that accompanies diabetes mellitus.

SEVERE LIVER DAMAGE. The chief storage organ for excess carbohydrate is the liver. When the liver is severely damaged by disease or by poisons (such as phosphorus, chloroform, or carbon tetrachloride) carbohydrate cannot be stored in adequate amounts. Since carbohydrate is not available for oxidation, fat is burned at a rapid rate and ketosis results.

KETOGENIC DIETS. Ketosis can be produced by giving a diet high in fat and low in carbohydrate. This type of diet is called a *ketogenic diet.* Ketosis occasionally is produced by this method as a means of treating infections in the urinary tract (kidneys and bladder). Many of the bacteria causing disease in the urinary tract cannot live and multiply in the presence of the ketone bodies. Of course, this treatment must be stopped before the patient is harmed by the acidosis that accompanies ketosis.

TRANSPORT OF LIPIDS FROM THE INTESTINE TO THE TISSUES

Following digestion, fatty acids, monoglycerides, cholesterol, cholesterol esters, and phospholipids accumulate for a time in intestinal cells. The pool of lipids is augmented to some extent by synthesis of lipids in these cells. Most of the fatty acids and monoglycerides are converted to triglycerides (fats). The glycerol required for this conversion is derived partly from the process of digestion and part is synthesized from carbohydrate. This group of lipids then is combined with a small amount of protein to form a complicated group of substances known as lipoproteins. These lipoproteins and water are secreted into lymph vessels, which convey them as microscopic droplets *(chylomicrons)* to the subclavian vein, where they enter the bloodstream. Chylomicrons are removed from the blood mainly by the liver, although some enter adipose tissue, approximately 50 percent of which is located just beneath the skin. Most of the other adipose tissue surrounds the abdominal organs and the connective tissue of muscles.

CHANGES IN THE LIVER

Under normal circumstances the liver does not store much lipid, although, by means of hydrolysis and new synthesis, this organ converts lipids, in part at least,* to lipids characteristic of the species. These lipids

*The properties of the fats stored in adipose tissue do reflect to some degree those of the fats present in foods.

are combined with protein to form lipoproteins, in which form they are soluble in water and can be transported to the tissues.

Lipoproteins have highly variable compositions. They can be separated into two groups known as α-lipoproteins and β-lipoproteins by electrophoresis (see page 354), carried out on paper, starch, or silica gel.* The lipoproteins in chylomicrons are low in protein: an average composition is, in percent, proteins, 2; phospholipids, 7; cholesterol esters, 6; unesterified cholesterol, 2; and triglycerides, 83. Other lipoproteins are composed in percent of proteins, 9 to 57; phospholipids, 18 to 29; cholesterol esters, 14 to 38; unesterified cholesterol, 3 to 8; and triglycerides, 5 to 50. The α-lipoproteins account for 3 percent and the β-lipoproteins, 5 percent, of the proteins found in normal plasma.

In some pathological conditions, the liver can store large amounts of fat, resulting in an enlarged "fatty liver." This can happen in starvation; uncontrolled diabetes mellitus; malnutrition, including that associated with alcoholism; and in poisoning caused by toxic chemicals, such as carbon tetrachloride.

CHANGES IN ADIPOSE TISSUE

Adipose tissue contains about 15 percent water; most of the remainder is fat, together with smaller amounts of other lipids. Fat constantly is being formed and hydrolyzed in adipose tissue. The fatty acids required for synthesis are derived from food and from synthesis in the body from precursors (pyruvate and acetate) derived from carbohydrate. Both glucose and insulin (see page 263) are necessary for the normal synthesis of fat. One reason is that α-glycerophosphate (phosphoglyceric acid), a necessary intermediate, is not produced in adipose tissue; it must come from glycolysis (see page 257).

The fatty acids required by other tissues are derived mainly by hydrolysis of fats in adipose tissue. The glycerol formed can be converted to glycogen in the liver (see page 257). The "free fatty acids" (FFA) released into the bloodstream from adipose tissue, although they are not esterified (that is, not combined chemically with glycerol), really are *not* free; they are solubilized by combination with protein (serum albumin; see page 353). Most of the fatty acids utilized by the body tissues are furnished by this albumin–fatty acid complex.

FUNCTIONS OF PHOSPHOLIPIDS

Very little is known about the functions of the phospholipids of the body. *Sphingomyelins* appear to be necessary for the formation of the myelin sheaths surrounding many of the nerve fibers. *Lecithins* furnish a part of the phosphoric acid necessary for building new cells, and, indeed, it is more than likely that the entire lecithin molecule takes a part in cell building. *Cephalins* are necessary for blood clotting and probably also take part in the manufacture of the protoplasm and membranes of the cells.

The first step in the synthesis of a lecithin in the tissues involves the addition of a phosphate group from adenosine triphosphate (ATP; see page 209) to one of the 3 OH groups of glycerol (see page 223).

*α-Lipoproteins move with the α-globulin fraction; β-lipoproteins accompany the β-globulins.

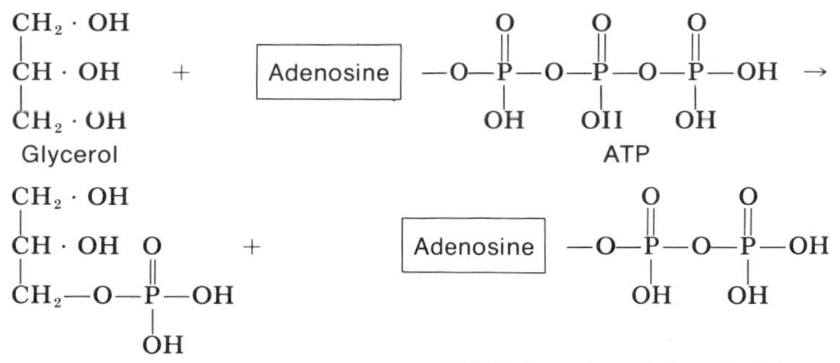

$$CH_2 \cdot OH$$
$$CH \cdot OH \quad + \quad \boxed{Adenosine} \ -O-\overset{\overset{O}{\|}}{\underset{OH}{P}}-O-\overset{\overset{O}{\|}}{\underset{OH}{P}}-O-\overset{\overset{O}{\|}}{\underset{OH}{P}}-OH \ \rightarrow$$
$$CH_2 \cdot OH$$

Glycerol \qquad\qquad\qquad ATP

$$CH_2 \cdot OH$$
$$CH \cdot OH \quad O \quad + \quad \boxed{Adenosine} \ -O-\overset{\overset{O}{\|}}{\underset{OH}{P}}-O-\overset{\overset{O}{\|}}{\underset{OH}{P}}-OH$$
$$CH_2-O-\overset{\overset{\|}{}}{P}-OH$$
$$\underset{OH}{}$$

ADP (adenosine diphosphate)

In the second step 2 fatty acid molecules are linked as esters to the other 2 OH groups of glycerol. Before the reaction occurs the fatty acids are "activated" by combination with coenzyme A (see page 211). During the reaction phosphoric acid splits off.

$$CH_2 \cdot OH$$
$$CH \cdot OH \quad O \qquad + 2\ CH_3 \cdot (CH_2)_{14} \cdot CO \cdot SCoA + H_2O \ \rightarrow$$
$$CH_2-O-\overset{\overset{O}{\|}}{P}-OH$$
$$\underset{OH}{}$$

Palmityl CoA

$$CH_2-O-CO \cdot (CH_2)_{14} \cdot CH_3$$
$$CH-O-CO \cdot (CH_2)_{14} \cdot CH_3 + H_3PO_4 + 2\ CoASH$$
$$CH_2 \cdot OH$$

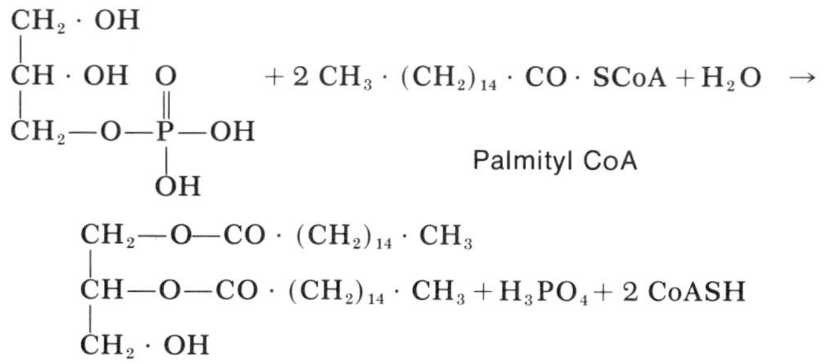

In the final step a complex compound known as cytidine* diphosphocholine reacts with the remaining OH group of the glycerol.

$$CH_2-O-CO \cdot (CH_2)_{14} \cdot CH_3$$
$$CH-O-CO \cdot (CH_2)_{14} \cdot CH_3 + \boxed{Cytidine} \ -O-\overset{\overset{O}{\|}}{\underset{OH}{P}}-O-\overset{\overset{O}{\|}}{\underset{OH}{P}}-O-CH_2-CH_2-\overset{+}{N}\!\!<^{OH^-\ CH_3}_{CH_3\ CH_3} \rightarrow$$
$$CH_2 \cdot OH$$

Cytidine diphosphocholine

$$CH_2-O-CO \cdot (CH_2)_{14} \cdot CH_3$$
$$CH-O-CO \cdot (CH_2)_{14} \cdot CH_3 \qquad\qquad + \boxed{Cytidine} \ -O-\overset{\overset{O}{\|}}{\underset{OH}{P}}-OH$$
$$CH_2-O-\overset{\overset{O}{\|}}{\underset{OH}{P}}-O-CH_2-CH_2-\overset{+}{N}\!\!<^{OH^-\ CH_3}_{CH_3\ CH_3}$$

Lecithin \qquad\qquad\qquad Cytidine monophosphate

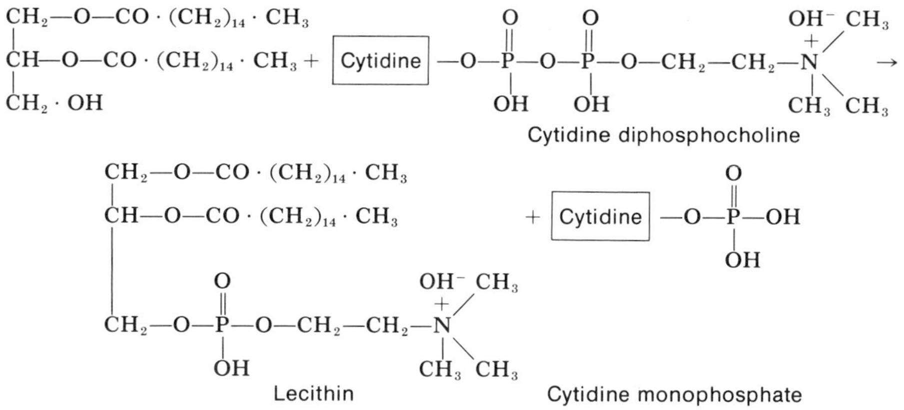

Molecules of lecithin may have different combinations of fatty acids present in them, but probably all of them are formed by the above reactions.

PHOSPHOLIPIDS AND CELL MEMBRANES. More than half the lipid present in most cells is phospholipid. Almost all of this phospholipid is located in the cell membrane. In the membrane, the phospholipid molecules are so arranged that their fatty acid tails point toward each other. The water-soluble heads, facing outward toward the inner and outer surfaces of the membrane, are attached loosely to sheets of protein. The membrane thus resembles in a rough way a "peanut butter sandwich" in which

*Cytidine is a nucleoside (see page 299) that yields cytosine and ribose on hydrolysis.

the fatty acid interior is the peanut butter. Numerous enzymes are imbedded in the membrane.

CHOLESTEROL METABOLISM

Every living organism investigated chemically has been found to contain sterols. The chief animal sterol is *cholesterol,* which is found in every cell and fluid in the body. Cholesterol enters the intestinal cells as free cholesterol, but most of it is combined chemically with fatty acids to form cholesterol esters. As already explained (page 233), the free and esterified cholesterol is incorporated into lipoproteins and enters the blood in the chylomicrons. But even more cholesterol is synthesized in the body, mainly in the liver and intestine. The rate of synthesis in the liver (though probably not in the intestinal cells) is lowered by diets high in cholesterol, by fasting, and by anything that interferes with intestinal absorption (lack of bile acids due to fistulas or obstruction of the bile ducts, for example). Fasting probably results in a lowered level of enzymes required for synthesis, and bile acids are necessary for intestinal absorption.

About 1 g of cholesterol is produced in the body each day from simpler molecules, especially acetate. Forty percent of this is converted to bile acids in the liver; the remaining 60 percent eventually is excreted in the bile as uncombined cholesterol. Thus in the liver cholesterol may be converted to bile acids, excreted in the bile, or incorporated into lipoproteins and distributed throughout the body. Some of the cholesterol excreted in the bile is reabsorbed. The compound sometimes crystallizes from bile in the gallbladder, producing *gallstones.* It is deposited, together with other lipids, in the walls of arteries in the condition known as *atherosclerosis,*

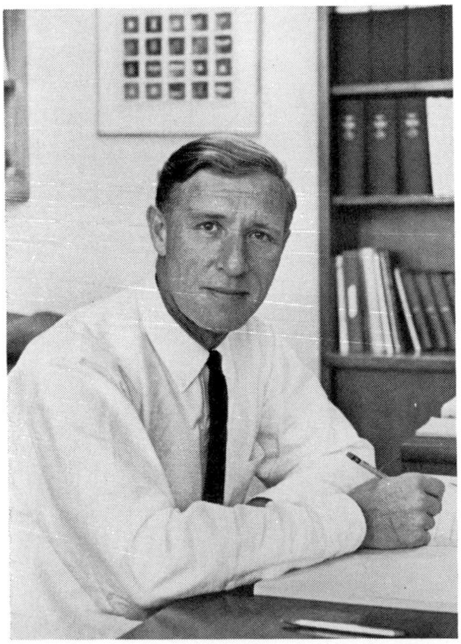

Fig. 22-3. Dr. Konrad Bloch of Harvard University received the Nobel Prize in medicine and physiology in 1964 together with Dr. Feodor Lynen of Max Planck Institute für Zellchemie for contributions to the knowledge of the complex pattern of cell reactions involved in the biosynthesis of cholesterol and fatty acids. Dr. Bloch's work was especially concerned with cholesterol, and that of Dr. Lynen, with fatty acids. Their work was closely interwoven. What is a sterol?

a type of arteriosclerosis or "hardening of the arteries." The level in the plasma is variable and in the United States ranges from about 150 mg per 100 ml to more than 300 mg per 100 ml.

The amount of cholesterol and other lipids in the blood is increased in diabetes mellitus. Sometimes small tumors or swellings, called *xanthomas*, will be found under the skin (particularly near joints) of patients with this disease. These tumors contain a large amount of cholesterol. The blood cholesterol also rises in any condition in which the plasma (the noncellular portion of the blood) does not contain enough protein. Plasma protein may be low either because the patient is not eating protein foods or because the proteins in the plasma are leaking out into the urine. We would expect the blood cholesterol to rise in *starvation* and in those *kidney diseases* (nephrosis and nephritis, among others) in which protein leaves the blood and passes out of the body in the urine. There appears to be some relation between the thyroid gland and the blood cholesterol level. Injection of thyroxine, the hormone of the thyroid gland, causes the amount of cholesterol in the blood to decrease, and in diseases such as cretinism and myxedema, in which the thyroid does not manufacture enough thyroxine, the blood cholesterol level is high. The blood cholesterol level usually increases in the later stages of pregnancy.

Most of the tissues of the body can synthesize cholesterol from acetic acid (CH_3COOH), although probably 97 percent is made in the liver and intestine. Some of the compounds thought to be formed during this synthesis are illustrated below.

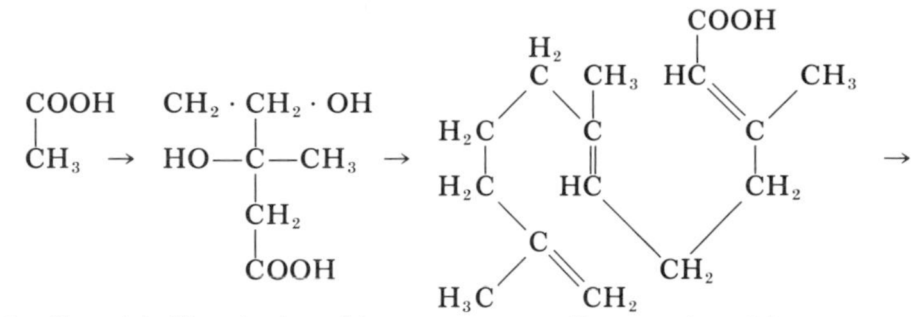

Acetic acid Mevalonic acid Farnesenic acid

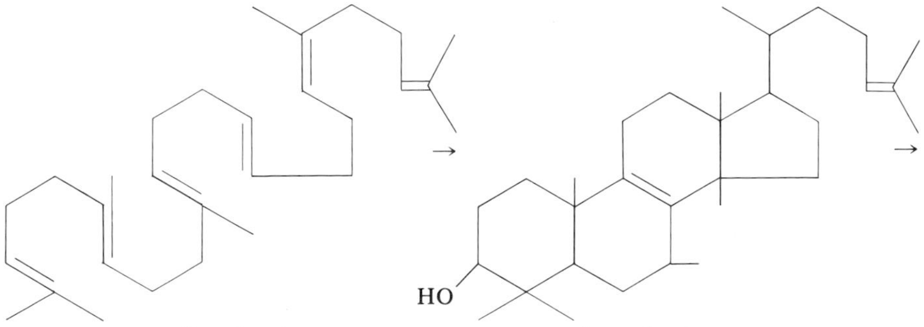

Squalene* Lanosterol

Continued.

*Each short line used in this skeleton formula is attached to a carbon atom. Sufficient hydrogen atoms are attached to each carbon atom to satisfy the 4 valences of carbon.

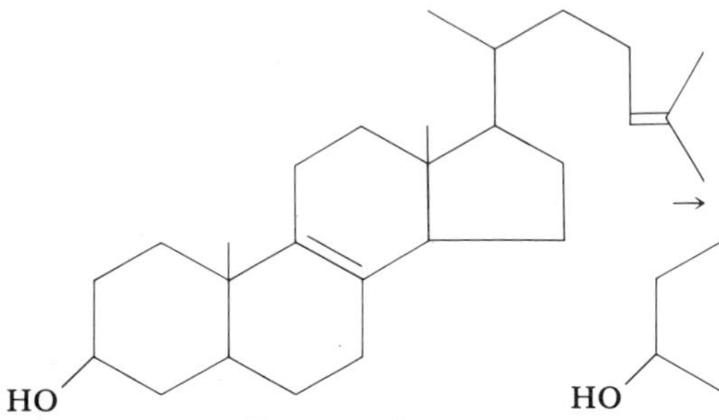

Zymosterol

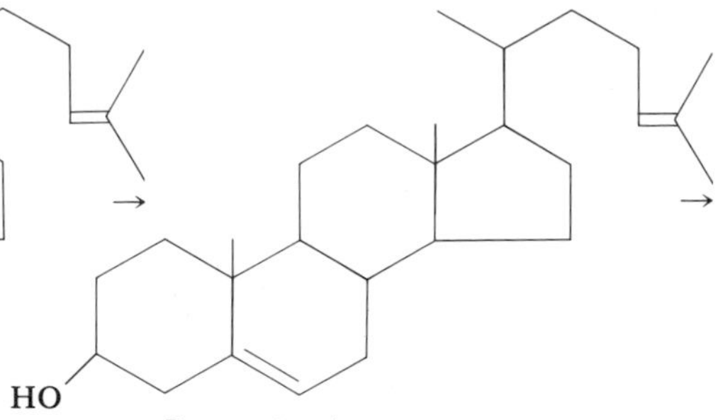

Dermosterol

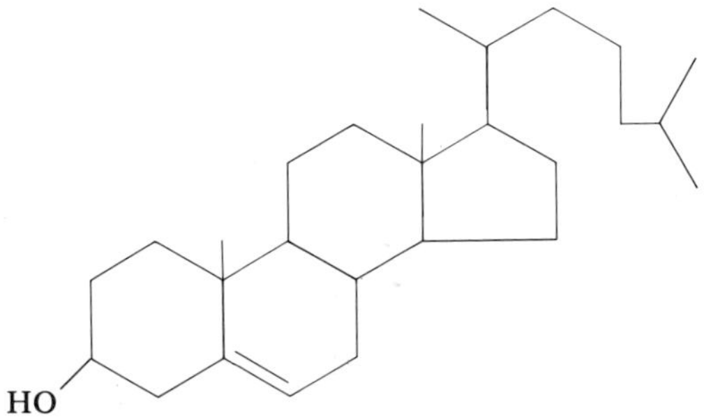

Cholesterol

Many medical scientists believe that high levels of cholesterol and triglycerides in the plasma predispose to the development of atherosclerosis. This disease usually involves the coronary arteries and coronary heart disease kills more Americans each year than any other single disease. Strokes (rupture of blood vessels in the brain) also usually are caused by atherosclerosis. These levels in turn are related to the diet. If more than 450 mg of cholesterol is present in the daily diet (which normally contains about 600 to 700 mg) some elevation of plasma cholesterol level results. Polyunsaturated fatty acids (that is, fatty acids whose molecules contain two or more double bonds) in the diet tend to lower the levels of plasma cholesterol and triglycerides, monounsaturated fatty acids have no effect, and saturated fatty acids tend to elevate them. A dietary plan designed to lower the level of these lipids in the plasma, and thus probably to protect against coronary heart disease and strokes, is described on page 470. Cholesterol levels also can be lowered by using appropriate drugs, but it is not yet certain that using them will decrease the incidence of atherosclerosis.

OBESITY

Obesity refers to the excess deposition of fat in the tissues and beneath the skin. In other words, *obese* people are *fat* people. A few cases of obesity are undoubtedly caused by disease of certain glands in the body—particularly the pituitary gland, the thyroid gland, and the gonads (sex glands). A large majority of obese individuals, however, are fat *because they eat more food than they burn up*. We have four main uses for food: (1) to make new cells (growth); (2) to replace worn-out cells and tissues; (3) to make certain special substances (such as hormones and enzymes) that are necessary for normal metabolism; and (4) to burn as a source of energy. Most adults need almost no food for growth and only a small amount for the production of hormones and enzymes. The replacement of worn-out tissues can be accomplished with surprisingly little food. It follows, then, that a large part of the food needed by adults is used for energy purposes. If very

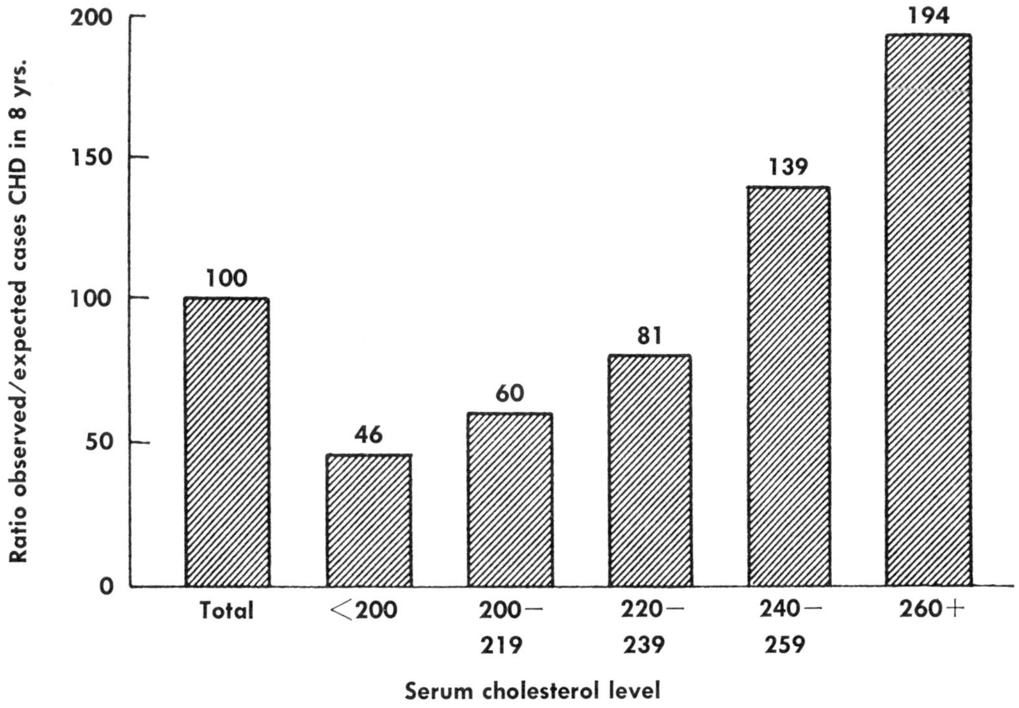

Fig. 22-4. Chart illustrating the correlation between level of cholesterol in the serum and the incidence of coronary heart disease (CHD) in men aged 30 to 59 at time of entry into study. Name some diseases in which the level of cholesterol is abnormally high. (Courtesy Dr. Thomas Dawber and Dr. William B. Kannel, National Heart Institute, National Institutes of Health; from Susceptibility to coronary heart disease, Mod. Conc. Cardiov. Dis. **30**:671, July 1961.)

much more carbohydrate and fat are present in the diet than are needed for energy requirements, the excess is stored as depot fat. Many people tend to become obese as they grow older. This results from a combination of two factors: (1) as a rule, they exercise less and so expend less energy; and (2) the rate at which foods are metabolized in the body becomes progressively less with advancing age. We expect, therefore, that a man 60 years of age will become obese if he eats the same amount of food as he did at 20 years of age.

LIPOIDOSES. Some diseases of enzymic defect involving abnormal storage of lipids in the tissues include the following.

Primary familial xanthomatosis with calcification of the adrenals. Cholesterol and triglycerides accumulate in cells in many organs and especially in the calcified adrenal glands. Death occurs at an early age.

Sulfatide lipoidosis. In this disease sulfatides (sulfur-containing lipids) accumulate in the nervous system and internal organs, especially in the kidney and biliary tract. In late stages violent muscular pains and weakness occur. The gallbladder is nonfunctioning. The clinical course is steadily downhill, although remissions occur.

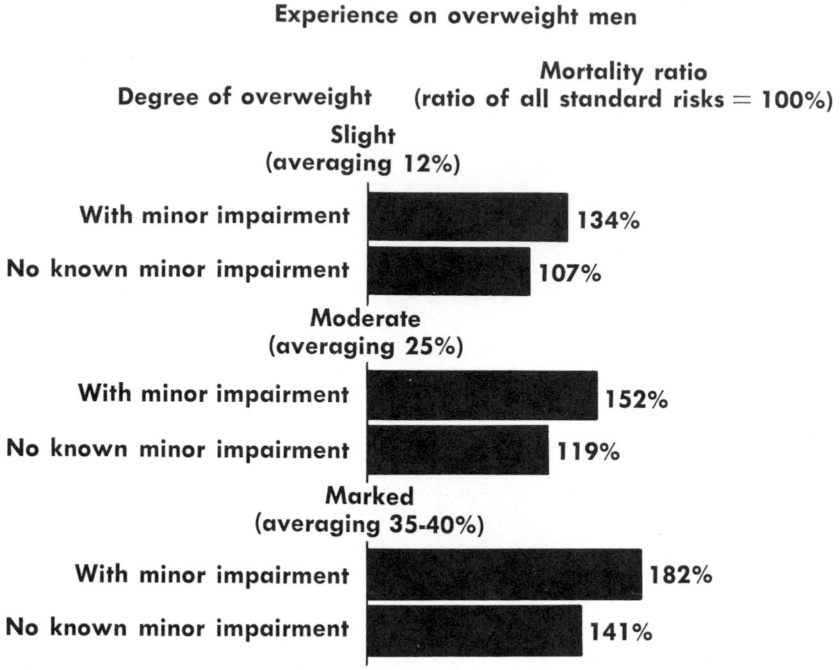

Fig. 22-5. Subsequent mortality among men, according to build classes, expressed as percentage of death rate of normal-weight men. This shows the influence of body weight on mortality, which is much increased by even minor impairments. (A minor impairment is defined as one which would not debar the applicant from obtaining Standard insurance—slight elevation of blood pressure, slight albuminuria, and psychoneurosis, for example.) Why do older people often tend to become obese? (Courtesy the Statistical Bureau of the Metropolitan Life Insurance Co.)

Familial neurovisceral lipoidosis (generalized gangliosidosis). There is a severe progressive cerebral degeneration that ends in death within the first 2 years of life. Glycolipids (lipids containing a sugar residue) accumulate in the brain, liver, spleen, and kidney. Patients show mental and motor retardation from infancy.

Angiokeratoma corporis universalis diffusum (syndrome of Fabry). Two abnormal lipids accumulate in the kidneys. There is a chronic kidney disease. Skin lesions appear in the lower trunk and genitals. There are eye symptoms, pain in the extremities, and sometimes edema. The leukocytes are deficient in the enzyme α-galactosidase.

Disseminated lipogranulomatosis. Patients have a hoarse voice and difficulty in eating and in respiration. There is an extreme involvement of joints and periarticular tissues with the development of a subcutaneous nodules and destruction of bony tissue. Foam cells (cells containing lipid droplets) occur in the pleura, liver, spleen, brain, and bone marrow.

Ceroid storage disease. An unknown pigmented lipid accumulates in the tissues. Cirrhosis of the liver and mental retardation are features of the disorder.

Tangier disease. There is enlargement of the liver, spleen, and lymph glands. The tonsils are much enlarged; they have an orange color and contain many foam cells packed with cholesterol. α-Lipoprotein, a protein normally present in the blood, is lacking. Another blood protein, β-lipoprotein, is doubled. The level of cholesterol in the blood is abnormally high.

Refsum disease. This disorder is characterized by polyneuritis, cerebellar ataxia (difficulty in walking), deafness, night blindness, retinitis pigmentosa (deposits of pigment in the retina of the eye), and ichthyosis (dry, harsh skin with adherent scales). There is a storage of 3,7,11,15-tetramethylpalmitic acid (a fatty acid derivative) in the tissues. The fatty acid level of the blood is elevated, as is the level of a copper-containing protein known as ceruloplasmin (see page 342).

STUDY QUESTIONS

1. What is meant by metabolism? Catabolism? Anabolism?
2. Briefly discuss the digestion and absorption of fat.
3. What are the two principal anabolic products of fatty acids? What is adipose tissue?
4. Name two functions of depot fat.
5. How much energy is obtained by the oxidation of 1 g of fat in the body?
6. What is meant by the theory of β-oxidation of fatty acids?
7. Name some of the types of compound formed during the catabolism of fatty acids.
8. What are the end products of fatty acid catabolism?
9. Name the ketone bodies.
10. Define ketosis.
11. What is the alkali reserve? What is acidosis? Is the blood acid in acidosis?
12. Explain how ketosis causes acidosis.
13. Name four causes of ketosis.
14. What is diabetic acidosis? Diabetic coma?
15. What are chylomicrons?
16. Explain how lipids reach the blood from the intestinal cells.
17. Is the liver an important storage site for fat?
18. What are lipoproteins?
19. Name some causes of a "fatty liver."
20. Is the fat in adipose tissue static or does it undergo constant change?
21. Name a hormone required for the synthesis of fat.
22. How are fatty acids transported from adipose tissue to other areas of the body?
23. Name a function for each of the following types of phosopholipid: lecithins, cephalin, sphingomyelins.
24. Is cholesterol found in all animals? Do you think it occurs in plants?
25. Name three factors that influence the rate of synthesis of cholesterol by the liver.
26. Where in the body is most cholesterol synthesized?
27. About how much cholesterol is made each day in the body?
28. What happens to cholesterol in the liver?
29. What are gallstones?
30. Name several pathological conditions associated with changes of the cholesterol level of the blood.
31. Why do many medical scientists believe that a high level of cholesterol in the plasma is undesirable?
32. What is the most common cause of obesity? Explain. Why do many adults gain weight as they become older?
33. Give four reasons why we need food.
34. Name and describe two diseases characterized by an abnormal storage of lipid in the tissues.

CHAPTER 23

Chemical nature of carbohydrates

DEFINITIONS

Carbohydrates are either simple sugars or substances that form simple sugars when they are hydrolyzed. Sugars decompose to form carbon and water when they are heated in the dry state. This tells us that each molecule of sugar contains carbon, hydrogen, and oxygen. Furthermore, each molecule contains twice as many hydrogen atoms as oxygen atoms. This explains why sugars so readily form water, since water also contains 2 hydrogen atoms for each oxygen atom. The simple sugars that interest us contain several alcohol (OH) groups and either a ketone or an aldehyde group in each molecule. Sugars whose molecules contain aldehyde (CHO) groups are called *aldoses*. *Ketoses* are sugars whose molecules contain ketone (CO) groups.

TYPES OF CARBOHYDRATE

The three principal types of carbohydrate are the *monosaccharides*, the *disaccharides*, and the *polysaccharides*. Monosaccharides are simple sugars and will not ordinarily react with water to form simpler substances. The two important types of monosaccharides are the *hexoses*, which contain 6 carbon atoms per molecule, and the *pentoses*, which contain 5 carbon atoms in each molecule. *Disaccharides* form monosaccharides when they are hydrolyzed, each disaccharide molecule forming 2 monosaccharide molecules.

$$\text{Disaccharide molecule} + H_2O \rightarrow 2 \text{ Monosaccharide molecules}$$

One molecule of polysaccharide yields *more than* 2 molecules of monosaccharide on hydrolysis.

HEXOSES

The three most important hexoses are *glucose, fructose*, and *galactose*. Notice that all three of these sugars have the same *empirical formula*, $C_6H_{12}O_6$, but each has a different *structural formula*. Glucose and galactose are aldoses; fructose is a ketose. Each of these monosaccharides exists when dissolved in water not only as the aliphatic molecule given above but also as cyclic molecules. An example is the cyclic form of glucose.

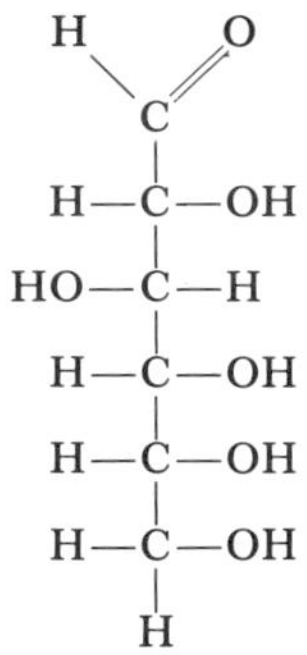

$C_6H_{12}O_6$
Glucose
(Aldose)

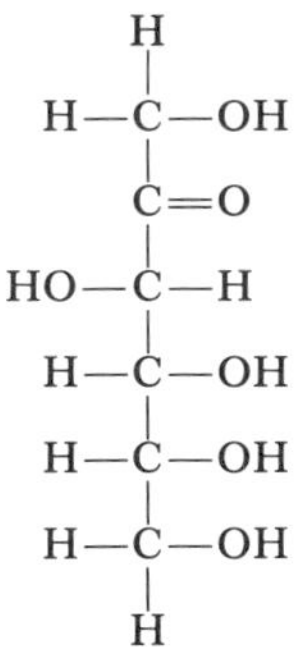

$C_6H_{12}O_6$
Fructose
(Ketose)

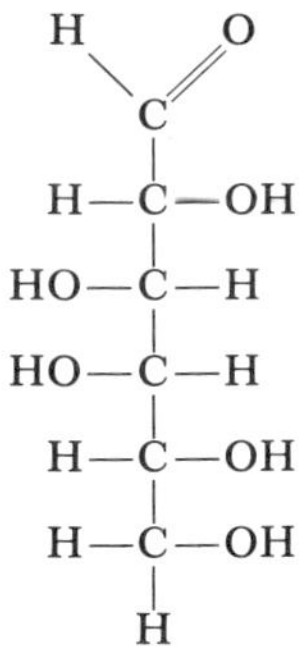

$C_6H_{12}O_6$
Galactose
(Aldose)

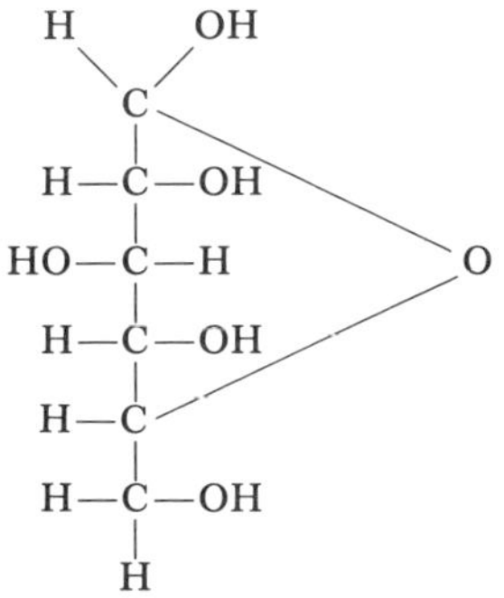

$C_6H_{12}O_6$
Glucose
(Cyclic form)

Glucose, also known as *dextrose* or *grape sugar,* is the most important hexose. In its pure state it is a white crystalline solid that readily dissolves in water. It is insoluble in most of the organic solvents. Most sweet fruits contain relatively large amounts of glucose. Ripe grapes, for example, contain 20 to 30 percent of this hexose. Glucose occurs normally in the blood and tissue fluids, and under certain abnormal conditions may occur also in demonstrable amounts in the urine. We shall discover later that the metabolism of carbohydrates is largely the metabolism of glucose because the other hexoses found in foods are converted to glucose in the body.

Glucose, in common with the other monosaccharides and with some disaccharides, is a *reducing agent.* We have already learned that aldehydes and ketones are reducing agents. Sugars owe their reducing power to the presence of these groups in their molecules. One test for the presence of glucose in blood and urine involves the reduction of copper with a valence of 2+ to copper with a valence of 1+. *Benedict's solution,* often used in testing urine for glucose, may be regarded as a solution of cupric hydroxide, $Cu(OH)_2$. In the presence of glucose the cupric hydroxide, $Cu(OH)_2$ (Cu^{++}), is reduced to cuprous oxide, Cu_2O (Cu^+), which precipitates as a brick-red or yellow solid. The test is usually carried out by heating 5 ml of Benedict's solution with 0.5 ml of urine. If the characteristic precipitate appears, we

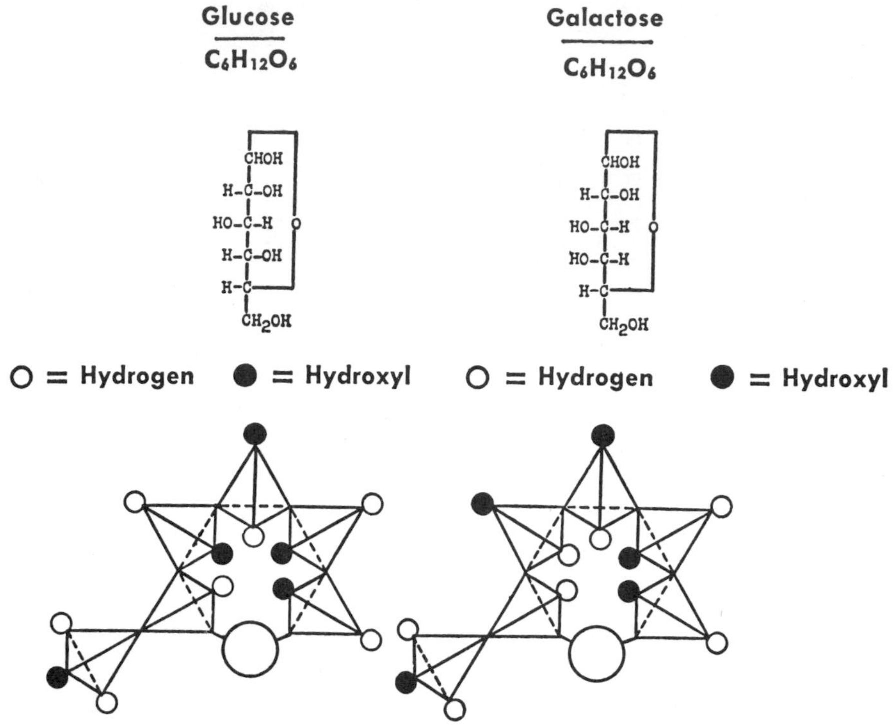

Fig. 23-1. Diagrams to show the cyclic structures of glucose and galactose. Carbon atoms have been represented as tetrahedrons (pyramids), each of the 4 corners of a tetrahedron representing one of the 4 carbon valences. How does the structural formula for glucose differ from that for galactose? (Courtesy Dr. Harold G. Loeb.)

know that a reducing agent, usually glucose, is present in the urine. Normal urine does not give a precipitate when treated in this way.

$CH_2OHCHOHCHOHCHOHCHOHCHO$	+	$2\ Cu(OH)_2$		$\rightarrow$
Glucose in pathological urine		Cupric hydroxide in Benedict's solution		
$CH_2OHCHOHCHOHCHOHCHOHCOOH$	+	$Cu_2O\downarrow$	+	$2\ H_2O$
Gluconic acid		Cuprous oxide (Brick-red or yellow precipitate)		

Fructose, often called *levulose,* is also found in sweet fruits. About half the sugar in honey is fructose, the other half being glucose. A mixture composed of equal parts of glucose and fructose is sometimes called *invert sugar.** Fructose is a ketose and will, therefore, reduce Benedict's solution.

*Sucrose, a disaccharide that yields fructose and glucose when hydrolyzed, is strongly dextrorotatory—that is, solutions of it rotate polarized light to the right. After hydrolysis, solutions of the resulting mixture of fructose and glucose rotate polarized light slightly to the left. Hence the direction of rotation of the polarized light has been inverted. This explains the origin of the term *invert sugar.*

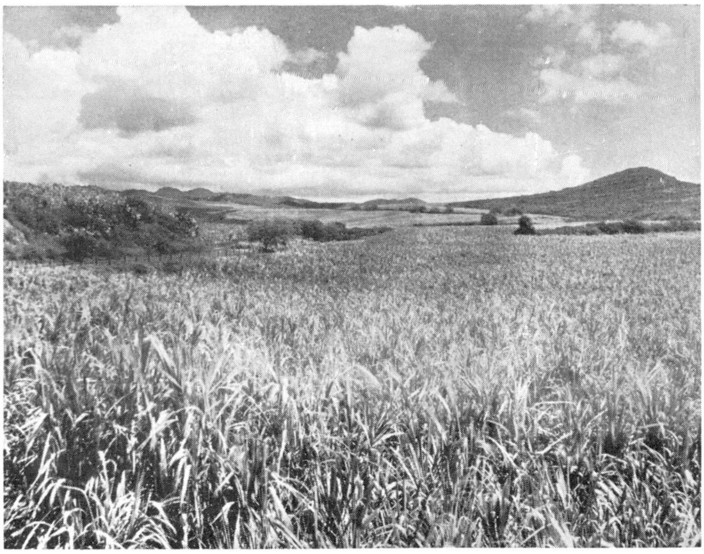

Fig. 23-2. Cane field in Hawaii. This is a typical field of sugar cane in the state of Hawaii, which normally produces about one-sixth of the nation's domestic supply. Does cane sugar differ from beet sugar? (Courtesy Pan-Pacific Press Bureau.)

Galactose is not found free in nature, but it is produced by the hydrolysis of lactose (milk sugar) in the digestive tract. It can also be prepared in the laboratory by the hydrolysis of certain polysaccharides.

FERMENTATION Glucose readily breaks down to form ethyl alcohol and carbon dioxide in the presence of a mixture of enzymes known as *zymase*.

$$\underset{\text{Glucose}}{C_6H_{12}O_6} \xrightarrow{\text{(Zymase)}} \underset{\text{Ethyl alcohol}}{2\ CH_3CH_2OH} + \underset{\text{Carbon dioxide}}{2\ CO_2}$$

The formation of alcohol and carbon dioxide from sugars in this way is called *fermentation*. Zymase is found in ordinary brewer's yeast (*Saccharomyces cerevisiae*). Most of the common hexoses and disaccharides undergo this reaction. Galactose and lactose, however, will not ferment when mixed with ordinary brewer's yeast, and are, therefore, exceptions to the general rule.

PENTOSES The pentoses are monosaccharides that have molecules containing 5 carbon atoms. Some plants contain small amounts of them in free form. They occur mainly, however, in chemical combination as polysaccharides. *Xylose* can be produced by the hydrolysis of woods and grains. *Arabinose* is produced when the gum of the cherry tree is hydrolyzed. *Ribose* and *deoxyribose* are constitutents of nucleic acids. Nucleic acids are compounds present in plant and animal cells (see page 297).

DISACCHARIDES Disaccharides have the empirical formula $C_{12}H_{22}O_{11}$. One molecule of disaccharide yields 2 molecules of hexose on hydrolysis. This hydrolysis is catalyzed by inorganic acids and by enzymes.

Sucrose is obtained commercially from sugar cane (cane sugar) and from sugar beets (beet sugar). It is the ordinary sugar we use on our dining tables. Glucose and fructose are formed on hydrolysis.

$$\text{Sucrose} + H_2O \rightarrow \text{Glucose} + \text{Fructose}$$

The mixture of glucose and fructose formed in this way is called invert sugar. The fermentation of sucrose in the presence of brewer's yeast involves two steps: (1) the hydrolysis of sucrose to form invert sugar, catalyzed by the yeast enzyme *invertase;* and (2) the fermentation of the invert sugar, catalyzed by *zymase.*

Sucrose does *not* reduce Benedict's solution. This means that sucrose does not have either an aldehyde or a ketone group. We explain this by supposing that the chemical linkage uniting the glucose with the fructose occurs between the aldehyde group of the glucose and the ketone group of the fructose. Thus, both these reducing groups are destroyed.

Lactose is the characteristic sugar of milk and is also called milk sugar. It is not as sweet as sucrose. One molecule of lactose yields 1 molecule of glucose and 1 molecule of galactose on hydrolysis.

$$\text{Lactose} + H_2O \rightarrow \text{Glucose} + \text{Galactose}$$

Lactose, unlike sucrose, *does not* ferment in the presence of brewer's yeast, and *does* reduce Benedict's solution. Certain bacteria make enzymes that catalyze the conversion of lactose to lactic acid. This conversion occurs when milk sours, and the characteristic taste of sour milk is from the presence of lactic acid.

Maltose (malt sugar) is found in germinating grains and in malt. It is one of the series of substances formed by the hydrolysis of starch.

$$\text{Starch} \xrightarrow{H_2O} \text{Dextrins} \xrightarrow{H_2O} \text{Maltose} \xrightarrow{H_2O} \text{Glucose}$$

On hydrolysis 1 molecule of maltose is changed to 2 molecules of glucose. Maltose has a free aldehyde group, since it reduces Benedict's solution. It undergoes fermentation in the presence of yeast enzymes.

Some of the properties of the important disaccharides are summarized in Table 23-1.

SOME IMPORTANT POLYSACCHARIDES

Cellulose is the polysaccharide that makes up the supporting tissue of plants. It has a molecular weight in the millions and forms glucose on complete hydrolysis. Cotton, linen, and filter paper are nearly pure cellulose. Like the other polysaccharides, cellulose will not reduce Benedict's

Table 23-1. Some properties of important disaccharides

Disaccharide	Fermentation with brewer's yeast	Reduction of Benedict's solution	Products of hydrolysis	Relative sweetness
Sucrose	Yes	No	Glucose Fructose	100
Lactose	No	Yes	Glucose Galactose	16
Maltose	Yes	Yes	Glucose Glucose	32.5

solution. It is not changed by any of the digestive enzymes secreted by the intestinal tract, and we are thus unable to digest it. Small amounts of acids and gases are formed from cellulose in the lower intestinal tract, this formation being catalyzed by bacterial enzymes. The intestinal tracts of ruminants (cows, sheep, goats, and so on) and some insects (termites) contain bacteria that can hydrolyze cellulose and thus make it available as food.

Many important substances are made from cellulose. Among these substances are the following:

1. *Pyroxylin* or *nitrocellulose*. When this is dissolved in a mixture of alcohol, ether, camphor, and castor oil the resulting product is called *flexible collodion*. Flexible collodion is used to cover small abrasions of the skin; when it dries it forms a flexible, protective covering ("new skin").
2. *Rayon*. A thick, yellow solution is formed by treating cellulose with sodium hydroxide and carbon disulfide. When this solution is forced through small holes into a sulfuric acid solution it solidifies to form threads of rayon (artificial silk).
3. *Cellophane*. This is made by several procedures. Its manufacture is nearly like that of rayon, except that the finished product is solidified in the form of sheets instead of threads.

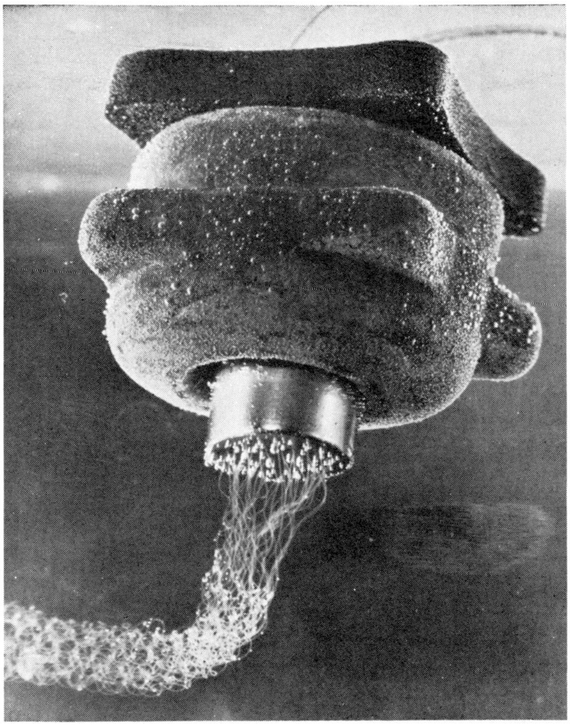

Fig. 23-3. A spinnerette in action. Viscose solution is being forced through tiny holes in the thimblelike nozzle into the surrounding acid-coagulating bath. All the filaments are collected to form a single thread, which after processing is ready for the manufacture of rayon fabrics. What type of chemical is rayon? (Courtesy Industrial Rayon Corp.)

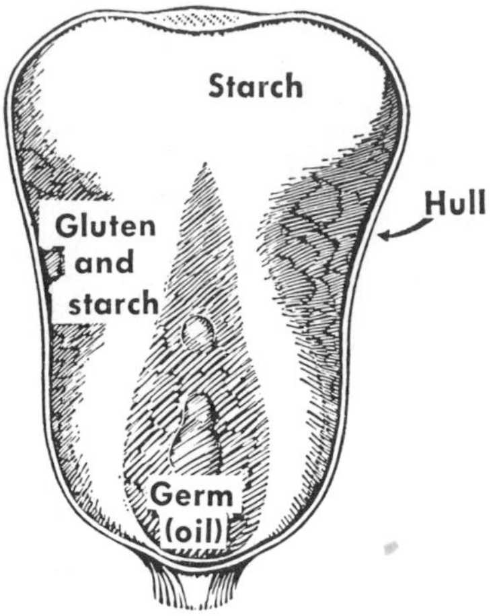

Fig. 23-4. Diagram showing the structure of the corn kernel. Starch is the principal component, the kernel containing about 60 percent of this substance. In the starch manufacturing industry the gluten and the hulls are made into feed for livestock. The germ contains a high percentage of oil, which, after purification, is used for salad oils and vegetable shortenings. What monosaccharide is formed by the hydrolysis of starch? (Courtesy Corn Industries Research Foundation.)

4. *Motion picture films.* The material used for making these films is prepared by treating cellulose with acetic acid. It is often called cellulose acetate.
5. *Gun cotton.* Gun cotton, or trinitrocellulose, contains more combined nitric acid than pyroxylin. As its name suggests, it looks very much like cotton. It is used in the manufacture of high explosives. One type of smokeless powder is made by treating gun cotton with acetone.

Starch is the characteristic polysaccharide storage food of plants and is widely distributed throughout the plant kingdom. It is an important animal food. Starch can be hydrolyzed by treatment with dilute inorganic acids or by mixing it with a solution of *diastase* (a general term for enzymes that hydrolyze starch). The diastases present in the digestive tract are called *amylases* (*amylum* is the Latin name for starch). Amylases catalyze the conversion of starch to a series of simpler substances: first to *dextrins,* then to *maltose.* Since the hydrolysis of maltose yields only glucose, we may suppose that the starch molecule is composed of an unknown number of glucose molecules combined chemically with each other. Its molecular weight in its native state is probably in the millions.

Starch exists in plants as small granules. It will not mix with water until these granules have been ruptured by heat or by grinding, after which it will form a colloidal solution. Starch reacts with iodine to give an intense blue color. This reaction is often used in testing for its presence. Most dextrins give a red color with iodine, but maltose gives no color at all.

Dextrins form sticky solutions in water. The mucilage used on postage stamps is made from dextrins.

Glycogen is present in all body tissues, particularly in the liver and muscles. It is the reserve carbohydrate food of the body. As we shall see later, it is formed in the cells by the chemical union of glucose molecules, a process called *glycogenesis*. The hydrolysis of glycogen, called *glycogenolysis* when it occurs in the body, yields glucose. Glycogen forms a substance having a red-brown color in the presence of iodine. Molecular weights of 270,000 to 100,000,000 have been reported for glycogen. The true value probably varies depending on the source of the glycogen, but probably is in the millions.

Dextrans are polysaccharides produced by certain bacteria growing in the presence of sucrose. They yield mainly or exclusively glucose when they are hydrolyzed. Specially processed dextran solutions are used as substitutes for blood plasma in the treatment of shock. They may play an important role in the production of tooth decay and dental disease (see page 319).

Pectins yield galactose, arabinose, and a sugar acid (galacturonic acid) on hydrolysis. They are present in fruits and berries. In the presence of sucrose and small amounts of acids they form jellies.

POLYSACCHARIDES AND IMMUNITY. When harmful bacteria invade the tissues, the body cells produce substances called *antibodies* that assist in destroying the invaders. When sufficient of these antibodies have been produced, the bacteria are not likely to be able to cause an infection, and a state of *immunity* is said to exist.

The bacteria that cause lobar pneumonia, tuberculosis, boils, gonorrhea, meningitis, and dysentery are known to contain specific polysaccharides. It has been shown that antibody formation is stimulated by the polysaccharide of the pneumococcus (which causes lobar pneumonia), and other bacterial polysaccharides are also important in this respect.

GLYCOSIDES

Substances that form carbohydrate and one or more other compounds on hydrolysis are called *glycosides*. Glycosides in which the sugar constituent is glucose are known as *glucosides*. Indeed, some authors use the term glucoside as a synonym for glycoside. The carbohydrate formed is usually, but not always, glucose. Digitoxin, digitalin, and gitoxin are glycosides found in digitalis (foxglove), a drug frequently used in the treatment of heart diseases. Strophanthus, another plant drug used in treating heart conditions, contains the two glycosides strophanthin and ouabain. Squill, a plant also known as sea onion, is used as an ingredient of cough syrups; in large doses it causes emesis (vomiting). It contains scillaren, a glycoside. The cerebrosides, which we have classified with the lipids, can also be considered glycosides because they yield galactose, a carbohydrate, on hydrolysis.

PHOTOSYNTHESIS

Only green plants have the ability to make carbohydrates. We know that fats can be made from carbohydrates and that the carbon necessary for protein formation also originates from them. Animals are, therefore, dependent on plants for life. Someone has said that *photosynthesis*, the name given to the process plants use to make carbohydrates, is the most important chemical reaction in the world. It has been estimated that photosynthesis involves the fixation of 400,000,000,000 tons of CO_2 annually.

Green plants contain a substance called *chlorophyll*. Apparently chlorophyll absorbs radiant energy from the sun, and this energy is used to cause carbon dioxide to combine with water to form carbohydrate.

$$\underset{\text{Carbon dioxide}}{6\,CO_2} + \underset{\text{Water}}{6\,H_2O} \rightarrow \underset{\text{Glucose}}{C_6H_{12}O_6} + \underset{\text{Oxygen}}{6\,O_2}$$

As the equation shows, oxygen gas is produced as a product of the reaction. From an energy point of view photosynthesis changes radiant energy into chemical energy; the chemical energy thus produced is the basis for nearly all plant and animal life. Photosynthesis is also important because it produces oxygen. Both animals and plants constantly use up oxygen in their metabolism, and our oxygen supply eventually would become exhausted if green plants did not make more for us.

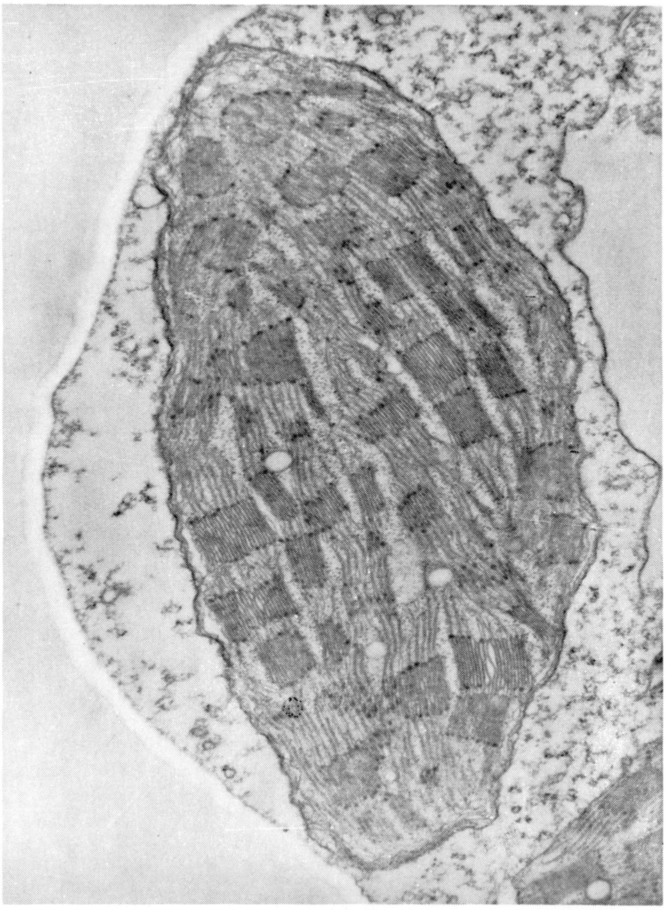

Fig. 23-5. A chloroplast in a maize cell is enlarged 40,000 diameters in this electron photomicrograph. The "light" reactions of photosynthesis take place within the rectangular "grana." What colored substance is contained in a chloroplast? (Courtesy Dr. A. E. Vatter, University of Colorado.)

In 1772, Joseph Priestley (often credited with the discovery of oxygen; see page 42) observed that a mouse placed under a bell jar soon suffocated unless a live green plant also was under the jar. This was evidence that oxygen was evolved by the plant. Jan Ingenhousz later (1779) found that plants produced oxygen only when they were exposed to light. In 1782, Jean Senebier showed that the reaction would not take place unless carbon dioxide was present. Finally, Nicolas Théodore de Saussure found that water was also essential, so that the overall reaction could be written:

$$CO_2 + H_2O \xrightarrow[\text{(chlorophyll)}]{\text{(light)}} \text{organic matter} + O_2$$

THE LIGHT REACTION OF PHOTOSYNTHESIS. As we have learned (see page 209), animal cells store up energy by making ATP. The process involves the production of electrons by the oxidation of carbohydrate and other foods. These electrons, as they travel down an electron transport chain, cause the formation of the ATP molecules and eventually create water from molecular oxygen and hydrogen ions.

In plant cells the electrons are created when visible light of a certain wavelength strikes chlorophyll, the green compound located in all higher plants (see page 191 for structure). In *cyclic photophosphorylation* the excited (high-energy) electrons thus created are captured by the first of a chain of electron carriers. One type of carrier molecule is believed to contain vitamin K (see page 443) and riboflavin (see page 424). Others appear to be cytochromes – compounds containing ring systems very similar to those in chlorophyll but with iron instead of magnesium. Eventually, the electrons return "home" to chlorophyll, which now is ready to be reactivated by light.

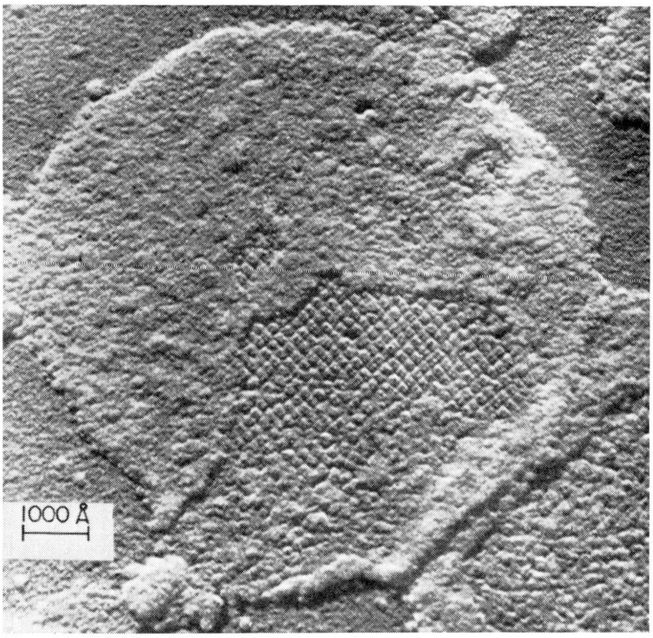

Fig. 23-6. Membranes containing chlorophyll taken from a spinach chloroplast. This chromium-shadowed preparation (magnified 187,000 times) shows that the membrane is composed of a highly ordered array of units called quantosomes. What is a granum? (Courtesy Dr. Roderic B. Park and Dr. John Biggins, University of California; from Quantosome: size and composition, Science **144:**1009, May 22, 1964. Copyright 1964 by the American Association for the Advancement of Science.)

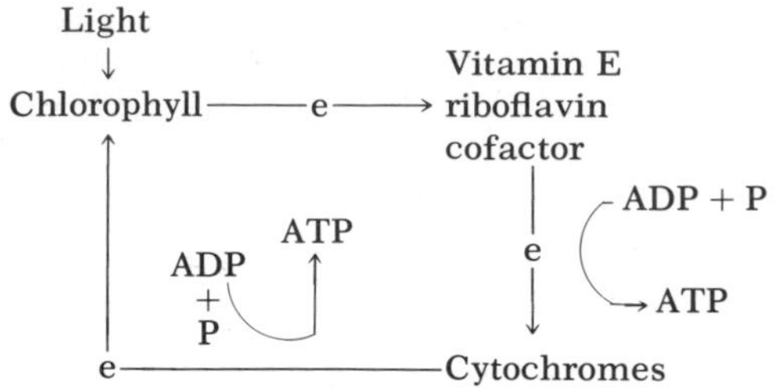

Another type of photosynthesis—*noncyclic photophosphorylation*—also occurs in the green plant. This reaction involves nicotinamide adenine dinucleotide phosphate ($NADP^+$), a coenzyme that differs from NAD^+ (see page 212) in having three, rather than two, phosphate radicals per molecule. Water also takes part in the reaction, and molecular oxygen is created.

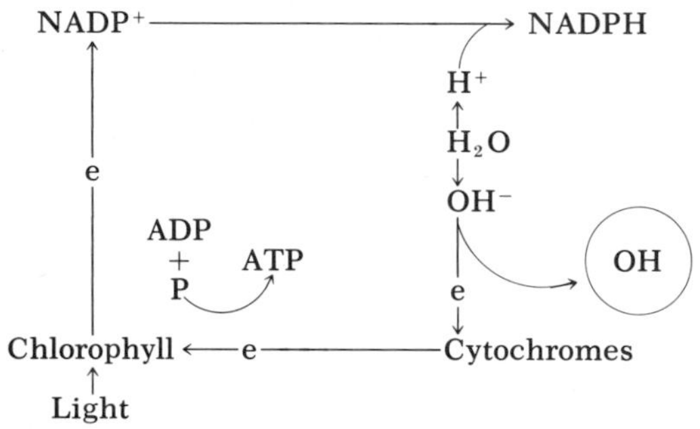

The OH radicals (shown in the circle) react with each other to form molecular oxygen and water.

$$4OH \rightarrow 2H_2O + O_2$$

The chlorophyll is located in minute structures known as chloroplasts. Within the chloroplast, like stacks of coins, are structures known as grana (see Fig. 23-5). Each granum is made up of stacked molecules of chlorophyll, sandwiched between membranes probably composed of protein and lipid. The chloroplast also contains the electron transport molecules.

THE DARK REACTION. The remaining reaction—the synthesis of glucose from CO_2 and H_2O—does not require light. It does require ATP and NADPH, however. Some of the compounds that take part in the reaction are illustrated in the following scheme:

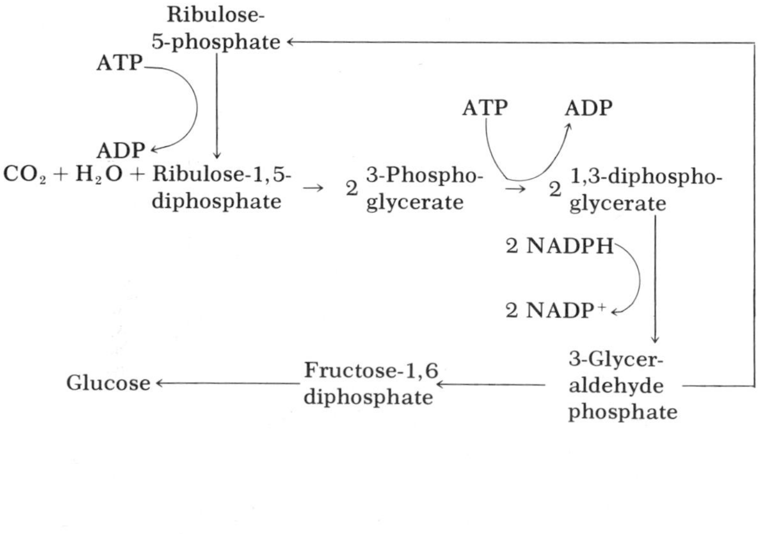

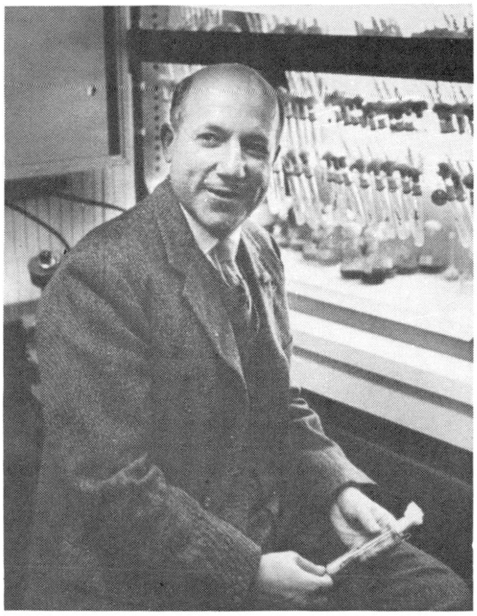

Fig. 23-7. Dr. Melvin Calvin of the University of California received the Nobel Prize in chemistry in 1961 for his elucidation of many of the complex processes involved in photosynthesis. What is meant by the "dark reaction"?

The cycle illustrated here is very much simplified—the cycle as presently known involves at least twelve distinct reactions Essentially, however, what happens is this: Five molecules of phosphoglycerate (3 C atoms per molecule) become transformed into compounds containing 3, 4, 6, and 7 carbon atoms; these in turn finally end up as 3 5-C atom molecules (ribulose diphosphate). More carbon dioxide reacts with these, and from them 6 phosphoglycerate molecules are formed. Thus the original 5 molecules of phosphoglycerate have become 6; in other words, 3 carbon dioxide molecules have been converted to phosphoglycerate. From this key intermediate carbohydrates, fats, and even amino acids and carboxylic acids are formed.

STUDY QUESTIONS

1. Make up a good definition for carbohydrate.
2. What are aldoses? Ketoses?
3. What are the three main groups of carbohydrates? Define each.
4. What are hexoses? Name three important hexoses.
5. What is the empirical formula for hexoses?
6. Give two other names for glucose.
7. Describe a test for the presence of glucose in urine. What is Benedict's solution?
8. What is another name for fructose? What is invert sugar?
9. Name one ketose and two aldoses.
10. What is fermentation? What is zymase? Name two sugars that do not undergo fermentation in the presence of brewer's yeast.
11. What are pentoses? Give three or four examples. Where are nucleic acids found?
12. What is the empirical formula for the disaccharides?
13. Give two other names for sucrose. What is invertase?
14. What is another name for milk sugar?
15. What chemical change occurs when milk sours?
16. What substances are formed by the hydrolysis of starch?
17. How could you use brewer's yeast and Benedict's solution to distinguish between sucrose, lactose, and maltose?
18. What are the products of hydrolysis of sucrose? Of lactose? Of maltose?
19. What substance is produced by the complete hydrolysis of cellulose? Of starch? Of glycogen?
20. Where is cellulose found in nature? Name some products made from cellulose.

21. What is a diastase? An amylase? What are dextrins? Dextrans?
22. What color does each of the following give with iodine: starch, dextrins, maltose, glycogen?
23. Why must starch be boiled or ground up before it will mix with water? Does starch form a true solution in water?
24. What is glycogen? Glycogenesis? Glycogenolysis?
25. What are pectins? Under what conditions will they gel?
26. What are antibodies? What is immunity? Why are polysaccharides thought to be important in immunity?
27. What is a glycoside? Name some glycosides used in medicine.
28. Explain how green plants use chlorophyll to make carbohydrates.
29. Give two reasons why photosynthesis is said to be the most important of all chemical reactions.
30. How does the "light reaction" differ from the "dark reaction"?

CHAPTER **24**

Metabolism of carbohydrates

SUMMARY OF CARBOHYDRATE DIGESTION

The saliva contains two enzymes that contribute to the digestion of carbohydrates. One of them, *salivary amylase,* catalyzes the formation of maltose by the hydrolysis of starch. The other, *salivary maltase,* catalyses the hydrolysis of maltose to glucose. The mixture of salivary amylase and salivary maltase is frequently called *ptyalin.* Salivary digestion is not very important because the food stays in the mouth only a short time. When the food is swallowed, the action of the salivary enzymes soon ceases because they are not active at the low pH of the gastric (stomach) juice. No enzymes concerned with carbohydrate digestion are present in gastric juice, but some hydrolysis of disaccharides probably occurs as a result of catalysis by the hydrochloric acid that is present. *Pancreatic amylase (amylopsin),* an enzyme present in pancreatic juice, is the most important starch-digesting enzyme. Starch that reaches the intestinal tract is converted in its presence to maltose. Maltose is hydrolyzed to glucose in the presence of *pancreatic maltase* (in pancreatic juice) and of *intestinal maltase* (in intestinal juice). *Lactase,* present in both pancreatic juice and intestinal juice, catalyzes the hydrolysis of lactose to glucose and galactose. Pancreatic juice and intestinal juice also contain *sucrase* (invertase), which catalyzes the conversion of sucrose to glucose and fructose.

In summary, then, digestion of the ordinary carbohydrate foods results in the conversion of these foods to the monosaccharides: *glucose, fructose,* and *galactose.*

Lactose is hydrolyzed slowly in the intestinal tract. There is evidence that this sugar can diffuse into the intestinal cells and undergo hydrolysis there. Lactose in some way assists in the absorption of calcium, magnesium, barium, strontium, phosphorus, and perhaps other substances. It promotes the manufacture of several vitamins (biotin, riboflavin, folic acid) by intestinal bacteria.

FATE OF FRUCTOSE AND GALACTOSE

Fructose and galactose are absorbed directly into the bloodstream (portal vein). The liver then removes fructose from the blood and changes it to *glucose.* Apparently fructose can also be changed to glucose by the cells of the intestinal tract. Galactose is converted to glucose by an enzyme pres-

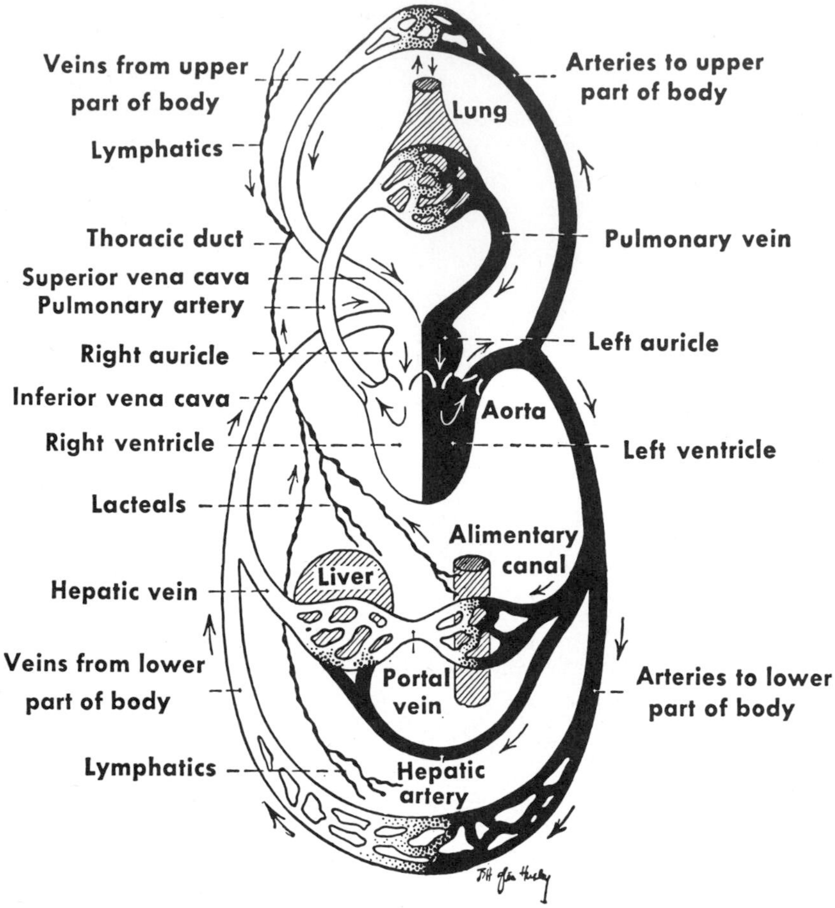

Fig. 24-1. Diagram illustrating the circulation of the blood. Notice that blood leaves the digestive tract (alimentary canal) through the portal vein. What is the first organ a glucose molecule reaches after it is absorbed from the digestive tract?

ent in normal red blood cells. It is obvious that the metabolism of carbohydrates is very largely the metabolism of *glucose*.

Galactosemia. Galactosemia ("galactose in the blood") or galactose diabetes is a metabolic disease of infancy. The disease is caused by an inherited lack of an enzyme (phosphogalactose uridyl transferase) found in normal red blood cells. This enzyme normally converts galactose to glucose. Infants with galactosemia cannot tolerate milk in any form. (Remember that the lactose present in milk is converted to glucose and galactose in the intestine.) Diarrhea, lack of appetite, weight loss, and jaundice are early signs. Cirrhosis (hardening) of the liver, mental retardation, blindness from cataracts, and death often follow.

GLYCOGEN FORMATION

Glycogen formation *(glycogenesis)* occurs chiefly in the liver and the muscles. The glucose formed during digestion is absorbed into the bloodstream (portal vein). The blood of the portal vein flows directly to the liver, where the excess glucose coming from the digestive tract is removed and stored as *glycogen*. Certain other substances can also be converted to glycogen in the liver. These substances include fructose, galactose, glycerol, some amino acids (from protein digestion), lactic acid, and fatty acids whose molecules have an odd number of carbon atoms. A large percentage of the protein of the diet can be converted to glycogen after digestion. This probably occurs only when the need for glycogen is urgent.

Muscles have the ability to remove glucose from the blood and to convert it to *muscle glycogen*.

BLOOD SUGAR LEVEL

Glucose is the normal sugar of the blood, and blood glucose is often called *blood sugar*. The average normal value for the glucose present in the blood of a fasting individual (fasting blood sugar) is 60 to 100 mg per 100 ml of blood. The liver is the most important organ in maintaining the level of blood sugar at this figure. When the blood sugar level rises, as it does following digestion, the liver removes the excess glucose and stores it as glycogen. When the level of glucose in the blood becomes too low, liver glycogen breaks down to glucose (*glycogenolysis*), which then enters the bloodstream. Liver glycogenolysis is almost constantly necessary because glucose is constantly being removed from the blood by the muscles and other tissues that burn it as a source of energy.

Glucose does not normally appear in the urine, at least not in amounts that can be detected with Benedict's solution. However, when the value of the blood sugar rises above a certain value, called the *renal threshold*, glucose "spills over," as it were, and appears in the urine. The value of the renal threshold is normally about 150 to 170 mg of glucose per 100 ml of blood. If too much carbohydrate is eaten and digested at one time the blood sugar level may exceed the renal threshold. This occurs also in certain diseases that involve carbohydrate metabolism and storage.

GLYCOLYSIS

The energy of carbohydrate oxidation is derived from a complex series of chemical reactions involving various compounds formed from glycogen (Fig. 24-2). The breakdown of glycogen to form these substances (glycolysis) requires the presence of phosphate radicals. For example, two of the products formed are glucose phosphate and fructose diphosphate. These sugar phosphates undergo cleavage to simpler products, with the formation of phosphopyruvic acid. Phosphopyruvic acid is then changed to *pyruvic acid* ($CH_3COCOOH$). If the oxygen supply to the muscle is abundant, a portion of this pyruvic acid (probably about one-fifth) is oxidized to CO_2 and H_2O, with the release of energy. The remainder is resynthesized to glycogen. If the oxygen supply is deficient (as it will be during severe exercise, for example), all or a part of the pyruvic acid is reduced to *lactic* acid ($CH_3CHOHCOOH$). Most of the lactic acid formed in this way is changed back to glycogen either in the muscle or, if the lactic acid escapes into the blood, in the liver. The other portion is reconverted to pyruvic acid, which is oxidized to CO_2 and H_2O, and energy is produced. It is evident, then, that when the muscle contraction is finished and the muscle has recovered, the only permanent change has been the loss of a portion of the glycogen originally present. This lost glycogen is replenished by a conversion of blood glucose to muscle glycogen.

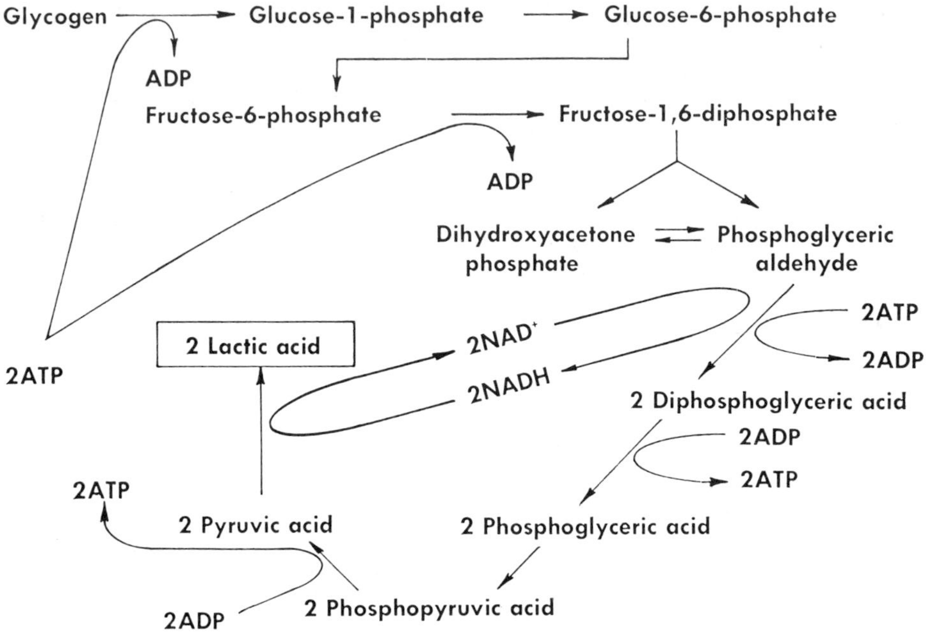

Fig. 24-2. Diagram illustrating the chemical changes that occur in glycolysis. Define glycolysis.

The phosphate radicals necessary for these changes are supplied by inorganic phosphate, *adenosine triphosphate,* and *creatine phosphate* (*phosphocreatine or phosphagen;* see page 285). The last two compounds contain nitrogen and are *not* carbohydrates. Most of the phosphate radicals lost by these compounds during the contraction are regained by them, with the result that the final products of glycogen breakdown (pyruvic acid, lactic acid, CO_2, and H_2O) do not contain phosphate.

If exercise (muscle contraction) is continuous and prolonged, lactic acid may accumulate faster than it can be oxidized, and a condition of *oxygen debt* is said to exist. After such exercise is finished the depth of respiration (breathing) is increased until enough extra oxygen has been carried to the tissues to oxidize the excess lactic acid and thus pay the oxygen debt.

$$\underset{\text{Lactic acid}}{CH_3CHOHCOOH} + \underset{\text{Oxygen}}{3\ O_2} \rightarrow \underset{\text{Carbon dioxide}}{3\ CO_2} + \underset{\text{Water}}{3\ H_2O}$$

The carbon dioxide formed by this oxidation escapes from the body through the lungs. Excess water is eliminated from the body partly through the lungs, partly from the skin (perspiration), and partly in the urine.

The end products of carbohydrate oxidation are always CO_2 and H_2O, regardless of which tissue the oxidation occurs in.

PENTOSE SHUNT The conversion of glucose to pyruvic acid can proceed by reactions other than those just discussed. The best known of these is termed the *pentose shunt*, or *hexose monophosphate shunt*. This pathway enables the tissues to make ribose-5-phosphate, a pentose phosphate utilized in the anabolism of nucleic acids (see Chapter 27). The reactions involved are summarized below:

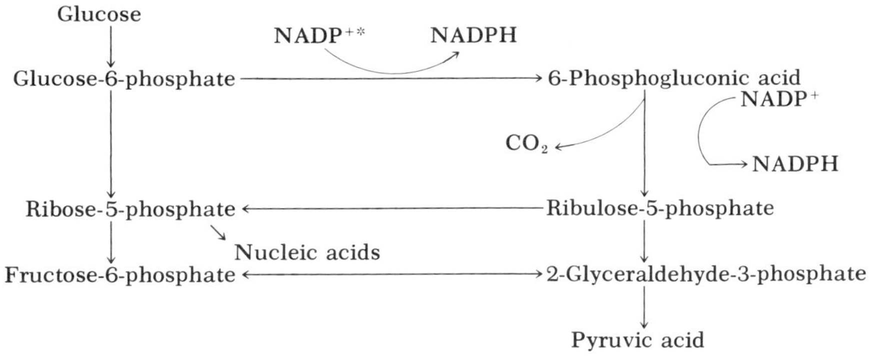

If this scheme is compared with the usual steps in glycolysis (see Fig. 24-2), it is clear that it really does represent a "shunt" around a portion of The reactions involved. The scheme as shown is highly simplified; it is necessary for the cycle to repeat at least six times before an accurate accounting for all the carbon atoms involved is possible.

TRICARBOXYLIC ACID CYCLE

The oxidation of pyruvic acid occurs mainly by way of the *tricarboxylic acid cycle*, known also as the Krebs cycle or the citric acid cycle. The various reactions that make up this cycle are as follows:

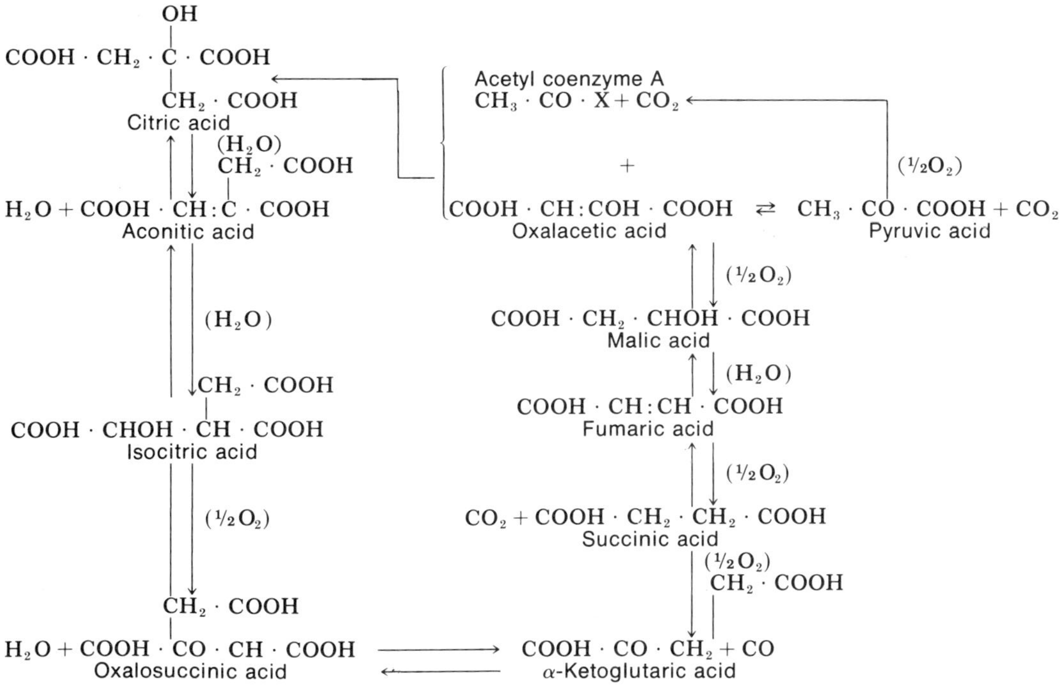

*$NADP^+$ differs from NAD^+ (see page 212) in having one more phosphate radical in its molecule.

Several interesting points should be noted in studying this cycle of reactions. Until recent years it was believed that CO_2 was entirely a waste product of animal metabolism, although it was known, of course, that plants use this gas to synthesize carbohydrate (see page 251). Studies with CO_2 containing heavy carbon, or radioactive carbon, have made it evident that carbon dioxide can and does enter into metabolic reactions in animal tissues. For example, as shown in the tricarboxylic acid cycle, CO_2 can combine with pyruvic acid to form oxalacetic acid.

An interesting feature of the cycle is the identity of the 2-carbon compound that combines with oxalacetic acid to form aconitic acid. This compound is an acetyl radical ($CH_3 \cdot CO$) attached chemically to a coenzyme known as coenzyme A (see page 211). Coenzyme A yields pantothenic acid (a vitamin; see page 435), adenine (see page 195), ribose, phosphoric acid, and mercaptoethylanolamine ($NH_2 \cdot CH_2 \cdot CH_2 \cdot SH$) on hydrolysis.

If a careful count is made of the oxygen used and of the CO_2 and H_2O produced during one complete cycle, it will be found that the overall reaction can be represented by the equation

$$CH_3 \cdot CO \cdot COOH + 2\tfrac{1}{2}O_2 \rightarrow 3CO_2 + 2H_2O$$

In other words, one molecule of pyruvic acid is oxidized completely to carbon dioxide and water in one complete cycle.

Although the tricarboxylic acid cycle first was investigated in connection with carbohydrate metabolism, it is evident that it is important also in the metabolism of fats and proteins. During the catabolism of fatty acids acetyl CoA is formed. The end stages of fatty acid catabolism can be identical with those of carbohydrate metabolism. It has been known for a long time that a large percentage of the amino acids

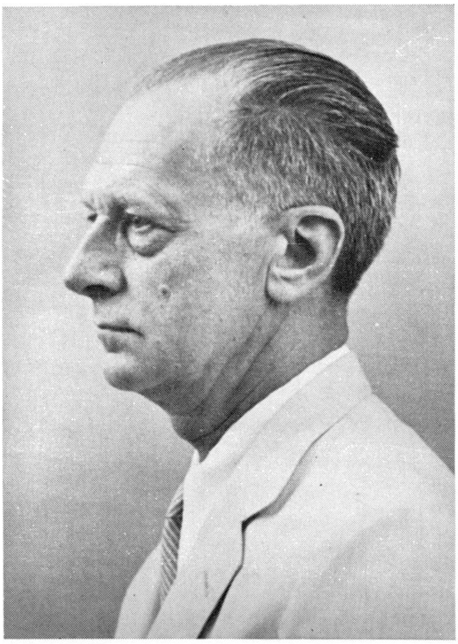

Fig. 24-3. Dr. Carl F. Cori, then at the Washington University School of Medicine, St. Louis, was awarded the Nobel Prize in medicine and physiology in 1947 for his work on the metabolism of glycogen. What compound is formed by the hydrolysis of glycogen?

present in proteins can be converted to carbohydrate and hence to pyruvic acid in the body. It is known also that glutamic acid, an amino acid found in proteins (see page 364), can be converted to α-ketoglutaric acid in the tissues. Hence, the tricarboxylic acid cycle is important in the catabolism of amino acids.

GLYCOGEN STORAGE DISEASES. In several diseases of enzymic defects (see page 215) there is an abnormal storage of glycogen in various tissues. Normal breakdown of glycogen is slowed or prevented because of the absence of an essential enzyme. Some of these diseases are listed in Table 24-1.

Hypoglycemia (low blood sugar) of marked degree occurs in the rare disorder known as *von Gierke's disease* (hepatonephromegalia glycogenica; type 1 glycogen storage disease). Glycogenolysis fails to occur normally in the liver and this organ becomes engorged with glycogen. The disease is hereditary.

McCardle's disease (type 5 glycogen storage disease) is characterized by a defect in the breakdown of muscle glycogen. Glycogenolysis in the liver is normal. Patients with the disease are unable to sustain exercise because of muscle cramps. They have difficulty in running and in climbing stairs.

METABOLISM OF NERVE TISSUE

Active brain and nerve tissues burn mainly carbohydrate to gain the energy necessary for the conduction of nerve impulses. The glycogen content of nerves is very low, and the tissues probably burn glucose directly without first converting it into glycogen. Pyruvic acid is formed and oxidized just as it is in muscle contraction. It is interesting that the burning of pyruvic acid requires the presence of a coenzyme composed of 2 molecules of phosphoric acid chemically combined with 1 molecule of thiamine. Thiamine is the chemical name for vitamin B_1.

CONVERSION OF CARBOHYDRATE TO FAT

All of us know that excess carbohydrates (sweets) in the diet can be changed to fat and stored as such in the body. It has been estimated that there is never more than a pound (454 g) of glycogen in the body at any one time. As we have learned, stored fat is burned as a source of energy in conditions where carbohydrate metabolism is impaired.

ENERGY OF CARBOHYDRATE OXIDATION

The oxidation of 1 g of carbohydrate in the body yields, on the average, 4 large calories of energy. Seventy-five to 80 percent of this energy is released in the form of heat. The remainder is used in allowing muscles to contract, glands to secrete, nerves to conduct impulses, and so on. As an engine, then, the body is only about 20 or 25 percent efficient, since only this percentage of the energy produced in the body can be used to do work. This compares favorably, however, with the efficiency of a gasoline engine.

Table 24-1. Glycogen storage diseases

Type	Organs involved	Deficient enzyme
1	Liver, kidneys	Glucose-6-phosphatase
2	Cardiac type (glycogen in all tissues)	α-Glucosidase
3	Liver, skeletal muscle, heart muscle	Amylo-1,6-glucosidase
4	Liver, reticuloendothelial system, kidneys, muscles, nervous tissue	Branching enzyme?
5	Skeletal muscles	Muscle phosphorylase
6	Liver	Liver phosphorylase

PROTEIN-SPARING ACTION OF CARBOHYDRATE

A large percentage of the protein of the diet can be converted to carbohydrate if the body is in urgent need of carbohydrate. If the carbohydrate food intake is too low, we will need more protein in the diet because a part of the protein will be converted to glucose and used for energy purposes. Carbohydrate is said to have a *protein-sparing action* since an abundant supply of carbohydrate food enables us to get by with a minimum of protein in the diet.

ACTION OF EPINEPHRINE

Epinephrine (adrenaline) is a compound (hormone) made in the adrenal glands, located one above each kidney (see page 397). Epinephrine causes a breakdown of glycogen. This results in an *increase* in blood sugar level and an increase in the lactic acid of the blood. After the effect of the epinephrine wears off, the excess glucose and lactic acid in the blood are converted back to glycogen in the liver. Some of the glucose may also be changed to muscle glycogen. Epinephrine has many other effects in the body. It is secreted into the blood in emotional states, and strong emotions, such as fear or anger, may cause the blood sugar level to rise above the renal threshold. If this occurs glucose appears in the urine.

FUNCTIONS OF INSULIN

Insulin is a substance (hormone) manufactured in the islands of Langerhans. The islands of Langerhans are small groups of cells located in the substance of the pancreas. Insulin is extremely important in carbohydrate metabolism. Its primary function is to promote the transfer of glucose across certain cell membranes. The transport of certain other sugars—D-galactose, D-xylose, L-arabinose, and D-mannose—also is facilitated. This is not true of L-xylose and D-arabinose, however.

Muscle cells (skeletal and cardiac), fibroblasts, and the cells of adipose tissue do not permit the passage of glucose without insulin, but the membranes of nerve cells, red blood cells, intestinal cells, and liver cells do.

Injection of a solution of insulin into the bloodstream causes: (1) a fall

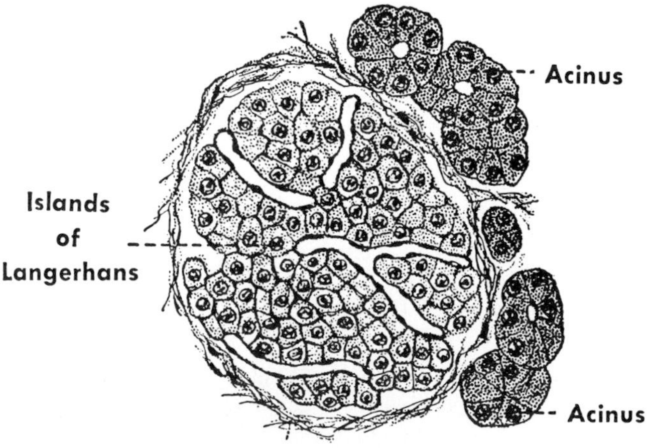

Fig. 24-4. A microscopic section of a normal pancreas to show a gland of internal secretion (island of Langerhans) and glands of external secretion (acinus). What products are manufactured by these two types of gland?

in the blood sugar level; (2) an increase in both muscles glycogen and liver glycogen; and (3) an increased rate of carbohydrate oxidation. The glucose that leaves the bloodstream apparently goes mainly into the muscles, where it is converted to muscle glycogen. Some of it may go into the liver, but there are reasons for supposing that the increase of liver glycogen may result from a decrease of liver glycogenolysis as well as from a conversion of lactic and pyruvic acids to glycogen in the liver. We know there is an increased production of these acids since the rate of carbohydrate burning is increased. The functions of insulin, then, may be summarized as follows:

1. It causes glucose to leave the bloodstream and enter the muscles (possibly the liver as well) where it is converted to glycogen.
2. It speeds up the rate of carbohydrate burning in the body.
3. It probably depresses glycogenolysis in the liver.
4. The liver of an animal from which the pancreas has been removed and which, therefore, has no source of insulin cannot convert carbohydrate to fat. Hence, it seems that one function of insulin is to catalyze the conversion of carbohydrate to fat.

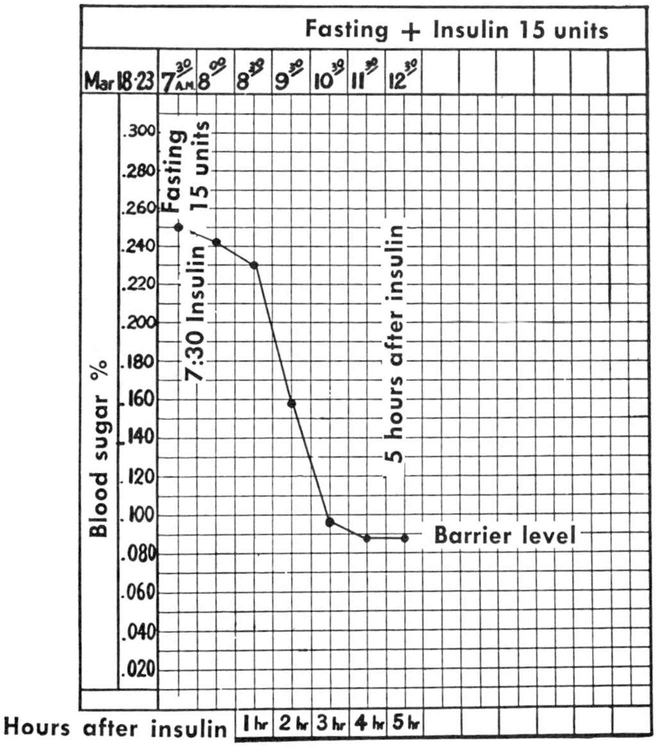

Fig. 24-5. Chart showing the effect of an insulin injection on the level of blood sugar. Notice that the blood sugar fell from a value of about 250 mg per 100 ml to a value of about 90 mg per 100 ml after the injection of 15 units of insulin (see Chapter 31). What is the average normal fasting value for the blood sugar level?

Diabetes mellitus. If the beta cells in the islands of Langerhans stop producing insulin, the disease known as diabetes mellitus ("sugar diabetes") results. It seems evident, however, that there are other causes as well. For example, insulin exists in the blood partly free and partly bound to protein. In some patients it is believed that all, or an excess amount, of the insulin is bound, so that it cannot act on cell membranes. In other cases substances that interfere with the action of insulin at cell membranes can be detected in the blood. Occasionally, patients appear to be making antibodies that neutralize insulin. Recently, it has been postulated that *chromium* is required for the activity of insulin and that some cases of diabetes mellitus may be caused by chromium deficiency.

Some patients, especially persons who develop diabetes mellitus late in life, can take synthetic drugs to control the disease. One type of drug appears to act by stimulating the beta cells to make more insulin. Another type acts by another mechanism that is not understood.

In the untreated disease the blood sugar level rises, sometimes to very high values, and sugar appears in the urine (because the renal threshold is exceeded). Carbohydrate oxidation is impaired and, as we might expect under these conditions, ketone bodies appear in large amounts in the blood and urine. This leads to the usual acidosis that accompanies ketosis. Untreated patients develop *diabetic coma* and finally die as a result of the profound acidosis. Insulin injections promptly alleviate the symptoms, and persons with diabetes can live many years quite normally if this substance is properly used. It must be remembered, however, that insulin is not in any sense a drug that will *cure* diabetes mellitus. Its use must ordinarily be continued as long as the patient lives. Insulin is a protein and is digested in the digestive tract. For this reason it must be injected by means of a hypodermic needle and cannot be given by mouth.

Glucose tolerance test. The *glucose tolerance test* is often used as an aid in diagnosing diabetes mellitus. The patient is required to fast for several hours, and

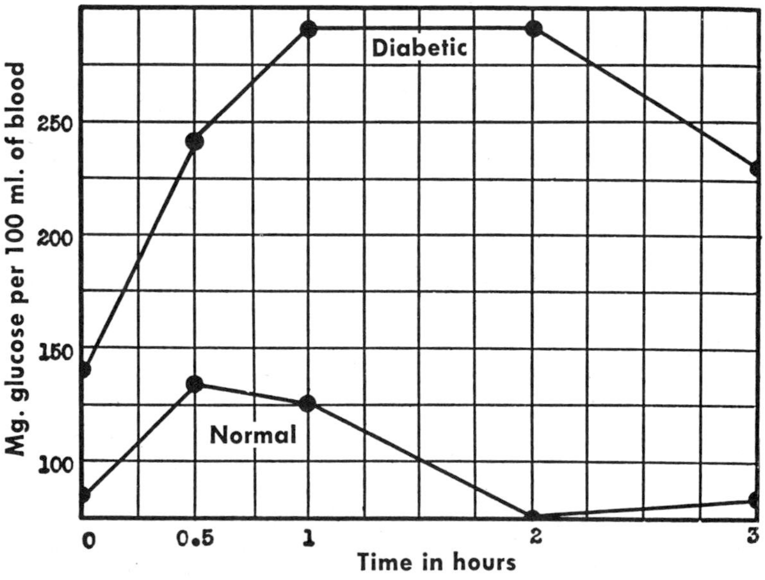

Fig. 24-6. Normal and diabetic glucose tolerance curves. Which of the following portions of the glucose tolerance curve do you think would be of most value in diagnosing diabetes mellitus: the rise, the peak, or the fall? Why?

the value of the blood sugar is determined at the beginning of the test. From 25 to 100 g of glucose is then given by mouth. Usually this is dissolved in a weak citric acid solution, which helps disguise the sweet taste of the glucose. Blood sugar determinations are then made at one-half hour, one hour, two hours, and three hours. Normally, the blood sugar level will rise to a peak at the one-half or one hour determination; in two hours it will be nearly back to the normal fasting value again (in some cases slightly lower than this value); and in three hours it will be approximately the same value as it was when the test was begun. It is supposed that the rising blood sugar stimulates the pancreas to produce insulin, which causes the glucose to leave the bloodstream. If the patient has diabetes mellitus, insulin is not secreted and the blood sugar level, which will be high even at the start of the test, does not return to its initial level for several hours. Fig. 24-6 illustrates the difference between normal and diabetic types of glucose tolerance curves.

A rough test consists in giving the patient glucose by mouth and testing the urine for the presence of glucose at half-hour intervals. Normal persons can ingest 100 or more g of glucose without any appearing in the urine; diabetics show glycosuria (glucose in the urine) with much less than this amount.

Lowered glucose tolerance (diabetic type of glucose tolerance curve) is found sometimes in old age, pregnancy, obesity, acromegaly (see page 405), hyperthyroidism (see page 392), uremia (see page 364), myocardial infarction (coronary attack), and liver disease.

INTRAVENOUS TOLBUTAMIDE TEST. Tolbutamide is a drug that lowers the level of blood sugar. It is used in the treatment of patients with mild diabetes mellitus. It can be used as an aid in the diagnosis of the disease.

A sample of blood is drawn and its level of blood sugar is determined. A solution containing 1 g of tolbutamide is then given intravenously over a period of 3 minutes. Samples of blood are taken at 20 minutes and at 30 minutes, and the levels of blood sugar in them are determined. If the level of sugar falls to less than 75 percent of the pretest level in 20 minutes, the patient does not have diabetes mellitus. If the fall in level in 20 minutes is 89 percent or more, diabetes mellitus can be diagnosed. Intermediate values are equivocal; the values at 30 minutes may be helpful in evaluating them.

GLUCAGON

The cells of the islands of Langerhans that make insulin are called the beta cells. Another group of cells present in the islands, known as the alpha cells, make a substance known as *glucagon*. Glucagon is a polypeptide (see page 270) whose molecules contain 29 combined amino acid residues. It's synthesis was announced in 1968. To some extent, at least, glucagon opposes the action of insulin, and injection of it into the blood causes a marked, though brief, rise in the level of blood sugar. The evidence at present is that glucagon increases the rate of glycogen breakdown in the liver and increases the rate of glycogen formation in muscle. Injection of glucagon also increases the level of free fatty acids in the plasma; it strengthens and slightly increases the rate of contractility of the heart. This effect on the heart is much less when the heart is damaged (chronic heart failure).

HYPOGLYCEMIA. The symptoms of hypoglycemia (low blood sugar) include weakness, trembling, rapid heartbeat (tachycardia), delirium, unconsciousness, and death in severe cases. These symptoms have been mistaken for those of epilepsy or brain disease. The symptoms of true hypoglycemia usually can be relieved promptly by giving sugar to the patient. If the patient is unconscious and unable to swallow, a glucose solution can be given by vein.

The most common cause of hypoglycemia is an overdose of insulin. Adenomas of the islands of Langerhans – that is, overgrowths of the cells that manufacture insulin

—represent another cause. Removal of the adenoma is the only permanent cure for this type of hypoglycemia. Severe liver disease may damage the liver to the extent that it cannot store sufficient glycogen to maintain the blood sugar level; hypoglycemia is a symptom of severe liver damage. Underactivity of the pituitary gland and underactivity of the cortex (outer portion) of the adrenal gland (Addison's disease) are frequently accompanied by some degree of hypoglycemia.

GLYCOSURIA. The presence of demonstrable amounts of glucose in the urine is called *glycosuria*. The most common *pathological* (abnormal) cause of glycosuria is diabetes mellitus, and this condition should be thought of when urinalysis reveals a positive test for sugar. It must be remembered, however, that a positive test is *not a diagnosis of diabetes mellitus* because other conditions can cause glycosuria. Some of the more common causes of glycosuria are diabetes mellitus, renal diabetes, alimentary glycosuria, emotional glycosuria, phlorhizin diabetes, liver damage, miscellaneous causes, and false glycosuria.

Diabetes mellitus. This diagnosis is made more probable if ketone bodies are also present in the urine. The glucose tolerance test will show a diabetic type of curve. The fasting blood sugar level will be high.

Renal diabetes. This is a condition characterized by an abnormally low renal threshold. The patient's urine always contains glucose, but the fasting blood sugar level is usually normal. The glucose tolerance test shows a normal curve.

Alimentary glycosuria. If a large amount of carbohydrate is taken into the digestive tract at one time, sugar will pass from the intestinal tract into the bloodstream more rapidly than the liver can remove it. In some cases the renal threshold will be exceeded and glycosuria will result. This type of glycosuria is only transitory.

Emotional glycosuria. We have already learned that epinephrine is secreted into the bloodstream in emotional states. This causes an elevation of the blood sugar level. Glucose appears in the urine if this elevation exceeds the renal threshold. Glycosuria, for example, sometimes is observed during routine physical examinations of student nurses. It is usually caused by the emotional state incident to the examination.

Phlorhizin diabetes. Phlorhizin is a glucoside obtained from the bark of the cherry tree. When it is injected into animals, it causes a lowering of the renal threshold and glycosuria. This type of glycosuria does not occur in patients, of course, but phlorhizin is often used in experimental work with animals.

Liver damage. Severe liver injury, as we have seen, leads to hypoglycemia. More moderate damage may result in a failure of the liver to remove glucose from the blood at a normal rate, and glycosuria appears if the renal threshold is exceeded. Liver damage is present in a number of conditions, including liver cirrhosis, phosphorus poisoning, and carbon tetrachloride poisoning.

Miscellaneous causes. Miscellaneous causes of glycosuria include morphine and strychnine poisoning, anesthesia, injury to the base of the brain, and asphyxia.

False glycosuria. Certain substances other than glucose may be present in the urine and may give a positive test with Benedict's solution. *Lactose* is sometimes present in urine in the last stages of pregnancy and during lactation (milk-production period). It can be distinguished from glucose with the aid of brewer's yeast. Glucose is destroyed in the presence of yeast (ferments), but lactose is not.

PENTOSURIA. This is a rare condition in which pentoses are excreted in the urine. Pentoses reduce Benedict's solution, but pentosuria can be distinguished from glycosuria with the use of another reagent, called *Bial's reagent*. This test is carried out by gently heating a mixture of Bial's reagent (1 ml) and urine (2 ml). Pentose is present if the solution becomes green.

Alimentary pentosuria occurs when large quantities of fruits or fruit juices are ingested. Idiopathic pentosuria is a disease of enzymic defect (see page 215) in which the pentose L-xylulose is excreted in the urine. There is no accompanying clinical syndrome, and the condition apparently is harmless.

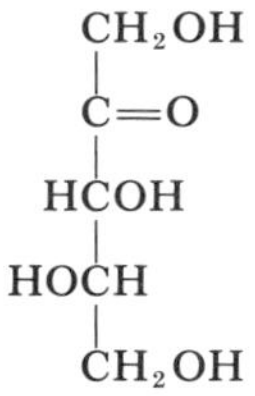

L-xylulose

Alkaptonuria. *Homogentisic acid*, a protein derivative, is present in the urine of patients who have *alkaptonuria*, and this acid may reduce Benedict's solution. Alkaptonuria, however, is such a rare condition that it seldom causes a mistaken diagnosis of glycosuria. Urine containing homogentisic acid turns black after standing several hours. In older people with alkaptonuria, tendons, cartilages, and fibrous tissues develop an abnormal pigmentation. This condition is referred to as *ochronosis*.

STUDY QUESTIONS

1. Make a table showing the enzymes concerned in carbohydrate digestion, their substrates, and the end products of digestion.
2. What is ptyalin? Amylopsin?
3. What is the fate of the galactose and fructose absorbed from the intestinal tract?
4. Where does glycogenesis occur in the body? Name six substances, or types of substance, that can be converted to glycogen in the liver.
5. What compound is formed by muscle glycogenolysis? By liver glycogenolysis?
6. What is the fate of the lactic acid formed in muscle contraction?
7. What is blood sugar? What is the normal fasting level of blood sugar?
8. How does the liver function to maintain a normal blood sugar level?
9. What is the renal threshold? What is the average value of the renal threshold in normal individuals?
10. What is glycolysis? How can it be prevented?
11. What is the cause of the low blood sugar in von Gierke's disease?
12. What chemical reactions are supposed to furnish the energy for muscle contraction?
13. About what percentage of the lactic acid formed in muscle contraction is burned to CO_2 and H_2O?
14. What is oxygen debt? Write an equation showing what happens when lactic acid unites with oxygen.
15. What are the end products of carbohydrate oxidation in the tissues? How much energy results when one gram of carbohydrate is burned in the body?
16. What are the end products of carbohydrate oxidation in brain tissue?
17. What vitamin is necessary for the oxidation of pyruvic acid in the brain and nerves? What is its chemical name?
18. How efficient is the body as a machine? What does this mean?
19. Explain what is meant by "the protein-sparing action" of carbohydrate.
20. Can carbohydrate be converted to fat in the body?
21. What are the functions of insulin? Where is insulin made?
22. What is the effect of an injection of epinephrine on the glycogen content of muscles and liver? On the blood sugar level?
23. What is another name for epinephrine?
24. What are some causes of diabetes mellitus? What are the chemical signs of this disease?
25. Is insulin a cure for diabetes mellitus? Explain.
26. What is glucagon?
27. Describe the glucose tolerance test. Draw curves illustrating normal and diabetic tests. What rough test is sometimes used?
28. Describe the intravenous tolbutamide test. What is its significance?
29. What are the symptoms of hypoglycemia? What is the commonest cause of it? Name some other causes.
30. Is glycosuria enough to warrant a diagnosis of diabetes mellitus? Name six causes of glycosuria.
31. What is false glycosuria? Name three causes of false glycosuria and tell how each might be distinguished from true glycosuria.

CHAPTER **25**

Chemical nature of proteins

Proteins are compounds of high molecular weight that yield *amino acids* on hydrolysis. All of them contain carbon, hydrogen, oxygen, and nitrogen; most of them contain sulfur; and a few contain phosphorus. The living cell contains 70 to 80 percent water; it has been estimated that about 90 percent of the remainder of the cell is formed by protein. All of us see protein material every day, since the entire external surface of the body—skin, hair, nails—is composed mainly of it. Although a large portion of the protein of the diet can be changed to carbohydrate in time of need, the chief function of protein is not to serve as a source of energy but to act as material for the building of new cells and the replacement of old cells in the tissues. Also, many compounds necessary for the normal functioning of the body—hormones, enzymes, pigments—are derived from the proteins in the food we eat.

TYPES OF PROTEIN

We define *simple proteins* as proteins that form only amino acids when they are hydrolyzed. This definition is probably not entirely correct because many of the proteins classified as simple proteins appear to contain small quantities of carbohydrates or lipids in their molecules. The most important simple proteins are the *albumins* and the *globulins*. Albumins are soluble in distilled water. Globulins will not dissolve in distilled water, but are soluble in dilute salt solutions. The other types of simple protein are listed in Table 25-1. Notice that their classification depends on (1) solubility and (2) whether or not they coagulate (precipitate) when they are heated in solution.

Conjugated proteins yield nonprotein substances as well as amino acids when they are hydrolyzed. For example, *nucleoproteins* yield nucleic acid and amino acids; *phosphoproteins* yield phosphoric acid and amino acids; *hemoglobin* yields heme (an iron-containing compound) and amino acids; and *glycoproteins* yield carbohydrates and amino acids. Nucleoproteins are found in all living cells. Most of the phosphate in our diet

Table 25-1. Classification of simple proteins

Type	Soluble in	Coagulation by heat	Examples
Albumin	Pure water Dilute salt solutions	Yes	Serum albumin (blood) Egg albumin (egg white) Lactalbumin (milk)
Globulin	Dilute salt solutions	Yes	Serum globulin (blood) Egg globulin (egg white) Fibrinogen (blood) Lactoglobulin (milk)
Glutelin	Dilute acids and bases	Yes	Glutenin (wheat) Oryzenin (rice)
Prolamin	70 to 80% alcohol		Gliadin (wheat) Zein (corn)
Albuminoid	No solvent (insoluble)		Keratin (hair and nails) Fibroin (silk) Collagen (bones and cartilage)
Histone	Water and dilute acid solutions; insoluble in ammonia solutions	Variable	Globin (from hemoglobin, the red protein of blood) Scombrone (from spermatozoa of mackerel)
Protamine	Pure water Ammonia solutions	No	Salmine (spermatozoa of salmon) Sturine (spermatozoa of sturgeon)

comes from such phosphoproteins as casein, the protein present in largest amount in milk, as well as from nucleoproteins. Mucin, the protein of saliva, is a glycoprotein.

Substances prepared by the action of heat, acids, alkalies, or enzymes on proteins are called *derived proteins*. The "scum" floating on the top of hot chocolate is a derived protein; it is formed by heating lactalbumin, one of the proteins in milk. The hydrolysis of proteins by enzymes yields substances made up of smaller molecules, called *proteoses;* then substances with still smaller molecules, called *peptones;* then compounds composed of several amino acids linked together, called *peptides;* and, finally, *amino acids*.

$$\text{Protein} \xrightarrow{(+H_2O)} \text{Proteoses} \xrightarrow{(+H_2O)} \text{Peptones} \xrightarrow{(+H_2O)} \text{Peptides} \xrightarrow{(+H_2O)} \text{Amino acids}$$

ISOELECTRIC POINT

Protein molecules are relatively huge. The molecular weights of most of the proteins found in the tissues range from about 17,000 to 700,000. At least one protein having a molecular weight close to 50,000,000 has been found in nature. Protein molecules in solution *ionize* and therefore have electric charges. Both positive and negative charges are produced by this ionization, and the large protein ions have both positive and negative charges. At a certain pH value, different for each protein, the number of positive charges on the protein ion equals the number of negative charges. When this is true the protein is said to be at the *isoelectric point* ("equal electric" point). At pH values above the isoelectric point the protein ion has more negative charges than positive charges; if the pH value is below the isoelectric point the positive charges outnumber the negative ones. It has been found that proteins are least soluble at or near the isoelectric point.

The isoelectric points of some common proteins are given in Table 25-2.

AMINO ACIDS

The building blocks of which protein molecules are made are *amino acids*. These amino acids contain an amino groups (NH_2) attached to the α-carbon atom; that is, to the carbon atom to which the acid (COOH) group is also attached.

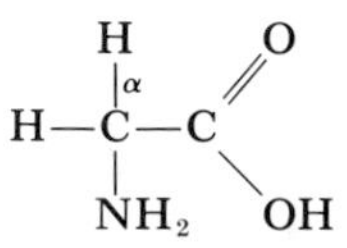

CH_2NH_2COOH
Glycine
(Amino acid)

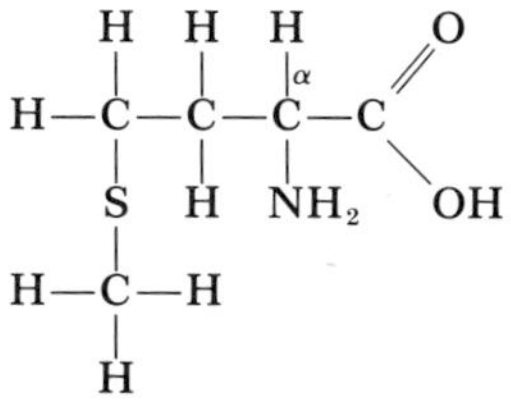

$CH_2(SCH_3)CH_2CHNH_2COOH$
Methionine
(Amino acid)

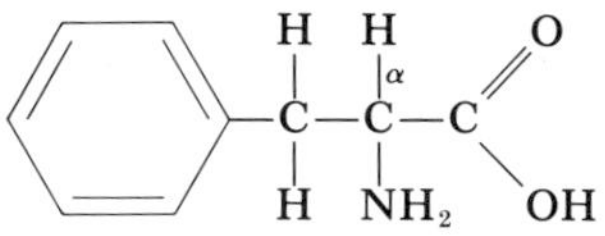

$C_6H_5CH_2CHNH_2COOH$
Phenylalanine
(Amino acid)

Inspection of the formulas in Table 4, page 481, will show that the amino acids (except glycine) contain an asymmetric carbon atom (see page 163) and hence can exist in two optically active forms. The amino acids found in animal and plant tissues have the L- configuration. Amino acids of the D-series occur in the capsules of some bacteria and in certain antibiotics.

Proteins are formed in tissues by the chemical union of amino acids. Only about 25 natural amino acids are known, but they can link themselves together in so many combinations that thousands of different kinds of protein molecules probably exist. When two amino acids unite with each other, they do so between the NH_2 group of one molecule and the COOH group of another.

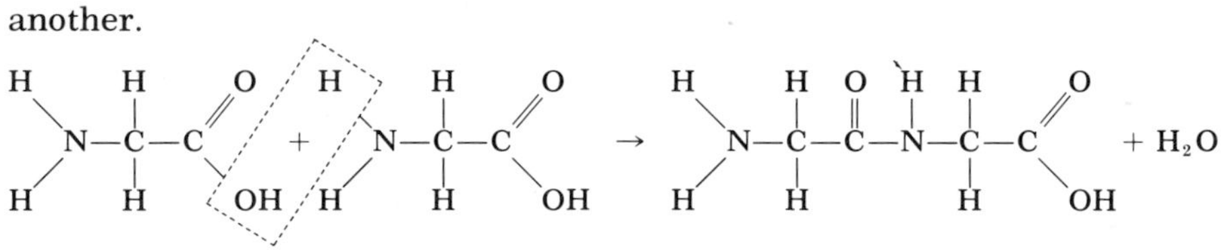

CH_2NH_2COOH Glycine (Amino acid) + CH_2NH_2COOH Glycine (Amino acid) → $CH_2NH_2CONHCH_2COOH$ Glycyl glycine (Dipeptide) + H_2O

The —CONH— linkage thus formed between the amino acids is called the *peptide linkage*. The compound formed by the linkage of two amino acids in this manner is called a *dipeptide*. If more than two amino acids unite in this way the compound is a *polypeptide*. Proteins are composed of extremely long polypeptides. Often, 1 protein molecule consists of 2 or more

Table 25-2. Isoelectric points of some familiar proteins

Protein	Isoelectric point at
Serum albumin (in blood)	pH 4.7
Serum globulin (in blood)	pH 5.4
Fibrinogen (in blood)	pH 5.6
Egg albumin (in egg white)	pH 4.6
Casein (in milk)	pH 4.7

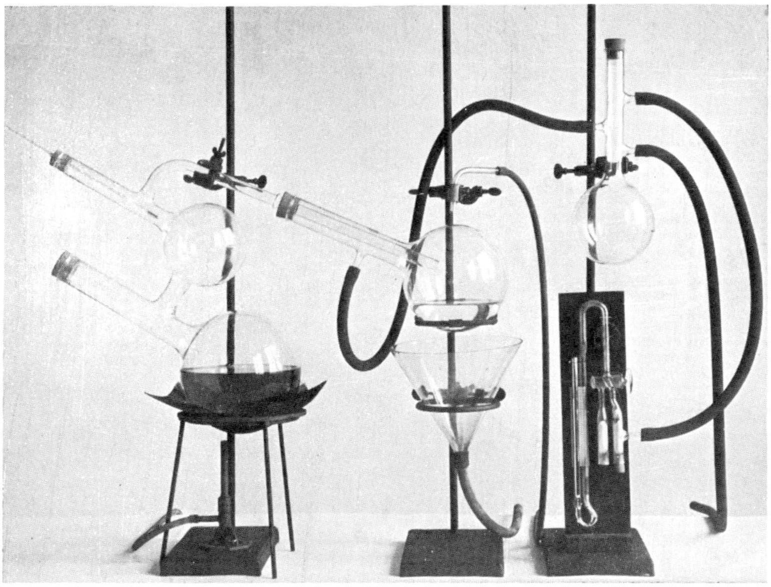

Fig. 25-1. Apparatus for distilling compounds under reduced pressure. Proteins often are hydrolyzed by heating them in the presence of hydrochloric acid, which acts as a catalyst. The hydrochloric acid is volatile and can be removed by distillation. This distillation must be carried out at a rather low temperature (30° to 50° C), however, to avoid destruction of some of the compounds formed from the protein. In order to cause the hydrochloric acid to distill at this temperature, most of the air in the apparatus must be removed. This is done by connecting the apparatus to a suitable pump (the rubber tubing at the right leads to a pump). Define amino acid. (Courtesy Eastman Kodak Company Research Laboratories.)

peptide chains linked chemically. Most of the protein molecules in the blood, for example, contain from 200 to 1,000 amino acid molecules linked by means of the peptide linkage.

We notice by inspecting the equation given above that water is formed when amino acids unite to form peptides and proteins. When this reaction is reversed – that is, when proteins are made to react with water (hydrolysis) – amino acids are formed. This is what occurs when proteins are digested, and amino acids (as well as peptides) are the end products of protein digestion.

In order to simplify the writing of formulas for peptides, shorthand symbols for the amino acids have been adopted. (See page 302.) When amino acids combine to form peptides, the carboxyl (—COOH) group of one reacts with the amino (—NH_2) group of the other. In the shorthand symbols the amino-acid residue (that is, combined amino acid) having a free carboxyl group is written on the right. For example,

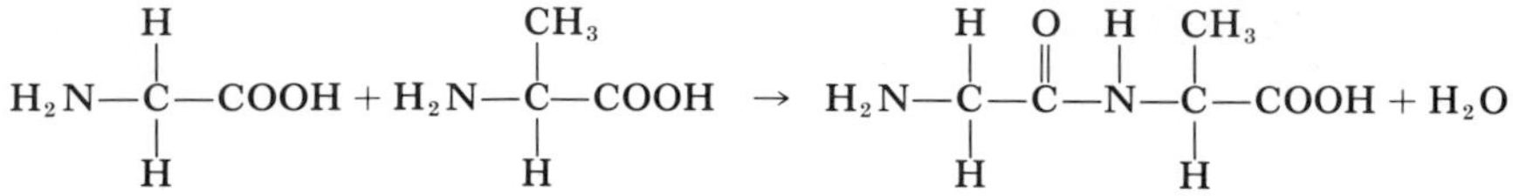

Glycine + Alanine → Glycylalanine
Shorthand: Gly   Ala   Gly - Ala + H_2O

If a third amino acid reacts with glycylalanine (to form a tripeptide), the new amino acid symbol will be written last (that is, on the right), since it will have the free carboxyl group.

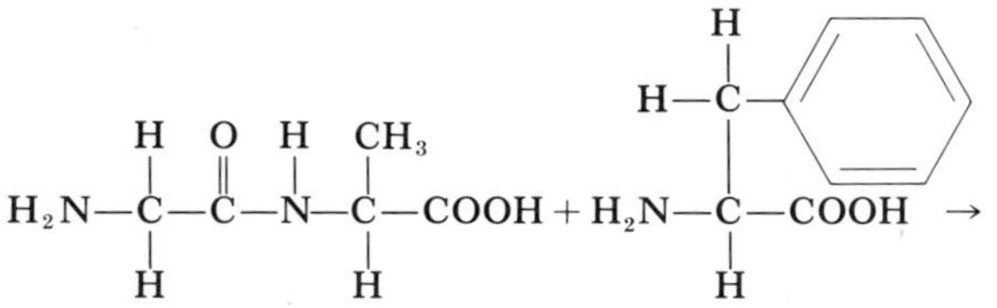

Glycylalanine + Phenylalanine →
Gly - Ala + Phe →

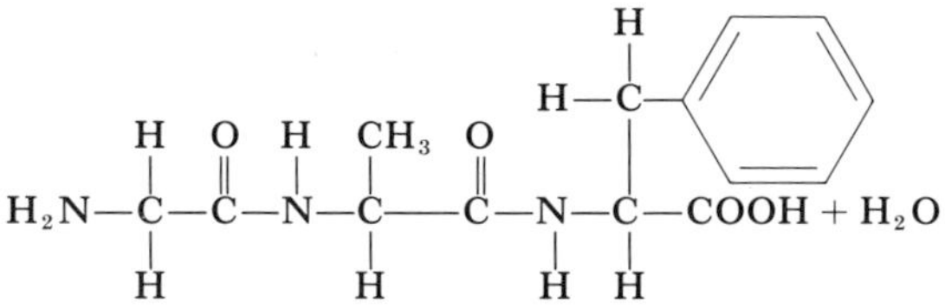

Glycylalanylphenylalanine
Gly - Ala - Phe + H_2O

Amino acids (and therefore proteins, which are made of them) are *amphoteric compounds* (see the discussion of amines on page 155). That is, they can neutralize both acids and bases.

$$\begin{matrix} CH_2COOH \\ | \\ NH_2 \end{matrix} + NaOH \rightarrow \begin{matrix} CH_2COONa \\ | \\ NH_2 \end{matrix} + H_2O$$

Reaction of an amino acid with a base

$$\begin{matrix} CH_2COOH \\ | \\ NH_2 \end{matrix} + HCl \rightarrow \begin{matrix} CH_2COOH \\ | \\ NH_3Cl \end{matrix}$$

Reaction of an amino acid with an acid*

The proteins of the blood are good buffers because they quickly neutralize either acids or bases that may enter the blood.

The amino groups of amino acids and proteins are destroyed when these substances react with formaldehyde, HCHO.

*Read "Coordinate Covalence," page 91.

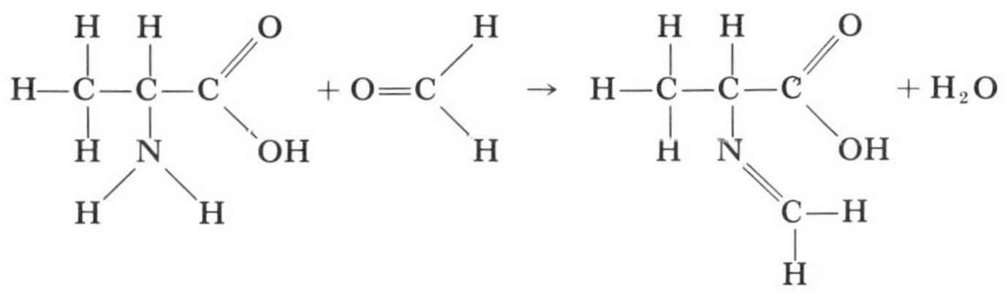

This reaction is used in preparing one type of *toxoid*. Some bacterial toxins are proteins. When they are treated with formaldehyde, they lose their toxicity and become harmless, but they still have the ability to cause the body to form antibodies against the original harmful toxin. These harmless proteins prepared from toxins are called toxoids. They can be injected into the bloodstream to increase the immunity of the body against the bacterial disease caused by the toxin from which the toxoid was made. Formaldehyde is used to inactivate the virus present in the Salk poliomyelitis vaccine.

STRUCTURE OF PROTEINS

The protein molecule is composed of one or more chains of amino acid residues (that is, one or more polypeptides). One of the smallest proteins, insulin (see page 401), consists of molecules made up of 2 polypeptide chains, one chain containing 21 amino-acid residues, and the other containing 30. The chains are held together by sulfur-sulfur (—S—S—) linkages. (See Fig. 32-15, page 402.)

The shape of a linear polypeptide can be represented by a structure known as the *α helix* (see Fig. 25-2). Each turn of this helix consists of 3.6 amino acid residues, so that each 5 turns contains exactly 18 residues. Each residue is linked to adjacent residues by hydrogen bonds (see page 92) between the nitrogen of the combined amino group and the oxygen of the combined carboxyl group of the other residue. The side chains of the amino acids (that is, all of the amino acid molecule except the $-\overset{\displaystyle H}{\underset{\displaystyle NH_2}{C}}-COOH$ portion) (see Table 4 on page 481) project at right angles to the helix.

Many of the fibrous proteins, such as those in hair, muscle, fingernails, and horn, consist of polypeptide chains (in the form of the α helix) that are twisted around one another like the strands in a piece of rope. Hair can be stretched to over twice its normal length under suitable experimental conditions. This involves breaking some of the hydrogen bonds between adjacent amino-acid residues. Silk fibers cannot be stretched very much since the polypeptide chains present are already in a stretched form. The chains in silk and probably in all other proteins are attached laterally to adjacent chains by hydrogen bonds. In some cases other linkages, such as sulfur-sulfur (—S—S—) or nitrogen-carbon $-\overset{\displaystyle H}{N}-\overset{\displaystyle O}{\overset{\|}{C}}-$, the peptide bond, are present.

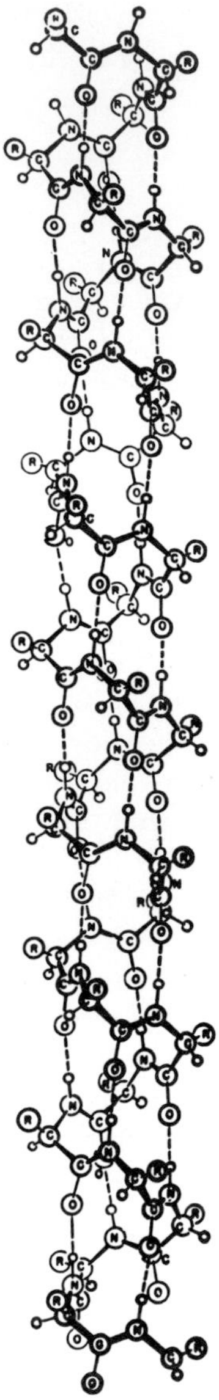

Fig. 25-2. Drawing illustrating the α-helix present in proteins. What is formed by the hydrolysis of a simple protein? (Courtesy Dr. Linus Pauling, Dr. Robert B. Corey, and Dr. H. R. Branson.)

METHODS OF MAKING PROTEINS INSOLUBLE

Many proteins that are not linear but rather are globular have been shown to exist as polypeptide chains having the α helix configuration. Insulin is such a protein. In these proteins the polypeptide helix is coiled and bent, probably at intervals of about 5 turns of the helix (that is, 18 amino-acid residues).

When proteins are changed so that they become insoluble at the isoelectric point they are said to be *denatured.*

SURFACE DENATURATION. Many proteins denature (become insoluble) at surfaces, particularly at surfaces between air and the protein solution.

Shaking a protein solution mixes air with the solution, and some of the protein precipitates.

HEAT DENATURATION. Practically all protcins become become denatured and precipitate when their solutions are heated. This is true also of bacterial proteins, and most of the instruments and clothing used in operating rooms are sterilized by heat. The denaturation of the bacterial protein kills the bacteria.

SALTING OUT. Most proteins are not soluble in concentrated salt solutions. Addition of some salt, such as ammonium sulfate, to protein solutions often causes the protein to precipitate, and this method is used in isolating proteins for study. If proper care is taken, the protein will not be denatured by this procedure and will dissolve again when the salt is removed by dialysis.

ALCOHOL. The prolamins are the only simple proteins soluble in alcohol-water mixtures of high alcohol content. Alcohol denatures other types of protein. Ordinary commercial alcohol is about 95 percent pure. This strength ordinarily is not used in sterilizing the skin, however, because it precipitates the protein at the surface of the bacteria so quickly that further penetration of alcohol is prevented; the bacteria are disabled, so to speak, but they are not killed. Better sterilization is obtained with 70 percent alcohol because its action is slow enough that it diffuses throughout the entire bacterium before the protein coagulates; when coagulation does occur it is complete, and the organism dies. Sterilization of the skin with 70 percent alcohol is commonly used before obtaining blood for blood transfusions, inserting a needle into a vein to inject drugs, and so on.

ALKALOIDAL REAGENTS. *Alkaloids* are complex organic plant substances that contain nitrogen and have the ability to neutralize acids. Many of them, such as morphine and codeine, are used as drugs. Certain organic

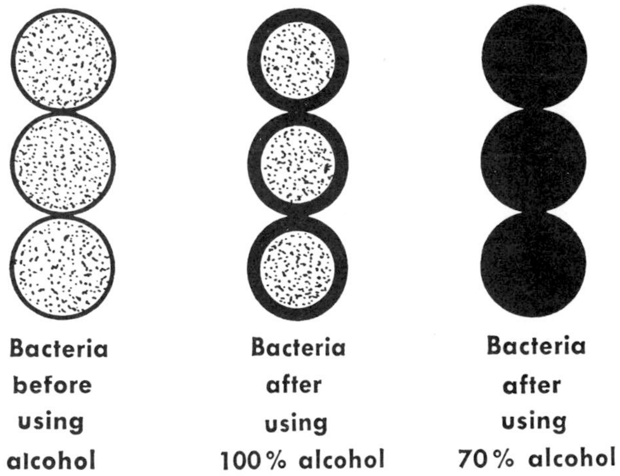

Fig. 25-3. Diagrams to show the effect of alcohol solutions on bacteria. Areas in solid black represent coagulated protein. Why is 70 percent alcohol more efficient than 100 percent alcohol in killing bacteria?

acids (for example, tannic acid and picric acid) combine with them to form insoluble salts. These acids, called *alkaloidal reagents,* also form insoluble compounds with proteins.

METALS. Certain metal salts, such as mercuric chloride (bichloride of mercury or corrosive sublimate) and silver nitrate (lunar caustic), precipitate proteins. They are used as antiseptics because they kill bacteria by their protein-combining action. They are poisonous if taken by mouth since they coagulate and destroy the body protein. Protein foods, such as eggs and milk, are used in the emergency treatment of heavy metal poisoning. They act by combining with the heavy metal, thereby saving the tissue proteins. An emetic (drug that induces vomiting) should always be given after the protein food is swallowed. If this is not done, the enzymes of the digestive tract will digest the protein food and release the heavy metal poison again. In other words, if vomiting is not induced the poisoning is only postponed – not prevented.

RADIANT ENERGY. Radiant energy (light energy), particularly that of ultraviolet rays and x-rays, is absorbed by proteins, and the energy produced causes most proteins in solution to become denatured. The protein (keratin) of the skin absorbs most of the ultraviolet rays of the sun and protects the cells of the tissues. X-rays are used to destroy cancer cells; one reason the cancer cell dies is because its protein is denatured. Fortunately, the protein of cancer cells is more sensitive to radiant energy than that of the normal tissue cells.

PROTEIN SOLVENTS

Proteins – with the exception of the prolamins, which dissolve in strong alcohol solutions – ordinarily will not dissolve in organic liquids. In general, we may say that the proteins in which we are most interested will all dissolve in dilute salt solutions. Strong alkalies and acids (except nitric acid) will dissolve proteins, and they are often used to put tissues into solution for chemical analysis. A 40 percent urea (NH_2CONH_2) solution is one of the best protein solvents we have. It is used sometimes to soak wounds; it probably owes its beneficial effect to its ability to dissolve and remove the dead tissue proteins in the wound. We must remember that dilute salt solutions are the only safe solvents if we do not want to denature the proteins; the other solvents usually denature them, as evidenced by the fact that they precipitate if the pH is adjusted to that of the isoelectric point and the solvent removed.

COLOR REACTIONS OF PROTEINS

The presence of proteins can be detected by adding reagents that produce characteristic colors with one or more of the amino acids or chemical groups present.

BIURET TEST.* This test is performed by adding the unknown solution to a weak solution of copper sulfate, $CuSO_4$, dissolved in strong sodium hydroxide. A violet color is produced in the presence of proteins. The test appears to depend on the presence of the peptide linkage.

MILLON TEST. Heating a protein solution in the presence of Millon's

*As the name of the test implies, it is positive for a compound known as biuret ($H_2N—CO—NH—CO—NH_2$).

reagent (mercury dissolved in nitric acid) causes the protein to precipitate; this precipitate has a brick-red color. The test depends on the presence of tyrosine and, to a lesser extent, tryptophan. Proteins that do not contain these amino acids will not give the test.

XANTHOPROTEIC ("YELLOW PROTEIN") TEST. Any of us who has spilled nitric acid on his skin has seen this test. Proteins assume a yellow color in the presence of concentrated nitric acid. If an excess of sodium hydroxide is now added so that the solution becomes alkaline, the yellow color turns to orange. Tyrosine, tryptophan, and phenylalanine are the amino acids responsible for the test.

HOPKINS-COLE TEST. This test is carried out by mixing the protein solution with a solution of glyoxalic acid (CHOCOOH), or its magnesium salt, and layering the mixture on top of concentrated sulfuric acid. A purple color will appear at the zone of contact of the two liquids if the protein contains tryptophan.

NINHYDRIN REACTION. The most widely used methods for the qualitative and quantitative detection of amino acids involve the use of ninhydrin and heat. The following reactions result in the formation of a pigment with a blue color.

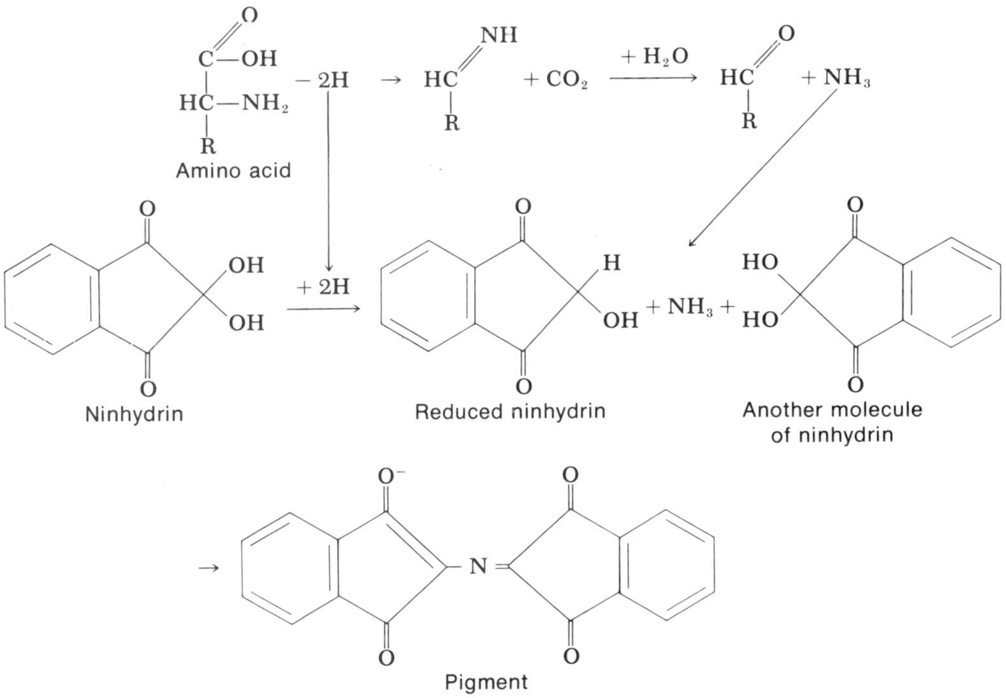

Thus, the amino acid is converted to the next lower aldehyde and CO_2. The reagent combines with the liberated NH_3 to form a pigment (ionized at the pH used for the reaction) that has a blue color.

HEMOGLOBIN

Hemoglobin is a conjugated protein present in the red blood cells. It is responsible for the red color of blood. The prosthetic (nonprotein) compound combined with protein (*globin*) to form hemoglobin is called *heme*.

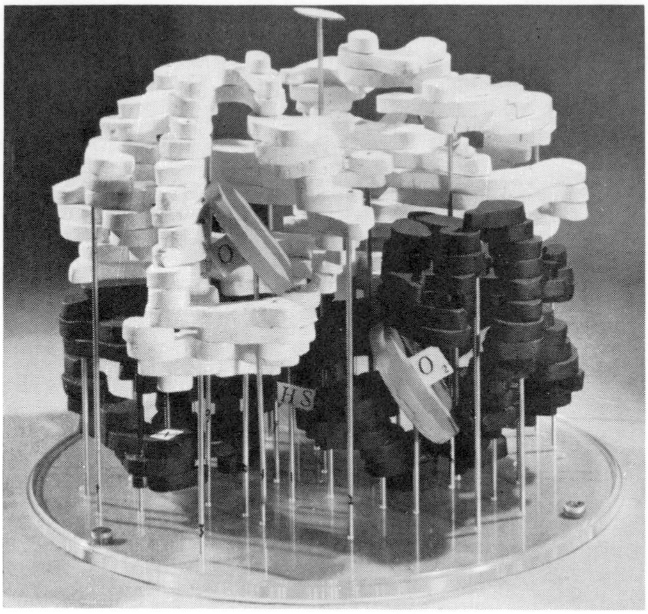

Fig. 25-4. Model of a hemoglobin molecule. The heme groups are indicated by gray disks. What is the function of hemoglobin? (Courtesy Dr. M. F. Perutz, British Medical Research Council; from X-ray analysis of hemoglobin, Science **140:**863, May 24, 1963. Copyright 1963 by the American Association for the Advancement of Science.)

Heme is an organic compound containing iron in chemical combination. This iron has a valence of 2+ (ferrous iron).

Several hemoglobin molecules are present in normal people. Each of them is composed of 4 subunits (peptide chains) bound chemically together. Two of these chains (α-chains) are identical and occur in all normal hemoglobins. The other 2 also are identical with each other; they may be β-chains, γ-chains, or δ-chains. Combined within the coiled chains are the 4 heme molecules. In part, the chains exist as the α-helix. In regions where bending takes place, however, the chains are linear.

Fetal hemoglobin (hemoglobin F) is (α, α, γ, γ,) in structure. Normal adult hemoglobin (hemoglobin A) is (α, α, β, β). Hemoglobin A_2, which occurs normally in small concentrations, is (α, α, δ, δ).

It is the function of hemoglobin to combine loosely with oxygen in the lungs and to take it to the tissues, where a part of this oxygen is released. One gram of hemoglobin can combine with about 1.3 ml of oxygen under ordinary conditions. Hemoglobin combined with oxygen is called *oxyhemoglobin*. We do not know just how this oxygen is combined. At least we know that it unites in such a way that the iron present is not oxidized; that is, the iron in oxyhemoglobin has a valence of 2+. It can be calculated that the number of oxygen molecules loosely combined in oxyhemoglobin is the same as the number of iron atoms.

Normally, about 15 or 16 g of hemoglobin is present in 100 ml of blood.

If the amount of hemoglobin is less than normal, the conditions is called *anemia*. The amount of hemoglobin is above normal in *polycythemia* (too many red blood cells). Polycythemia may be secondary to other conditions (such as heart disease); it may be the result of lowered oxygen content in the outside air (this occurs, for example, at high altitudes); or it may be present as a specific disease, called *polycythemia vera* (erythremia).

The finding of the abnormal hemoglobin S in sickle-cell anemia (see page 215) led to a search for other forms of hemoglobin that might differ from the usual hemoglobin A; a number have been found. The hemoglobin during fetal life, hemoglobin F, is especially adapted to receive oxygen from the maternal blood in the placenta. After birth it is replaced, over a period of four to six months, by hemoglobin of the adult type. More than 60 other hemoglobins have been found in normal and anemic people. The abnormal chains in these hemoglobins may differ from each other by only 1 amino acid residue in about 300 residues.

In *thalassemia (Cooley's anemia)* the red blood cells are small and flat and do not have the normal content of hemoglobin. There are 3 categories of thalassemia: the disease may be caused by underproduction of (never total lack of) any one of the chain types α, β, or δ. δ-Chain thalassemia does not cause illness, presumably because the resulting low level of hemoglobin A_2 is more than compensated for by the normal adult hemoglobin A. In the so-called major form of the disease the usual signs and symptoms of a severe anemia are present. Unless the disease is asymptomatic, it manifests itself during the first year of life.

METHEMOGLOBIN

When hemoglobin is heated in the presence of air or oxygen, it is changed to a brown substance called *methemoglobin*. Certain oxidizing agents will also cause this. The iron in methemoglobin has been oxidized and has a valence of 3+. This change occurs when meat is cooked and is responsible for the brown color of cooked meats. Certain drugs, such as sulfanilamide, also cause the formation of methemoglobin. Injection of methylene blue into the blood of patients with methemoglobin in their bodies converts the methemoglobin to hemoglobin.

CARBON MONOXIDE POISONING

Carbon monoxide, CO, combines with hemoglobin to form a compound called carbon monoxide hemoglobin (carbonyl hemoglobin). This compound is unable to combine with oxygen, and the patient dies of asphyxia (lack of oxygen) if too much hemoglobin combines with carbon monoxide. Carbon monoxide hemoglobin can be changed to oxyhemoglobin by means of oxygen, but it requires about 200 molecules of oxygen to replace 1 molecule of carbon monoxide. The only effective treatment we have is to make the patient breathe pure oxygen in the hope that enough carbon monoxide hemoglobin will be changed back to oxyhemoglobin to save the patient's life. Breathing pure oxygen also increases the amount of this gas dissolved in the blood and thereby increases the oxygen supply to the tissues.

MYOGLOBIN

Myoglobin, sometimes referred to as "muscle hemoglobin," is present in all muscles. It is responsible for most of the red color of fresh muscle. It is a conjugated protein composed of a protein (apomyoglobin) combined chemically with heme (also the prosthetic group in hemoglobin). Like hemoglobin, it combines reversibly with oxygen; its function is to act as a reservoir of oxygen in the muscle. When there is a lack of oxygen, it releases it; when oxygen is present in excess, it stores it. One molecule of myoglobin contains 1 combined heme molecule: hemoglobin molecules, as already noted, contain 4.

ROLE OF PROTEINS IN MUSCULAR CONTRACTION. Skeletal muscle (voluntary or striated muscle) contains at least 2 proteins that appear to play an important role in muscular contraction. *Myosin* exists in the muscle fiber in strands or fibers. *Actin* can exist as globular particles (G-actin) or as fibers (F-actin). When F-actin and myosin are mixed either *in vivo* (in the muscle) or *in vitro* (in the test tube), a fibrous protein complex known as actomyosin is formed. Actually, fibers of this protein complex can be prepared in the laboratory and serve as models of the fibers believed to exist in living muscle. When adenosine triphosphate is added to an actomyosin fiber under proper conditions, the fiber contracts to a fraction of its former length. It seems quite possible, then, that a reaction involving ATP and actomyosin is the immediate cause of muscular contraction.

STUDY QUESTIONS

1. What elements are found in proteins?
2. Make up a definition for protein.
3. Where are proteins found? What are their functions?
4. Name three types of protein and define each. What two kinds of simple protein are most important?
5. Where do we obtain most of the phosphate in our diet?
6. What are proteoses? Peptones? Peptides? Amino acids?
7. What is meant by the isoelectric point?
8. What kind of charge do proteins have if the pH is above the isoelectric point? Below the isoelectric point?
9. What kind of compound is produced by the complete hydrolysis of simple proteins?
10. Why are the acids obtained from proteins called amino acids?
11. Write an equation showing how two amino acids unite to form a dipeptide.
12. What occurs when proteins are digested?
13. What is an amphoteric compound?
14. Why are proteins good buffers?
15. What aldehyde is sometimes used in the preparation of toxoids? How does it work?
16. Name seven methods of making proteins insoluble. What is meant by denaturation?
17. Why is heat used in sterilizing instruments and clothing?
18. Why is 70 percent instead of 95 percent alcohol used in sterilizing the skin?
19. What is carbon monoxide hemoglobin?
20. What is the emergency treatment for heavy metal poisoning?
21. What protects our tissues from the ultraviolet rays of the sun?
22. Name some protein solvents.
23. Name and describe five color reactions for proteins.
24. What is hemoglobin?
25. What is the valence of iron in heme?
26. What is oxyhemoglobin?
27. How much hemoglobin is normally present in 100 ml of blood? What is anemia?
28. What is methemoglobin?
29. Why is carbon monoxide poisonous?
30. Discuss briefly the structure, distribution, and function of myoglobin.
31. What is myosin? Actin? Actomyosin? How does ATP affect a fiber of actomyosin?

CHAPTER 26

Metabolism of proteins

SUMMARY OF PROTEIN DIGESTION

The digestion of proteins begins in the stomach. The stomach glands secrete a substance called *pepsinogen*. Pepsinogen reacts with the hydrochloric acid of the gastric juice to form an enzyme, *pepsin*. Pepsin acts as a catalyst for the hydrolysis of proteins to proteoses and peptones. *Trypsinogen* and *chymotrypsinogen* are secreted by the pancreatic cells. Trypsinogen reacts with *enterokinase,* a substance found in the small intestin, to form *trypsin*. In the presence of trypsin, chymotrypsinogen forms *chymotrypsin*. Trypsin and chymotrypsin are enzymes that act as catalysts for the change of proteoses and peptones to polypeptides. A mixture of polypeptidases (erepsin) found both in pancreatic juice and in intestinal juice catalyzes the hydrolysis of polypeptides to amino acids. Amino acids and soluble peptides are the end products of protein digestion. These compounds are absorbed directly from the digestive tract into the bloodstream and are then distributed to the tissues.

ANABOLIC PRODUCTS OF AMINO ACIDS

Amino acids are used to build new body protein and to form essential nitrogen-containing compounds other than protein; some of them can be converted to glycogen in the liver (see page 257). Several amino acids are known to be capable of forming ketone bodies in the liver, and there is evidence that there are others that may also be able to undergo this change. We know that glucose can be converted to fat, and, of course, any amino acids that can form glucose (or glycogen) can later be changed to fat.

ESSENTIAL AMINO ACIDS

It has been found that growth cannot take place unless certain amino acids, called *essential amino acids,* are present in the diet. The essential amino acids are: threonine, valine, isoleucine, methionine, lysine, histidine, phenylalanine, tryptophan, and leucine.* Proteins that contain all these

*Arginine must also be in the diet to secure a *rapid* rate of growth. It has been found that histidine is not essential for the maintenance of nitrogen balance in adult human beings—a state in which the amount of nitrogen eaten equals the nitrogen lost from the body each day.

acids are called *adequate proteins*. Proteins from which one or more of the essential amino acids are missing are called *inadequate proteins*. Gelatin, an animal protein that lacks tryptophan, and zein, a plant (corn) protein that lacks tryptophan and lysine, are examples of inadequate proteins. Lactalbumin, a protein of milk, is a good example of an adequate protein.

AMINO ACID CATABOLISM

Those amino acids not used in the formation of new tissue protein are changed to other products in the liver and kidneys. The first change involves the removal of the amino group (a process called deamination), with the formation of ammonia (NH_3) and a keto acid. This change is referred to as *oxidative deamination*.

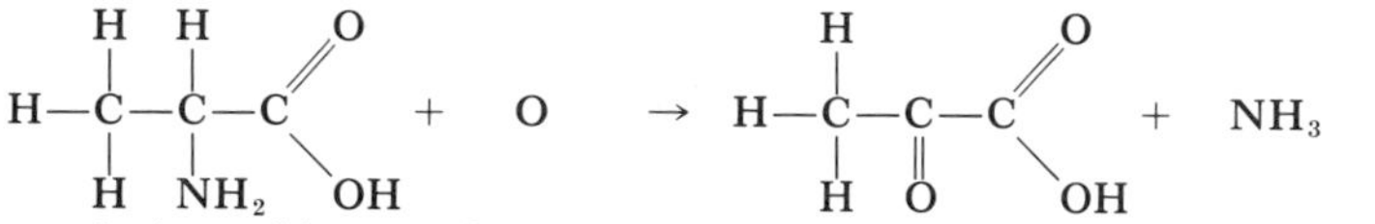

Amino acid — Oxygen — Keto acid — Ammonia

The keto acids formed by this process may be oxidized directly to carbon dioxide and water or they may be used to form glycogen and other anabolic products (hormones, pigments, etc.).

$$\underset{\text{Keto acid}}{2\,CH_3COCOOH} + \underset{\text{Oxygen}}{5\,O_2} \rightarrow \underset{\text{Carbon dioxide}}{6\,CO_2} + \underset{\text{Water}}{4\,H_2O}$$

The ammonia formed by oxidative deamination combines with carbon dioxide in the liver to form urea. This change involves the complex series of reactions shown on the opposite page.

There is a disease of enzymic defect caused by a lack of, or inhibition of, each of the enzymes catalyzing the numbered reactions in the ornithine cycle.

HYPERLYSINEMIA. The primary cause of this condition is a deficiency of the enzyme *lysine NAD oxidoreductase*. This causes an increase in the body content of the amino acid lysine. The high level of lysine inhibits the enzyme *arginase*, which catalyzes reaction (1) of the ornithine cycle. A patient with this disease, seen at 27 years of age, could not walk, talk, feed himself, or dress himself. He was not toilet trained. His physical development resembled that of a child 9 to 10 years old. He weighed 69½ pounds and was 52 inches tall.

CITRULLINEMIA. This condition is caused by a deficiency of the enzyme *argininosuccinic acid synthetase*. It is characterized by severe mental deficiency.

ARGININOSUCCINIC ACIDURIA is caused by a deficiency of the enzyme *argininosuccinic acid lyase*. It is characterized by vomiting, ataxia (inability to walk), epileptic fits, friable, tufted hair, and mental deficiency. In some cases there is liver damage.

HYPERAMMONEMIA (TYPE 1). This disorder is caused by a deficiency of the enzyme *ornithine transcarbamylase*. One patient, 6 years old, gave a history of attacks beginning in the third year of life. They were characterized by vomiting, screaming, headaches, slurring of speech, and confusion. These attacks were followed by lethargy, stupor, and ataxia. There were physical and mental retardation. The level of blood ammonia was elevated during the attacks.

HYPERAMMONEMIA (TYPE 2). Type 2 results from a deficiency of the enzyme *carbamyl phosphate synthetase*. A patient seen at 3 months of age had typical attacks that began at 10 days of age. They were characterized by vomiting, lethargy, dehydration, and flaccidity (relaxation of muscles). The attacks occurred whenever milk

These reactions are known as the *ornithine cycle*, the *ornithine-urea cycle*, the *urea cycle*, and the *Krebs-Henseleit urea cycle*.

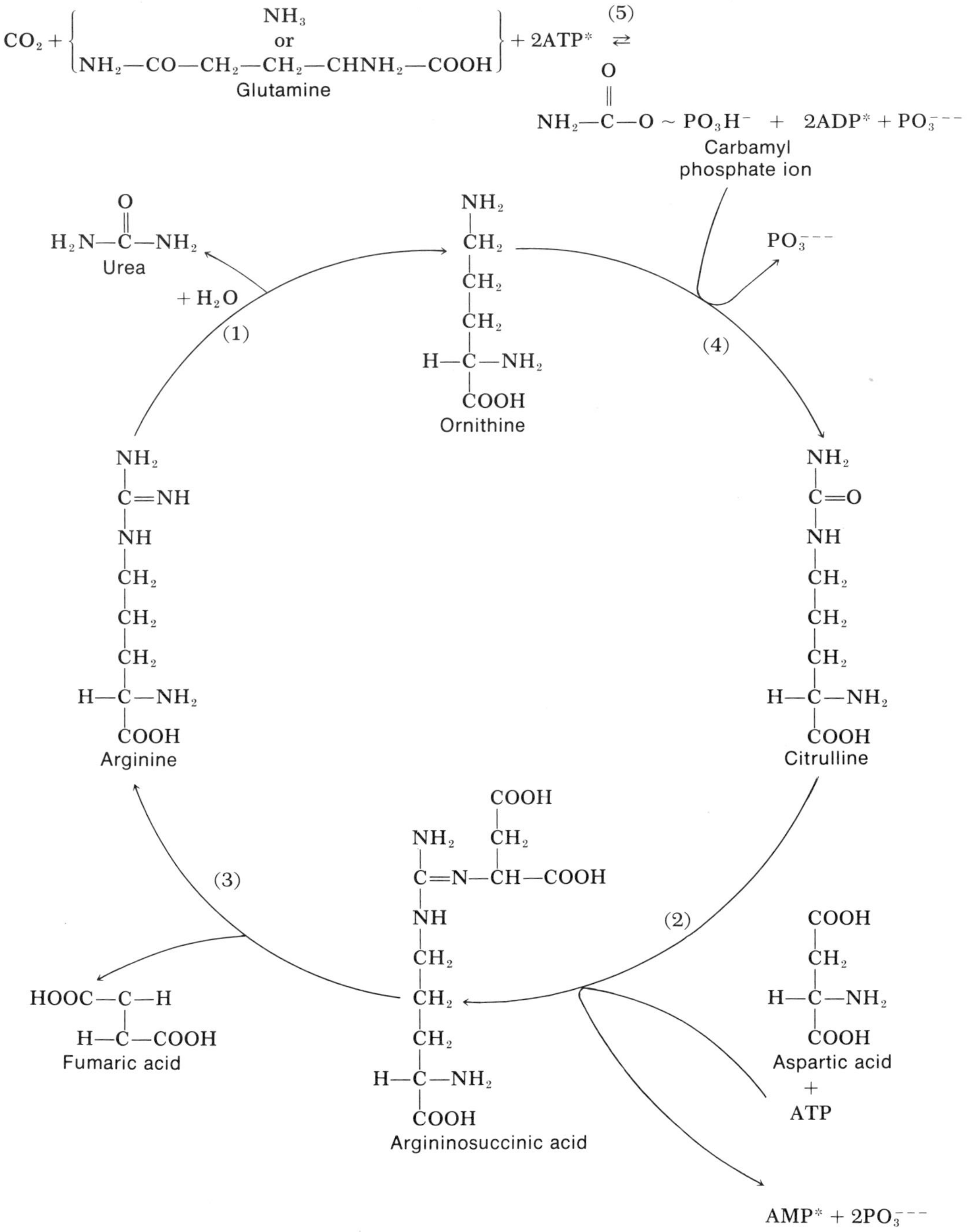

*ATP = adenosine triphosphate; ADP = adenosine diphosphate; AMP = adenosine monophosphate.

or products derived from it were fed. They subsided when the infant was given a diet low in protein. The level of blood ammonia was high during attacks.

FATE OF UREA

Urea is one of the end products of amino acid catabolism, the other end products being CO_2 and H_2O. After its formation in the liver urea enters the blood. It is removed from the blood by the kidney, which excretes it in the urine. Small amounts are excreted in the saliva and sweat.

FORMATION OF AMMONIUM SALTS BY THE KIDNEYS

When ketone bodies and other acids are excreted by the kidney, sodium is lost from the blood because these acids are largely excreted as sodium salts. This loss of sodium, if severe, decreases considerably the ability of the blood to form sodium bicarbonate, one of the chief buffers against acids. In other words, the loss of sodium causes *acidosis*. The kidney helps prevent this acidosis by forming *ammonium salts*, such as ammonium bicarbonate. The ammonium salts then react with the sodium salts of the harmful acids.

$$CH_3CHOHCH_2COONa + NH_4HCO_3 \rightarrow CH_3CHOHCH_2COONH_4 + NaHCO_3$$

Sodium hydroxybutyrate	Ammonium bicarbonate	Ammonium hydroxybutyrate	Sodium bicarbonate

Most of the sodium bicarbonate formed in this reaction diffuses back into the bloodstream, and the ammonium salt of the harmful acid is excreted in the urine. This, of course, partly prevents the loss of sodium from the blood, and so partly prevents acidosis.

It seems likely that the ammonium salts made in the kidney are formed mainly from glutamine, a compound related to the amino acid glutamic acid.

AMMONIUM SALTS IN BLOOD

All of the active organs in the body appear to form small amounts of ammonium salts in their metabolism. Some of these escape into the blood. The liver promptly converts ammonium salts to urea, however, and the concentration of these compounds in the blood is very low—between 0.01 and 0.1 mg per 100 ml of blood. Ammonium salts in the diet are likewise converted to urea in the liver.

The amount of ammonia in the blood increases greatly in the presence of hepatic coma, a serious disorder caused by severe damage to the liver.

ENERGY OF PROTEIN CATABOLISM

When we examine the formula for urea, we find that the nitrogen is present as amino groups, just as it is in amino acids.

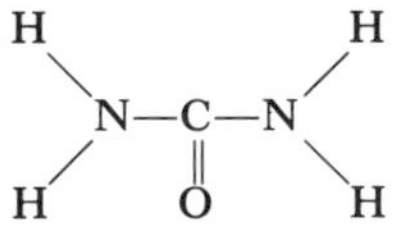

NH_2CONH_2

Urea

The nitrogen of amino acids, therefore, is not oxidized in metabolism since no change in valence of the nitrogen has occurred. In other words, we do not gain any energy from the nitrogen present in proteins. However, the remainder of the amino acid combines with oxygen (is oxidized) to form carbon dioxide and water. On the average, 1 g of protein yields 4 large calories of heat when it is burned in the body. This is the same energy value that carbohydrates have (4 large calories per gram), but is less than that of fats (9 large calories per gram).

CREATINE AND CREATININE

Creatine is one of the substances cells need. It contains nitrogen and is, therefore, made from the protein of the diet (since carbohydrates and fats do not contain nitrogen). Creatine is changed in the body to *creatinine*, which is then excreted in the urine.

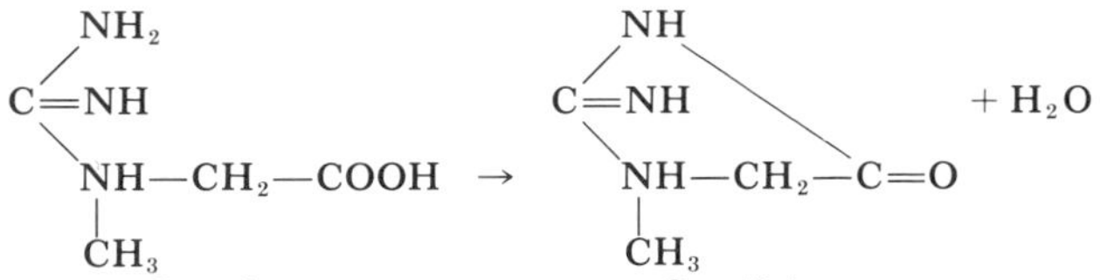

Creatine → Creatinine

Creatine is synthesized in the body from the amino acids glycine, arginine, and methionine.

Much of the creatine in muscle cells is present as the phosphate ester. The phosphate radical is combined as an energy-rich bond and can be used to regenerate ATP from ADP.

$$\text{Creatine} \sim \text{phosphate} + \text{ADP} \rightarrow \text{Creatine} + \text{ATP}$$

CREATINURIA. Creatinuria refers to the excretion of appreciable amounts of creatine in the urine. This is normal in children up to the age of puberty and it may occur normally during menstruation and in some cases of pregnancy. Creatine is found in small amounts in the urine of normal adults. It occurs in abnormally large amounts in conditions accompanied by failure to burn carbohydrate, conditions accompanied by excessive tissue breakdown, and diseases of muscles.

1. *Conditions accompanied by failure to burn carbohydrate.* Such conditions include starvation, diabetes mellitus, and severe liver disease. We are not yet able to explain why creatine occurs in the urine in the conditions.

2. *Conditions accompanied by excessive tissue breakdown.* When cells, particularly muscle cells, disintegrate rapidly, the creatine in them enters the bloodstream and is excreted in the urine. Fevers of long duration, wasting diseases, and exophthalmic goiter are conditions in which destruction of tissue is more rapid than normal. They are accompanied by creatinuria.

3. *Diseases of muscles.* Muscle cells contain more creatine than any other cells in the body. When these cells break down as a result of disease, creatine appears in the urine. Muscular dystrophies and myasthenia gravis are examples of muscle disorders. Muscular atrophy (shrinking), usually caused by a disease of the nerves that supply the muscle, is characterized by a loss of muscle tissue. Creatinuria is often present in muscular atrophy.

SIGNIFICANCE OF CREATININE EXCRETION. In general, it has been found that the amount of creatinine excreted each day in the urine is fairly constant for a given individual. The amount excreted appears to depend mainly on the amount of muscle tissue present in the individual's body. The amount excreted per day by males is usually higher than that excreted by females, probably because the average male has more muscle than the average female. The creatinine present in blood (about 0.8 to 1.5 mg in 100 ml) increases in severe uremia.

ANABOLISM OF HEMOGLOBIN

While the fetus is still in the uterus a large share of the hemoglobin in the blood is made in the liver and spleen. In adult life, however, the normal production of hemoglobin and the formation of the red blood cells is exclusively a function of *bone marrow* (the soft inner portion of bones).

CATABOLISM OF HEMOGLOBIN

The synthesis and catabolism of hemoglobin proceeds as illustrated by the following scheme.

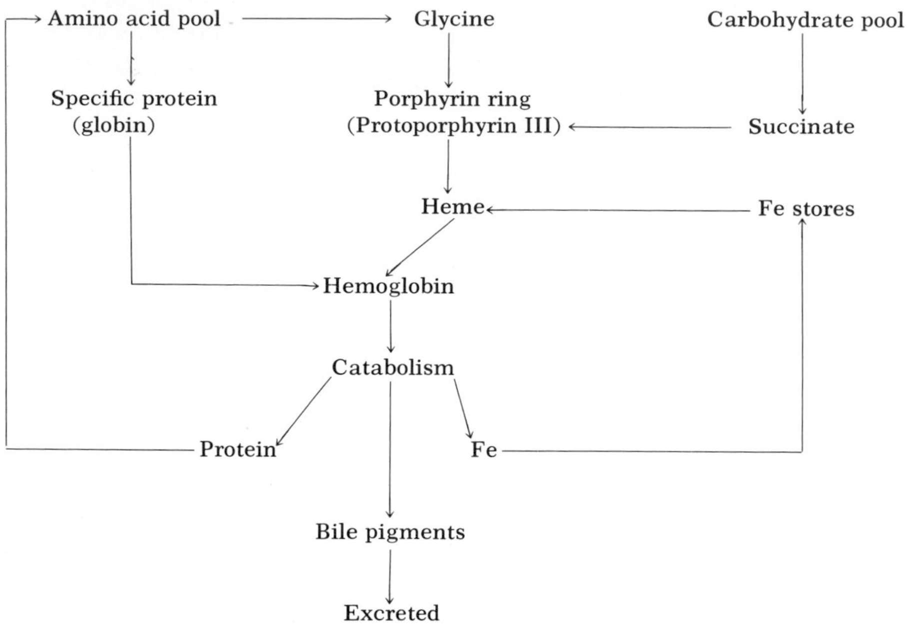

It is estimated that red blood cells live about 120 days, after which they disintegrate. The hemoglobin released when this occurs is then catabolized. The globin (protein) part of the molecule is metabolized like other proteins. *Heme* breaks down chiefly in the spleen and the liver. One of its breakdown products is *bilirubin* (a yellow-brown pigment). Bilirubin passes out of the blood, through the liver into the bile ducts, and finally enters the small

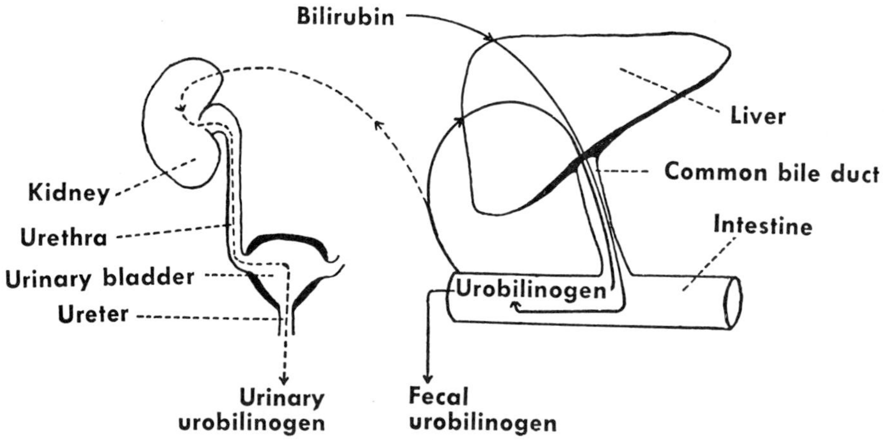

Fig. 26-1. Diagram to show the source and fate of urobilinogen. Normally, most of the urobilinogen absorbed from the intestine enters the intestine again in the bile. Under what circumstances would an increased amount of urobilinogen follow the route indicated in the diagram by the dotted line?

intestine with the bile. In the intestinal tract a part of the bilirubin is *oxidized* to other bile pigments, such as biliverdin (a green pigment) and bilicyanin (a blue pigment). In the lower intestinal tract bacterial enzymes catalyze the *reduction* of bilirubin to *mesobilirubinogen* (colorless). A portion of the mesobilirubinogen is then *oxidized* to *urobilin*. Urobilin has a brown color and is responsible for part of the color of normal feces (stool). In some cases of diarrhea there is insufficient time for urobilin to be formed, and the stools may have a green color from their content of biliverdin. Some of the color of normal feces is from *stercobilin*, a compound very similar to urobilin, which is formed from bilirubin.

Some of the important catabolic products of hemoglobin are indicated in the following diagram (adapted in part from a scheme suggested by Dr. C. J. Watson):

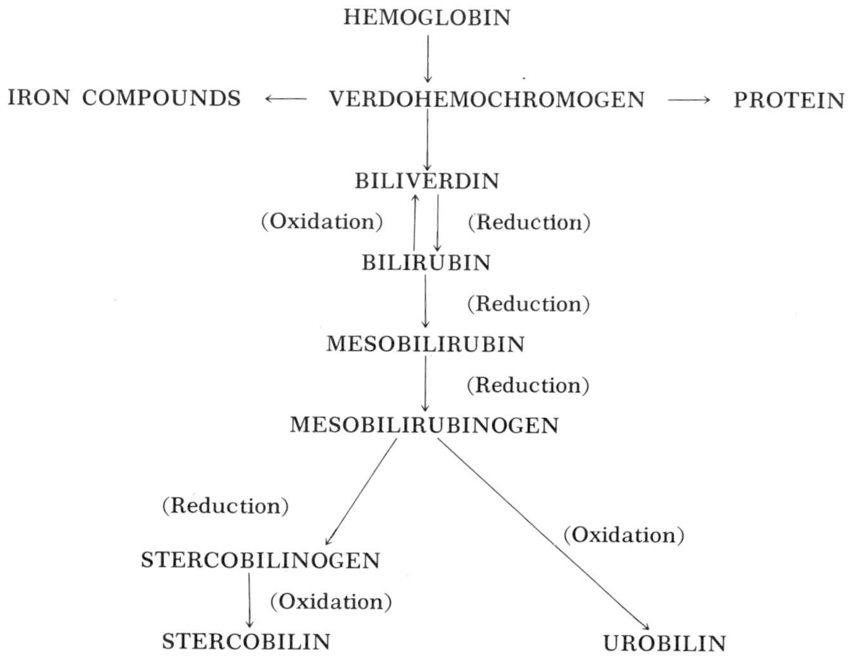

Mesobilirubinogen, urobilin, stercobilinogen, and stercobilin usually are determined chemically as a group, and the number of milligrams of all these compounds is reported as "mg of urobilinogen." In other words, the term *urobilinogen* is used in medicine as a name for this whole group of substances.

JAUNDICE. An increase in the normal amount of bilirubin in the blood is called *jaundice (icterus)*. The skin of patients with jaundice has the characteristic yellow-brown color of bilirubin. Jaundice is usually one of two types: (1) *Obstructive jaundice* is caused by some obstruction, such as a gallstone, that prevents the entrance of bile into the intestinal tract. White or clay-colored stools are seen in this type because the brown urobilin cannot be made in the absence of bilirubin. Increased amounts of bilirubin appear in the urine. (2) *Hemolytic jaundice* is caused by an increased rate of destruction of red blood cells. This causes an increased catabolism of hemoglobin, and, therefore, an increased production of bilirubin. Jaundice results when the bilirubin is produced more rapidly than the liver can excrete it. Bilirubin does not appear in increased amounts in the urine in this type of jaundice nor are the stools clay colored.

SIGNIFICANCE OF UROBILINOGEN. Most of the urobilinogen formed in the intestinal tract is eliminated in the feces. A certain amount, however, passes from the intestinal tract into the bloodstream. Most of this is removed from the blood by the liver, which returns it to the intestinal tract by way of the bile. In severe liver disease the damaged liver is unable to remove these compounds from the blood and they are then excreted in the urine. *An increase in the amount of urobilinogen excreted in the urine (normally less than 3 mg per day) usually indicates liver damage.**

It is apparent that the amount of urobilinogen in the feces will be *less than normal* when the patient has obstructive jaundice because the bilirubin from which it is made cannot get into the intestinal tract in normal amounts in this condition. The urobilinogen content of feces will be *increased* in hemolytic jaundice because bilirubin is being poured into the intestinal tract at an increased rate.

MYOGLOBINURIA. *Myoglobin* is an iron-containing protein found in muscle (see page 279). Chemically, it resembles one of the peptide chains found in hemoglobin and has a molecular weight (about 17,000) that is approximately one-fourth that of hemoglobin. It contains combined heme. It appears in the urine following extensive muscle damage (crush injuries, burns, electric shock, physical beating, arterial thrombosis). An infectious disease (Haff disease) results in myoglobinuria. Occasionally myoglobinuria is present for no apparent cause (idiopathic paroxysmal myoglobinuria).

PORPHYRIA. Porphyrins are complex cyclic compounds composed of four pyrrole units linked together by methine (—CH=) bridges to form a large ring structure. One of these, protoporphyrin III, combines with iron to form heme.

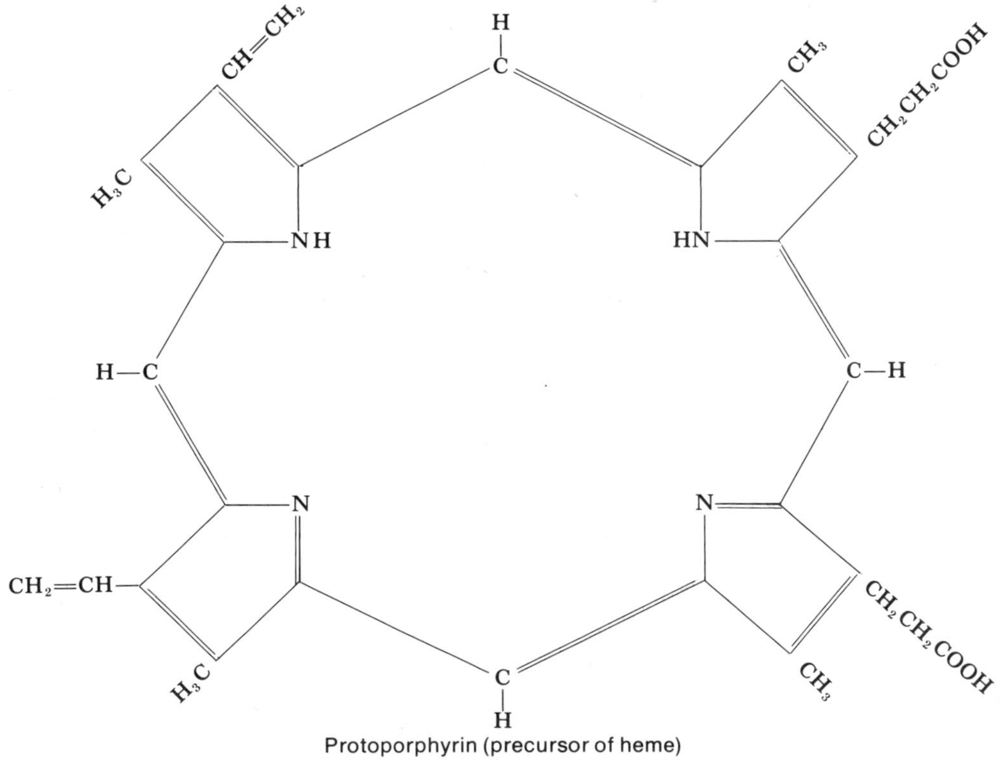

Protoporphyrin (precursor of heme)

*An increase in urinary urobilinogen may be found also in some cases of hemolytic jaundice.

Porphyria is a condition in which excessive amounts of porphyrins (known as uroporphyrins when they occur in urine and as coproporphyrins when they occur in feces) are excreted. The disease can be congenital (that is, present at birth) or acquired. Important signs and symptoms include sensitivity of the skin to light, a purplish complexion, gastrointestinal complaints, and nervous and mental symptoms. Typically, the urine, on standing, develops a pink or red color.

Porphyria may be latent (inapparent) for years, the clinical disease appearing after some inciting occurrence (alcoholism, use of barbiturates, liver disease).

PROPERDIN. Properdin is a protein found in normal serum in trace amounts (6 to 12 μg per milliliter). In the presence of a mixture of substances present in blood (known collectively as complement) and magnesium ions it acts as a normal defense mechanism of the body. Under suitable conditions the properdin system (properdin, complement, and magnesium ions) will kill certain bacteria, neutralize some viruses, and lyse (disrupt) certain abnormal red blood cells. The disease known as paroxysmal nocturnal hemoglobinuria (PNH) is a rare type of anemia in which the patient's red blood cells are hemolyzed by his own or other normal sera. However, sera devoid of properdin will not cause hemolysis. Properdin has been found to be protective against radiation illness of animals after their exposure to x-rays.

Special transformations of certain amino acids in the body

GLYCINE

Glycine, NH_2CH_2COOH, is the simplest amino acid. It combines with the benzoic acid present in some fruits (cranberries, plums, and prunes) and other foods to form *hippuric acid*. Hippuric acid is a normal component of the urine. *Glycocholic acid*, whose salts are found in the bile, is formed by the reaction between glycine and an organic acid called cholic acid. Glycine, arginine, and methionine are required for the synthesis of creatine. Glycine also is a precursor of heme, cholesterol, and purines.

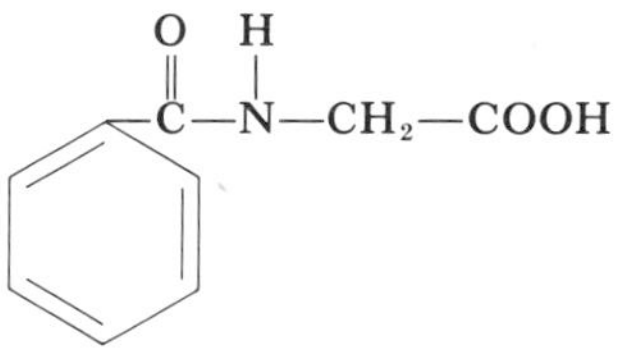

Hippuric acid

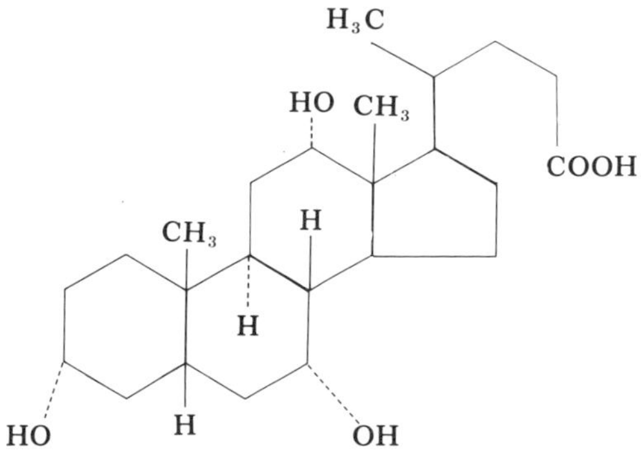

Cholic acid

CYSTINE

Taurocholic acid is another bile acid. It is formed by the reaction between taurine and cholic acid. Taurine is formed from cystine in the body. Cystine crystals (which look like the symbol for the benzene ring) are found in urine sediments in cases of the rare disease known as *cystinuria*.

CYSTINURIA. Patients with this disease excrete abnormally large quantities of the amino acids cystine, lysine, arginine, and ornithine in the urine. The loss of these substances from the body does not cause any known harmful effects. Three of the 4 amino acids are soluble and cause no difficulty in the urinary tract. However, cystine is not very soluble and precipitates with the formation of kidney and bladder stones. The formation of these stones is the only known pathology in cystinuria. *Penicillamine* (see page 158) is useful in the therapy of this condition; it reacts

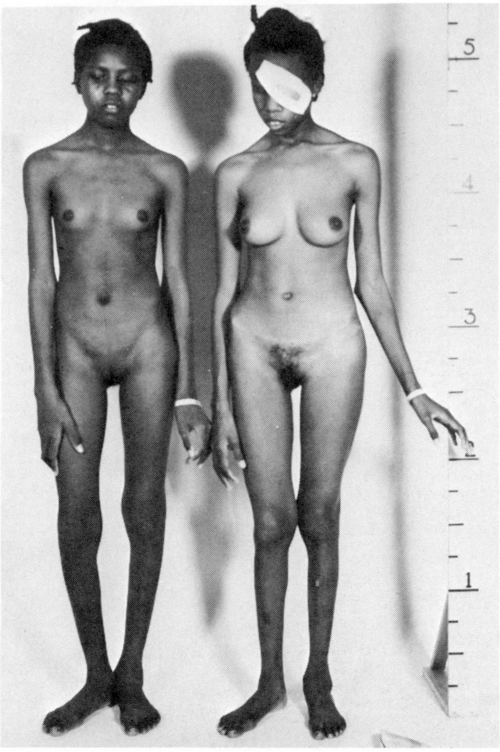

Fig. 26-2. Two patients with homocystinuria. What enzyme is deficient in this disorder? (From Thomas, R. P., and others: Homocystinuria and ectopia lentis in Negro family, J.A.M.A. **198:**561, 1966.)

chemically with cystine in the body to form 2 soluble substances. This prevents the formation of the cystine kidney and bladder stones.

Homocystinuria. This disease is caused by the absence of the enzyme *cystathionine synthetase.* Brain damage and mental retardation are variable; 60 percent of the patients have low intelligence. Dislocation of the lens of the eye usually occurs. The hair is fine and sparse. Skeletal deformities are common. There is a characteristic shuffling gait caused by a knock-knee deformity. Homocystine occurs in the urine. Diets low in the amino acid methionine and high in the amino acid cystine are beneficial if they are started early in life.

$$
\begin{array}{l}
\qquad\qquad\qquad\quad NH_2 \\
\qquad\qquad\qquad\quad | \\
S—CH_2—CH_2—CH—COOH \\
| \qquad\qquad\qquad\quad | \\
S—CH_2—CH_2—CH—COOH \\
\qquad\qquad\qquad\quad | \\
\qquad\qquad\qquad\quad NH_2
\end{array}
$$

Homocystine

TRYROSINE *Epinephrine,* the hormone of the medulla of the adrenal gland, and *thyroxine,* the hormone of the thyroid gland, are made from tyrosine in the body. *Melanin,* the brown pigment of the hair and skin, is also formed from this amino acid. Persons with *albinism* (lack of normal pigmentation

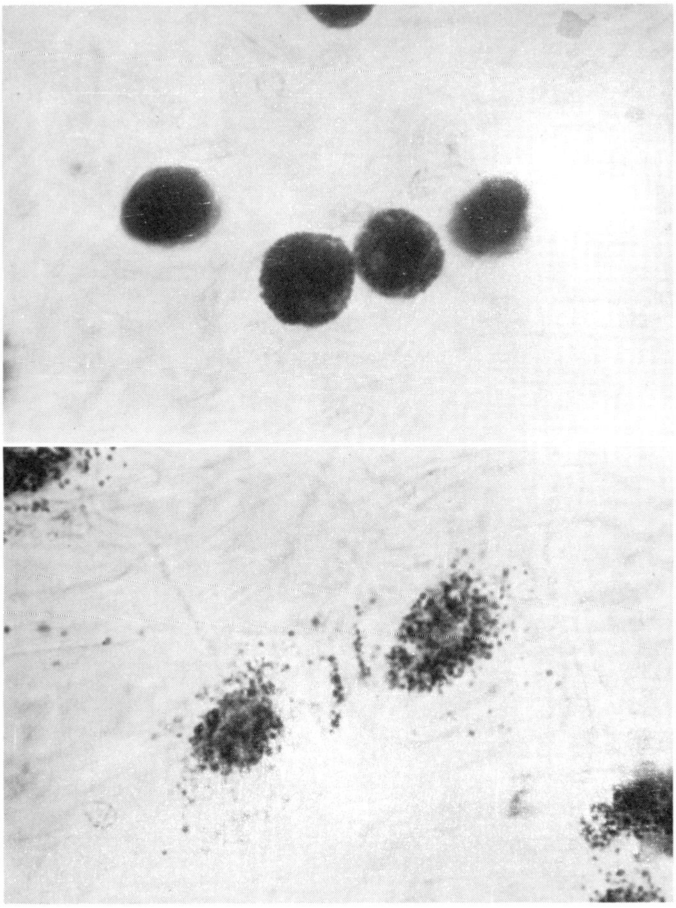

Fig. 26-3. Animal tissues contain many mast cells. (The German word *Mast* means feeding or fattening.) **A,** Within these cells are numerous granules that contain histamine (and, in some animals, serotonin) in bound, nonreactive form; **B,** in an allergic reaction, in which a foreign antigen reacts with an antibody, the mast cells are disrupted, and their granules are released. This process is accompanied by the release of active histamine, which is responsible, at least in part, for the signs and symptoms of the allergic reaction. From what amino acid is histamine formed in the body? (Courtesy Dr. J. H. Humphrey, National Institute for Medical Research, London; from Humphrey, J. H., and White, R. G.: Immunology for students of medicine, 1963, Philadelphia, F. A. Davis Co.)

of skin, hair, and eyes) lack an enzyme system required for the synthesis of melanin. *Phenylpyruvic acid,* which is made from phenylalanine in the body, is found in the urine of some feeble-minded children (see page 215). *Homogentisic acid,* a breakdown product of tyrosine, occurs in the urine in the condition called alkaptonuria. It will be remembered that homogentisic acid sometimes reduces Benedict's solution (see page 267). Urine that contains this compound turns black after standing several hours.

TYROSINEMIA is a rare disease caused by a lack of the enzyme *p-hydroxyphenyl pyruvic oxidase*. The level of tyrosine in the plasma is high. Clinically, there is liver and kidney damage. Slight mental retardation is observed in some, but not all, patients. Half of the patients have fever. Most have anorexia (lack of apetite), vomiting, diarrhea, and abdominal distention. An odor resembling cooked or rotten cabbage emanates from the body and from the urine. A diet low in phenylalanine and tyrosine is beneficial if started early in life. (Tyrosine can be formed from phenylalanine in the body.)

HISTIDINE

Histamine is a substance found in traces in many tissues in the body. It is made from the amino acid *histidine*. Histamine causes a fall in blood pressure and it stimulates secretion of gastric juice and contraction of the stomach muscles. Small amounts (0.5 to 1 mg) of histamine are sometimes injected into patients to cause a flow of gastric juice, usually when gastric juice is desired for chemical analysis.

HISTIDINEMIA. In this disease, histidine increases in the blood and in the urine. The only clinical abnormality has been a speech defect (slowness in learning to talk) in some, but not all, children. One clinician has referred to it as "a defect in search of a disease." Its major importance may be that a common test for the detection of phenylketonuria (see page 215) also is positive in this disorder (that is, in both conditions a wet diaper turns blue when ferric chloride is applied). The missing enzyme is histidase, whose function is to catalyze the deamination of histidine.

MAPLE SYRUP URINE DISEASE. This is a disease of enzymic defect. Its name is derived from the characteristic odor of the urine. The basic defect is the absence of the enzyme system that catalyzes the decarboxylation of the branched chain amino acids leucine, isoleucine, and valine. These amino acids and their keto-derivatives are increased in both blood and urine. This results in damage to the brain, with serious mental deficiency. The disease may be dormant in infancy, only to appear in late childhood.

METHIONINE

Methionine, one of the essential amino acids, has in its molecule a methyl ($-CH_3$) group that is readily transferred to certain other compounds in the tissues. This methyl group transfer often is referred to as *transmethylation*. Creatine and choline are two metabolic compounds whose methyl groups are derived from methionine.

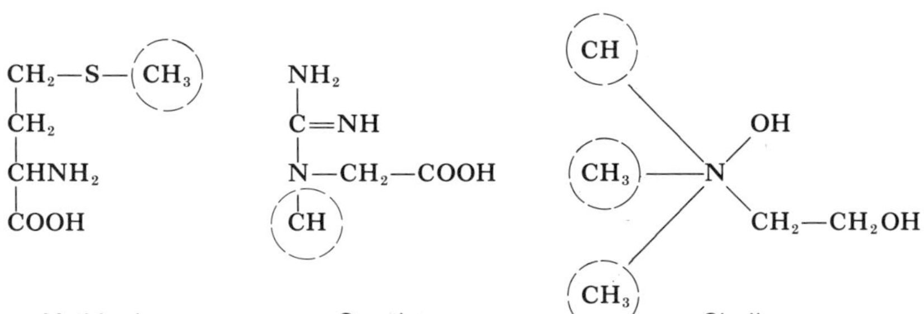

Methionine Creatine Choline

SEROTONIN. It has been known for years that clotted blood contains a substance capable of causing small arteries to constrict and the smooth muscle of the intestine to contract. This substance, chemically 5-hydroxytryptamine, is known as *serotonin*. It is made in the body from the amino acid tryptophan and exists preformed in blood platelets (see page 346).

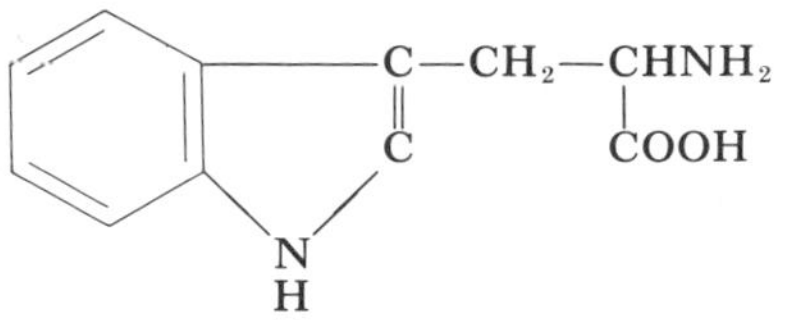

Tryptophan

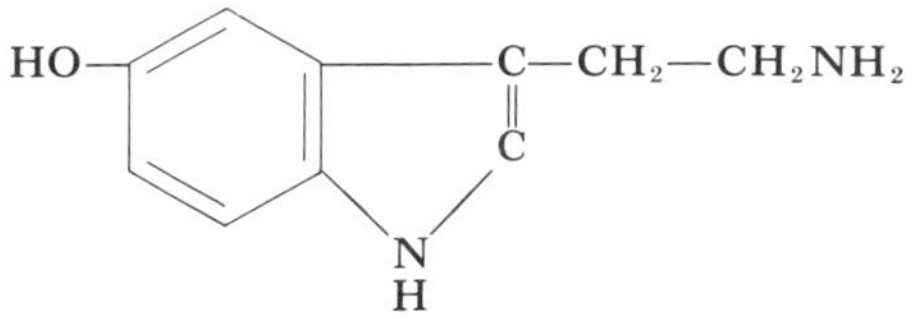

Serotonin (5-hydroxytryptamine)

Serotonin is found in serum (but not in plasma, see page 346), intestine, spleen, and especially in the brain. It is present also in urine.

Lysergic acid diethylamide (LSD), when injected into human beings in tiny doses (of the order of 30 μg, or 0.03 mg), causes a temporary state resembling schizophrenia, a common mental disease in which visual hallucinations often occur. In laboratory experiments it has been found that LSD inhibits or abolishes the biological

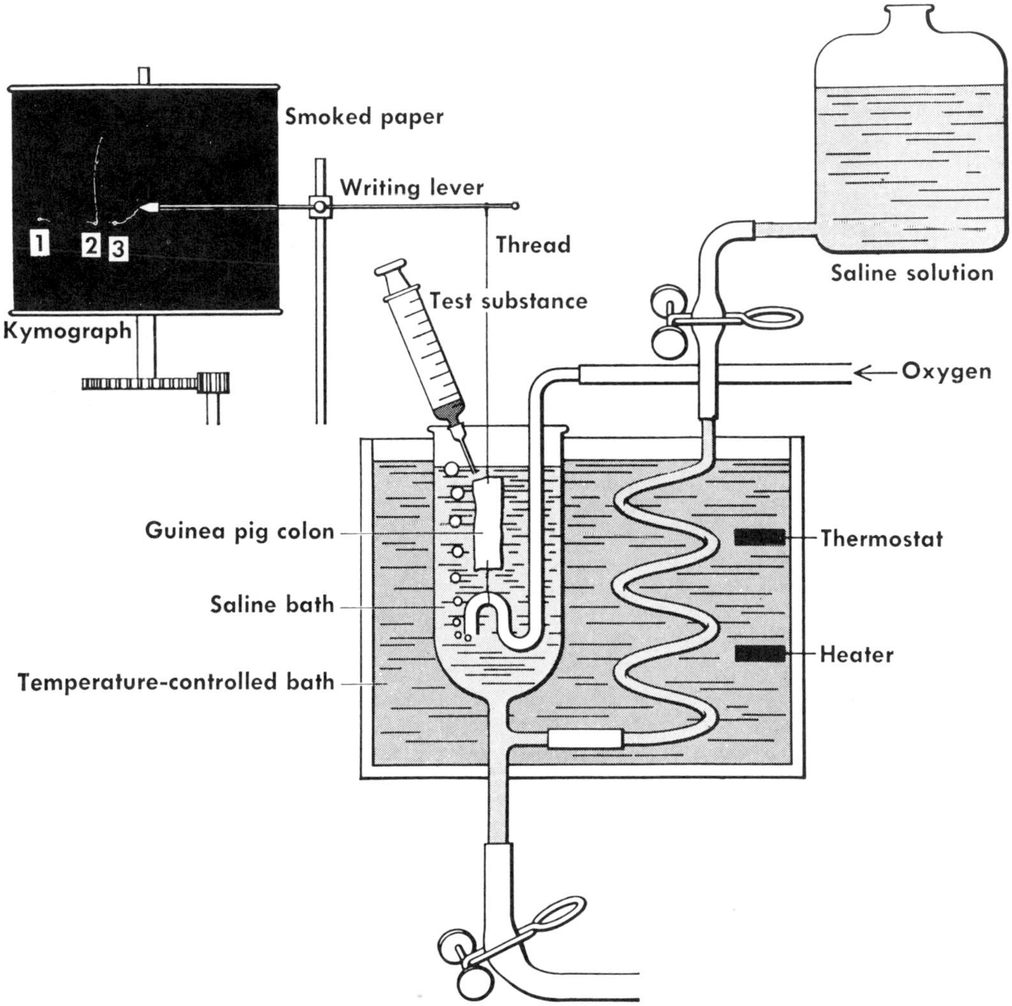

Fig. 26-4. Diagram illustrating apparatus used for the assay of bradykinin. From what is this peptide formed in the body? (Courtesy Dr. H. O. J. Collier; from Kinins, Sci. Amer. **207:** 111, August 1962.)

effects of serotonin (such as stimulation of smooth muscle contraction). This has led to speculation that serotonin may have something to do with conduction along nerve pathways in the brain, and that some mental illness may be caused by an abnormality of serotonin metabolism. This possibility has been strengthened by the finding that reserpine, a drug capable of calming violent mental patients, causes a release of serotonin from the brain into the blood.

BRADYKININ. Blood contains an enzyme known as *kallikrein*. Usually it is combined with an inhibitor and is, therefore, inactive. The active enzyme can be released from its inhibitor experimentally by a number of devices: acidification, dilution with salt solution, addition of acetone or papain (a mixture of enzymes present in the papaya plant), or simply by allowing the blood to come in contact with glass. Tissue injury that results in an inflammatory reaction (redness, swelling, local heat, and pain) also activates kallikrein.

TEST OBJECT	ACTION	DOSE OR CONCENTRATION
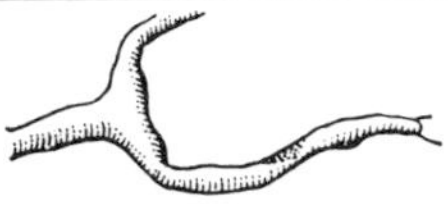 Isolated rat uterus	Smooth-muscle contraction	.1 nanogram per milliliter
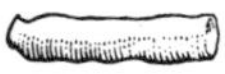 Isolated rat duodenum	Smooth-muscle relaxation	.8 nanogram per milliliter
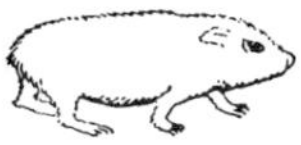 Whole guinea pig	Constriction of bronchioles	.5 microgram per kilogram (intravenous)
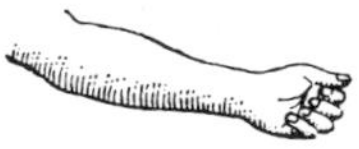 Human forearm	Dilation of blood vessels	100 nanograms (intra-arterial)
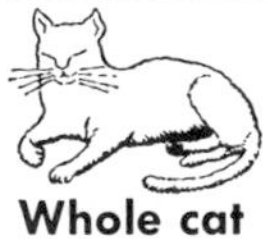 Whole cat	Lowered blood pressure	400 nanograms per kilogram (intravenous)
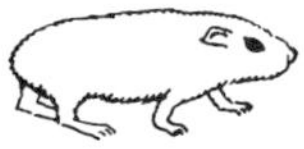 Guinea pig skin	Increased capillary permeability	.1 to 1 nanogram (intradermal)
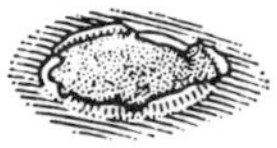 Human blister base	Pain	.1 to 1 microgram per milliliter

Fig. 26-5. The potency of pure bradykinin is shown by the extremely small dosages or highly dilute concentrations needed to evoke its principal effects in a variety of test objects. What is the derivation of the word bradykinin? (Courtesy Dr. H. O. J. Collier; from Kinins, Sci. Amer. **207**:111, August 1962.)

When active kallikrein is formed in blood, it acts on the α-globulin fraction of the plasma proteins (see page 354) to form a peptide known as *kallidin II*. An enzyme present in blood (aminopeptidase) causes a molecule of the amino acid lysine to split off the end of the kallidin II. This results in the formation of the peptide bradykinin (also known as *kallidin I*).

Arg–Pro–Pro–Gly–Phe–Ser–Pro–Phe–Arg
Bradykinin

Bradykinin causes the various smooth muscles of the body to contract or to relax. For example, it causes contraction of the smooth muscle of the isolated rat uterus, guinea pig bronchioles, and isolated guinea pig colon. It relaxes the smooth muscle of the isolated rat duodenum and causes dilation of blood vessels. This peptide also increases capillary permeability and lowers blood pressure. When it is injected into the skin, it produces the classic signs and symptoms of acute inflammation (redness, swelling, heat, and pain).

One assay for bradykinin consists in measuring its ability to cause constriction of a strip of guinea pig colon (see Fig. 26-4). Another biologically active substance, histamine (see page 292) also responds to this test but acts more quickly than does bradykinin. This explains the derivation of the name bradykinin (from the Greek words *bradys*, meaning "slow," and *kinein*, meaning "to move").

It seems probable that the release of bradykinin in the tissues is one cause of the acute inflammatory process. It is interesting that aspirin, long known to be effective in relieving the signs and symptoms of acute inflammation, can neutralize some of the biological effects produced by bradykinin. For example, the administration of aspirin can prevent the constriction of guinea pig bronchioles that follows the intravenous injection of bradykinin. When bradykinin is injected intraperitoneally into mice, the animals exhibit a phenomenon known as writhing—that is, they press their abdomens down against the floor of the cage in a characteristic fashion. Relatively small doses of aspirin abolish this behavior.

Bradykinin exists for only a short time after it is formed in the tissues—although long enough to produce its powerful biological effects. A tissue enzyme (carboxypeptidase) that catalyzes the splitting off of arginine inactivates it.

STUDY QUESTIONS

1. Make a table showing the enzymes concerned in protein digestion, their substrates, and the end products of digestion.
2. What is pepsinogen? Trypsinogen? Enterokinase? Chymotrypsinogen?
3. Can a large percentage of the protein in the diet be converted to glycogen in the body? (See Chapter 24.)
4. Can ketone bodies be formed from amino acids?
5. What are essential amino acids? Name five of them.
6. What are adequate proteins? Inadequate proteins? Give an example of each.
7. What is oxidative deamination? What kind of substances are formed by it in the liver?
8. What is the fate of the keto acids formed in the liver?
9. What is the fate of the ammonia formed by oxidative deamination?
10. What are the end products of the catabolism of amino acids?
11. Under what conditions does the kidney form ammonium salts? How does this help prevent acidosis?
12. What is the fate of ammonium salts that enter the blood?
13. How much energy is derived from the burning of 1 g of protein in the tissues? What part of the amino acid molecule does not furnish any energy?
14. Name three abnormal types of conditions in which creatinuria occurs. Is creatine ever found normally in the urine? When?
15. What does the amount of creatinine excreted in the urine seem to depend on? Why do men excrete more creatinine than women? Name a condition in which the creatinine in the blood is higher than normal. What is the function of creatine phosphate?
16. Where is hemoglobin made in the body? What materials are required for its manufacture? Describe the structure of the hemoglobin molecule.

17. Draw a diagram showing the chief products formed by the catabolism of hemoglobin.
18. From what compound are mesobilirubinogen and urobilin made? Where are they made? What compounds are responsible for the brown color of normal feces?
19. What is jaundice? What are the two principal types of jaundice? How do you think they might be distinguished?
20. Is an increased amount of bilirubin found in the urine in obstructive jaundice? In hemolytic jaundice?
21. What do clay-colored stools indicate? Green stools?
22. What is the significance of an increased excretion of urobilinogen in the urine?
23. What change in the amount of urobilinogen excreted in the feces occurs in hemolytic jaundice? In obstructive jaundice? Why?
24. What is the significance of myoglobinuria?
25. What is the chemical nature of myoglobin?
26. Which porphyrin is a precursor of heme?
27. What are the chief signs and symptoms of porphyria?
28. What is hippuric acid? Glycocholic acid? What amino acid is necessary for their manufacture?
29. Name some important properties of properdin.
30. Name a substance made from cystine in the body. In what disease do cystine crystals appear in the urine?
31. Name two hormones made from tyrosine in the body. What is melanin?
32. What substance occurs in the urine in some cases of feeble-mindedness? In alkaptonuria?
33. For what purpose is histamine used in medicine? From what amino acid is it made?
34. What is histidemia?
35. Discuss maple syrup urine disease.
36. What is meant by transmethylation?
37. Why is serotonin thought to play a role in mental disease?
38. Name and describe several diseases of enzymic defect involving amino acids.

CHAPTER 27

Nucleic acids and the code of life

When an egg is fertilized by union with a living spermatozoan, the resulting single cell contains within itself all of the information required to produce a living, functioning organism. Moreover, this new organism has characteristics inherited from its parents and had the potentiality of transmitting certain of these inherited characteristics to its offspring. From the point of view of biochemistry, this means that somewhere in every living cell there is a code—the genetic code or code of life—that enables the cell to produce the enzymes required for the synthesis and metabolism of the essential chemical substances and structures of living things. Since all enzymes are proteins, the coded information must specify the sequence in which amino acids are joined together to make proteins of specific composition, size, and linear structure.

The code of life exists in a series of huge linear molecules known collectively as *deoxyribonucleic acid*, or *DNA*. If it were possible to splice together the DNA molecules in one human cell to form a single thread, it would be about a yard in length and would weigh about 6 picograms. (One billion picograms equals 1 milligram.) The familiar *chromosomes* are strands of DNA. A human cell normally contains 46 of them. *Genes* are regions in the DNA threads that contain the coded information required for the synthesis of a single specific protein. A virus particle, the smallest structure known to contain the genetic code, probably contains from a few to several hundred genes. A bacterial cell may contain 1,000 or so genes; a human cell probably contains a million or more.

THE CHEMICAL STRUCTURE OF NUCLEIC ACIDS

The various products obtained by the hydrolysis of nucleic acids are shown in the following diagram:

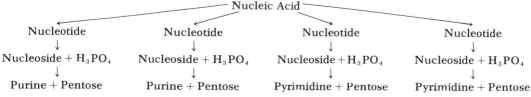

Nucleic Acid

Nucleotide	Nucleotide	Nucleotide	Nucleotide
↓	↓	↓	↓
Nucleoside + H_3PO_4	Nucleoside + H_3PO_4	Nucleoside + H_3PO_4	Nucleoside + H_3PO_4
↓	↓	↓	↓
Purine + Pentose	Purine + Pentose	Pyrimidine + Pentose	Pyrimidine + Pentose

The final products obtained by this hydrolysis are *phosphoric acid, pentoses, purines,* and *pyrimidines.*

Two kinds of nucleic acid are recognized. One of these, deoxyribonucleic acid (abbreviated DNA) occurs almost exclusively in the nuclei of cells. The other, ribonucleic acid (abbreviated RNA) is found both in the nucleus and in the cytoplasm.

The hydrolysis products of DNA are *adenine* and *guanine* (purines; see page 195); *cytosine* and *thymine* (pyrimidines; see page 194); *phosphoric acid;* and *deoxyribose* (a pentose; see page 242)

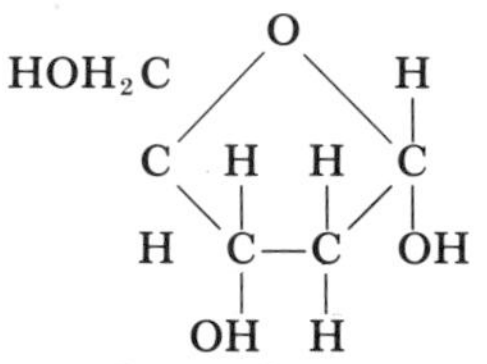

Deoxyribose

The corresponding products formed by the hydrolysis of RNA are *adenine* and *guanine* (purines); *cystosine* and *uracil* (pyrimidines); *phosphoric acid;* and *ribose* (a pentose).

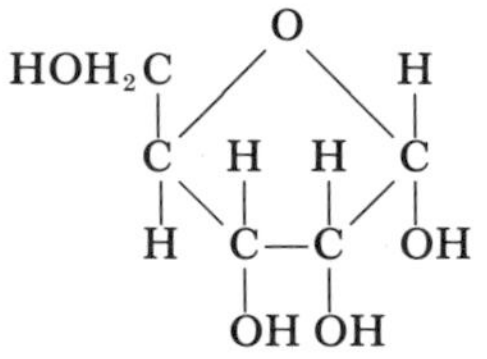

Ribose

NUCLEOSIDES AND NUCLEOTIDES

Nucleosides are composed of purines or pyrimidines chemically combined with ribose or deoxyribose. They have names derived from the bases (that is, purines or pyrimides).* The names of those derived from pyrimdines end in -idine; those derived from purines have names ending in -osine.

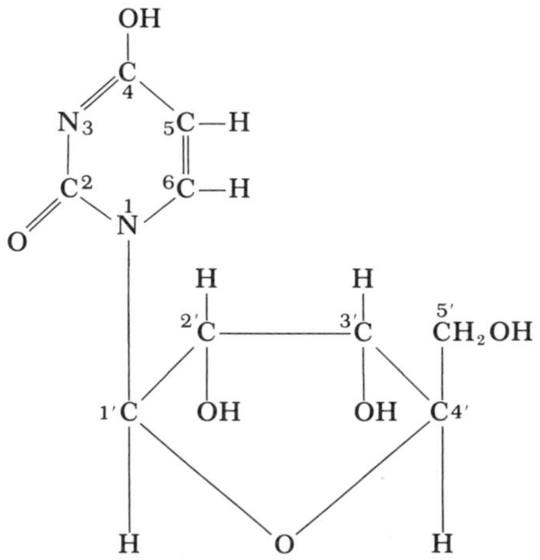

Uridine, a nucleoside

*Purines and pyrimidines often are referred to as bases since they can combine with acids to form salts.

Nucleotides are phosphoric acid esters in which the phosphoric acid is combined with the pentose of a nucleoside at the 5′ position.

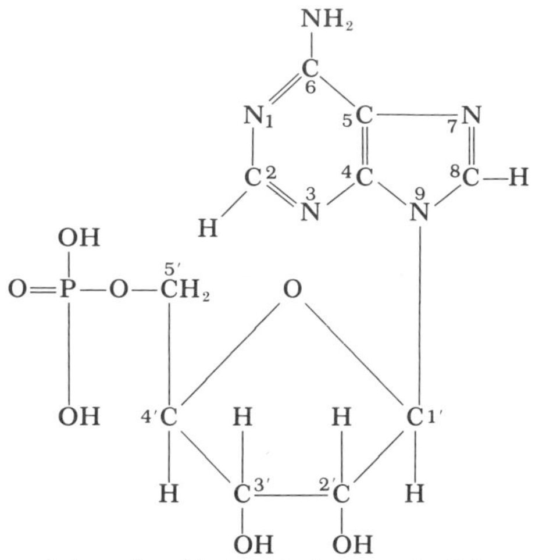

Adenosine-5′-phosphate, a nucleotide

In addition to their role as components of the nucleic acids, some of the nucleotides have important functions in metabolism. For example, adenosine phosphate can combine with additional phosphoric acid to form adenosine diphosphate (ADP) and adenosine triphosphate (ATP). These compounds are important in storing and releasing the energy required for numerous metabolic reactions. (See Fig. 20-4 on page 213.)

THE STRUCTURE OF DNA

Within the nucleus of resting (that is, nondividing) cells DNA usually exists as two long chains or threads coiled around each other as are the strands in a piece of rope. This coiled structure often is referred to as a *helix* (see page 300). The long axis of each coil is formed by the deoxyribose and phosphoric acid (see Fig. 27-2). The coils are held together by hydrogen bonds (see page 92) between the purines and pyrimidines. The spatial relationships are such that *adenine and thymine always are paired, as are cytosine and guanine.*

During cell division the DNA helical molecules uncoil, probably from one end, much as a zipper does when it is unfastened. As this takes place,

Table 27-1. Names of nucleosides and nucleotides

Base	Nucleoside	Nucleotide
Cytosine	Cytidine	Cytidine-5′-phosphate
Uracil	Uridine	Uridine-5′-phosphate
Thymine	Thymidine	Thymidine-5′-phosphate
Adenine	Adenosine	Adenosine-5′-phosphate
Guanine	Guanosine	Guanosine-5′-phosphate
Hypoxanthine (see page 313)	Inosine	Inosine-5′-phosphate

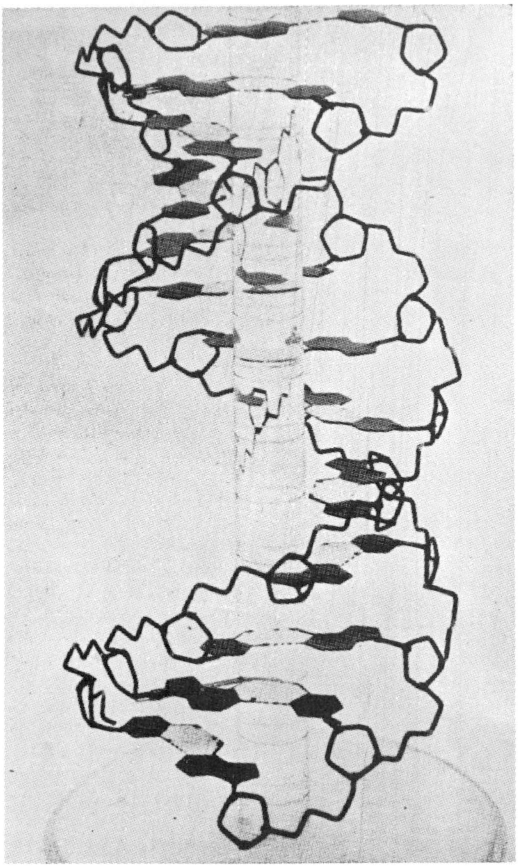

Fig. 27-1. Structural model showing a pair of DNA chains wound as a helix about the fiber axis. The pentose sugars (5-sided figures) can be seen plainly. From every one on each chain protrudes a base (purine or pyrimidine) linked to an opposing base at the same level by a hydrogen bond. These base-to-base links act as horizontal supports holding the chains together. What is a hydrogen bond? (From Crick, F. H. C.: The structure of the hereditary material, Sci. Amer. **151**:56, 1954.)

each coil acts as a template, or mold, around which a new coil is formed. When division is complete, each daughter cell has a double-stranded DNA helix identical with that of the parent cell. Stated in the terminology of genetics, the number of chromosomes doubles during cell division so that each daughter cell has the same number as did the mother cell.

The major enzyme mediating the replication of DNA is known as *duplicase*.

MESSENGER RNA

The coded information required for the synthesis of proteins resides in the DNA of the nucleus. Since, however, protein synthesis occurs in the cytoplasm, and not in the nucleus, it is obvious that this information must be transmitted to the sites of protein synthesis. The first step in this transfer is the synthesis in the nucleus of a strand of RNA, known as *messenger RNA*. DNA acts as a template for this synthesis, according to the following

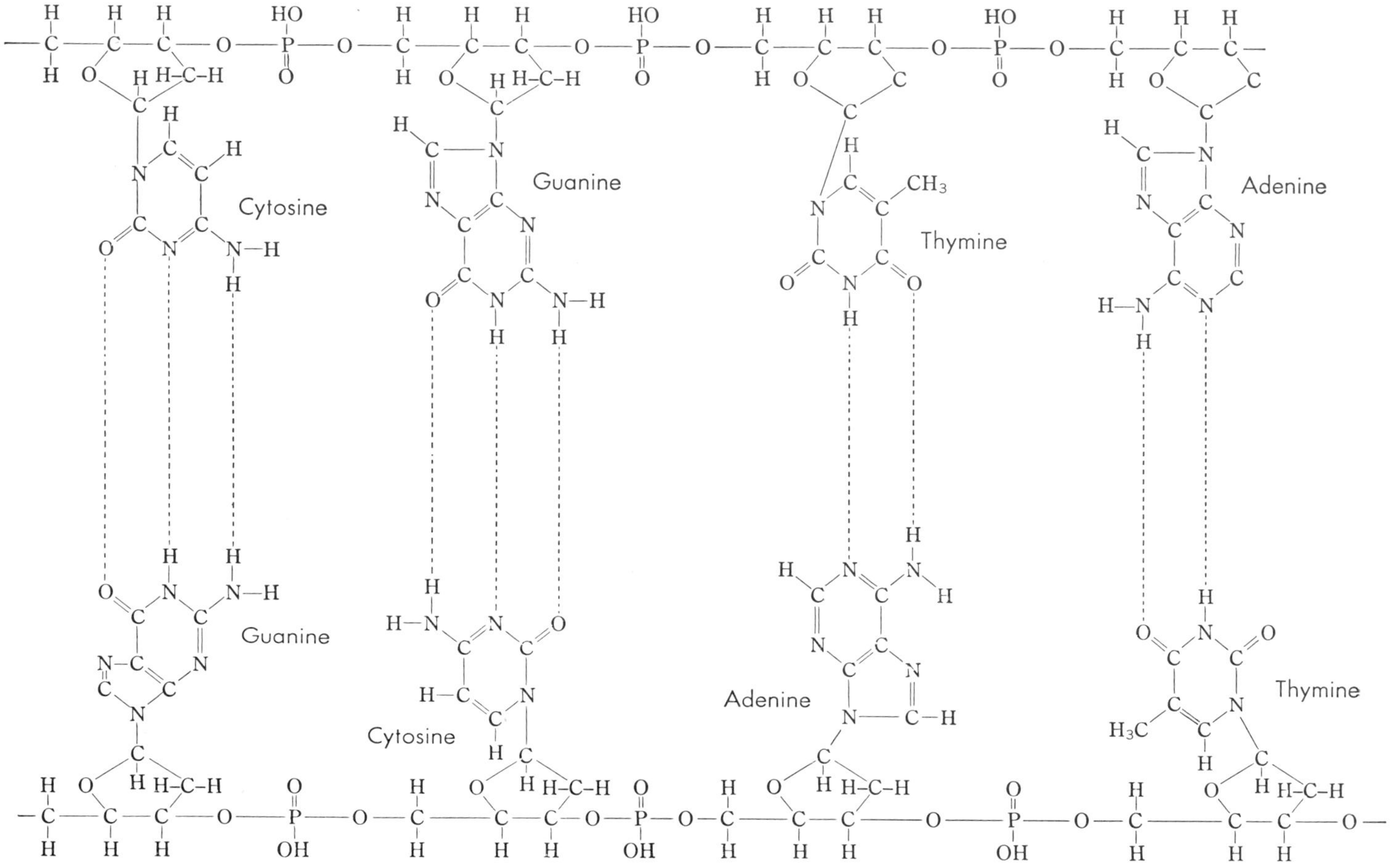

Fig. 27-2. Diagram showing the chemical linkages along a portion of a DNA chain. The dotted lines represent hydrogen bonds. What are the products of hydrolysis of DNA?

rule: adenine in the DNA molecule always pairs with uracil in the forming RNA molecule; thymine in DNA pairs with adenine in RNA; and cytosine always pairs with guanine. Synthesis probably begins at a region of the DNA molecule representing the code for the first amino acid in a specific protein and proceeds along the chain. As this occurs, the newly formed RNA "peels off" much as a zipper separates when it is unfastened. If we use A for adenine, G for guanine, C for cytosine, T for thymine, and U for uracil, the process can be illustrated diagrammatically:

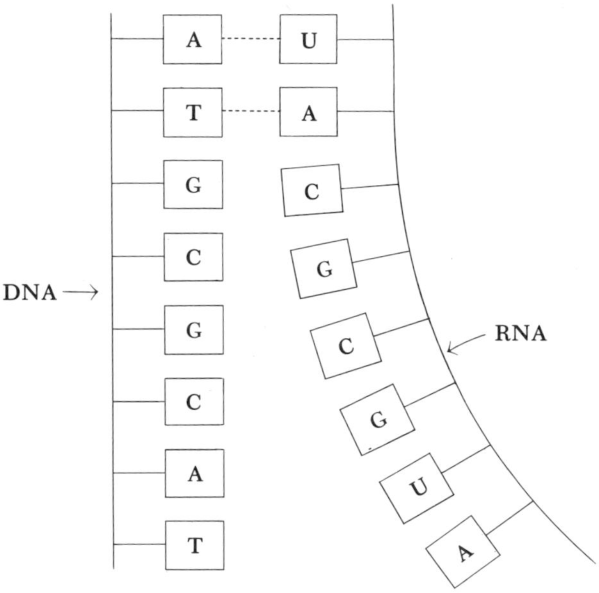

We shall find later that three bases are required to furnish the code "word" for a single amino acid. This "word" is called a *codon*. Thus, there are DNA codons and messenger RNA codons.

If the messenger RNA molecule is designed to carry information that will result in a protein containing two hundred amino acid residues, ob-

Table 27-2. Amino acids required for protein synthesis

Amino acid	Abbreviation	Amino acid	Abbreviation
Alanine	Ala	Glutamic acid	Glu
Arginine	Arg	Glutamine	Gln
Asparagine	Asn	Glycine	Gly
Aspartic acid	Asp	Histidine	His
Cysteine	Cys	Isoleucine	Ile
Leucine	Leu	Lysine	Lys
Methionine	Met	Phenylalanine	Phe
Proline	Pro	Serine	Ser
Threonine	Thr	Tryptophan	Trp
Tyrosine	Tyr	Valine	Val

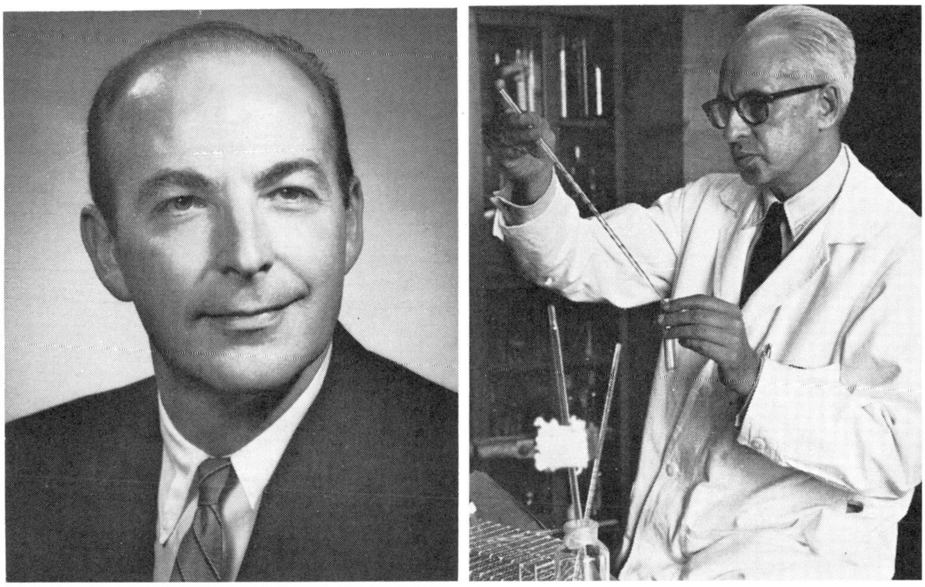

Fig. 27-3. Dr. Arthur Kornberg (left) of Stanford University and Dr. Severo Ochoa (right) of New York University were awarded the Nobel Prize in medicine and physiology in 1959 for their work on the synthesis of nucleic acids by enzymatic reactions in test tubes. Dr. Kornberg synthesized DNA and Dr. Ochoa synthesized RNA. How do these types of nucleic acid differ?

viously it must be long enough to possess six hundred bases. In general, then, messenger RNA molecules have high molecular weights.

Messenger RNA, after its formation in the nucleus, migrates into the cytoplasm, where it takes part in the synthesis of the specific protein for which it carries the code.

NATURE OF THE GENETIC CODE

It has been determined that twenty different amino acids are involved in protein synthesis. Some proteins contain other amino acids, but these are formed by chemical reactions that take place after protein synthesis has occurred. These twenty amino acids are listed in Table 27-2.

If the code for the amino acids is carried by the bases in the messenger RNA, obviously these four bases must arrange themselves into *at least* twenty different combinations. If four bases are arranged in pairs, only sixteen arrangements are possible. Therefore the assumption was made that the code for one amino acid must be in a combination of at least three bases. When the four bases are arranged in groups of three, sixty-four combinations are possible (see Table 27-3). It is evident also that some amino acids are specified by more than one arrangement of three bases, since there are sixty-four base triplets and only twenty amino acids.

The first experiment that led to the discovery of a code word for an amino acid was carried out in 1961. By using the proper enzyme system, it was possible to make an artificial nucleic acid molecule from just one nucleotide: uridine-5′-phosphate. In other words, a series of these molecules were coupled together to form a long

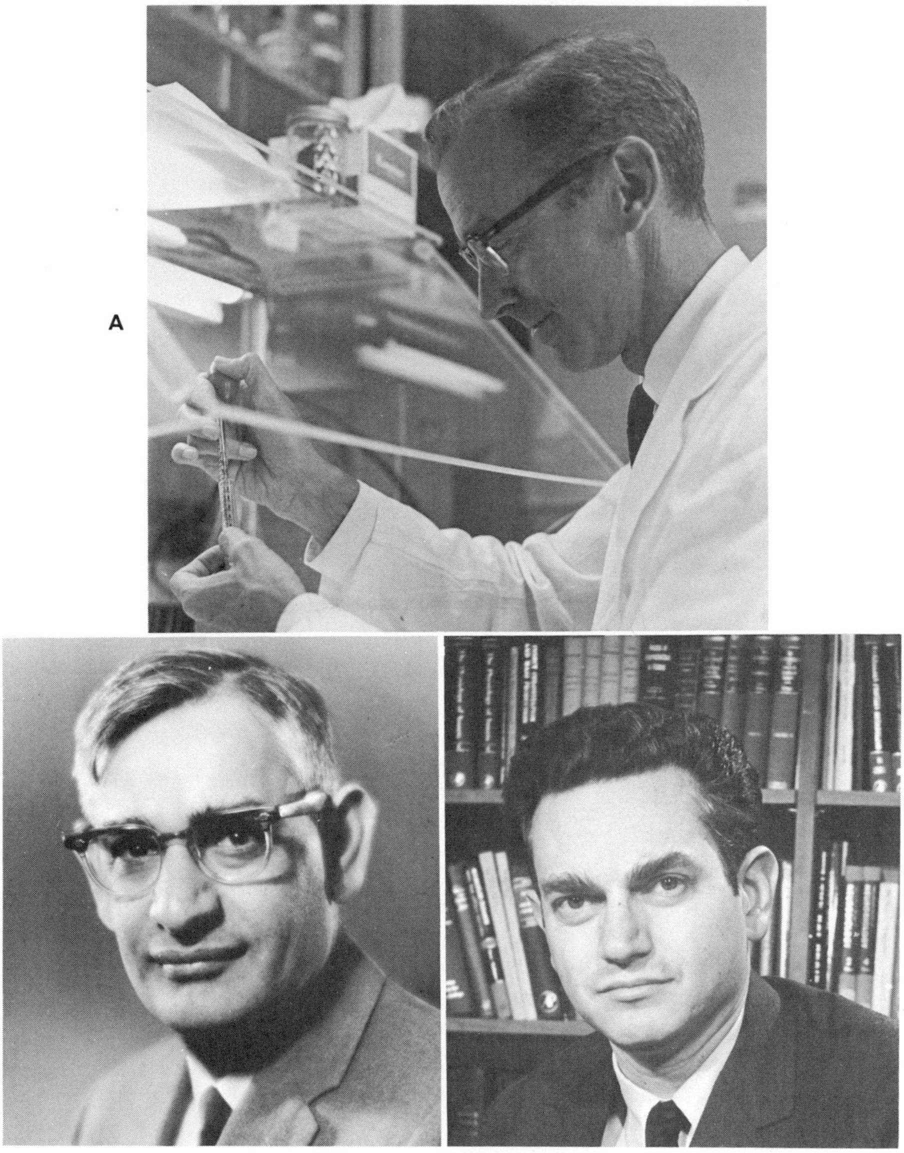

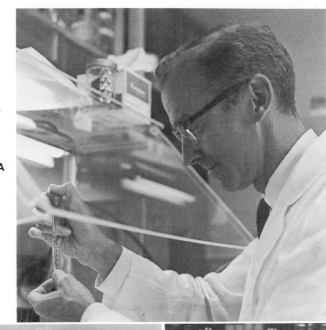

Fig. 27-4. Dr. Robert W. Holley **(A),** Dr. Har Gobind Khorana **(B),** and Dr. Marshall W. Nirenberg **(C)** were awarded the Nobel Prize in medicine or physiology for 1968 for their pioneering work that played a major role in solving the mystery of the genetic code. Dr. Holley's work was carried out at Cornell University, Dr. Khorana's at the University of Wisconsin, and Dr. Nirenberg's at the National Heart Institute. What is the function of a "nonsense codon"?

Table 27-3. Messenger RNA codons—the genetic code*

Amino acids	Codons	Amino acids	Codons	Amino acids	Codons	Amino acids	Codons
Phe	UUU	Ser	UCU	Tyr	UAU	Cys	UGU
Phe	UUC	Ser	UCC	Tyr	UAC	Cys	UGC
Leu	UUA	Ser	UCA	N_2†	UAA	N_3†	UGA
Leu	UUG	Ser	UCG	N_1†	UAG	Trp	UGG
Leu	CUU	Pro	CCU	His	CAU	Arg	CGU
Leu	CUC	Pro	CCC	His	CAC	Arg	CGC
Leu	CUA	Pro	CCA	Gln	CAA	Arg	CCA
Leu	CUG	Pro	CCG	Gln	CAG	Arg	CGG
Ile	AUU	Thr	ACU	Asn	AAU	Ser	AGU
Ile	AUC	Thr	ACC	Asn	AAC	Ser	AGC
Ile	AUA	Thr	ACA	Lys	AAA	Arg	AGA
Met	AUG	Thr	ACG	Lys	AAG	Arg	AGG
Val	GUU	Ala	GCU	Asp	GAU	Gly	GGU
Val	GUC	Ala	GCC	Asp	GAC	Gly	GGC
Val	GUA	Ala	GCA	Glu	GAA	Gly	GGA
Val	GUG	Ala	GCG	Glu	GAG	Gly	GGG

*U = uracil; A = adenine; C = cytosine; and G = guanine.
†N_1, N_2, and N_3 sometimes are referred to as *nonsense codons* because they do not code amino acids. Instead, they act as "periods" and signal the termination of a peptide chain.

chain. When this artificial nucleic acid was substituted for messenger RNA in a cellular extract system that was capable of synthesizing protein, the resulting product was a long chain of phenylalanine molecules combined with each other; that is, a protein containing a single amino acid was formed. This was not surprising, because the only codon possible was UUU, since uridine was the only base in the artificial messenger RNA. Hence, it was established that one codon for phenylalanine is UUU.

In other experiments, various ratios of nucleotides were used to make artificial nucleic acids. For example, when a ratio of 5 U to 1 A was used, it could be calculated by statistical mathematical methods that the resulting nucleic acid should have the following proportions of codons: UUU = 25, UUA = UAU = AUU = 5, AAU = AUA = UAA = 1, AAA = 0.2. In the protein formed by this artificial messenger RNA, it was found that phenylalanine, tyrosine, and asparagine were present in ratios of 25:5:1. It could easily be surmised that for phenylalanine a codon was UUU; for tyrosine it was UUA, UAU, or AUU; and for asparagine it was AAU, AUA, or UAA. Experiments of this type have led to our present knowledge of the code.

TRANSFER RNA

The next important problem to discuss is the mechanism that allows messenger RNA to participate in the actual synthesis of a protein. In the cytoplasm there are molecules of RNA that contain about seventy bases. There is at least one that is specific for each of the twenty amino acids—and probably there is one for each of the sixty-four possible triplets. These RNA molecules exist in the form of a bent helix, illustrated diagrammatically in Fig. 27-5. At one end of the helix, there are three bases that are unpaired. The other end contains the bases adenine, cytosine, and cytosine, in sequence. Each transfer RNA can combine with a specific amino acid, as illustrated in Fig. 27-6. The code triplets present in the transfer RNA molecules are known as *decodons* or *anticodons*.

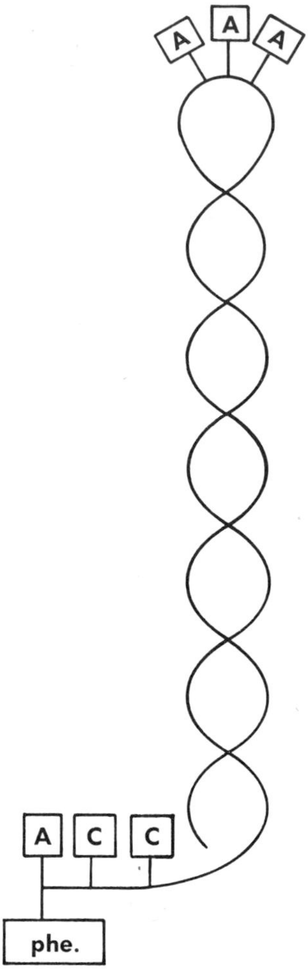

Fig. 27-5. Diagram of a molecule of transfer RNA. What is the function of transfer RNA? (Drawing by James Skillman.)

In the actual synthesis of protein, the transfer RNA becomes attached to the messenger RNA by hydrogen bonds. If, as an example, the three unpaired bases of the transfer RNA are AAA, this molecule will attach itself at a region of the messenger RNA where the code sequence UUU occurs. (Remember that A always bonds with U; see page 302.) Since UUU in the messenger RNA is the code word for phenylalanine, this particular transfer RNA carries this amino acid. Imagine that a series of these transfer RNAs attach themselves along the messenger RNA chain. This would result also in a series of amino acids in a definite sequence and in close proximity to each other (see Fig. 27-6). In the presence of enzymes in the cytoplasm these amino acids unite with each other by forming peptide bonds (see page 270), and the result is the formation of a protein.

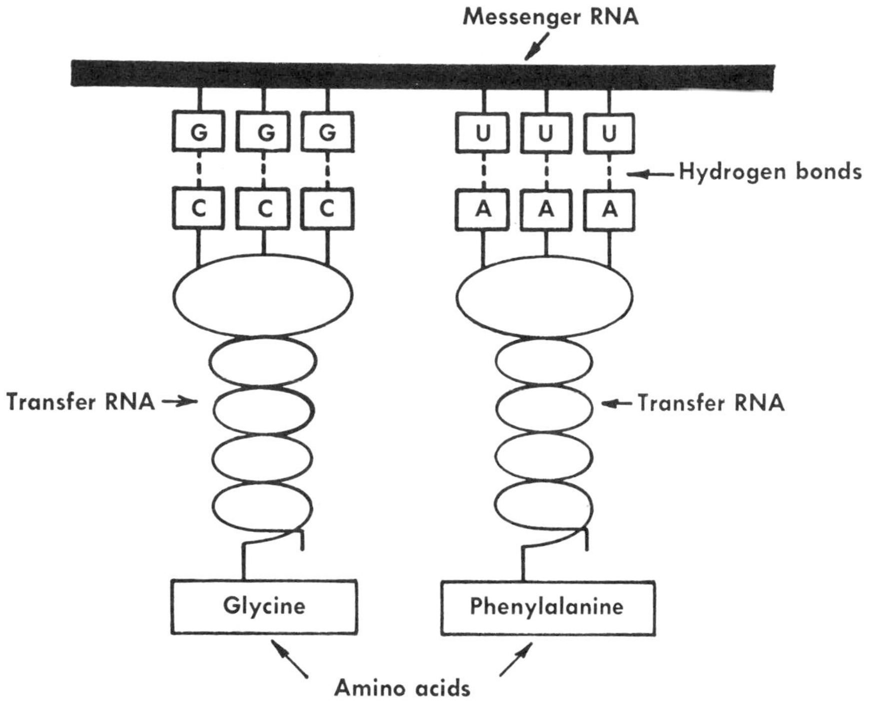

Fig. 27-6. Diagram illustrating the attachment of transfer RNA molecules to a molecule of messenger RNA. What type of bond is involved in this attachment? (Drawing by James Skillman.)

RIBOSOMES

The actual union of the amino acids with each other takes place on structures in the cytoplasm known as *ribosomes*. These ribosomes consist of about 40 percent protein and 60 percent RNA. According to present ideas, a ribosome moves along a strand of messenger RNA much as a pulley can be made to move along a horizontally stretched rope. As each triplet code comes in contact with the ribosome, it combines with the corresponding triplet in a transfer RNA. As the next triplet reaches the ribosome, this is repeated, and the two amino acids thus brought together combine with each other. In this way, as the ribosome continues to pass along the messenger RNA strand, the string of amino acids becomes longer and longer until, finally, the complete protein is formed, each amino acid in its proper sequence.

After one ribosome begins its journey along the messenger RNA strand, another can begin the same journey, and a single strand of messenger RNA can have several (indeed as many as sixty in the case of poliomyelitis virus RNA) ribosomes attached to it at a single instant of time. Each of these will make one molecule of protein, each identical, since the same strand of messenger RNA is used (see Fig. 27-7).

Ribonuclease is an enzyme that catalyzes the hydrolysis of RNA to produce nucleoside-3′-monophosphate. In certain, though not all, cells it is located almost

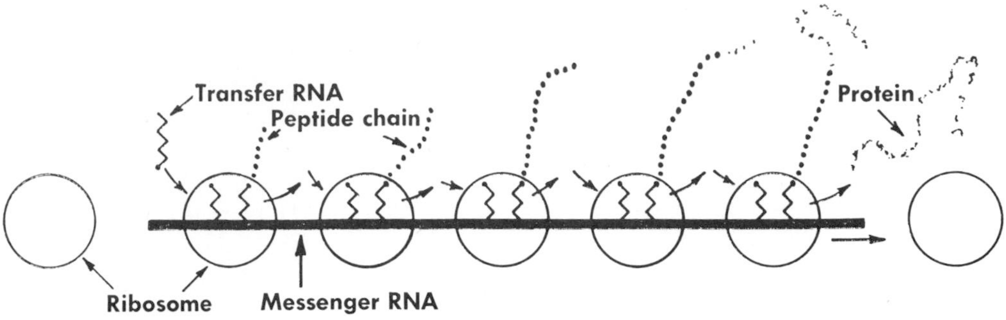

Fig. 27-7. Diagram illustrating the formation of a protein molecule. How are ribosomes involved in this synthesis? (Drawing by James Skillman.)

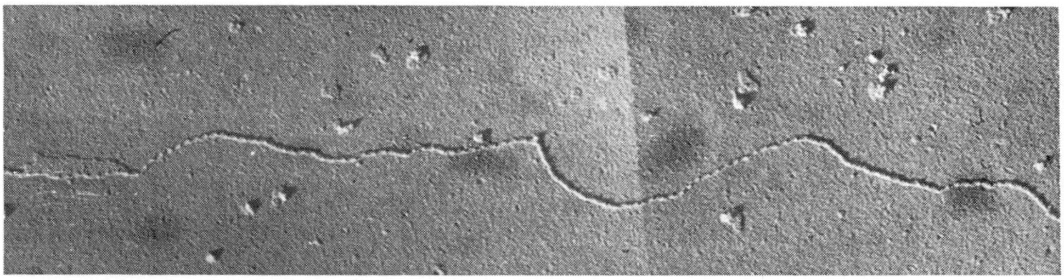

Fig. 27-8. Electron photomicrograph showing a long polyribosome (series of ribosomes —also called a polysome) isolated from rat skeletal muscle tissue. This polysome contained about 115 ribosomes on the chain. What is the chemical composition of a ribosome? (Courtesy Dr. C. B. Breuer, Dr. M. C. Davies, and Dr. J. R. Florini, Lederle Laboratories; from Biochemistry **3:**1713, November 1964. Copyright the American Chemical Society.)

exclusively in the ribosomes. It has been postulated that the function of the ribonuclease in the ribosomes is to inactivate messenger RNA, thus removing it from the ribosomes. This would free the ribosomes to interact with other messenger RNA strands, including those with codes for protein synthesis different from that of the degraded messenger RNA.

GENETIC REPRESSORS

A specific gene—sometimes more than one—is required for the synthesis of a specific protein, such as an enzyme or structural protein (for example, the keratin in fingernails). Although every cell of an individual's body contains identical DNA, obviously various cells differ both morphologically and functionally. Thus, there must be mechanisms that prevent the incorporation of some genes in a specific molecule of RNA, which, of course, carries information leading to the formation of specific proteins. One known mechanism involves proteins known as *genetic repressors.* A repressor binds directly to a site on the DNA molecule at the point where the code for a gene begins; this site is known as an *operator*. This prevents the enzyme RNA polymerase from incorporating this genetic information into RNA and thus eliminates this gene. Each gene, or set of genes that work together, is controlled by a specific repressor. In some cases, the re-

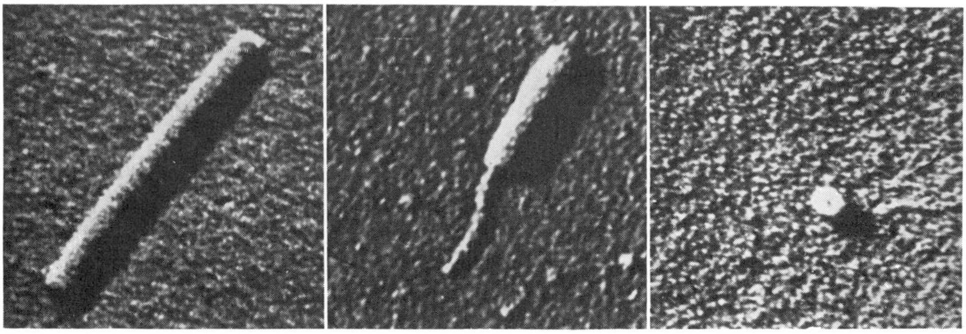

A B C

Fig. 27-9. A display of tobacco mosaic virus (TMV) substructures. **A,** An intact TMV particle; **B,** a partially degraded particle from which the RNA remains as a coaxial filament; **C,** a short portion of RNA-free protein, seen end on, and exhibiting a central hole. (×125,000.) Which portion of the tobacco mosaic virus is responsible for the infection of the tobacco plant? (Arranged by R. C. Williams, Virus Laboratory, University of California, Berkeley; from Hart, R. G.: Electron-microscopic evidence for the localization of ribonucleic acid in the particles of tobacco mosaic virus, Proc. Nat. Acad. Sci. U. S. A. **41**:261, 1955.)

pressor can combine with a small molecule known as an *inducer*. When this occurs, the repressor no longer can attach itself to the operator and the repressed gene thus will be manufactured again. In other cases, the repressor is not active (cannot attach itself to the operator) until it is activated by combining with a small molecule known as a *corepressor*.

For example, some bacteria can use lactose as food. They must manufacture lactase (β-galactosidase), which is required for the conversion of lactose to glucose and galactose. But if the culture medium in which they are growing does not contain lactose, the gene required for the synthesis of lactase is not needed and its synthesis is switched off by a specific repressor known as the *lac* repressor. If lactose is added to the medium, a breakdown product formed from it acts as an inducer, which combines with the repressor, rendering it incapable of combining with the operator. Thus the DNA now transmits the appropriate code for the synthesis of lactase to RNA. When all the added lactose is used up, the repressor again becomes active, attaches itself to the operator portion of the DNA molecule, gene formation is suppressed, and lactase no longer is manufactured.

VIRUSES

Viruses are particles of matter made up of a protein shell (sometimes called a capsid) and a core of nucleic acid. The nucleic acid is RNA for some viruses and DNA for others; no virus contains both types. There has been much philosophic discussion as to whether viruses should or should not be regarded as living organisms. The problem arises because viruses are dependent on host cells (living cells that they can invade) both for energy and for the building blocks to create new particles of virus. Moreover, many of them have been isolated in the form of crystals, and in this respect they resemble organic molecules.

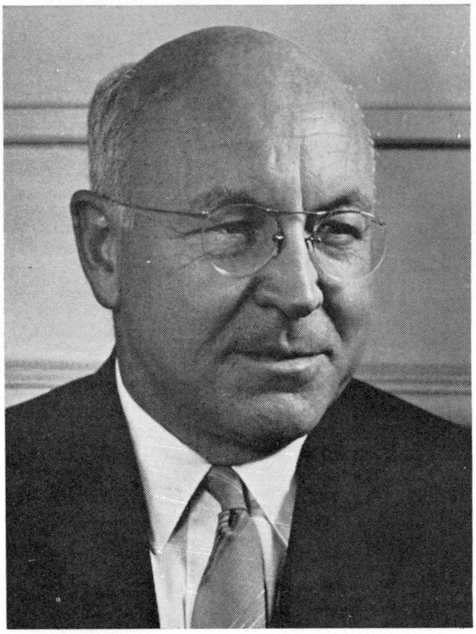

Fig. 27-10. Dr. Wendell M. Stanley, then at the Rockefeller Institute, received the Nobel Prize in chemistry in 1946. He was the first scientist to isolate a virus in crystalline form. He shared the prize with Dr. John H. Northrop, who crystallized many enzymes, and Dr. James B. Sumner, who first crystallized an enzyme (urease). Is a virus alive?

When a virus particle invades the cell, its nucleic acid, in effect, displaces the nucleic acid of the cell, and hence the genetic code of the virus is imposed on the living cell. As a result, the cell produces numerous new virus particles, often resulting in disruption of the cell and release of the newly formed virus particles. Each of these particles can invade a new host cell, and in this way a viral infection spreads and progresses.

If the virus contains DNA, its nucleic acid acts as a template for the synthesis of messenger RNA. If it contains RNA, its nucleic acid acts as messenger RNA, and the viral RNA acts as a template for the synthesis of additional identical molecules, which act as messenger RNA.

INTERFERON. When viruses grow in cells, a defense mechanism comes into play. The infected cells produce a protein capable of inhibiting the growth of the infecting virus. This protein is known as *interferon*. One interferon that has been well studied has a molecular weight between 20,000 and 34,000. Interferon can be used experimentally to prevent the infection of cells by a virus, but it has not been useful in stopping the growth of the virus after infection has been established.

Interferons are *species specific*. That is, each species of animal, including the human, makes its own definite interferon. Hence, it would not be anticipated that interferons isolated from lower animals would be useful in preventing viral infections in humans. However, there is experimental work in animals that offers hope that substances capable of stimulating the body to make more of its own interferon may be developed in the future. There is some evidence that interferon stimulates the body to produce a specific protein (translation inhibition protein, TIP) that actually is the active agent that interferes with replication of viruses in the tissues.

Interferon also is active against chlamydiae ("psittacosis group organisms") and some protozoa (organisms causing malaria, toxoplasmosis, and leishmaniasis).

ANABOLISM OF PURINES

The tissues are capable of synthesizing purines (and hence nucleosides and nucleotides). The different molecules utilized in the synthesis are aspartic acid, glycine, carbon dioxide, glutamine, and formic acid. The first purine formed exists as the nucleotide inosinic acid. From this substance adenosine-5′-phosphate and guanosine-5′-phosphate can be formed.

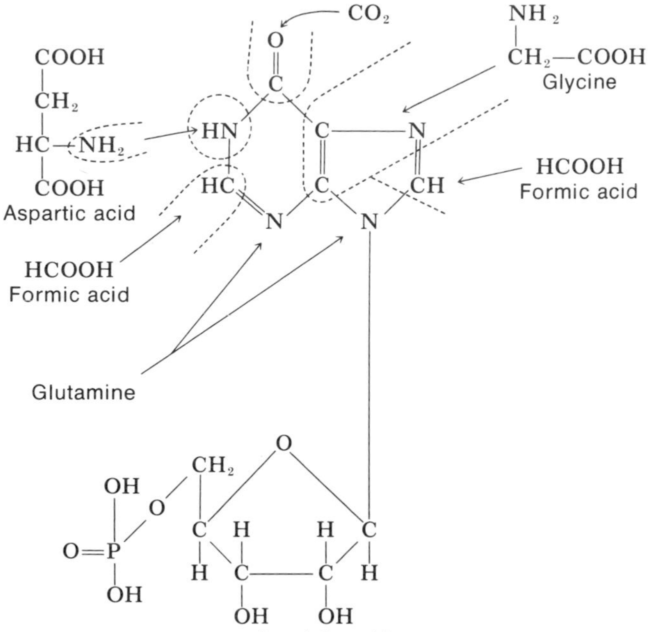

Inosinic acid

COENZYME F. Formic acid is very reactive chemically and does not exist free in the tissues. Instead it occurs as part of a complex molecule related chemically to folic acid (a vitamin, see page 432) and known as coenzyme F, CoF, or "active formate."

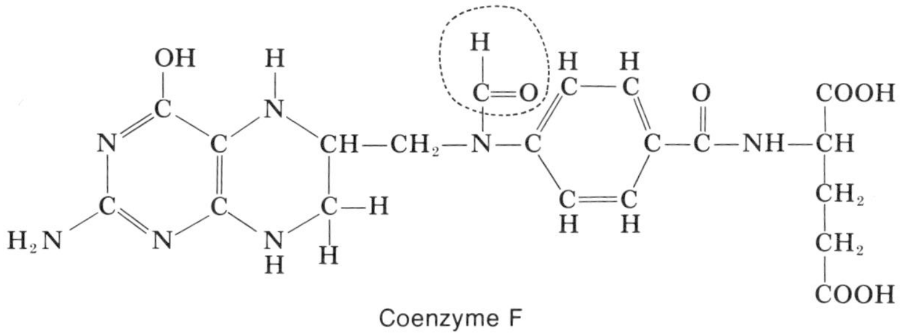

Coenzyme F

SYNTHESIS OF ADENINE AND GUANINE

Inosinic acid combines with aspartic acid to form an intermediate compound, which loses fumaric acid to yield adenosine-5′-phosphate. If we abbreviate ribose by Rib and phosphate by (P), the reactions can be visualized as follows:

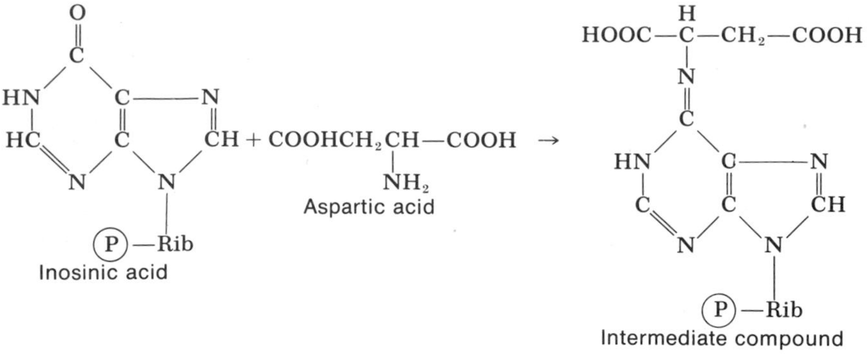

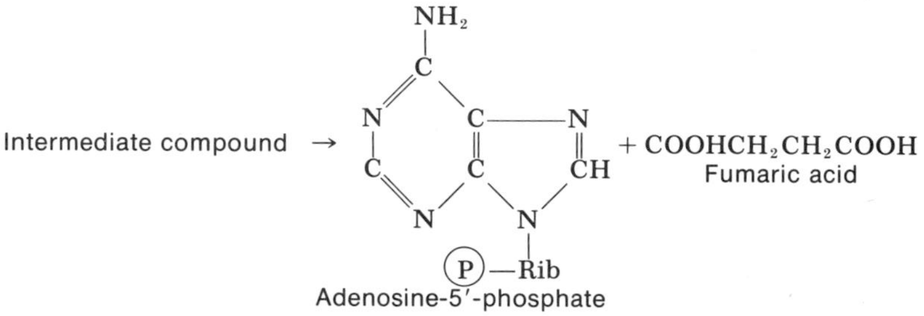

Adenosine-5′-phosphate can hydrolyze to form adenine (see page 195), ribose, and phosphoric acid.

Inosinic acid can combine with water and lose hydrogen to form an intermediate compound. When this compound reacts with glutamine, guanosine-5′-phosphate and glutamic acid are formed.

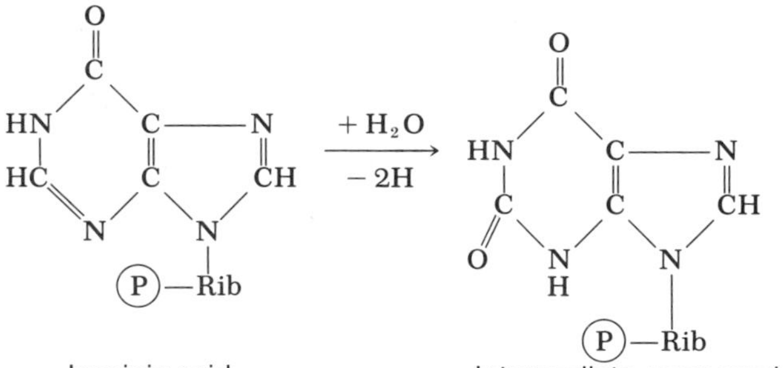

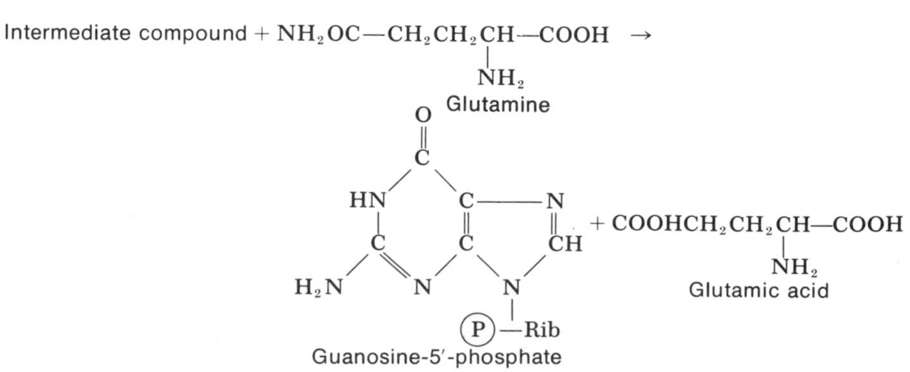

Guanosine-5′-phosphate can be hydrolyzed to form guanine (see page 195), phosphoric acid, and ribose.

CATABOLISM OF ADENINE AND GUANINE

Both adenine and guanine are converted to uric acid, which, in the human, is eliminated in the urine as a waste product. Most mammals (man, the apes, and the Dalmatian coach dog are exceptions) convert the uric acid to allantoin, which then is the final product excreted in the urine.

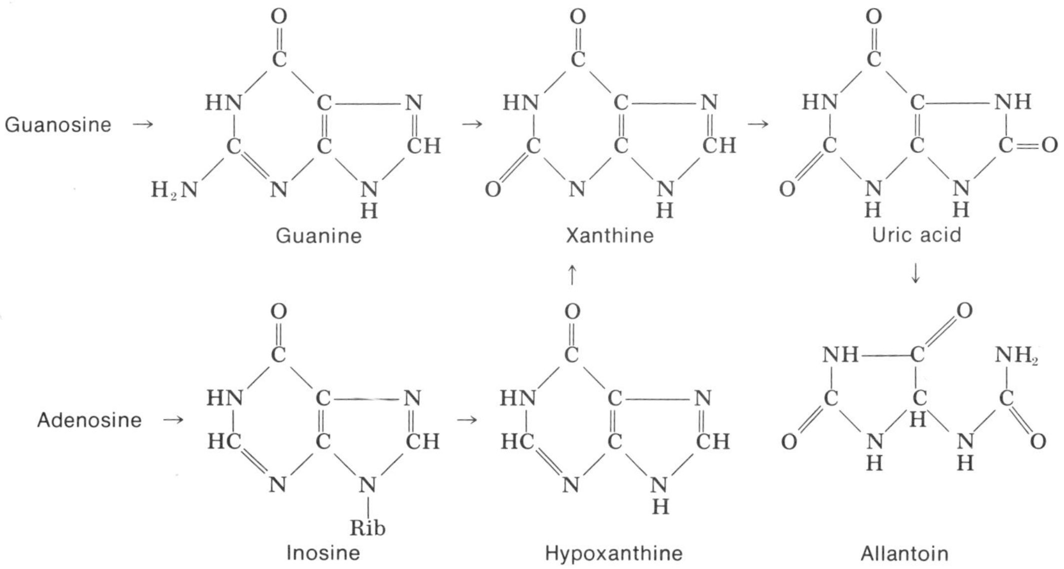

GOUT. Persons with the disease of enzymic defect (see page 215) known as *gout* produce excessive amounts of uric acid. In the early stages of the disease, deposits of sodium urate form, at intervals, in the cartilage around joints, and this causes an extremely painful, local red and swollen lesion. Cartoons would have us believe that the big toe is the joint involved, and often, but not always, this is true. As the disease progresses, a type of chronic arthritis (gouty arthritis) may develop, in which permanent deposits of sodium urate, known as tophi, form at various joints and interfere with motion.

Several drugs that increase the elimination of uric acid from the body have been developed. When patients with gout take one of these daily, often the acute attacks can be prevented, and, in some cases, the tophi of chronic gouty arthritis become smaller or disappear altogether.

Another drug, allopurinol, inhibits xanthine oxidase, the enzyme that catalyzes the formation of uric acid from xanthine. This drug thus inhibits the formation of uric acid in the body and is used in the management of patients with gout.

In some patients with gout there is a deficiency of the enzyme *hypoxanthine-guanine phosphoribosyltransferase* (HGPRT). This enzyme is involved in the synthesis of purines that are precursors of uric acid. This deficiency does not appear to be the only cause of gout, however.

LESCH-NYHAN SYNDROME. This is a disease of enzymic defect occurring in children in which the level of blood uric acid is elevated and there is a marked increase in the excretion of uric acid in the urine. Clinically, patients exhibit mental retardation, spastic cerebral palsy, choreoathetosis (irregular, continuous, slow involuntary movements of the muscles of the extremeties and the face), and aggressive, self-mutilating behavior. Only males have this disease, but it can be transmitted by the mother.

This disorder of children apparently is caused by a deficiency of an enzyme con-

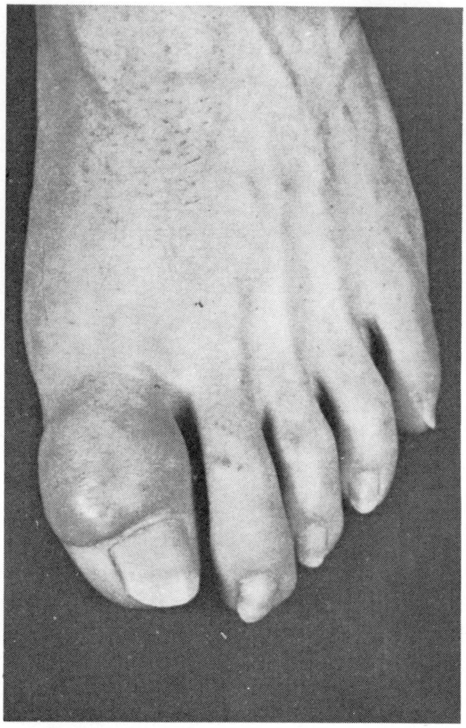

Fig. 27-11. Photograph of the big toe of a patient with an acute attack of gout. What body metabolite is connected with gout? (Courtesy Dr. John H. Talbott; from the Merck Sharp & Dohme Seminar.)

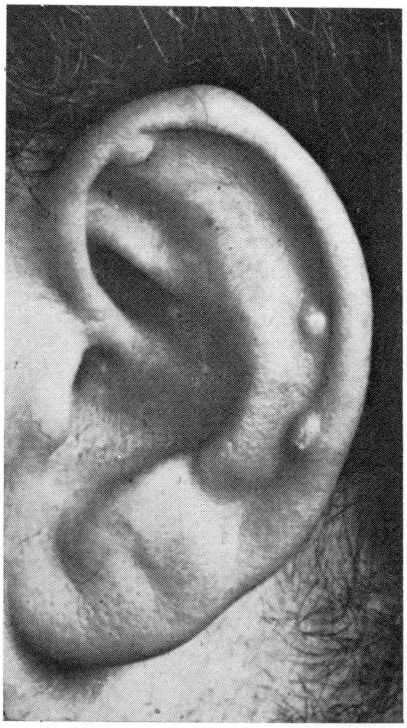

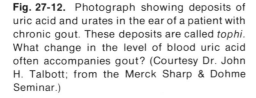

Fig. 27-12. Photograph showing deposits of uric acid and urates in the ear of a patient with chronic gout. These deposits are called *tophi*. What change in the level of blood uric acid often accompanies gout? (Courtesy Dr. John H. Talbott; from the Merck Sharp & Dohme Seminar.)

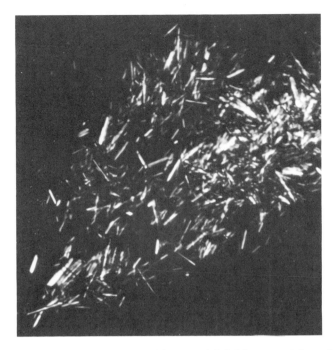

Fig. 27-13. Sodium urate crystals found in synovial fluid removed from the knee of a patient suffering from acute gout. Is gout a disease of enzymic defect? (From Good, A. E., and Frishette, W. A.: Crystals in dried smears of synovial fluid, J.A.M.A. **198:**80, 1966.)

cerned in purine metabolism known as *hypoxanthine-guanine phosphoribosyltransferase*. As already mentioned, this same deficiency may be involved in some cases of gout in adults.

ANABOLISM OF PYRIMIDINES

The synthesis of a pyrimidine nucleotide in the body can be illustrated as follows.

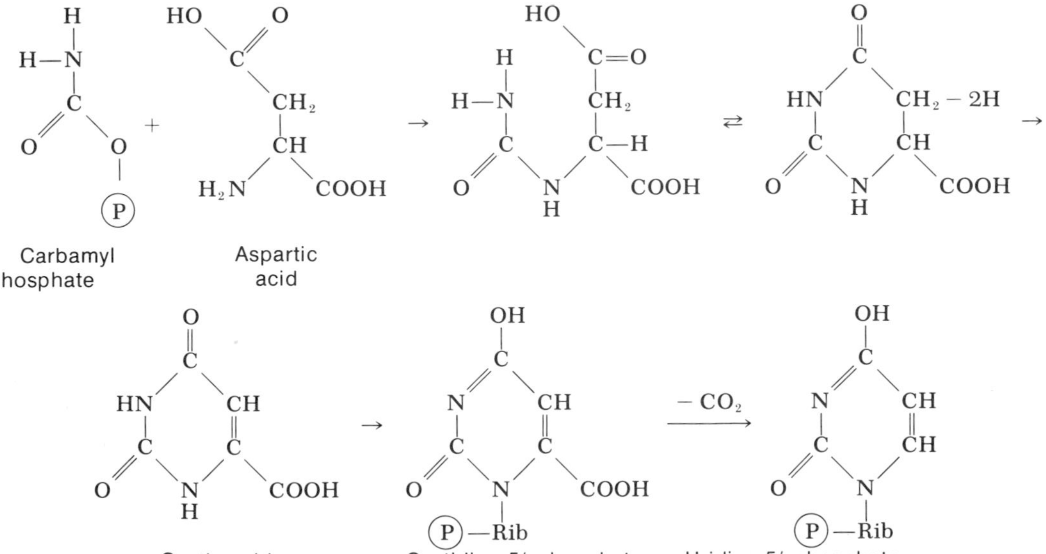

Carbamyl phosphate

Aspartic acid

Orotic acid

Orotidine-5′ phosphate

Uridine-5′-phosphate

Nucleotides containing cytosine and thymine are formed by a similar series of reactions.

CATABOLISM OF PYRIMIDINES The process of degradation of the pyrimidine nucleotides is almost the reverse of the synthetic reactions. Note, however, that the —COOH group that is lost when uridine-5′-phosphate is formed is not part of the resulting compounds, and so aspartic acid is not formed. Instead, β-alanine (which may be thought of as aspartic acid minus a —COOH group) is formed.

$$NH_2CHCH_2COOH$$
β-alanine

The resulting carbamyl phosphate and β-alanine can be converted to carbon dioxide, water, phosphate, and urea. The end products of pyrimidine catabolism, then, are CO_2, H_2O, and urea (see page 282).

STUDY QUESTIONS

1. What type of information is contained in the genetic code present in a fertilized egg?
2. From the point of view of the biochemist, what are chromosomes?
3. What is the chemical name of the substance abbreviated as DNA? As RNA?
4. How many chromosomes are present in a normal human cell?
5. Chemically speaking, what is a gene?
6. How many genes are estimated to be present in a virus particle? In a bacterial cell? In a human cell?
7. What are nucleic acids?
8. Name the types of compound formed when a nucleic acid molecule is hydrolyzed.
9. What type of nucleic acid is found only in the nucleus?
10. What are the specific products of hydrolysis of DNA? Of RNA?
11. Define nucleotide. Nucleoside.
12. What is the name of the nucleoside that contains adenine?
13. What is the name of the nucleotide that contains uracil?
14. Do nucleotides have any function apart from their importance as structural units of nucleic acids?
15. What is ATP?
16. Describe the DNA helix.
17. What type of chemical bond holds the strands of the DNA helix together? Describe this bond in your own words.
18. What molecules are paired in the DNA helix?
19. Explain how the DNA in a cell becomes doubled during cell division.
20. What is messenger RNA?
21. Where and how is messenger RNA synthesized?
22. Do messenger RNA molecules have large or small molecular weights?
23. How many amino acids are involved in the synthesis of proteins?
24. How many different codons are present in messenger RNA?
25. How many purine or pyrimidine bases are required to form one codon? One anticodon?
26. Describe the first experiment that led to the discovery of a code word for phenylalanine.
27. What is transfer RNA?
28. About how many bases are present in a single transfer RNA molecule?
29. How many different types of transfer RNA are there?
30. Explain how messenger RNA and transfer RNA interact in protein synthesis.
31. What are ribosomes?
32. What is the role of ribosomes in protein synthesis?
33. Define: genetic repressor; operator; inducer; corepressor. Explain in your own words how a repressor functions to prevent the manufacture of a specific enzyme.
34. What are viruses?
35. Do you think viruses should be classed as living organisms? Why?
36. How does a virus particle multiply?
37. What is interferon?
38. Name several substances that take part in the synthesis of a purine.
39. What is coenzyme F?
40. How is adenosine-5′-phosphate formed from inosinic acid?
41. What are the hydrolysis products of adenosine-5′-phosphate?
42. How is guanosine-5′-phosphate formed from inosinic acid?

43. What are the products of hydrolysis of guanosine-5′-phosphate?
44. What is the end product of purine catabolism in man?
45. What animals excrete allantoin instead of uric acid?
46. What is gout?
47. What amino acid is involved in the synthesis of uridine-5′-phosphate?
48. Why is β-alanine, rather than aspartic acid, formed during the catabolism of uridine-5′-phosphate?
49. What are the end products of purine catabolism?

CHAPTER **28**

Chemistry of the digestive tract

The digestive tract is a tube that passes through the body. In a technical sense materials in this tube are not inside the body at all. The various structures that make up this tract include the mouth, pharynx (throat), esophagus, stomach, small intestine, large intestine, rectum, and anus. It is a function of the digestive tract to convert the food to substances that can pass from the small intestine into the body proper, where they undergo the various changes we have already discussed.

TEETH The cavity (central portion) of a tooth is called the *pulp cavity*, and it contains the blood vessels and nerves of the tooth. The main body of the tooth is made of a substance resembling bone, called *dentin*. Outside of the dentin and above the gums is the familiar white *enamel*. Below the gum line the dentin is surrounded by a material called *cement*. Both dentin and enamel are chemically very similar to bone. They are made of hard inorganic material embedded in a protein matrix. It is estimated that one-fourth of the weight of these materials is protein. The other three-fourths is a mixture of inorganic compounds. These compounds are similar to the minerals known as fluorapatite, chlorapatite, and dahllite. Small amounts of magnesium phosphate, iron oxide, and sodium salts are also present.

$CaF_2[Ca_3(PO_4)_2]_3$	$CaCl_2[Ca_3(PO_4)_2]_3$	$CaCO_3[Ca_3(PO_4)_2]_3$
Fluorapatite	Chlorapatite	Dahllite

Enamel contains much less protein than do dentin and cement and is the hardest material found in the body. It also contains more fluorine; it is estimated that about 20 percent of the weight of enamel is due to the presence of material resembling fluorapatite.

The hardness of enamel is correlated, up to a certain point, with the amount of fluorine present. If insufficient fluorine is present, the enamel is too soft. However, excessive amounts of fluorides in drinking water cause a large increase in the fluorine content of the enamel and this

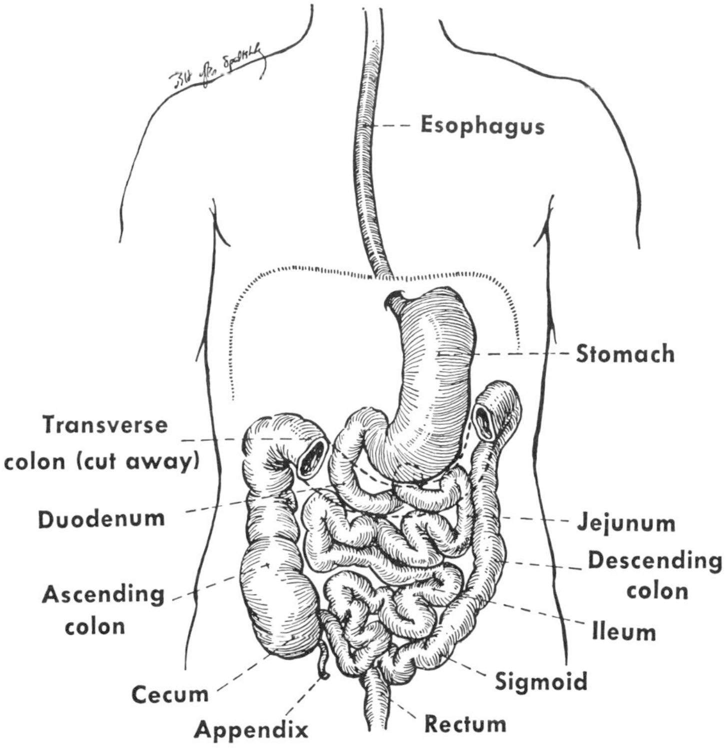

Fig. 28-1. The digestive tract. What is the purpose of digestion?

results in the condition known as *mottled enamel (mottled teeth)*. In this condition the enamel prisms (small particles of which enamel is composed) do not lie close enough together and even have a tendency to fall apart. Mottled enamel is therefore brittle. Instead of the glistening white of normal enamel, mottled enamel has a flat, chalky appearance. It is readily stained by pigments in the diet.

Shortly after the teeth are cleaned by brushing, deposition of a material known as *plaque* begins on the surfaces of the teeth. It is formed by the growth of bacteria that produce filamentous strands. It causes the "furry" feel to the tongue that is familiar to everybody. Probably dextrans (see page 249) made by bacteria from sucrose act as the "glue" that causes the plaque to adhere firmly to the surfaces of the teeth.

The immediate cause of *dental caries (decayed teeth)* is the local production of acid from sugar, especially sucrose, by bacteria. The microorganisms responsible for this grow well in plaque, and it is important to remove them by brushing the teeth frequently, especially after eating.

There is a growing opinion that the plaque and the bacteria growing in it in older people are different from the plaque and bacteria found in childhood and early adult life. Caries are much more common in the latter age group. On the other hand, periodontal disease, which is the major cause of the loss of teeth, occurs much more commonly in older age groups.

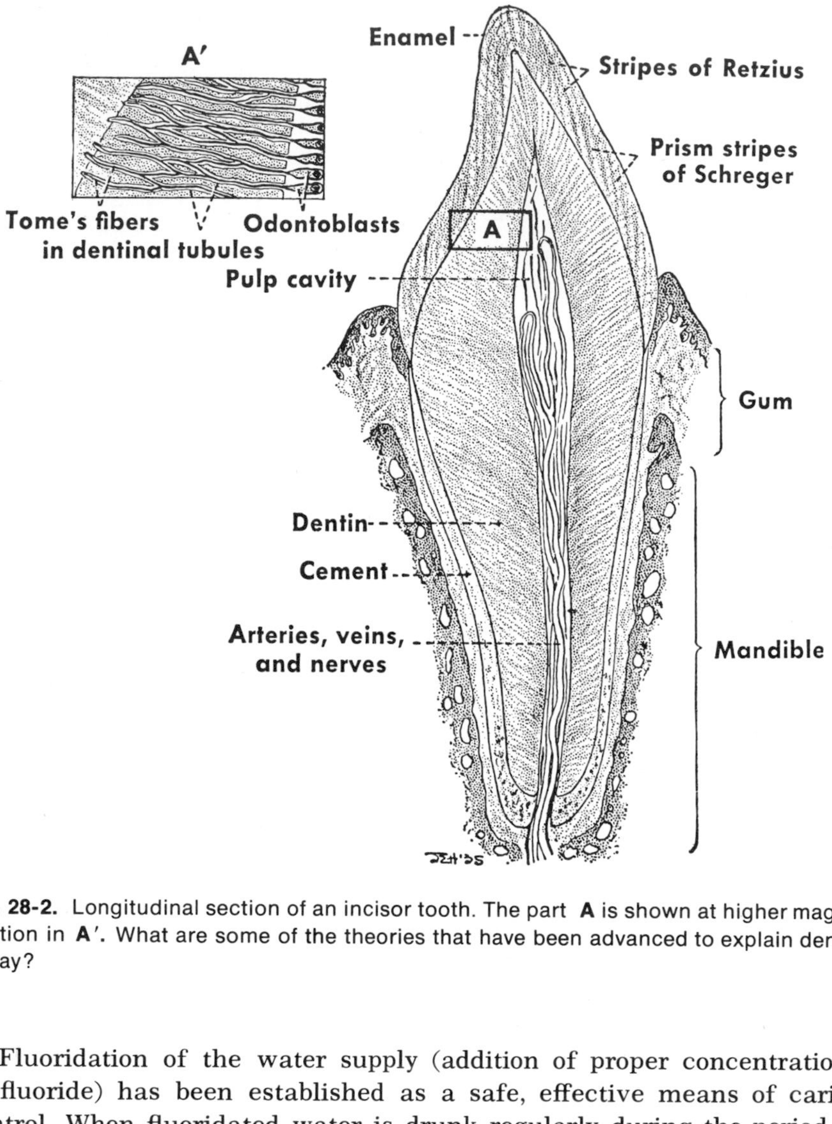

Fig. 28-2. Longitudinal section of an incisor tooth. The part **A** is shown at higher magnification in **A′**. What are some of the theories that have been advanced to explain dental decay?

CARIES CONTROL BY FLUORIDATION

Fluoridation of the water supply (addition of proper concentrations of fluoride) has been established as a safe, effective means of caries control. When fluoridated water is drunk regularly during the period in which teeth are developing, the reduction in amount of caries in later life may amount to as much as 60 percent. The amount of fluoride added to the drinking water for this purpose varies from about 0.7 parts per million (ppm) in hot climates to about 1.2 ppm in cooler climates.

Fluorine is deposited in the teeth as fluorapatite. This type of apatite is resistant to the attack of acid that forms in the dental plaque as a result of bacterial metabolism. This probably explains its effectiveness in reducing the incidence of caries.

PLAQUE AND CALCULUS. If plaque is not removed by regular cleaning, calcium apatite forms in the filamentous network and results in the deposition of a hard material, known as calculus, or tartar, on the teeth. If this extends down between the gums and the teeth, it may result in periodontal disease. Also, bacteria that

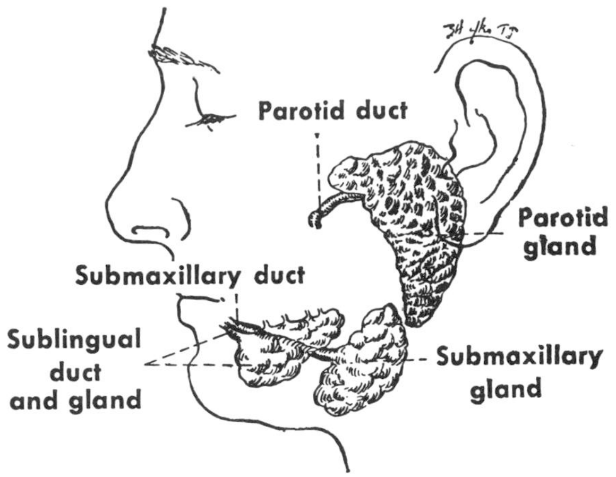

Fig. 28-3. The salivary glands. What is the most important enzyme found in saliva?

produce acid, and which probably are the immediate cause of caries, can grow in plaque.

PERIODONTAL DISEASE. This term is used to describe several diseases of the tissues surrounding the teeth. In some cases it exists as a simple gingivitis, or inflammation of the gums. In more serious disease pus pockets may form deep around the roots of the teeth. Finally, there may be atrophy (wasting away) of the bony socket, so that the teeth become loose. Periodontal disease, most common in older people, is the usual cause of loss of teeth. Many unproved theories have been advanced to account for this disease. Regardless of what the true cause may be, dentists agree that regular removal of calculus can prevent it in the great majority of cases.

SALIVA

Saliva is a fluid secreted into the mouth cavity by the various salivary glands. It is more than 99 percent water. It contains various inorganic salts, a small amount of urea, mucin (a glycoprotein), and enzymes.

Ptyalin is a term that refers to the salivary enzymes concerned with the digestion of starch: *salivary amylase,* which catalyzes the hydrolysis of starch to dextrins and, finally, to maltose; and *salivary maltase,* which catalyzes maltose hydrolysis, with the production of glucose. However, digestion in the mouth is not of much importance. The pH of saliva is about 6.8 to 7.2, and its enzymes work best at this pH. The food placed in the mouth is soon swallowed, and when it becomes mixed with the acid gastric juice, the salivary enzymes cease to be effective.

Traces of enzymes that catalyze the digestion of proteins and fats are also present in saliva. It seems likely that the salivary enzymes are of importance only because they may digest food particles lodged between the teeth. Such particles, if not removed, serve as media in which harmful bacteria can grow and multiply.

It is the function of saliva to moisten the mouth and food and to lubricate the food so that it can be swallowed more easily. The lubricating properties of saliva are due to the presence of mucin.

GASTRIC JUICE

Gastric juice is the fluid secreted by the glands of the stomach. Its secretion is caused by the sight, smell, or even the thought of appetizing foods. A substance (hormone) called *gastrin* is made by the pyloric end (near where the stomach joins the small intestine) of the stomach. Gastrin causes a flow of gastric juice and an increased motility of the stomach. Gastrin also causes the pancreas to secrete pancreatic juice, probably by stimulating the vagus nerve.

It has been possible to isolate two peptides from hog stomach mucosa that have the activity of gastrin. They have been named gastrin I and gastrin II. The structure of gastrin II is

$$\text{Glu–Gly–Pro–Try–Met–(Glu)}_5\text{–Ala–}\underset{}{\overset{\displaystyle SO_3H \atop |}{\text{Try}}}\text{–Gly–Try–Met–Asp–Phe–NH}_2$$

Surprisingly, it has been found that a peptide containing only the last four amino acids has one-fifth the activity of gastrin itself. Even more startling, perhaps, is the finding that the addition of a fifth amino acid to the tetrapeptide (that is, peptide consisting of four amino acid residues) gives a pentapeptide that has activity equal to gastrin.

Pepsinogen is a proenzyme secreted in the gastric juice. It reacts with the hydrochloric acid of the gastric juice to form the active enzyme *pepsin*. Pepsin catalyzes the hydrolysis of proteins with the formation of *proteoses* and *peptones*. Pepsin has the ability to make proteins, particularly casein, insoluble. Both pepsinogen and pepsin have been isolated in pure crystalline form.

Pepsinogen has a molecular weight of 43,000. Below pH 5 it splits to form pepsin (molecular weight 36,000), 5 small peptides, and a polypeptide capable of inhibiting the activity of pepsin (pepsin inhibitor). The pepsin molecule has only 4 basic amino acid residues and 36 amino acid residues with free acid groups (groups capable of yielding hydrogen ions in water). This unusual distribution of acid and basic residues accounts for its stability even at pH 1; it is denatured above pH 6. Pepsin has a broader specificity (will split more different peptide bonds) than any other protease (enzyme catalyzing the hydrolysis of the peptide bonds of proteins).

A second protease, *gastricsin,* also is present in gastric juice.

Gastric juice also contains *lipase,* a fat-splitting enzyme. It is not certain whether this enzyme is secreted with the gastric juice or whether it is regurgitated into the stomach from the small intestine. At any rate, gastric lipase is not of much importance in the digestion of fats. The stomach does not contain any mechanism or substance that will emulsify fats, and, as we shall see, fats that are not emulsified are not easily digested. Fats already emulsified before they are eaten are partly hydrolyzed to *fatty acids* and *glycerol* in the presence of gastric lipase. For example, the emulsified fats of egg yolk and milk are partly digested in the stomach.

Hydrochloric acid is a normal component of gastric juice and is present to the extent of about 0.4 percent. This amount of hydrochloric acid gives the gastric juice a pH of about 1.0 when it is freshly secreted. Alkalies in the food, however, may raise the pH as high as pH 3 or 4. Hydrochloric acid assists in denaturing food proteins and probably kills many of the bacteria swallowed with the food.

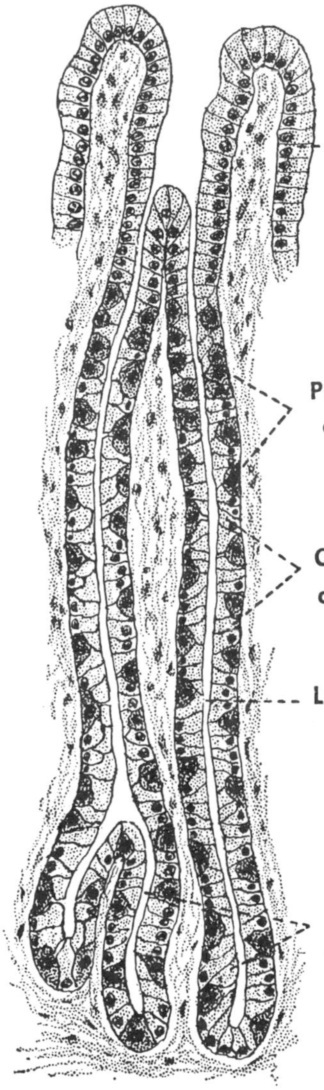

Fig. 28-4. A microscopic section of the lining of the stomach to show the gastric (stomach) glands. Hydrochloric acid is secreted by the parietal cells, and pepsinogen is secreted by the chief cells. What converts inactive pepsinogen to active pepsin?

It is estimated that hydrochloric acid is absent in about 5 percent of normal young and middle-aged people. The amount of hydrochloric acid in gastric juice is zero in pernicious anemia, and it is usually decreased in cancer of the stomach and in old age. Cancer of the stomach sometimes obstructs the passage of food into the intestine. Because the amount of hydrochloric acid is low or absent in this condition, certain bacteria are able to grow in the stomach contents. These bacteria catalyze the formation of lactic acid from the lactose in the food. If it is found that the stomach empties slowly, that the hydrochloric acid content is low or absent, and that relatively large quantities of lactic acid are present, cancer of the stomach should be suspected.

The stomach manufactures a substance called the *intrinsic factor* that is necessary for the proper absorption of vitamin B_{12} (see page 430). If the stomach lining (mucosa) shrinks and ceases to function, the vitamin B_{12} present in the diet is not well absorbed, and the disease called *pernicious anemia* results. Hydrochloric acid is not present in the stomach in this condition because the cells that make it are in the nonfunctional stomach lining. Pernicious anemia is treated with vitamin B_{12} or with liver extracts that contain it.

Hypochlorhydria is a term used to indicate an abnormally low concentration of hydrochloric acid in gastric juice. *Achlorhydria* refers to a complete absence of hydrochloric acid from this fluid.

Hyperchlorhydria means an increase in the hydrochloric acid content of the stomach. It is commonly present in acute gastritis (inflammation of the stomach lining) and in cases of duodenal ulcer. Hyperchlorhydria usually does not accompany gastric ulcer, an area in the stomach in which the lining has been destroyed, leaving the underlying tissues exposed. Highly nervous or emotional individuals may have hyperchlorhydria.

Rennin is an enzyme found in the stomach of the calf and of the kid. It catalyzes the change of casein, the principal protein of cow's milk, to paracasein. In the presence of calcium salts calcium paracaseinate is then formed. This substance is insoluble and precipitates. Crude extracts of calf stomach containing rennin are known as rennet. Dietitians often employ rennet in preparing milk foods and custards.

Many textbooks state that rennin occurs in the stomach of human beings. However, there is no convincing evidence for this statement, and, indeed, there is considerable evidence to the contrary. Human gastric juice will clot milk, as do extracts containing rennin, but this clotting appears to be caused by the pepsin present in the juice.

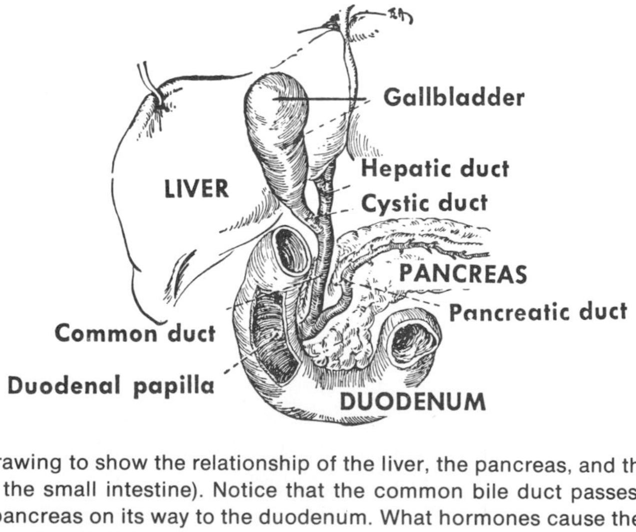

Fig. 28-5. Drawing to show the relationship of the liver, the pancreas, and the duodenum (first part of the small intestine). Notice that the common bile duct passes through the head of the pancreas on its way to the duodenum. What hormones cause the pancreas to secrete its digestive fluid?

SECRETIN AND CHOLECYSTOKININ-PANCREOZYMIN

Prosecretin is a substance manufactured by the cells of the duodenum (first portion of the small intestine). When food passes from the stomach into the duodenum, some hydrochloric acid is carried with it. This acid reacts with prosecretin to form *secretin,* a hormone. Secretin enters the bloodstream, which takes it to the pancreas. It is interesting that secretin was one of the first hormones to be discovered. W. M. Bayliss and E. H. Starling announced its discovery in 1902. Epinephrine, another hormone, had been isolated in 1901.

Secretin causes mainly the secretion of bicarbonate and water from the pancreas. A second substance, *cholecystokinin-pancreozymin,* stimulates the secretion of the pancreatic digestive enzymes. It is released from the duodenal mucosa after the duodenal mucosa has been exposed to protein, fat, and carbohydrate.

PANCREATIC JUICE

It is estimated that 500 to 800 ml of pancreatic juice are secreted into the duodenum each day. This fluid is slightly alkaline since it contains sodium bicarbonate. It will be remembered that sodium bicarbonate hydrolyzes slightly in water to form small quantities of the *strong base* sodium hydroxide and the *weak acid* carbonic acid. Since sodium hydroxide ionizes almost completely and carbonic acid ionizes only very slightly, sodium bicarbonate solutions are slightly alkaline.

$$\begin{array}{ccc} NaHCO_3 + H_2O & \rightleftarrows & NaOH + H_2CO_3 \\ & & \downarrow\uparrow \\ & & Na^+ + OH^- \end{array}$$

Pancreatic juice contains several important enzymes and proenzymes. *Trypsinogen* is a proenzyme in pancreatic juice. It reacts with *enterokinase,* a substance produced in the duodenum, to form active *trypsin.* Trypsin catalyzes the hydrolysis of proteins, proteoses, and peptones to form *polypeptides.* About one-seventh of the total protein in pancreatic juice is trypsin. It only catalyzes the hydrolysis of peptide bonds in which the amino acid contributing the —CO— group is lysine or arginine.

Chymotrypsinogens A and B occur in pancreatic juice. Chymotrypsinogen A has been investigated thoroughly. It has a molecular weight of 25,000 and an isoelectric point near pH 9.1. It is composed of a single polypeptide chain.

Both trypsin and chymotrypsin catalyze the formation of a family of chymotrypsins from the chymotrypsinogens. They account for about 32 percent of the total proteolytic (protein-digesting) activity of bovine (cow) pancreatic juice. α-Chymotrypsin, derived from chymotrypsinogen A, has been widely studied. Its molecule is composed of 3 peptide chains linked together by —S—S— bridges. The chymotrypsins catalyze the formation of polypeptides from proteoses, peptones, and proteins.

Carboxypeptidases A and B together constitute about 26 percent of the total proteolytic activity of pancreatic juice. They are formed in the intestine from zymogens (active enzyme precursors) present in pancreatic juice. They catalyze the hydrolysis of peptides to amino acids. Amino acids and soluble peptides are the end products of protein digestion. They are absorbed directly into the bloodstream.

Pancreatic amylase (amylopsin) catalyzes the formation of *maltose* from *starch*. *Maltase, lactase,* and *sucrase (invertase)* are enzymes that act as catalysts for the hydrolysis of the disaccharides maltose, lactose, and sucrose. These sugars are absorbed intact into the intestinal cells, and digestion occurs either within, or on the surface of, these cells. Maltose yields glucose; lactose yields galactose and glucose; and sucrose yields fructose and glucose. The end products of carbohydrate digestion, then, are *glucose, galactose,* and *fructose*. These monosaccharides are absorbed directly into the bloodstream and undergo the various reactions in the tissues described in Chapter 24.

Sucrase can catalyze the hydrolysis of both sucrose and maltose.

Fats cannot be digested efficiently unless they are emulsified. The digestive enzymes will dissolve in water but not in fat. The enzymes can only catalyze fat hydrolysis at the *surface* of a fat drop, where the water in which they are dissolved touches the fat. The amount of surface can be increased by breaking large fat drops up into small ones. A fat drop, for example, that has a diameter of 10 mm has a surface of 314 sq mm. If we divide this drop into drops that have diameters of 1 mm, the area of each drop will be smaller, *but the total surface area of all the drops will be 3,140 sq mm*. In other words, we have increased the surface at which digestion can take place by ten times. Emulsions contain very small drops of fat suspended in water, and digestion of fat in this form is much more rapid than digestion of large particles of fat.

Fats in the intestinal tract are emulsified by *bile*. They are then digested (hydrolyzed) in the presence of *pancreatic lipase (steapsin)*, yielding *fatty acids, glycerol,* and *monoglycerides* (compounds whose molecules yield 1 molecule of glycerol and 1 molecule of fatty acid on hydrolysis) as end products.* The glycerol is water soluble and is absorbed directly into the cells lining the intestine and into the bloodstream. The fatty acids and monoglycerides become incorporated into submicroscopic droplets known as *micelles*. They are about 40 to 100 angstroms in diameter (1 cm = 1,000,000 angstroms), and are water clear. Bile acids (see page 289) surround them. One portion of the bile salt molecule is water insoluble and is directed inward. The other part is water soluble and is directed outward. As the micelle approaches the villi (see Fig. 28-7), the bile salts are dropped off and the fatty acids and monoglycerides are absorbed into the villi by direct diffusion. This absorption occurs in the upper part of the small intestine. Most of the liberated bile salts are absorbed in the lower part of the small bowel.

The intestinal cells convert the absorbed glycerol, fatty acids, and monoglycerides into fats. This fat is incorporated into *chylomicrons*. These droplets have a core of fat (triglyceride), cholesterol, and cholesterol esters. The outside layers of the chylomicron consist of phosphatides, especially

*Under some circumstances fats can be absorbed directly without undergoing hydrolysis (see page 228).

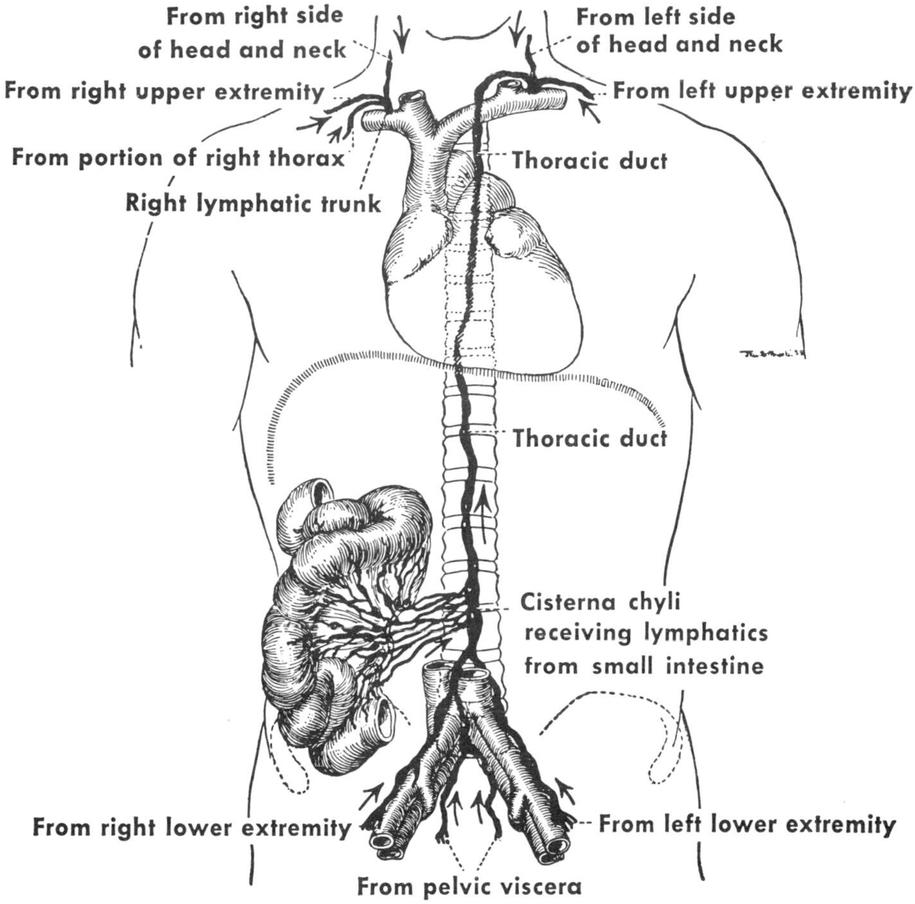

Fig. 28-6. Diagram to show the circulation of the lymph. How does lymph from the intestine reach the bloodstream?

phosphatidyl choline (lecithin). Small amounts of free cholesterol and protein also are present in this envelope.

Following a meal, chylomicrons pass into the lacteals (lymph vessels of the intestine). The lymph vessels take them to the bloodstream, which distributes them to the various tissues of the body.

Food contains both free cholesterol and cholesterol esters. Hydrolysis of cholesterol esters to cholesterol and fatty acids is catalyzed by the pancreatic enzyme *cholesterol esterase*. Free cholesterol, together with bile acids, monoglycerides, and fatty acids, is solubilized in microscopic droplets (micelles), which then are absorbed into the intestinal cells. In man, less than 10 percent of the cholesterol fed is absorbed. The remainder is excreted in the stool as such or as other sterols, mainly coprosterol, made from cholesterol by intestinal bacteria.

Phospholipids, in part at least, are absorbed without hydrolysis.

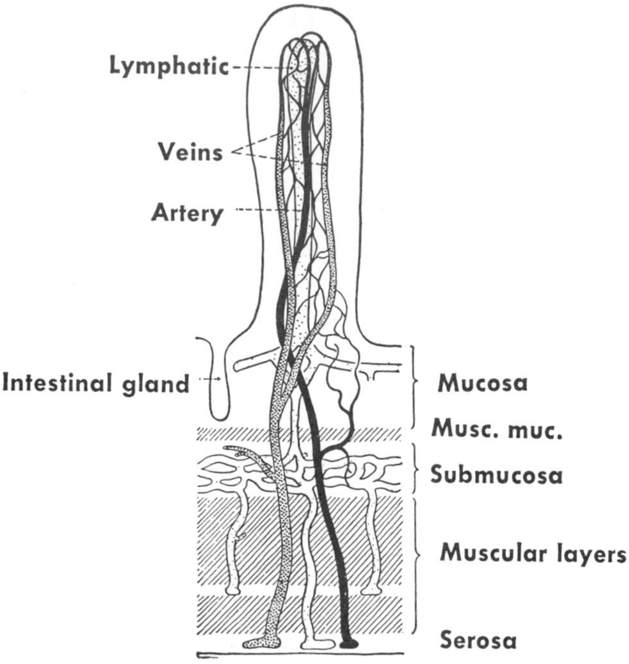

Fig. 28-7. One of the intestinal villi showing the mechanism for the absorption of digested foods. A villus is a minute, club-shaped structure that projects from the mucous membrane that lines the intestine. The artery is black, the vein is heavily stippled, and the lymphatic vessel (lacteal) is lightly stippled. What foods are absorbed into the bloodstream after digestion? Into the lacteals after digestion?

BILE The bile is manufactured in the liver and is then stored for a time in the gallbladder, in which organ it becomes concentrated by a loss of water to the bloodstream. When fat enters the small intestine, a substance (hormone) called *cholecystokinin-pancreozymin*, made by the small intestine, enters the bloodstream. The cholecystokinin portion of the molecule causes contraction of the gallbladder. This forces the stored bile to enter the duodenum. The pancreozymin part of the molecule stimulates pancreatic secretion.

Bile is a yellow-brown or green liquid with an alkaline reaction and an intensely bitter taste. During the time that the bile is stored in the gallbladder, sodium bicarbonate diffuses back into the blood, and the pH decreases to a value between 5.5 and 7. Bile contains *no* digestive enzymes but, as we have seen, it is nevertheless important in the digestion of fats and in the absorption of fatty acids. Several substances, including cholesterol and bile pigments, are excreted in the bile.

The bile salts are responsible for the emulsifying power of bile. The chief bile salts are *sodium glycocholate* and *sodium taurocholate*. These substances lower surface tension to a remarkable degree and are excellent emulsifying agents (see page 61). Bile salts are unable to enter the duodenum at a normal rate in obstructive jaundice and are found in the urine in this condition. Urine containing bile salts can be recognized by its unusually low surface tension. If a small amount of powdered sulfur is sprinkled carefully on the surface of normal urine, the surface tension is high enough so that the sulfur does not sink. If bile salts are present, the surface tension is abnormally low and sulfur sinks at once (Hay's test).

Bilirubin is the chief bile pigment. As we have seen, biliverdin and bilicyanin are formed by its oxidation. Mesobilirubinogen and urobilin are produced from bilirubin by the action of intestinal bacteria (see page 287).

Cholesterol (see pages 227 and 236) is excreted from the body by way of the bile. Hard precipitates, known as gallstones, sometimes form in the gallbladder. They are usually composed mainly of cholesterol, with variable amounts of bilirubin, calcium salts and other inorganic materials.

INTESTINAL JUICE

Intestinal juice, also known as *succus entericus,* is secreted by the cells of the small intestine. It has been said that a substance known as *enterocrinin* (supposedly made in the intestine) stimulates the secretion of this fluid. The intestinal juice is alkaline because of its content of sodium bicarbonate. However the upper portions of the intestinal tract are ordinarily slightly acid (pH 6.8) because of the strong hydrochloric acid that enters with the chyme (material from the stomach).

Intestinal juice, contains a mixture of peptidases (erepsin), *maltase, sucrase,* and *lactase.* Various enzymes concerned with the digestion of nucleic acid are also present. These enzymes are listed in Table 28-1.

LACTASE DEFICIENCY. Patients with this disease of enzymic defect have a deficiency of the enzyme lactase and thus do not digest lactose completely. Lactose is poorly absorbed and its osmotic activity within the intestinal tract causes a large influx of water, leading to cramps and diarrhea. When the lactose reaches the lower intestinal tract, bacteria act on it to form CO_2 and organic acids that cause distention and increase the diarrhea. Most patients with this disease cannot tolerate more than one glass of milk per day. (Lactose is the sugar present in milk.) The disease is most common in Negroes, but the incidence in white people also is high.

The *lactose tolerance test* can be used as an aid to diagnosis. The patient swallows 50 g per square meter of body surface area of lactose dissolved in 400 ml of water.* (One quart of milk contains approximately 50 g of lactose.) Blood samples are taken at 0, 20, 30, 60, 90, and 120 minutes. A rise of the level of blood glucose (a digestive product of lactose) that is less than 25 mg per 100 ml at all of these time periods suggests that the patient has lactase deficiency. This diagnosis is strengthened if the patient exhibits clinical signs of lactase deficiency after swallowing the lactose. The test is not perfect since some patients who show no signs or symptoms after ingesting large volumes of milk also exhibit a "flat" lactose tolerance test.

GLUTEN ENTEROPATHY. This disease has been known in the past as nontropical sprue, celiac disease, ideopathic steatorrhea, and malabsorption syndrome. It is characterized by faulty intestinal absorption resulting from inflammation and atrophy of the intestinal villi. Usually it is observed in childhood but it may appear for the first time in adult life.

The changes in the villi are caused by *gliadin,* a prolamin (see page 269) present in the protein mixture known as gluten. Gluten (and hence gliadin) occurs in wheat,

*A patient who is 5 feet 3 inches tall and who weighs 115 pounds has a body surface area of 1.5 square meters. See Fig. 34-1 on page 450.

Table 28-1. Enzymes concerned with the digestion of nucleic acid

Enzymes	Substrate	End products*
Polynucleotidases (nucleinases)	Nucleic acid	Nucleotides
Nucleophosphatases (nucleotidases)	Nucleotides	Phosphoric acid, H_3PO_4 Nucleosides
Nucleosidases	Nucleosides	Pentoses Purines Pyrimidines

*Final products of nucleic acid digestion = phosphoric acid, pentoses, purines, and pyrimidines.

Table 28-2. The digestive enzymes

Enzymes	Substrates	End products
Saliva:		
Salivary amylase	Starch	Dextrins, maltose
Salivary maltase	Maltose	Glucose
Gastric juice:		
Pepsin	Proteins	Proteoses, peptones
Gastric lipase	Emulsified fats	Fatty acids, glycerol
Pancreatic juice:		
Trypsin	Proteins, proteoses, peptones	Polypeptides
Chymotrypsin	Proteins, proteoses, peptones	Polypeptides
Pancreatic amylase (amylopsin)	Starch	Dextrins, maltose
Pancreatic maltase	Maltose	Glucose
Pancreatic sucrase (invertase)	Sucrose	Glucose, fructose
Pancreatic lactase	Lactose	Glucose, galactose
Pancreatic lipase (steapsin)	Fats	Fatty acids, glycerol
Pancreatic polypeptidases	Polypeptides	Peptides, amino acids
Cholesterol esterase	Cholesterol esters	Cholesterol, fatty acids
Intestinal juice:		
Intestinal polypeptidases	Polypeptides	Amino acids
Intestinal maltase	Maltose	Glucose
Intestinal sucrase (invertase)	Sucrose	Glucose, fructose
Intestinal lactase	Lactose	Glucose, galactose
Polynucleotidases (nucleinases)	Nucleic acid	Nucleotides
Nucleophosphatases (nucleotidases)	Nucleotides	Phosphoric acid, nucleosides
Nucleosidases	Nucleosides	Pentoses, purines, pyrimidines

barley, oats, and rye. The probable immediate cause of the disease is a lack of a pepdidase in the intestinal mucosal cells that hydrolyzes gliadin. Gluten enteropathy thus is a disease of enzymic defect.

The disorder is characterized by poor absorption of the products of digestion of fats, carbohydrates, and proteins. There is also malabsorption of vitamin D and calcium (see page 438), vitamin K (see page 443); folic acid and iron (see page 432), and fluid and electrolytes.

The malabsorption of fats and the products of fat digestion usually causes steatorrhea (fatty, foul-smelling, abundant stools), diarrhea, and weight loss. Failure to absorb vitamin D and calcium may result in hypocalcemia (low level of calcium in the plasma; see page 338 and, occasionally, tetany (intermittent muscular contractions accompanied by pain). If this condition is long-lasting, osteomalacia (see page 440) accompanied by pains in the bones and susceptibility to fractures may result.

When vitamin K is malabsorbed, a bleeding tendency may develop. This causes hematuria (blood in the urine).

Failure to absorb folic acid and iron may cause iron deficiency anemia and macrocytic anemia (red cells deficient in number but larger than normal).

Patients usually are free of symptoms and signs of the disease if they do not eat foods containing gliadin.

ENTEROGASTRONE

A substance called *enterogastrone* is secreted by the intestinal cells in the presence of fats and sugars. This substance inhibits the secretion of gastric juice and stops contractions of the stomach, which are our "hunger pangs." It is common experience that sweets "ruin the appetite" and abolish the sensation of hunger. It has been suggested that the presence of the sugar in the sweets causes a secretion of enterogastrone, which allays the sensation of hunger by preventing contractions of the stomach muscles.

BACTERIAL ACTION IN THE INTESTINE

Large numbers of bacteria live and reproduce in the lower intestinal tract. They live on the materials of the diet that escape digestion. *Ptomaines* (review Amines in Chapter 17) are formed from amino acids in the presence of the intestinal bacteria. Carbon dioxide gas is also produced by this reaction.

$$\underset{\substack{\text{Alanine}\\\text{(Amino acid)}}}{CH_3CHNH_2COOH} \rightarrow \underset{\substack{\text{Ethyl amine}\\\text{(Ptomaine)}}}{CH_3CH_2NH_2} + \underset{\substack{\text{Carbon}\\\text{dioxide}}}{CO_2}$$

Some common ptomaines include tyramine (from tyrosine), histamine (from histidine), cadaverine (from lysine), and putrescine (from arginine). Hydrogen sulfide (H_2S) and small amounts of methane (CH_4) are also produced from amino acids by bacterial action.

Another group of bacteria form lactic and acetic acids from carbohydrates. Indigestible carbohydrates, such as cellulose, agar, pectins, and gum arabic (acacia), form the bulk of the bacterial carbohydrate food, but any digestible carbohydrates that reach the lower intestine are also changed partly to organic acids. Some gases, particularly methane, are produced along with the acids. The acids stimulate the intestinal musculature and probably are responsible for most of the laxative action of cereals, agar, psyllium seed, and similar carbohydrate materials.

FECES

Between one-half and one-fourth of the dry material of the feces is composed of dead and living bacteria. Indigestible material from the diet, such as cellulose and scleroproteins, mucin, waste materials from the intestinal cells, and calcium and magnesium soaps, are also present. *Coprosterol* is a sterol excreted in the feces; it is made from cholesterol in the intestinal tract. The color of normal feces is from *urobilin* and *stercobilin,* pigments derived from bilirubin. The odor of feces is mainly from *skatole* and *indole,* two substances produced by the action of bacteria on the amino acid tryptophan.

Abnormal colors of the feces are sometimes significant in pathological conditions:

1. Green-colored stools usually indicate that the food has passed through the

intestinal tract so rapidly that the normal pigments have not been formed. The green color is from biliverdin. Certain drugs may also impart a green color to feces.

2. Clay-colored or acholic ("no bile") stools mean that bile is prevented from entering the intestinal tract. This color is characteristic of obstructive jaundice.
3. Bloody stools indicate bleeding in the lower intestinal tract. They are present in hemorrhoids (piles), cancer of the rectum, rectal polyps (small tumors attached to the lining of the rectum), dysentery, and ulcerative types of colitis (inflammation of the colon, or large intestine).
4. Black, or "tarry," stools frequently indicate bleeding high up in the intestinal tract. The color is from methemoglobin, formed from hemoglobin by oxidation in the intestine. This type of stool is found in bleeding from the mouth and lungs (if coughed up blood is swallowed) in some cases, but is more common if gastric ulcer, duodenal ulcer, or cancer of the stomach is present. Certain drugs, particularly those containing iron, may also cause tarry stools.

Some samples of feces contain amounts of blood too small to be detected by direct observation. This blood may be from blood in the diet or from bleeding in the intestinal tract. It is called occult ("hidden") blood. It can be detected with the benzidine test (see page 208) or with a modification of this test in which an alcoholic solution of gum guaiac is used instead of benzidine (guaiac test).

Urobilinogen* is present in increased amounts in hemolytic jaundice. Its excretion is diminished in obstructive jaundice. An excretion of less than 5 mg per day is almost certain evidence that a cancer is present in the neighborhood of the bile duct, usually in the head of the pancreas. Apparently this is almost the only type of obstruction that can prevent *completely* the entrance of bile into the duodenum.

*The urobilinogen determined clinically is really made up of mesobilirubinogen, urobilin, stercobilinogen, and stercobilin.

STUDY QUESTIONS

1. Why do we say that materials in the digestive tract are not really in the body?
2. What is the function of the digestive tract?
3. What elements make up the inorganic phase of dentin and enamel? Do dentin and enamel contain protein?
4. What is the hardest material found in the body?
5. How does the composition of enamel differ from that of dentin?
6. What effect does fluorine have on the hardnes of enamel? What condition is caused by an excess of fluorine in the drinking water?
7. Is fluoridation of drinking water useful? Explain.
8. What is dental plaque?
9. What is calculus?
10. Discuss periodontal disease.
11. Name four possible causes of dental caries (decayed teeth). Why does a pregnant woman require an extra amount of calcium and phosphorus in her diet?
12. Does brushing the teeth *prevent* tooth decay? Explain your answer. Why is mouth cleanliness important?
13. Name the substrates and end products for salivary amylase and salivary maltase. What is ptyalin?
14. In what way is salivary digestion important?
15. What is mucin?
16. What compound is present in greatest abundance in saliva?
17. Name some functions of saliva.
18. What factors cause a secretion of gastric juice? What is gastrin?
19. What is rennin? Rennet?
20. What is pepsinogen? How is it converted to pepsin? Name the substrate and end products for pepsin.
21. How important is gastric lipase?
22. How much HCl is present in 100 ml of gastric juice, on the average? What is the pH of freshly secreted gastric juice? How is this pH altered by the entrance of food into the stomach?
23. Name three functions of HCl in gastric juice.
24. In what conditions does achlorhydria or hypochlorhydria occur? What percentage of normal young people have no hydrochloric acid in their stomachs?

25. Under what conditions do relatively large amounts of lactic acid occur in the stomach?
26. What is the intrinsic factor?
27. What vitamin is used in the treatment of pernicious anemia? Why is achlorhydria characteristic of this disease?
28. Name two conditions in which hyperchlorhydria is found. What is gastric ulcer?
29. How is secretin formed from prosecretin? What is the function of secretin? What is pancreozymin?
30. What substance accounts for the alkalinity of pancreatic juice? Are the contents of the upper intestinal tract usually alkaline? How do you explain this?
31. Name the enzymes found in pancreatic juice, giving the substrates and end products for each.
32. What is trypsinogen? Chymotrypsinogen? What activates each?
33. What are the end products of fat digestion? Protein digestion? Carbohydrate digestion?
34. What is amylopsin? Steapsin?
35. Why cannot fats be digested efficiently unless they are emulsified? What fluid emulsifies fats in the intestine?
36. Since fatty acids are not soluble in water, how are they absorbed? Do they pass directly into the blood from the intestinal tract?
37. What is cholecystokinin? What type of food is most effective in causing its secretion?
38. What organ manufactures the bile? What organ concentrates it?
39. Are enzymes found in the bile? Name some substances excreted in the bile.
40. What compounds in bile are responsible for its emulsifying power? Name two of them. Why are they good emulsifying agents?
41. Describe Hay's test for bile salts in urine. In what condition is this test positive?
42. What is the chief bile pigment? From what is it formed in the body?
43. What are gallstones? What substances do they usually contain?
44. Name the enzymes found in intestinal juice, giving the substrates and end products for each one.
45. What is enterocrinin? What is its supposed function?
46. What is enterogastrone? What is its function? What foods cause its secretion?
47. How may eating candy stop the sensation of hunger?
48. Discuss lactose deficiency.
49. What is the cause of gluten enteropathy?
50. List and explain 4 clinically important results of gluten enteropathy.
51. What are ptomaines? Give several examples.
52. What acids are formed from undigested carbohydrate foods by bacterial action?
53. Why are cereals laxative?
54. Name a sterol found in feces.
55. What substances are responsible for the normal color of feces? For the odor of normal feces?
56. Name some pathological conditions associated with each of the following types of stool: acholic stools; green stools; tarry stools; bloody stools.
57. What is occult blood? What two tests are used to detect it?
58. How is the fecal excretion of urobilinogen altered in hemolytic jaundice? In obstructive jaundice? In cancer of the head of the pancreas?

CHAPTER **29**

Inorganic metabolism

WATER We can appreciate better the tremendous importance of water in metabolism when we recall that water is by far the most abundant compound in living tissues. At six weeks of intrauterine ("in the uterus") life the human embryo is about 97.5 percent water. The newborn baby is 71 to 72 percent water, and 58 to 65 percent of an adult is water.* In general, the younger and more active the tissues are, the more water they contain. Infants, for example, need far more water in proportion to their body weight than do adults.

Water is the best of all solvents, and most of the chemical reactions of the tissues could not take place in its absence. The water of the bloodstream distributes heat uniformly throughout the body, and the evaporation of water from the lungs and skin is a major factor in temperature regulation. Water has a higher surface tension than the other chemical substances in the body. We have already learned that surface-active substances collect at boundaries between water and materials with lower surface tension. This high surface tension of water enables the surface-active enzymes to collect at the boundary between the water in which they are dissolved and the food to be digested. The important inorganic ions of the body fluids are present only because water allows ionization.

The body water is obtained from several sources and is eliminated by several routes. Some of these are:

Sources of water	*Excretion of water*
Water drunk or injected	Excreted in the urine
Water present in foods	Excreted in the feces
Water formed in chemical reactions in the tissues	Insensible loss from the lungs and skin
Water released by destruction of body tissues	Water lost in sweating

*More modern techniques for measuring body water (see page 128) give a figure somewhat lower than this—from 51 to 55 percent.

Considerable water is formed by chemical oxidations in the tissues. It is estimated that approximately 12 g of water are produced for each 100 large calories of heat. As a rule, about two-thirds of the normal loss from the body is by way of the urine. When the body is at rest, 25 percent of the heat lost from it is accounted for by the evaporation of water from the lungs and skin. Most of this is insensible ("unconscious") perspiration since sweating does not occur until a skin temperature of 30° C is reached. Insensible perspiration and respiration together result in a loss of approximately 50 g of weight per hour. This is because the carbon dioxide and water lost from the body weigh more than the oxygen absorbed.

The amount of water used in metabolizing some common food products is shown in Table 29-1 (after Dr. Irving McQuarrie). This water is used mainly in dissipating the heat of oxidation and in excreting end products of catabolism.

It is estimated that 0.75 g of water is required during vigorous exercise for each extra large calorie of heat produced.

If the protein and inorganic contents of the diet are increased, an increased amount of water is needed to eliminate the products of metabolism. Diseases accompanied by *dehydration* (excessive loss of water) also require an increased water intake. Indeed, death occurs if more than one-fifth of the body water is lost without being replaced. If the water stores are lowered, dehydration fever results because the water necessary for adequate dissipation of body heat is not available. Dehydration will accompany vomiting or diarrhea, fever, acidosis, and diabetes insipidus unless the water intake is increased.

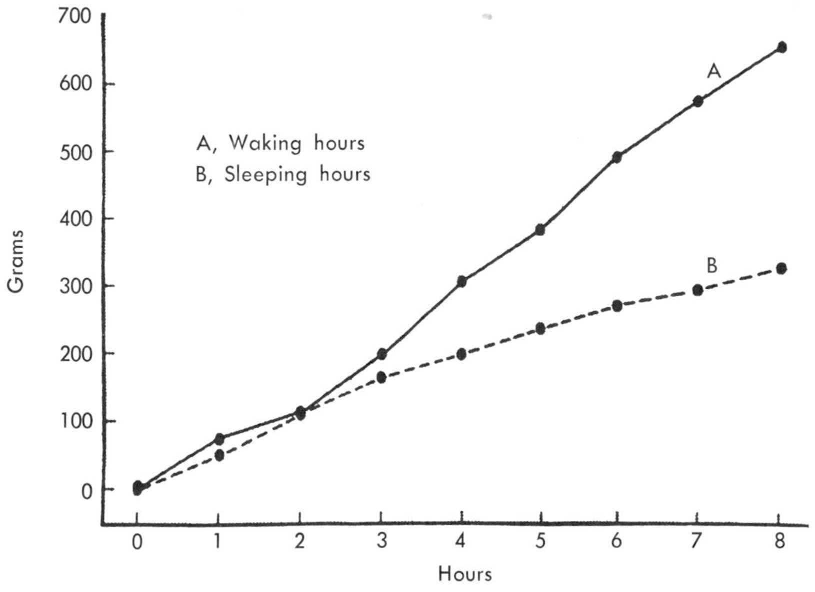

Fig. 29-1. Insensible water loss during sleeping and waking hours. What do you suggest is the reason for the lower values during sleep? (From Bradham, B., Thompson, N. J., and Reynolds, J. C.: The use of a metabolic scale, J.A.M.A. **198**:746, 1966.)

Table 29-1. Grams of water required to metabolize 100 grams of food

Food	Grams of water
Protein	350
Starch	46
Fat	48
Beef, sirloin	143
Eggs	156
Milk	43
Bread	102

When vomiting is present, water must often be administered under the skin, by way of a vein, or by rectum. Of course, the rectal route cannot be used in the presence of diarrhea.

The rate of heat production in the body increases about 13 percent for each degree Centigrade, or about 7 percent for each degree Fahrenheit, rise in body temperature. Extra water is needed for dissipation of this extra heat.

Acidosis favors loss of water from the body—in contrast to alkalosis, which favors its retention. Patients with diabetes mellitus, for example, excrete three or four times as much urine per day as do normal people.

Diabetes insipidus is a condition characterized by a high rate of excretion of dilute urine. For example, one of Dr. McQuarrie's patients gave a history of having excreted as much as 16 kg of urine in one day, even though the patient (a 4-year-old boy) weighed only 11 kg. This condition is treated by giving extracts of the posterior lobe of the pituitary gland.

The elimination of water is decreased if the thyroid gland does not secrete sufficient amounts of its hormone, thyroxine. One symptom of underactivity of this gland is a peculiar edema of the skin, called *myxedema*. Injection of insulin, the hormone manufactured by the islands of Langerhans in the pancreas, favors the retention of water by the body.

Water retention decreases resistance to infectious diseases, and patients with edema are more susceptible to infections. The irritability of the nervous system is increased when water is retained. Patients with epilepsy (a disease of the nervous system characterized by convulsions) have fewer attacks if the water intake is kept at a low level.

If more than 50 ml of water per kilogram of body weight is taken into the body each hour, a condition known as *water intoxication* results. The symptoms of this condition include restlessness, muscle tremors, vomiting, diarrhea, prostration, convulsions, and finally death if water administration is continued. The best antidote for water intoxication is a solution of sodium chloride (10 percent). This leads us to suspect that the condition may be caused by a dilution of the sodium chloride of the body fluid. A similar set of symptoms results when marked sweating occurs ("miners' cramps" or "stokers' cramps"). Sweat contains about 0.7 percent sodium chloride, and excessive sweating causes a loss of this substance from the body. Drinking plain water will not relieve this condition, but dilute sodium chloride solution (0.7 percent) promptly relieves the symptoms.

SODIUM BICARBONATE

We have already found that sodium bicarbonate is one of the important buffer salts of the blood. Its concentration in the bloodstream is lowered in acidosis and raised in alkalosis. Diarrhea and vomiting have a marked effect on the sodium bicarbonate level of the blood.

Diarrhea causes a lowering of the blood sodium bicarbonate and, therefore, acidosis. All of the secretions (pancreatic juice, bile, intestinal juice) of the intestinal tract contain sodium bicarbonate. Under normal circumstances most of this is absorbed again. In diarrhea the sodium bicarbonate present in the intestine is lost in the stools, and a lowering of the sodium bicarbonate level of the blood results.

Vomiting causes a rise in the blood sodium bicarbonate and, therefore, alkalosis. The formation of the hydrochloric acid in gastric juice involves the removal of chlorine from the sodium chloride of the blood and the removal of hydrogen from water. The sodium and hydroxyl radicals set free in this process react with carbon dioxide to form sodium bicarbonate. In other words, the secretion of hydrochloric acid into the stomach causes a simultaneous increase of the sodium bicarbonate of the blood. Under normal circumstances the secretion of gastric hydrochloric acid is greatest just after a meal. After meals, therefore, the blood becomes more alkaline from an increase of sodium bicarbonate, and since a part of this is excreted in the urine, the urine becomes more alkaline also. This alkalinity of the urine after meals is often called the "alkaline tide." During vomiting the hydrochloric acid of the stomach is continually being lost, and the stomach cells continue to make more. If this process keeps up, the amount of sodium bicarbonate in the blood increases faster than it can be eliminated, and alkalosis results.

The blood sodium bicarbonate level is lowered in any condition in which acids enter the blood. For example, it is low in ketosis and after severe exercise (from lactic acid). Eclampsia, which is characterized by serious convulsions and which sometimes accompanies pregnancy, is a condition in which the alkali reserve (mainly $NaHCO_3$) is low. Uremia (see page 364) is accompanied by an acidosis since acid phosphates and sulfates cannot be eliminated from the body at a normal rate in this condition.

SODIUM CHLORIDE

An average adult eats about 10 g of sodium chloride each day and excretes about the same amount in the urine. The excretion in the urine is very low during starvation; it is increased in Addison's disease (due to lack of the hormone of the cortex of the adrenal gland), making the sodium chloride level of the blood low. Persistent vomiting also decreases the blood sodium chloride since chloride is continually being removed from the blood to form hydrochloric acid in the stomach. Excessive vomiting is also accompanied by an increase in blood sodium bicarbonate, as we have seen, and by some degree of dehydration uremia. The administration of sodium chloride solution by vein builds up the low sodium chloride level, overcomes the dehydration, and combats the alkalosis (high $NaHCO_3$) by increasing the elimination of sodium bicarbonate in the urine. The vomiting that accompanies intestinal obstruction and the pernicious vomiting that may accompany pregnancy are perhaps the most common causes of low levels of blood sodium chloride.

An excessive amount of sodium chloride in the diet causes edema. Patients with edema are usually given a diet very low in this substance.

CALCIUM

Calcium has a number of important functions in the body: (1) It is necessary for the coagulation of blood; (2) it is necessary for the formation of bones and teeth; (3) it is necessary for the maintenance of a proper rhythm of the heartbeat; (4) it is a normal component of milk and is necessary for proper milk formation; (5) calcium ions are *depressing ions* and assist in maintaining a balance between the depressing and stimulating ions of the blood.

Calcium makes up about 2 percent of the body weight; 97 percent of it is located in the bones and teeth; 9 to 11.5 mg of calcium are present normally in 100 ml of blood plasma. The red blood cells do not contain this element. Approximately half of the blood calcium is present as calcium ions; the remainder is united mainly to the blood proteins.

Calcium in the diet is not equally well absorbed from the digestive tract; for example, the calcium in milk is well absorbed, but the calcium in vegetables is not. Sugars in the diet favor calcium absorption, while fats and phosphates reduce it.

Calcium salts are excreted both by way of the intestinal tract and in the urine. Some of the calcium in feces has passed through the intestinal tract without absorption, but a portion of it has probably been excreted into the small intestine. If the urine is alkaline, the majority of calcium is being excreted by way of the intestinal tract. When the urine is acid, as it usually is on a normal diet, calcium excretion is mainly by the urinary route.

The level of blood calcium is controlled primarily by the parathyroid glands—four small structures located in the neck, back of the thyroid gland. If these glands are removed, the level of blood calcium falls. This results in a removal of the depressing effect of calcium ions, and the patient has *tetany*, or convulsions. When the parathyroid glands are overactive or when the hormone of these glands (parathormone) is injected into the blood, the blood calcium level rises. If this rise is high enough, the depressing action of the calcium ions causes *coma*.

Absence of adequate amounts of calcium from the diet may be the cause of *osteoporosis*, a condition in which the hard material of the bones is thin and porous. This condition is sometimes accompanied by tetany because the blood calcium level is too low. *Spasmophilia*, or *infantile tetany*, a disorder of childhood, is also accompanied by a low blood calcium level. It appears that vitamin D enables us to absorb and utilize calcium salts efficiently, and rickets (see page 439) and spasmophilia are found in children suffering from a deficiency of this vitamin.

Fifteen to 50 percent of people of age 65 or older have some degree of osteoporosis. There are at least 4 million persons in the United States with severe osteoporosis. The incidence is four to six times greater in women than in men. The cause really is not known with certainty, although many physicians attempt treatment with sex hormones or large daily intakes of

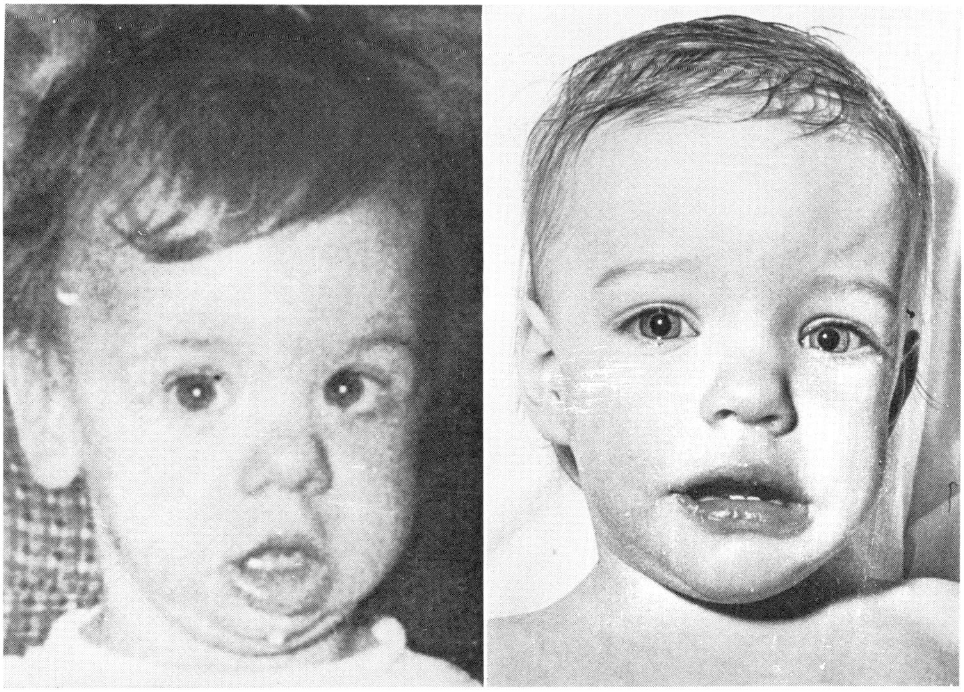

Fig. 29-2. Two children with idiopathic hypercalcemia. Note the pinched, snub nose with nostrils pointing forward, underdevelopment of the bridge of the nose and mandible, prominent epicanthal folds, squint, loose upper lip, open mouth, hanging lower lip, narrow temples, large ears, and rounded forehead. Why is a diet low in vitamin D used in therapy? (See page 338.) (From O'Brien, D., Pepper, T. D., and Silver, H. K.: Idiopathic hypercalcemia of infancy, J.A.M.A. **173:**1106, 1960.)

calcium. In rats, osteoporosis can be produced by long-term feeding of diets low in calcium. The experimental disease can be reversed by feeding diets high in calcium.

Idiopathic hypercalcemia of infancy is a disease characterized by physical and mental retardation. The level of calcium in the plasma varies from 12 to 18 mg per 100 ml. Treatment consists in giving diets low in calcium and in vitamin D and in the administration of an active adrenal steroid such as hydrocortisone. Treatment often is unsatisfactory, and many of these young patients die before the age of 5 years. Spontaneous remissions (periods during which the patient is apparently free of disease) sometimes occur.

PHOSPHORUS

Most of the phosphorus of the body is found in the bones and teeth. The functions of phosphorus compounds in the body include: (1) the formation of bones and teeth; (2) the formation of phospholipids, nucleic acid, and other organic phosphorus compounds; (3) the formation of phosphate salts, which act as buffers in blood and urine; (4) esters of phosphoric acid are formed in the breakdown of muscle glycogen to lactic acid; (5) phosphorus is a normal constituent of the milk protein casein; (6) glucose must unite with phosphoric acid before the glucose can pass from the blood into muscles and liver, and from the kidney tubules into the blood; this union, as well as the formation of bone, is catalyzed by a group of enzymes known collectively as *phosphatase*. ATP, NAD^+, $NADP^+$, creatine phosphate, and nucleic acids are important compounds that contain phosphorus.

Inadequate amounts of phosphorus and calcium in the diet cause *rickets* (see page 439). The utilization of phosphorus (as well as calcium) is much better in the presence of vitamin D, and unless the phosphorus and calcium intakes are very low, adequate amounts of this vitamin will prevent rickets. The level of acid-soluble phosphorus in the blood plasma is lowered in rickets. The level of blood alkaline phosphatase (see page 364) is increased in this condition, as well as in certain other diseases of bones. Since alkaline phosphatase is excreted in the bile, the amount of this enzyme also increases in obstructive jaundice.

About two-thirds of the phosphorus excretion is by way of the urine, the other one-third leaving the body with the feces. Almost all the phosphorus in urine is in the form of inorganic phosphates. It seems likely that the phosphorus in the feces represents phosphorus that was never absorbed.

Most of the phosphates in the diet come from the phosphoproteins and nucleoproteins of the protein foods. Smaller amounts come from phospholipids, phosphoric acid esters, and other organic phosphorus compounds.

POTASSIUM

Potassium salts are found characteristically *inside* of cells; sodium salts occur chiefly in fluids that *surround* cells. Red blood cells, for example, are almost devoid of sodium salts, whereas the plasma has only a very low concentration of potassium salts. In Addison's disease the level of plasma potassium rises. It has been supposed that the lack of the hormone of the

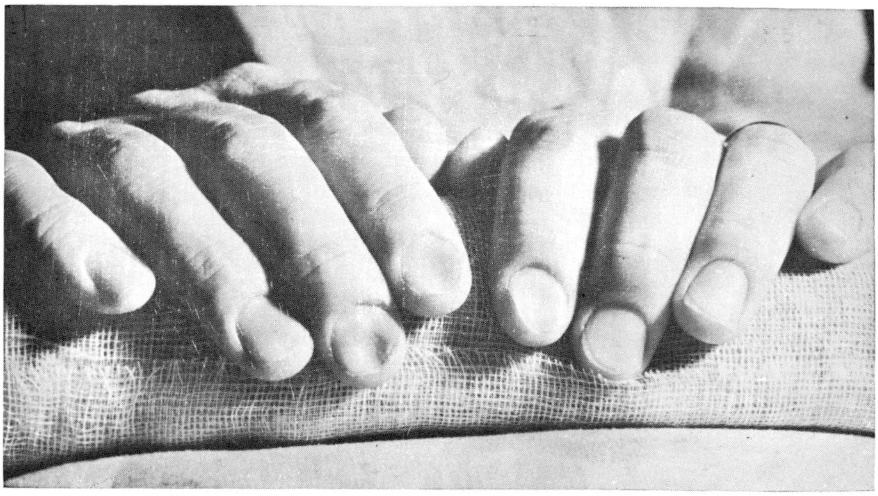

Fig. 29-3. Photograph of the fingers of a patient with microcytic (small red blood cell) anemia with achlorhydria. Note the spoon-shaped nails with pronounced concavity. What element can be used in the therapy of this type of anemia?

adrenal cortex (and it is this lack that causes Addison's disease) changes the cell membranes so that potassium is able to escape from them into the tissue fluids. The normal adult body contains between 125 and 155 g of potassium.

If a large amount of potassium salt is given by mouth, it is excreted in the urine in a short time. Some extra sodium salt is also excreted along with the potassium salt. Potassium salts have a diuretic effect (increase the flow of urine) and formerly were used as diuretics in medicine.

One cause of potassium deficiency is stress (that is, illness, surgery, trauma), resulting in an increased activity of the adrenal gland (see page 400). Severe deficiency leads to periodic attacks of paralysis. Clinical manifestations disappear promptly following administration of 1 to 8 g of KCl orally or a smaller quantity intravenously. Vomiting and diarrhea cause a loss of body potassium. The use of laxatives and diuretics also may lead to excess potassium excretion.

IRON

The adult human body contains, on the average, about 3.5 to 4 g of iron. Approximately 2.5 to 3 g of this is combined in hemoglobin. The remaining gram or so is stored in the liver, spleen, and bone marrow.

Most iron is transported in the plasma as ferric iron combined with a specific protein. This iron-protein is known as *transferrin,* and the average normal concentration of transferrin is 250 mg per 100 ml of plasma. The amount of iron present in 100 ml of plasma varies normally from 50 to 180 μg per 100 ml.

In addition to its obvious function in forming hemoglobin and transporting oxygen, iron is required for the synthesis of myoglobin (see page 279) certain enzymes (peroxidases, catalase), and the cytochromes.

Excessive intake of iron (for example, after numerous blood transfusions) causes a deposition of extra iron in the liver and other tissues—a condition known as *siderosis*. In the disease of unknown origin known as *hemochromatosis* enormous amounts of iron (as much as 50 g) may be deposited in tissues other than red cells. Deposits occur mainly in the liver, pancreas, and lymph nodes.

Meat and green vegetables are the richest food sources of iron, but most of the natural foods contain this element. Milk and white bread are deficient in iron. A newborn baby has enough iron stored in his body for about 6 months and can live on milk alone during this period.

Since iron is needed to build hemoglobin in the body, iron deficiency results in *anemia* because the body is unable to build sufficient hemoglobin in the absence of this element. Copper appears to be a necessary catalyst for hemoglobin formation, but only traces are required and true copper deficiency in human beings is extremely rare.

FERRITIN. Many tissues of the body, and particularly the liver, spleen, and intestinal mucosa, contain a colorless protein known as apoferritin. Under physiological conditions apoferritin combines with iron (probably as $Fe(OH)_3$) to form a conjugated protein known as *ferritin*. Crystalline ferritin contains approximately 23 percent iron, all in the ferric state. There is increasing evidence that much, if not all, of the stored iron of the body (that is, iron not present in active molecules such as hemoglobin, tissue enzymes, and transferrin) is present as ferritin.

IODINE Thyroxine, the hormone secreted by the thyroid gland, is 65 percent iodine. If iodine is missing from the diet, thyroxine cannot be formed, and a condition of *hypothyroidism* (underactivity of the thyroid gland) is said to exist. In iodine deficiency the thyroid gland increases in size, and this enlarged gland is called a *goiter*. The different types of hypothyroidism will be described in Chapter 32. The addition of iodides to table salt has greatly reduced the incidence of goiter in those regions where such iodized salt is used.

FLUORINE Fluorine, as we have seen, is present in relatively high concentration in the enamel of the teeth. An excess of fluorine in the drinking water causes *mottled enamel*. The remaining enamel of decayed teeth seems to have a lower fluorine content than normal enamel.

In regions in the United States where the level of fluoride in the drinking water is high (4 to 5.8 ppm), the prevalence of osteoporosis and the accompanying collapsed vertebrae (most common in older women) is reduced. In addition, there is evidence that there is a reduction in calcification of the aorta in both sexes in high-fluoride areas.

COPPER Only traces of the copper in the diet are absorbed; probably 85 to 99 percent of the quantity eaten is eliminated in the feces. In the blood about half is present in the red blood cells and half in the plasma.

Almost all of the copper in the plasma exists as a constituent of a blue protein known as *ceruloplasmin*. The normal copper concentration of plasma is 65 to 165 μg per 100 ml in adult humans. The adult body contains about 100 mg of copper. Most of it is incorporated in enzymes. A small amount is complexed with RNA.

In the disease known as *Wilson's disease (hepatolenticular degeneration)*, the level of ceruloplasmin (normally 20 to 50 mg are present in 100 ml of plasma) is extremely low. Probably as a result of this (that is, lack of the protein to transport copper) abnormal deposits of copper occur in various tissues, and this results in tissue damage. The disease is characterized by progressive brain damage, liver injury, and kidney lesions.

Penicillamine (see page 158) forms a chelate with copper. This chelate is excreted in the urine, thus decreasing the amount of copper in the body. Penicillamine is used in the treatment of Wilson's disease.

Patients with Wilson's disease, under treatment with penicillamine, have a reduction in sensitivity to salt, sweet, sour, and bitter tastes. Taste sensitivity becomes normal if they are given 5 to 15 mg of copper as copper sulfate by mouth daily. Thus, copper may play a role in taste.

Copper is an essential constituent of tyrosinase, an enzyme necessary for the synthesis of skin pigment (melanin). It is necessary for the formation of hemoglobin.

Copper deficiency has seldom been observed in humans (see page 341). Severe copper deficiency causes swayback disease in lambs; bone defects in dogs, pigs, and chickens; and loss of hair color in sheep and rats. Copper deficiency also causes a reduction in the formation of hemoglobin and anemia in experimental animals.

In pigs copper deficiency can cause a weakening of the walls of the blood vessels, notably the aorta. This may cause rupture of the vessel and death. The specific cause seems to be related to a lack of a copper-containing enzyme named amine oxidase. This enzyme is necessary for the oxidation of the amino acid lysine and for the eventual production of desmoline, a substance that forms "cross links" responsible for the elasticity and stability of elastin, the major protein of the wall of the aorta.

Some mollusks (snails and octopuses) and arthropods (horseshoe crabs and scorpions) have blue blood. The color is due to a copper-containing protein that serves these animals as a carrier of oxygen (instead of hemoglobin). Although this protein does not contain heme, it is known as *hemocyanin.*

TRACE METALS. Probably much harm or much good can be done by minute changes in the concentration of metals that occur in trace amounts in the tissues.

Cobalt is an integral part of vitamin B_{12} (see page 430). It is necessary for red blood cell formation. The usual diet supplies an abundance of the metal.

Zinc is required for the growth and functions of blood cells, liver, kidneys, and other organs, probably including the male gonads. It occurs as an essential part of enzymes (for example, the enzyme that catalyzes the breakdown of ethyl alcohol in the liver). The amount of zinc in the liver is low in diseases of that organ, and the kidney content falls in chronic kidney disease. The amount present in white blood cells is low in some types of leukemia. Ordinarily, drinking water contains sufficient zinc to supply nutritional needs.

Zinc deficiency has been observed in males studied in Iran and Egypt. The clinical features included dwarfism, testicular atrophy, retardation of skeletal maturation, and a low level of the enzyme alkaline phosphatase (see page 364) in the serum. The diet of these patients was mainly bread and beans. The level of zinc was decreased in the plasma, red blood cells, and hair. The excretion of zinc in the urine and feces was less than in control subjects.

Six patients given supplemental zinc grew 5 to 8 inches in height in a year. Three other patients ingesting the same diet, but not given zinc, grew only 2 to 3 inches in the same period.

The earliest biochemical "lesion" in zinc deficiency is a failure of RNA synthesis, followed by decreased formation of protein and DNA. It has been suggested that zinc may protect RNA from destruction by the enzyme RNA-ase.

Manganese and *molybdenum* are required for normal metabolism, bone formation, and body growth.

Chromium is required for the optimal activity of insulin.

STIMULATING AND DEPRESSING IONS

Certain ions normally found in the blood have a *stimulating* effect and others have a *depressing* effect: OH^-, Na^+, and K^+ ions are stimulating ions; Ca^{++}, Mg^{++}, and H^+ are depressing ions. Ordinarily there are just sufficient concentrations of these various ions so that neither overstimulation nor overdepression occurs. In acidosis, the H^+ concentration increases and the OH^- concentration decreases. This results in a depression, as in *coma,* a characteristic symptom of acidosis. An increase of OH^- and a decrease in H^+ occur in alkalosis; here tetany (convulsions) is the characteristic finding. When calcium ions increase in the blood, coma results; when calcium ions are decreased, tetany is produced. Magnesium salts are sometimes injected into the bloodstream to combat convulsions.

CATION BALANCE IN BODY FLUIDS

In the plasma of all animals, including man, the concentration of Na^+ is much greater than the concentration of K^+; also the concentration of Ca^{++} exceeds the concentration of Mg^{++}. Inside the body cells of most animals (the cow is an exception), these ratios are reversed: K^+ concentration is higher than that of Na^+; and the concentration of Mg^{++} greatly exceeds that of Ca^{++}. Indeed some cells apparently have no Ca^{++}. The total amount of all of these ions inside cells is about equal to the total amount of them in the plasma and extracellular fluid of the body.

Cells that have high metabolic activity—for example, heart muscle cells—have a higher ratio of K^+ to Na^+ and a higher ratio of Mg^{++} to Ca^{++} than do less active cells—for example, cells in the outer layer of the skin.

Abnormalities in the concentrations of Mg^{++} and K^+ tend to occur together. For example, plasma levels of both are high in adrenal insufficiency and low in spontaneous hypopotassemia (low level of K^+ in the plasma) and magnesium deficiency.

STUDY QUESTIONS

1. What percentage of a newborn baby is water? What percentage of an adult?
2. Name several functions of water in the body.
3. Name four sources from which tissues obtain water.
4. Name four ways in which water is lost from the body.
5. How much water is produced chemically in the body for each 100 large calories of heat produced?
6. How do you explain the fact that we lose weight by breathing?
7. At what temperature does sweating begin? What is insensible perspiration?
8. What is dehydration? How much of the body water can be lost without producing death?
9. Name four diseases, or types of disease, accompanied by dehydration unless extra water is given to the patient.
10. How much is heat production in the body increased for each rise of one degree Centigrade in body temperature?
11. What material is used to treat diabetes insipidus?
12. What effect do you think dehydration would have on epilepsy?
13. What is water intoxication? How much water would *you* have to drink per hour to produce this condition? What is the best antidote for water intoxication?
14. What is the cause of stokers' cramps? How is this condition prevented?
15. How is the concentration of $NaHCO_3$ in the blood altered in vomiting? In diarrhea? Explain.
16. What is the alkaline tide?
17. Name four conditions in which the $NaHCO_3$ content of blood is lower than normal.
18. How much NaCl is eaten by an average adult in one day? How much of this is excreted in the urine?
19. Name two causes of low blood NaCl. Why is NaCl solution injected into the veins of patients with intestinal obstruction?
20. What inorganic substance is given only in small amounts to patients with edema? Why?
21. Name five functions of calcium salts in the body.
22. Where is most of the calcium of the body located? Why do you think we use plasma or serum, rather than whole blood, for calcium determinations?
23. What important food contains calcium in a form easily absorbed from the digestive tract?
24. What type of food assists calcium absorption? What type inhibits it?
25. Where are calcium salts excreted from the body? How does the pH of the urine influence the route of calcium excretion?
26. What gland controls the level of calcium in the blood? What symptoms would you expect from underactivity or removal of this gland? From overactivity of this gland?
27. What conditions are caused by low calcium intake or absorption? How does vitamin D help prevent these conditions?
28. Name five functions of phosphorus in the body.
29. What disease is caused by a low phosphorus intake? Why is this disease most common when vitamin D is not present in normal amounts in the diet?
30. What is phosphatase? Name some conditions in which the level of phosphatase in the blood is elevated.
31. What types of food furnish phosphates to the body?
32. How do potassium and sodium differ with respect to where they occur in the body?
33. In what disease does the level of blood potassium rise? What explanation has been given for this?
34. What types of food are richest in iron? Lowest in iron?

35. Where does a baby obtain his iron during the period in which he lives entirely on milk?
36. Why do we need iron? How does iron deficiency produce anemia?
37. What metal acts as a catalyst for the production of hemoglobin?
38. Why does a lack of iodine in the diet cause an underactivity of the thyroid gland?
39. What is a goiter?
40. What is the cause of mottled enamel? How does the fluorine content of the enamel of decayed teeth differ from that of normal teeth?
41. What is ceruloplasmin?
42. What is the apparent cause of Wilson's disease?
43. Name a function of copper.
44. Is copper well absorbed from the intestinal tract?
45. Name one function of each of the following: zinc, cobalt, manganese, molybdenum, chromium.
46. Name three stimulating and three depressing ions found in the blood. Explain why convulsions occur in alkalosis and in low blood calcium. Why is coma a symptom of acidosis and of high blood calcium?
47. Discuss the distribution of Na^+, K^+, Ca^{++}, and Mg^{++} in the body.

CHAPTER 30

Blood

Approximately one-twelfth of the normal adult human body is blood. The average blood volume is 30 ml per lb for males and 27.5 ml per lb for females. This essential body fluid is slightly heavier and more viscous than water. It consists of a suspension (about 45 percent) of *formed elements* (red blood cells, white blood cells, and platelets) in a fluid known as *plasma* (about 55 percent).

Normally there are approximately five million red blood cells (erythrocytes) in each cubic millimeter of blood. If the number found is appreciably above this figure the patient is said to have polycythemia (see page 279). A significant decrease in the number found indicates anemia (see page 279).

The number of white blood cells (leukocytes) present in a cubic millimeter of blood normally varies between 5,000 and 10,000. These cells occur in several well-recognized forms (granulocytes–neutrophils, eosinophils, basophils; lymphocytes; monocytes), and a *differential count* (that is, a count indicating the percentage of each type of leukocyte present in a sample of blood) often is of value as a diagnostic procedure. In general the white cell count rises sharply in acute infections, although there are important exceptions (for example, typhoid fever). The count may reach enormous proportions in some types of the disease known as *leukemia*.

Platelets (thrombocytes) are small fragments of tissue (about one-third the diameter of a red blood cell); there are approximately 200,000 to 400,000 present in each cubic millimeter of normal blood. This number may be lowered markedly in various disease complexes (purpuras) accompanied by capillary bleeding. The role of platelets in blood clotting will be discussed later in this chapter.

The circulating blood is the "great highway" of the body. It transports oxygen to the tissues and carbon dioxide from the tissues to the lungs. It transports food, waste products, and various chemical substances important in metabolism. The circulating water of the blood is extremely important in the regulation of body temperature. Its white blood cells and antibodies are active antagonists of invading microorganisms. Its plasma proteins play an important role in the transport of fluids across the capillary

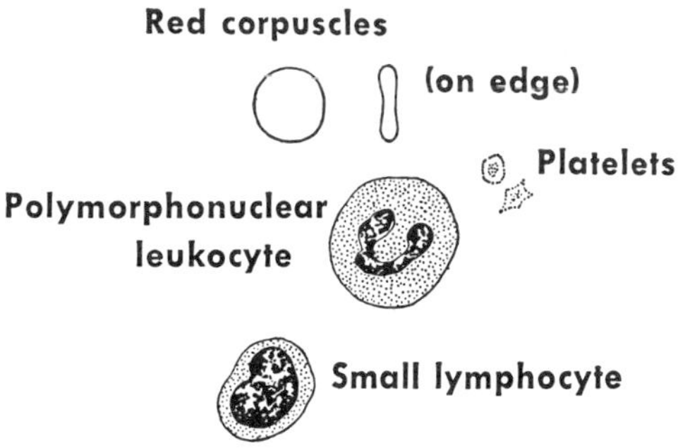

Fig. 30-1. The "formed elements" of blood. "Leukocyte" is a synonym for white blood cell. A lymphocyte is one kind of white blood cell. Polymorphonuclear leukocytes are also called "pus cells" because of their presence in large numbers in pus. Which of the cells illustrated contains hemoglobin? What is a function of the blood platelets?

membrane (see page 356) and its buffers serve to maintain the pH of the body at a value compatible with life.

Some of the important chemical substances found in blood are listed in Table 30-1.

The chemistry and metabolism of *hemoglobin* have been discussed in Chapters 25 and 26.

TRANSPORT OF OXYGEN TO THE TISSUES

In the short space of one minute under average conditions a normal adult absorbs about 350 ml of oxygen and eliminates about 315 ml of carbon dioxide. Less than 2 percent of this oxygen is carried from the lungs to the tissues in simple solution. The remainder diffuses from the air in the lungs into the red blood cells. In these cells it combines with hemoglobin (see page 278). In the tissues hemoglobin releases a part of its oxygen and returns to the lungs for a fresh supply.

One gram of hemoglobin is capable of combining loosely with 1.34 ml of oxygen. The tension or partial pressure of the oxygen in the alveoli (air sacs) of the lungs is relatively high—about 100 mm of Hg. As blood passes through the lungs, this pressure causes oxygen to diffuse into it and to combine with hemoglobin. Although a molecule of hemoglobin is in contact with alveolar oxygen a relatively short time (all the blood in the body—about 5 to 7 liters—passes through the lungs once each minute), the hemoglobin in the blood leaving the lungs is 95 percent saturated with oxygen. One hundred milliliters of this oxygenated blood, which contains about 15 g of hemoglobin, thus contains approximately 20 ml of loosely combined oxygen. In the tissues the oxygen tension is only 30 to 40 mm of Hg, and some of the oxyhemoglobin (see page 278) changes to reduced hemoglobin (that is, hemoglobin without loosely bound oxygen). The venous blood returning to the lungs after its passage through the tissues contains about 13 or 14 ml of loosely combined oxygen in each 100 ml.

As we have just noted, the low oxygen tension of the tissues favors the loss of oxygen from oxyhemoglobin. Two other factors also favor this loss:

1. The conversion of oxyhemoglobin to reduced hemoglobin is accelerated and made more complete by carbon dioxide. The relatively high carbon dioxide tension of the tissues increases the loss of oxygen from the blood.
2. The amount of oxygen with which hemoglobin will combine at low tensions of oxygen is reduced if the pH of the blood is lowered. The pH of the blood changes from approximately 7.43 (arterial blood) to about 7.25 (venous blood) as it

Table 30-1. Some chemical components of human blood

Blood component	Normal range	Pathological conditions in which abnormal values occur	
		Increased in	**Decreased in**
Hemoglobin	14 to 16 g per 100 ml of whole blood	Polycythemia (erythremia); dehydration	Anemias
Nonprotein nitrogen (npn)	25 to 35 mg per 100 ml of whole blood	Nephritis; eclampsia; metal poisoning; intestinal obstruction; prostatic obstruction; Addison's disease; dehydration; hemorrhage	
Blood urea nitrogen (bun)	10 to 15 mg per 100 ml of whole blood	(same as npn)	
Creatinine	1 to 2 mg per 100 ml of whole blood	Nephritis	
Uric acid	3 to 6 mg per 100 ml of serum	Gout; leukemia; kidney damage, primary or secondary	
Amino acid nitrogen	3 to 6 mg per 100 ml of serum	Nephritis; acute yellow atrophy of the liver; leukemia	After insulin injection
Total plasma proteins	6.5 to 8.2 g per 100 ml of serum	Anhydremia; multiple myeloma	Nephrosis; malnutrition; liver disease
Albumin	3.5 to 4.5 g per 100 ml of serum	Anhydremia	Nephrosis; malnutrition; liver disease
Globulin	1.5 to 3.0 g per 100 ml of serum or plasma	Nephrosis; uremia; multiple myeloma; kala-azar; liver disease; malignancy; anaphylaxis; chronic infections	
Fibrinogen	0.2 to 0.5 g per 100 ml of plasma	Acute infections	Cirrhosis of the liver; chloroform or phosphorus poisoning; severe anemias; typhoid fever
Fatty acids	9 to 14 millimoles per liter; 250 to 390 mg per 100 ml of whole blood	Ether narcosis; diabetes; pneumonia; nephritis; anemias	
Cholesterol	150 to 230 mg per 100 ml of plasma or serum (1/3 free; 2/3 esterified)	Nephrosis; lipemia; diabetes; hypothyroidism; biliary obstruction; pregnancy; high lipid diet; perhaps atherosclerosis	Hyperthyroidism; pernicious anemia; liver disease; low ratio of esterified cholesterol in liver damage

Table 30-1. Some chemical components of human blood—cont'd

Blood component	Normal range	Pathological conditions in which abnormal values occur	
		Increased in	**Decreased in**
Icterus index	4 to 7*	Hemolytic anemia; obstructive jaundice; liver disease	
Bilirubin	0.3 to 1.1 mg per 100 ml of plasma or serum	Hemolytic anemia; obstructive jaundice	
Glucose	70 to 100 mg per 100 ml of venous whole blood (fasting)	Diabetes; severe nephritis; pancreatic disease; hyperthyroidism; some liver diseases; hyperfunction of adrenal cortex· asphyxia; cerebral lesions	Hyperinsulinism; Addison's disease; some liver diseases; hypothyroidism
CO_2 combining power	53 to 64 ml of CO_2 per 100 ml of plasma†	Alkalosis; hyperpnea; vomiting; excess intake of alkali	Acidosis; uncontrolled diabetes; nephritis; diarrhea; asphyxia
Inorganic phosphorus	3 to 4 mg per 100 ml of plasma or serum (4 to 6 in children)	Renal rickets; uremia; nephritis; hypoparathyroidism	Infantile rickets; celiac disease; hyperparathyroidism
Chloride	98 to 106 mEq‡ per liter of plasma or serum; 570 to 620 mg (as NaCl) per 100 ml of plasma or serum	Nephritis; cardiac conditions; prostatic obstruction; eclampsia	Fever; burns; pneumonia; Addison's disease; diabetes; vomiting; anaphylaxis
Protein-bound iodine	4 to 8 μg per 100 ml of serum	Hyperthyroidism; pregnancy	Hypothyroidism; nephrosis
Calcium	4.5 to 5.7 mEq per liter; 9 to 11.5 mg per 100 ml of serum	Hyperparathyroidism	Hypoparathyroidism; infantile tetany; severe nephritis; celiac disease; renal rickets; osteomalacia; nephrosis; steatorrhea
Sodium	130 to 143 mEq per liter; 300 to 330 mg per 100 ml of plasma or serum	Overactivity of the adrenal cortex	Pregnancy; Addison's disease; intestinal obstruction; severe nephritis
Potassium	3.5 to 5.0 mEq per liter; 14 to 20 mg per 100 ml of plasma or serum	Acute bronchial asthma; uremia; Addison's disease; uncontrolled diabetes; intestinal obstruction	Familial periodic paralysis; hyperinsulinism

*See page 385.
†See page 353.
‡Milliequivalents (see page 366).

Table 30-1. Some chemical components of human blood—cont'd

Blood component	Normal range	Pathological conditions in which abnormal values occur	
		Increased in	Decreased in
Alkaline phosphatase	2.0 to 4.5 units* per 100 ml of serum (5 to 12 units in children)	Paget's disease; rickets; hyperparathyroidism; some bone diseases; some liver diseases	
Acid phosphatase	0 to 1.1 units† per 100 ml of serum	Carcinoma of the prostate with metastases	
Glutamic oxalacetic aminopherase (transaminase)	5 to 40 units‡ per 100 ml of serum	Acute myocardial infarction; infectious hepatitis; infectious mononucleosis; serum hepatitis; toxic hepatitis	

*Bodansky units (mg of phosphorus—as phosphate—liberated on incubation of serum with buffered glycerophosphate at pH 8.6 under standard conditions).

†Units as defined in the preceding footnote, except that the buffered glycerophosphate has a pH of 5.0 (Shinowara, Jones, and Reinhart method).

‡Wroblewski, Felix, and LaDue, John S.: Serum glutamic oxalacetic aminopherase (transaminase) in hepatitis, J.A.M.A. **160**:1130, 1956. For a definition of unit, see Karmen, Arthur: A note on the spectrophotometric assay of glutamic-oxalacetic transaminase in human blood serum, J. Clin. Invest. **34**:131, 1955.

circulates through the body. This change results in part from the small quantities of carbonic acid (H_2CO_3) formed when carbon dioxide enters the blood ($CO_2 + H_2O \rightleftarrows H_2CO_3$) and partly from the diffusion from the tissues into the blood of organic acids (such as lactic and pyruvic acids) formed in metabolism.

TRANSPORT OF CARBON DIOXIDE TO THE LUNGS

Most of the potassium of the blood is inside the red blood cells; most of the blood sodium is in the plasma. With the exception of hydrogen ions, cations (positively charged ions) do not readily diffuse across the red blood cell membrane. At the pH of the blood, oxyhemoglobin is negatively charged, and a part of this negative charge is neutralized by potassium ions. We shall represent the resulting potassium oxyhemoglobinate molecule by the shorthand symbol $KHbO_2$.

When arterial blood reaches the capillaries, oxygen splits off, leaving, for a short time, reduced potassium hemoglobinate.

$$KHbO_2 \rightarrow KHb + O_2$$

Some of the carbon dioxide entering the blood from the tissues (under a pressure of about 47 to 50 mm of Hg) diffuses into the red blood cells. Inside the red blood cells there is a rapid conversion of carbon dioxide to carbonic acid. This reaction is catalyzed by an enzyme known as *carbonic anhydrase*.

$$CO_2 + H_2O \rightarrow H_2CO_3$$

Carbonic acid then reacts with potassium hemoglobinate, forming reduced hemoglobin, potassium ions, and bicarbonate ions.

$$KHb + H_2CO_3 \rightarrow HHb + K^+ + HCO_3^-$$

As the concentration of bicarbonate ions inside the red blood cell increases, there is a marked tendency for these ions to diffuse out into the plasma. If we recall that potassium ions do not readily diffuse from the interior of the cells to the plasma, it becomes evident that bicarbonate ions cannot pass across the red blood cell membrane *unless some anion (negatively charged ion) in the plasma simultaneously passes into the cell.* That is, positively charged ions cannot move very far away from negatively charged ones (in this case the negatively charged hemoglobin molecule) because of the marked attraction of the opposite electrical charges. Hence, as bicarbonate ions enter the plasma from the red blood cells, anions (chiefly chloride ions) pass into the cells. When this diffusion process reaches an equilibrium, about 60 percent of the bicarbonate ions is in the plasma; the other 40 percent is in the red blood cells. This passage of chloride ions into the red blood cells when carbon dioxide enters the blood is called the *chloride shift.*

A small amount of the carbon dioxide entering the red blood cells combines directly with the free amino (NH_2) groups of the hemoglobin to form *carbamate* linkages.

$$HHbNH_2 + CO_2 \rightarrow HHbNHCOOH$$

In summary, the carbon dioxide entering the blood from the tissues is transported to the lungs partially in simple solution in the plasma (about 5 percent of the total), partially as carbamate (about 10 percent), and chiefly as bicarbonate (about 85 percent).

When blood enters the capillaries of the lungs, most of the reduced hemoglobin is converted to oxyhemoglobin.

$$HHb + O_2 \rightarrow HHbO_2$$

$HHbO_2$ has a greater tendency to form salts with potassium ions than has HHb. The reactions that took place in the tissues, therefore, are reversed, with the rapid formation of $KHbO_2$ and H_2CO_3 inside the red blood cells. In the presence of carbonic anhydrase this H_2CO_3 quickly forms CO_2 and H_2O. (Remember that an enzyme catalyzes a reversible reaction in both directions.) The carbon dioxide tension of the alveoli (air sacs) of the lungs is about 40 mm of Hg. This is less than that of the blood, and the carbon dioxide formed in the red blood cells diffuses first into the plasma and then into the lungs. As the bicarbonate ions of the red blood cell disappear, bicarbonate ions and chloride ions again diffuse across the cell membrane—this time bicarbonate ions into the cells and chloride ions into the plasma. These reactions are sufficiently rapid so that about 10 to 15 percent of the free and combined carbon dioxide is removed during the passage of the blood through the lung capillaries.

Potassium oxyhemoglobinate, in contrast to reduced hemoglobin, has little tendency to form carbamates, and much of the carbon dioxide found as carbamate splits off as free gas, which escapes into the alveoli of the lungs.

ACID-BASE BALANCE The capacity of the blood to resist large changes in pH is due mainly to its content of carbonic acid, bicarbonates, phosphates, and proteins.

(Review the discussion of buffers on page 88.) The most important of these buffer systems is that composed of the bicarbonates (chiefly $NaHCO_3$) and carbonic acid. At the pH of blood there are present about 20 bicarbonate ions for each molecule of carbonic acid. When an acid (for example, pyruvic acid, $CH_3COCOOH$) enters the blood, it is neutralized almost immediately by the bicarbonate present.

$$NaHCO_3 + CH_3COCOOH \rightarrow H_2CO_3 + CH_3COCOONa$$

The carbonic acid formed ionizes only slightly, and thus a large change in pH is prevented. Conversely, alkalis that gain entrance into the blood are neutralized by carbonic acid.

$$NaOH + H_2CO_3 \rightarrow NaHCO_3 + H_2O$$

The term *alkali reserve* refers to the amount of bicarbonate stored in the blood. Until most of this reserve is used up the body can protect itself against foreign or metabolic acids. *Acidosis* (page 232) results whenever there is a significant decrease in the amount of alkali reserve or a significant increase in the amount of carbonic acid in the blood. Conversely, *alkalosis* results from a significant increase in alkali reserve or a marked decrease in carbonic acid.

Metabolic acidosis is caused by a loss of available fixed base (such as $NaHCO_3$) or by an increase in acids other than carbonic. The acidosis is said to be *compensated* if respiratory adjustments (that is, increased loss of carbonic acid as CO_2 in the lungs) prevent a lowering of the pH of the blood. In *uncompensated acidosis* there is a significant lowering of pH.

Some common causes of metabolic acidosis are as follows:

1. Excessive ingestion of acid salts such as ammonium chloride.
2. Ketosis (see page 232).
3. Severe dehydration. Continued loss of water may reduce blood volume to such a degree that renal blood flow is diminished, with the result that metabolic acids are not excreted and accumulate in the body.
4. Diabetes mellitus, because of the accompanying ketosis. (See page 233.)
5. Types of liver disease in which carbohydrate metabolism is impaired. The resulting increase in fatty acid catabolism results in ketosis (see page 233).
6. Advanced kidney disease. The acidosis is caused by retention of acids (such as phosphoric and sulfuric) that normally are excreted as acid salts by the kidney.

Respiratory acidosis is caused by pulmonary insufficiency (decreased exchange of gases in the lungs). Usually anoxemia (lack of sufficient oxygen in the blood) and cyanosis (bluish skin color from an increased amount of dark reduced hemoglobin in the blood) are present. The retained carbon dioxide forms carbonic acid and causes the acidosis. Some disorders in which respiratory acidosis may occur are morphine poisoning, pneumonia, pulmonary edema, and emphysema.

Metabolic alkalosis is caused by a loss of acid in excess of base, or by the ingestion of large quantities of alkaline salts, such as sodium bicarbonate. Excessive vomiting is a common cause. Infants who lose large amounts of acid salts as a result of severe diarrhea may develop metabolic alkalosis. Metabolic diseases (such as Cushing's disease, page 406) that result in a loss of potassium salts in the urine may be complicated by the development of alkalosis. Another cause is the prolonged use of potent diuretics, since most of these cause an increased loss of potassium salts in the urine. The mechanism whereby excessive excretion of potassium salts results in alkalosis is not known. Metabolic alkalosis may be compensated (no change of blood pH) or uncompensated (rise of blood pH).

Respiratory alkalosis usually results from the excessive loss of CO_2 in the expired air as a result of hyperventilation (overbreathing). This may be caused by an organic lesion in the respiratory center of the brain. Other causes include anoxemia, high fever, infections, drug intoxication (for example, from salicylates or sulfonamides), and respiratory neurosis. Usually, the kidneys compensate by excreting sodium bicarbonate in the urine.

One of the physiological disadvantages of acidosis is the inability of the blood to transport the normal amount of carbon dioxide from the tissues to the lungs because of the unavailability of sufficient cations (mainly Na^+) to form the necessary amount of bicarbonate. Normally, each 100 ml of plasma can transport approximately 53 to 64 ml of carbon dioxide as carbonic acid and as bicarbonate. The estimation of the *carbon dioxide combining power (CO_2 combining power)* is carried out in the laboratory by obtaining a sample of the patient's plasma (using special precautions to avoid diffusion of CO_2 from the blood and diffusion of bicarbonate into the red blood cells prior to separation of the plasma) and equilibrating it with a gas mixture containing the concentration of CO_2 normally present in the alveoli of the lungs. One way of doing this is by blowing alveolar air from a normal individual through the plasma. After this the plasma is placed in a special apparatus (usually the Van Slyke apparatus is used) and is treated with an excess of acid. The acid makes the dissolved CO_2 very insoluble and converts bicarbonates to salts and carbon dioxide gas. For example, if HCl is added to plasma, the $NaHCO_3$ present reacts with it and CO_2 is formed:

$$HCl + NaHCO_3 \rightarrow NaCl + H_2O + CO_2 \uparrow$$

The total volume of CO_2 released from a known amount of plasma is then measured, and the number of milliliters of CO_2 calculated to be present in 100 ml of the plasma is the CO_2 combining power of the plasma. As stated above, values of 53 to 64 ml per 100 ml are normal. Higher values indicate alkalosis, and lower values indicate acidosis. For example, a value for the CO_2 combining power of 20 volumes percent (that is, 20 ml per 100 ml of plasma) indicates serious acidosis.

Renal regulation of acid-base balance. Ordinarily, the amount of nonvolatile acid (that is, acids other than carbonic) eaten and produced by the tissues each day exceeds the intake of available base. This excess of acid is buffered by anions (such as Na^+) with, however, a resulting loss of bicarbonate, which leaves the body as CO_2. Eventually, the alkali reserve of the body would be exhausted if the $NaHCO_2$ thus lost were not regenerated in some way. This is accomplished by the kidneys, which, on the usual diet, excrete an excess of acid, so that normally the urine is slightly more acid than is blood (pH 7.4 for normal arterial blood and about pH 6 for normal urine). The pH of the urine can vary over a large range of values (4.5 to 8.2), depending on the excess acid that must be excreted to maintain acid-base balance.

Plasma Proteins

A large number of different proteins are present in plasma. Many of them have been isolated and purified. From our point of view, however, the plasma proteins can, in most cases, be grouped into four major fractions: *serum albumin, serum globulin, fibrinogen,* and *prothrombin.* Serum albumin is particularly important in regulating the passage of fluid across the capillary walls; this will be discussed later in this chapter. Most of the antibodies are found in the globulin fraction. The globulins also combine loosely with many insoluble substances (such as lipids, iron, copper, and hormones) and transport them throughout the body. Fibrinogen and prothrombin are necessary for blood clotting. Numerous enzymes occur in the plasma.

The concentration of serum albumin (normally about 4 g per 100 ml)

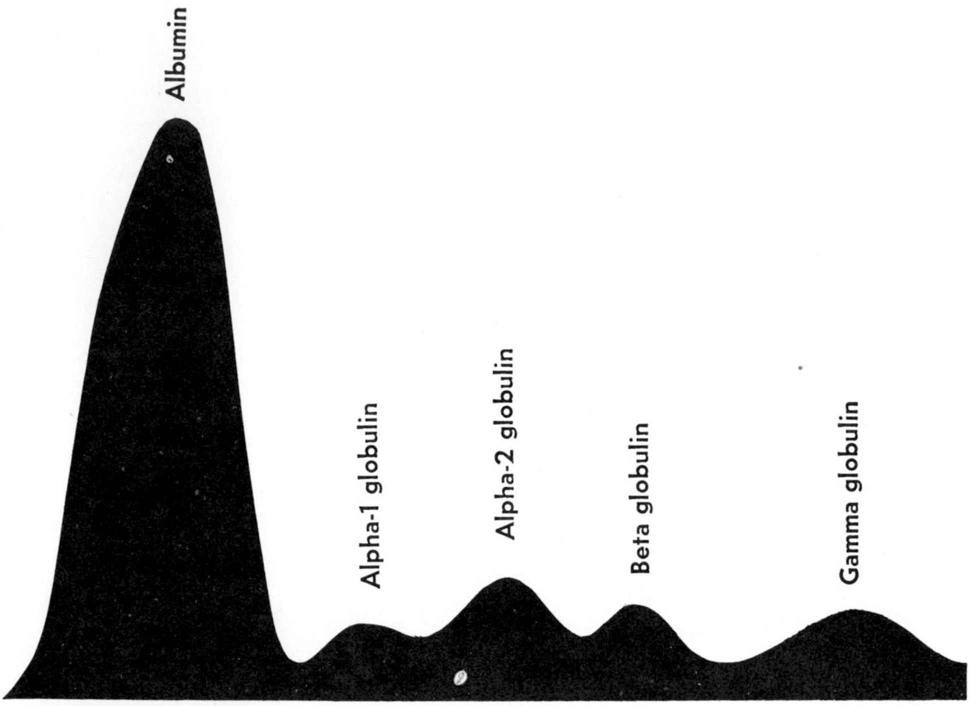

Fig. 30-2. An electrophoretic pattern of human serum. Why is fibrinogen not shown? (Courtesy Dr. George Phillips.)

is increased in dehydration (loss of body water). It is lowered in liver disease since this organ is the site of its formation. It is lowered also in nephrosis (a disease in which much albumin escapes into the urine) and in malnutrition. It is used in the treatment of shock (a condition accompanied by a leakage of fluid across the capillary walls into the tissues with a resultant loss of blood volume, fall of blood pressure, and collapse; it often accompanies accidental or surgical injury). It can be used also to control certain types of edema ("waterlogging" of the tissues) and is used as food by the body.

The concentration of serum globulins normally is approximately 1.5 to 3.0 g per 100 ml of plasma. This level is increased in a number of abnormal conditions (nephrosis, uremia, multiple myeloma, syphilis, pneumonia, kala-azar, anaphylaxis). Low levels rarely are encountered and usually accompany a general lowering of the concentration of plasma protein in conditions such as marked atrophy of the liver.

If plasma is examined in a special kind of apparatus, known as an electrophoresis apparatus, the globulin fraction can be separated into three subgroups: α-globulins, β-globulins, and γ-globulins. In the electrophoresis machine the plasma is placed in an electric field, and the charged protein molecules migrate toward the positively charged electrode (since they exist as negatively charged ions in plasma). They move at different speeds, depending on shape and charge, and after a time become separated partially or completely from each other. A special optical device is used to detect the protein boundaries since, of course, they are colorless and hence invisible

Table 30-2. Human immunoglobulin polypeptide chains

	Heavy chains				Light chains	
	IgG	**IgA**	**IgM**	**IgD**	**Type K**	**Type L**
Molecular weight	55,000	65,000	70,000	?	22,500	22,000
Carbohydrate	2%	10%	10%	?	?	?
Antigen	γ (gamma)	α (alpha)	μ (mu)	δ (delta)	κ (kappa)	λ (lambda)

to the unaided eye. γ-*Globulin,* also called *immune serum globulin* or *immunoglobulin,* contains numerous antibodies; it is used widely to give passive immunity against measles and infectious hepatitis. Its value in preventing poliomyelitis has been established.

Structure and nomenclature of the immunoglobulins. Since each immunoglobulin molecule presumably is an antibody molecule, there must be literally thousands of different ones. However, immunologists have classified them into 4 major types, known as IgG (γ-G), IgA (γ-A), IgM (γ-M), and IgD (γ-D). (The Ig is an abbreviation for immunoglobulin.)

Each IgG molecule is made up of 2 identical heavy polypeptide chains (molecular weight about 55,000) and 2 identical light polypeptide chains (molecular weight about 22,500). The heavy chains in IgG are called γ-chains (gamma-chains); the light chains are either κ-chains (kappa-chains) or λ-chains (lambda-chains). Molecules containing κ-chains are called type K molecules; molecules containing λ-chains are type L molecules. The 4 chains are connected by —S—S— bridges: one between a light chain and a heavy chain; and 1, 2, or 3 between the 2 heavy chains. In the following diagram of an IgG molecule, H means heavy chain and L means light chain. The dotted bridges may or may not be present in a particular molecule.

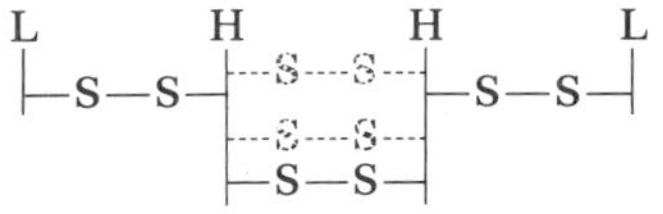

Normal serum contains from 12 to 14 mg of IgG per ml. The antigenic specificity (that is, ability to act as a specific antibody) is determined by the heavy chain of the immunoglobulin molecule, which is unique for each antibody. IgG molecules can combine with 2 molecules of antigen. Healthy adults synthesize from 2 to 5 g of IgG daily. Synthesis may be increased as much as 700 percent in response to pathologic conditions.

IgA molecules exist as molecules similar to IgG molecules, or as 2, 3, or 4 such molecular units linked together by —S—S— bridges between single heavy chains in adjacent units. Normal serum contains from 2 to 4 mg of IgA per ml. IgA is unique in that it is secreted in tears, saliva, the respiratory tract, and the intestinal tract.

IgM often is the first γ-globulin fraction to increase after immunization. Its molecule consists of 4 monomers (molecules similar to IgG molecules) connected by —S—S— bridges between adjacent heavy chains. Serum normally contains about 1 mg per ml. It is the chief γ-globulin in the fetus.

IgD has been recognized only recently. There is approximately 0.03 mg per ml of normal serum. Its molecules are monomers, similar in structure to the IgG molecules.

Diseases of enzymic defect involving immunoglobulins. Three diseases involving defects of immunoglobulins are discussed below.

Agammaglobulinemia (Bruton's disease). In this inherited disorder, only traces of IgG are present in the blood, and the synthesis of IgA and IgM also is defective.

Lymph follicles and plasma cells (which manufacture γ-globulins) are absent. The usual lymphatic tissue in the pharynx is lacking. Patients (usually children) are highly susceptible to infections.

Alymphoplasmacytic agammaglobulinemia. In this disease the total γ-globulin in the serum is less than 25 percent of normal. The number of circulating lymphocytes is reduced as is the number of these cells in lymphoid tissue. Death from infection usually occurs before 2 years of age.

Dysgammaglobulinemia. This disorder is characterized by a selective deficiency of specific γ-globulin fractions. Usually IgG and IgA are deficient (type A). In type B disease, IgG and IgM are deficient.

CERULOPLASMIN. One of the proteins in the γ-globulin fraction is colored blue, and is known as *ceruloplasmin.* (The Latin word *caeruleus* means dark blue.) This protein contains most of the copper present in plasma. In *Wilson's disease (hepatolenticular degeneration)* there is a marked decrease in the content of ceruloplasmin in the plasma. The disease is characterized by large deposits of copper in the liver and brain. Signs and symptoms include those of liver damage (not present in all patients), incoordination, and tremors of the limbs (see page 342).

C-REACTIVE PROTEIN (CRP). This protein is not present normally in the blood of humans but does occur in the presence of some inflammatory and necrotic disease processes. It derives its name from the fact that it forms a precipitate with the C-polysaccharide of the pneumococcus. Some of the diseases in which this protein appears in the blood are bacterial infections, acute rheumatic fever, acute myocardial infarction, and widespread cancer.

HAPTOGLOBINS. The haptoglobins are a group of serum proteins that have the peculiar ability to combine with hemoglobin. Decreased levels of haptoglobin accompany many anemias and liver diseases. Increased levels occur in a variety of inflammatory diseases.

MUCOPROTEINS. These serum proteins have chemically bound carbohydrate (galactose and mannose) as a part of their molecules. They are increased in many clinical diseases—cancer, tuberculosis, pneumonia, rheumatic fever, active rheumatoid arthritis, burns, myocardial infarction, gout, and various disorders accompanied by fever. Lowered levels are found in some types of liver disease, nephrosis, and endocrine (hormone) disorders. Clinically, the level of mucoprotein can be used as an indicator to follow the course of active rheumatoid arthritis. As the acute episode subsides, the level of mucoprotein decreases. The laboratory report indicates the concentration of mucoprotein in terms of the amount of galactose and mannose. The normal value is 8 to 14 mg of galactose-mannose per 100 ml of serum.

EDEMA. Fluid leaves and enters the bloodstream through the walls of the *capillaries,* the small vessels connecting the arteries with the veins. If fluid leaves the blood faster than more fluid enters it, the tissues become "waterlogged." This "waterlogged" condition is called edema. There are four important causes of edema: low plasma proteins, increased venous pressure, capillary damage, and blockage of lymphatics.

Low plasma proteins. Fig. 30-3 is a diagram of a capillary. At the arterial end of the capillary the blood pressure is about 32 mm of Hg; at the venous end it is about 12 mm of Hg. This pressure is forcing fluid out of the capillary into the tissues. Normally, there is little or no protein in the fluid (lymph) around the capillary. The proteins in the plasma, therefore, exert an osmotic pressure that tends to force fluid into the capillary. We see that the capillary blood pressure and the protein osmotic pressure (often called the colloid osmotic pressure, because protein molecules are so large they act like colloidal particles) oppose each other. At the arterial end of the capillary the blood pressure is higher than the osmotic pressure, and fluid *leaves* the capillary as the arrows in the diagram show. At the venous end, on the other hand, the osmotic pressure is higher than the blood pressure, and fluid *enters* the capillary. Now, if the protein concentration in the blood becomes low, the osmotic pressure is lowered, and much more fluid will leave the capillary than will enter it. This results in *edema.*

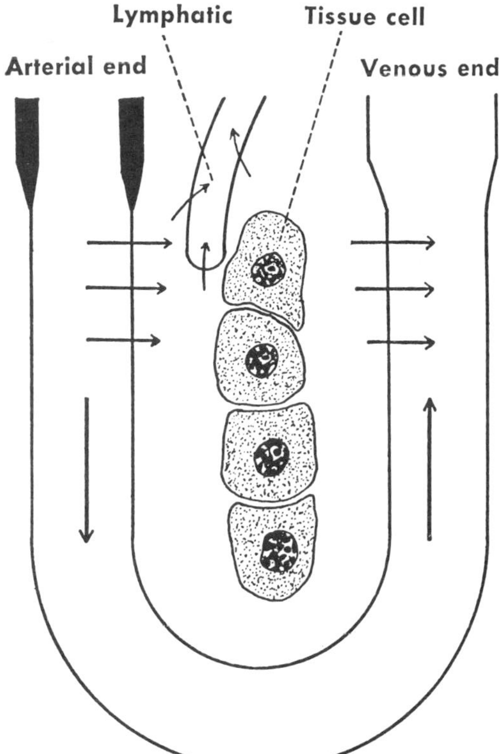

Fig. 30-3. Diagram of a capillary loop. The arrows indicate the normal direction of fluid movement. Name one type of edema in which you would expect the fluid to contain fairly large amounts of protein.

Serum albumin is more important than serum globulin in preventing edema because (1) there is more of it in the plasma (3.5 to 4.5 g of albumin and 1.5 to 3.0 g of globulin in 100 ml of plasma), and (2) the molecules of albumin are smaller so that a given weight of albumin contains more molecules than a given weight of globulin. If we recall that the osmotic pressure depends on the *number* of molecules, or particles, and not on their size we realize that a given weight of albumin causes a higher osmotic pressure than the same weight of globulin.

Increased venous pressure. When the pressure in the veins increases, this pressure is transmitted to the capillaries, and the capillary blood pressure also rises. This means that the pressure forcing fluid out of the capillaries is increased, and edema results. Increased venous pressure occurs in heart disease. It also occurs when large veins are obstructed. For example, a cancer in the abdominal cavity may obstruct the large vein (interior vena cava) that returns the blood from the lower limbs, causing marked edema of the legs.

Capillary damage. When the capillary walls are damaged, the plasma proteins are able to pass through them into the tissue spaces outside the capillary. In a short time the concentrations of protein inside and outside the capillary are the same. Since there is then no longer any difference in concentration across the capillary membrane, the protein osmotic pressure becomes zero. This leaves the capillary blood pressure unopposed, and edema results. This is probably the cause of the early edema of the face that occurs in acute glomerulonephritis, a kidney disease.

Blockage of lymphatics. Even under normal circumstances slightly more fluid

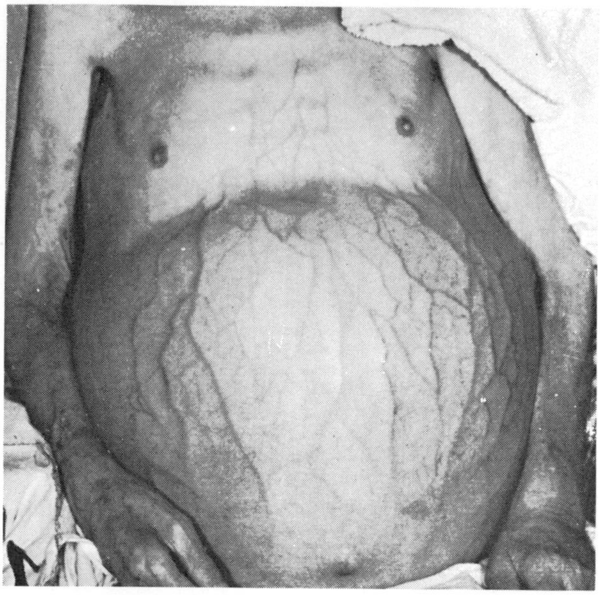

Fig. 30-4. Photograph of an alcoholic person who has increased venous pressure as a result of cirrhosis (hardening) of the liver. Note the abdomen enlarged from ascites (fluid in the abdominal cavity) and the dilated skin veins. What is the cause of this patient's ascites? (From Davidson, C. S.: Some considerations in the diagnosis and treatment of liver disease, Med. Sci. **5**:726, May 25, 1959.)

leaves the capillaries than enters them again. This excess fluid, called lymph, enters small vessels, called *lymphatics* or *lymph vessels*. The lymphatics travel along with the blood vessels and finally collect into one vessel that empties into the subclavian vein in the neck. If these lymphatics become obstructed, this drainage cannot take place, and fluid gradually accumulates in the tissues, causing edema. This type of edema occurs in the tropical disease known as filariasis or elephantiasis. This condition is caused by small worms *(Filaria)* that enter the body and live in the lymphatics. They are especially likely to obstruct the lymphatics that drain the lower limbs; these limbs then swell to huge proportions as a result of edema.

BLOOD CLOTTING

If blood is taken from a vein and placed in a test tube, it will become firm in a few minutes so that it will not run out of the tube, even when it is inverted. We say the blood has clotted. The blood clot gradually shrinks, and a clear yellow fluid, called *serum*, exudes from it.

The clotting of blood involves the conversion of the soluble fibrinogen to insoluble fibrin. Fibrin precipitates in long threads, which cluster together to make a spongelike structure. This fibrin mass entraps the blood cells and platelets and thus forms the clot. Many theories that attempt to explain how fibrinogen is converted to fibrin have been advanced. We must confess that we still do not know the complete story.

The first step in blood coagulation (clotting) is a disintegration of the platelets. These structures are fragile and readily disintegrate when blood comes in contact with tissue. This breakdown of platelets results in the formation of *thromboplastin*, a cephalin-protein complex. Thromboplastin then reacts with *calcium ions* and *prothrombin* to form a protein called *thrombin.*

$$\text{Thromboplastin} + Ca^{++} + \text{Prothrombin} \rightarrow \text{Thrombin}$$

Finally, thrombin reacts with fibrinogen to form insoluble fibrin, which precipitates and forms the blood clot.

$$\text{Thrombin} + \text{Fibrinogen} \rightarrow \text{Fibrin}$$

Calcium *ions* are necessary for normal clotting. Blood commonly is prevented from clotting by adding some compound that *removes calcium ions.* Sodium or potassium citrate can be used; these salts react with calcium to form calcium citrate, an organic salt that *does not ionize.* Sodium citrate (or a mixture containing sodium citrate, citric acid, and dextrose—ACD, or acid citrate dextrose solution) ordinarily is used to prevent clotting during blood transfusions. *Oxalates* and *fluorides* form insoluble salts with calcium, and also are used to prevent clotting.

Stage 1 of blood clotting requires about three to five minutes for completion. This is the time required for the formation of plasma thromboplastin from its precursors. Activity begins when the platelet factor is released and reacts with the antihemophilic factor (AHF) and other substances present in plasma.

Antihemophilic factor (AHF)
Plasma thromboplastin component (PTC) $\xrightarrow[\text{Factor V}]{Ca^{++}}$ Plasma thromboplastin
Platelet factor
Stuart-Prower factor (X)
Plasma thromboplastin antecedent (PTA)
Hageman factor (XII)

Various tissues of the body contain thromboplastins that apparently exist in an active form. When a tissue thromboplastin is added to blood, clotting occurs in a few seconds.

A classic bleeding disease, hemophilia, in which plasma thromboplastin is formed very slowly, has been recognized for years. It is caused by a deficiency of AHF. This disorder now is know as hemophilia A. Similar, much rarer, bleeding disorders are caused by a deficiency of PTC (hemophilia B or Christmas disease—the first patient recognized as having the disease was named Christmas) and by a deficiency of PTA (hemophilia C). Hemophilia A and B exist mainly in males, but are transmitted by the mother. The other form of hemophilia occurs equally in both sexes.

In *stage 2* inactive prothrombin is converted to active thrombin. The time required for this is eight to fifteen seconds.

$$\text{Prothrombin} \xrightarrow[\text{Accessory factors}]{\text{Thromboplastin} + Ca^{++}} \text{Thrombin}$$

The accessory factors required for tissue thromboplastin are factor V, factor VII, and factor X. Factors V and X, but not factor VII, also are required for plasma thromboplastin.

Stage 3, the conversion of fibrinogen to fibrin, is almost instantaneous.

$$\text{Fibrinogen} \xrightarrow{\text{Thrombin}} \text{Fibrin (blood clot)}$$

Thrombin is an enzyme; it catalyzes the conversion of fibrinogen to insoluble fibrin and some peptides (fibrinopeptides). The newly formed fibrin forms soft, easily dispersible aggregates (soft clots). In the presence of calcium ions, thrombin then activates an enzyme known as fibrin-stabilizing factor (FSF). This active enzyme then catalyzes cross linking between fibrin molecules, producing a final, hard clot.

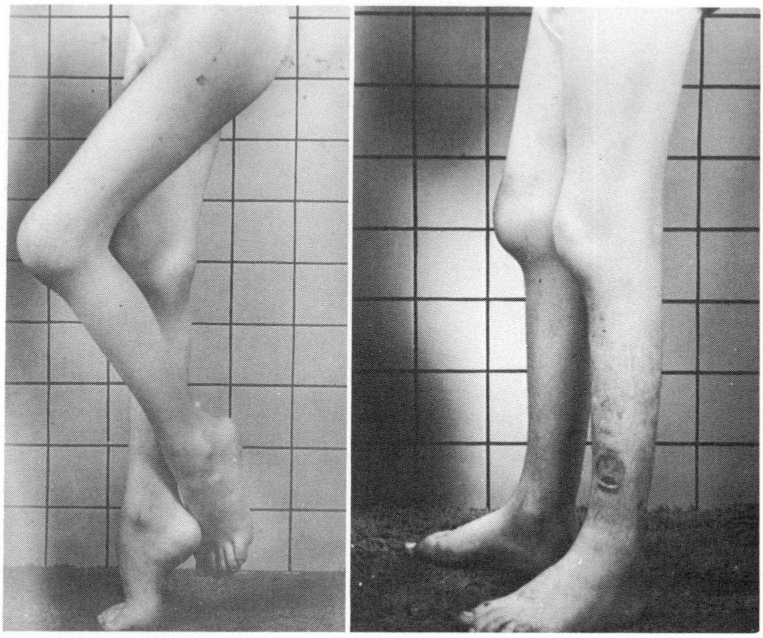

A B

Fig. 30-5. Photograph showing legs of a patient with hemophilia. **A,** Preoperative deformities; **B,** postoperative correction. The preoperative deformities resulted from bleeding into the joints. Is hemophilia more common in males or in females? (Courtesy Dr. William F. Enneking.)

$$\boxed{\text{Fibrin}}-\overset{\overset{\displaystyle O}{\|}}{C}-\boxed{OH + H}-\underset{\underset{\displaystyle H}{|}}{N}-\boxed{\text{Fibrin}} \rightarrow \boxed{\text{Fibrin}}-\overset{\overset{\displaystyle O}{\|}}{C}-\underset{\underset{\displaystyle H}{|}}{N}-\boxed{\text{Fibrin}} + H_2O$$

Soft clots → Hard clots

Tissues and blood contain substances known as *plasminogen activators*. These substances can react with a protein complex in blood, *plasminogen*, to convert it into an active proteolytic enzyme known as *plasmin* or *fibrinolysin*. The situation is complicated by the fact that blood also contains *plasmin inhibitors*. As blood circulates through the blood vessels, if fibrin (a clot) is encountered, any free plasmin present is adsorbed to the fibrin. This separates the plasmin from the inhibitors in the blood, and the active plasmin digests (liquefies) the fibrin. Probably there is a continuous formation of tiny clots in the body as a result of small injuries. The plasmin system tends to protect the blood vessels from becoming permanently closed by these clots.

$$\text{Fibrin} \xrightarrow[\text{(Fibrinolysin)}]{\text{Plasmin}} \text{Lysis}$$

The names of the various factors well recognized as being necessary for normal blood clotting, and the multiple names used for certain of them, are as follows:

Factor I: Fibrinogen
Factor II: Prothrombin
Factor III: Thromboplastin (tissue); Thrombokinase
Factor IV: Calcium

Table 30-3. Diseases of enzymic defect involving blood clotting factors

Factor deficient or lacking	Disease
Factor I. Fibrinogen	Afibrinogenemia (absence of fibrinogen) Hypofibrinogenemia (abnormally low level of fibrinogen)
Factor II. Prothrombin	Hypoprothrombinemia (abnormally low level of prothrombin)
Factor V. Proaccelerin	Parahemophilia
Factor VII. Proconvertin	Hypoproconvertinemia (abnormally low level of proconvertin)
Factor VIII. AHF	Hemophilia A
Factor IX. PTC, Christmas factor	Hemophilia B
Factor XI. PTA	Hemophilia C
Factor XIII. FSF	Thrombopathia hemophilica

Factor V: Labile factor; proaccelerin; plasma Ac (accelerator) globulin
Factor VI: Not assigned
Factor VII: Stable factor; proconvertin; SPCA (serum prothrombin conversion accelerator); co-thromboplastin; auto-prothrombin I
Factor VIII: Antihemophilic factor (AHF); thromboplastinogen; platelet cofactor I; plasma thromboplastic factor A
Factor IX: Plasma thromboplastin component (PTC); Christmas factor; platelet cofactor II; plasma thromboplastic factor B; autoprothrombin II
Factor X: Stuart-Prower factor
Factor XI: Plasma thromboplastin antecedent (PTA)
Factor XII: Hageman factor
Factor XIII: Fibrin stabilizing factor (FSF)

The cascade scheme of blood clotting. An alternative scheme to diagram the steps involved in blood clotting is known as the *cascade* or *waterfall sequence.*

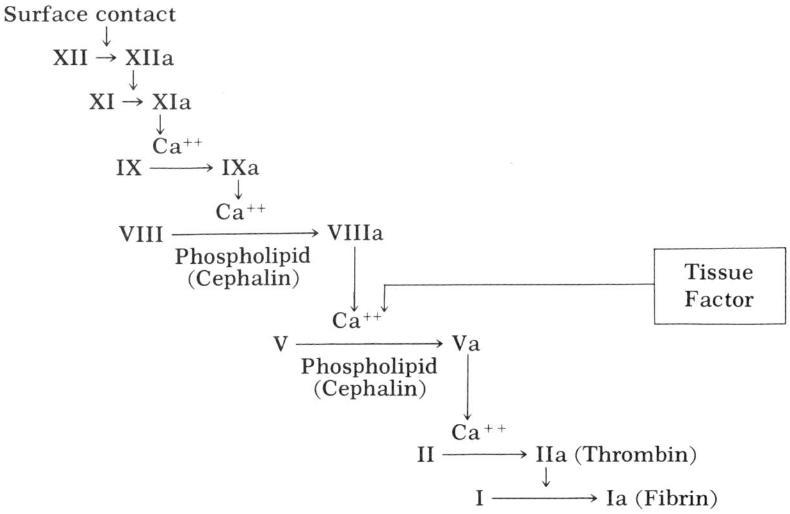

This scheme assumes that the process of blood coagulation is a series of enzyme-catalyzed reactions, each enzyme activating the next one in the sequence.

Other factors. Heparin is an organic compound that has been isolated from the liver and other tissues. Small amounts occur in blood. Heparin prevents blood clotting. It is supposed that the small amount in the blood helps prevent the coagulation of the blood in the blood vessels. There is not enough, however, to prevent clotting when platelets disintegrate in large numbers as they do during hemorrhage (bleeding). Heparin is used in the management of patients in whom there is danger of thrombosis (formation of thrombi, or clots, inside the blood vessels themselves).

Plasma normally contains about 0.2 to 0.5 g of *fibrinogen* in 100 ml. The concentration of *prothrombin* is extremely low and is not known accurately. Both of these proteins are made in the liver and both are deceased in severe liver disease. Almost any infection causes an increase in the concentration of fibrinogen. Fibrinogen also is high during menstruation and pregnancy. It has been found that prothrombin, as well as factors VII, IX, and X; cannot be made in the liver in the absence of *vitamin K*. This vitamin is not absorbed from the intestinal tract in the absence of bile, and bleeding (due to low prothrombin level) easily occurs in conditions in which bile is prevented from reaching the small intestine (obstructive jaundice, biliary fistula). Occasionally, babies have a low prothrombin level at birth and may bleed severely after slight injuries.

The estimation of prothrombin level is done most simply by mixing standardized amounts of oxalated plasma, thromboplastin suspension, and calcium ions. The time required for clotting is measured and is reported as the *prothrombin time*. The time indicating a normal amount of prothrombin in the plasma varies depending on the reagents and conditions under which the test is carried out, but in general, for a given laboratory, it has a rather definite value somewhere between ten seconds and twenty seconds. An *increase* in prothrombin time indicates a *decrease* in the

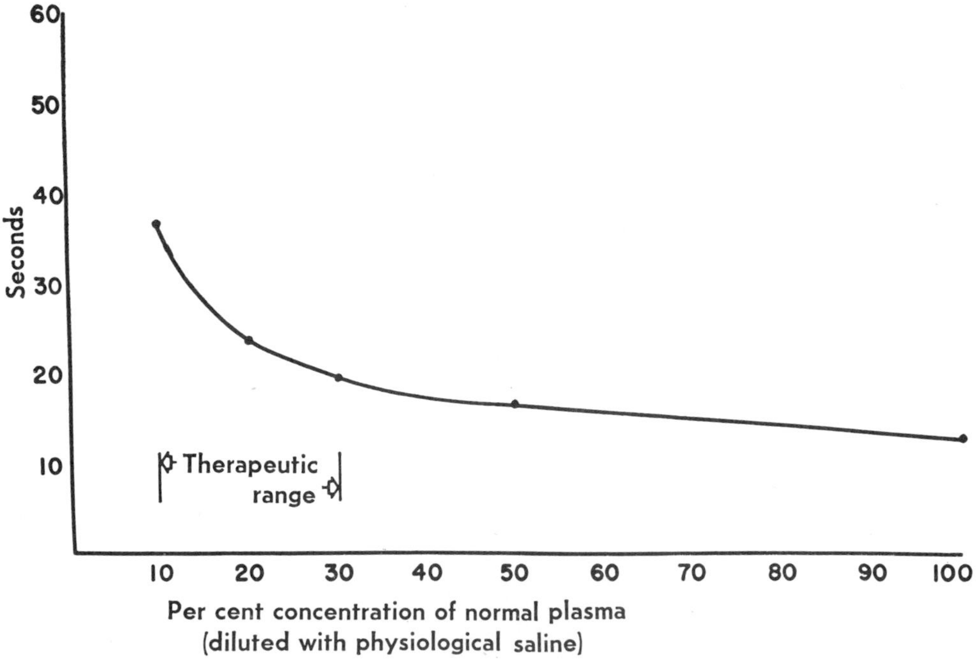

Fig. 30-6. Typical prothrombin activity curve. For what purpose is this curve used? (Courtesy Dr. George Phillips and Mrs. Jane Lenahan.)

concentration of prothrombin in the plasma and suggests that vitamin K should be given to the patient.

Many patients who have had a coronary thrombosis or other illness involving intravascular clotting are given a drug that tends to inhibit clotting as a prophylactic measure. One of the first of these drugs to be used successfully was bishydroxycoumarin (trademark: Dicumarol), a substance first isolated from spoiled sweet clover hay. (The spoiled hay caused a bleeding disease of cattle.)

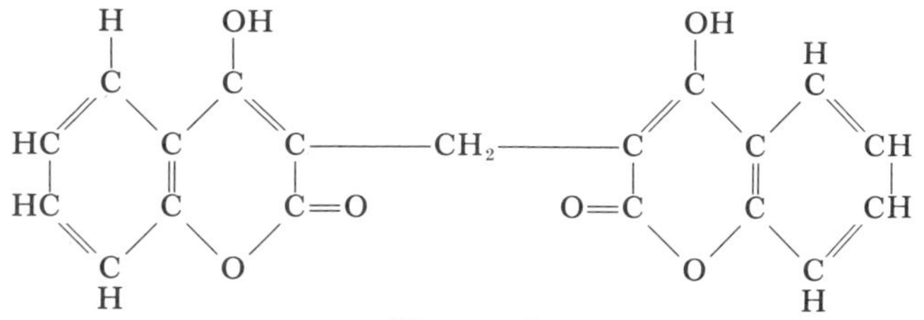

Dicumarol

Dicumarol and similar drugs act to inhibit the formation of prothrombin, factor VII, and factor X by the liver. It is customary to give the patient sufficient drug to lower the activity of these factors to 10 to 25 percent of normal. This corresponds to a prothrombin time of twenty to forty seconds, as the test is carried out by most clinical laboratories.

Platelets and arterial wall damage. When there is a tear in the wall of an artery, bleeding usually occurs. The tearing exposes the media (layer of the arterial wall beneath the intima, or inner lining) of the artery to the blood. The media, like other types of supporting tissue, contains a protein known as *collagen* (see page 269). Platelets adhere to this collagen. The attached platelets then release ADP (see page 209), which reacts in some way with platelet membranes. This causes several layers of platelets to adhere to those attached to the collagen. This forms a platelet plug, which seals the lesion. The ADP also activates a contractile protein (similar to the contractile protein of muscle), leading to its contraction or shortening. This in turn decreases the average size of each platelet and leads to closer packing.

The immobilized platelets intitiate the formation of fibrin (by means of the clotting mechanism; see page 358), which forms a seal around the platelet plug.

Much research is underway based on the hypothesis that this same sequence of events can be detrimental by causing the formation of the thrombus (blood clot) that is responsible for coronary artery occlusion—the major cause of death in persons more than 45 years of age. This might occur if a crack developed in the wall of a coronary artery, this exposing collagen in the media of the vessel to the blood. The events described above then should occur. If now the blood clotting initiated by the immobilized platelets resulted in a sizeable (relative to the diameter of the artery) clot around and on the platelet plug, the artery would be occluded and a coronary attack would occur.

Sedimentation rate. If a sample of oxalated or citrated blood is drawn into a long capillary tube and the tube then is maintained in a vertical position, the red blood cells slowly settle downward, leaving a clear zone of plasma at the top of the tube. The normal rate of settling differs in different laboratories, depending on the anticoagulant used, the shape and size of the capillary tube, and the temperature; and each laboratory should standardize the procedure used with samples of blood from normal people. The *sedimentation rate (erythrocyte sedimentation rate, ESR)* is reported in millimeters per hour. It is increased in pregnancy, menstruation, certain chronic infections (for example, tuberculosis), some acute infections (for example, rheumatic fever), some chronic metabolic diseases (for example, rheumatoid arthritis), and in many cases of cancer. This cause of the increased rate of sedimentation in these conditions is an increased tendency to the red blood cells to clump together, forming aggregates that settle more rapidly than do single cells. Variations in the plasma globulins and perhaps also in the fibrinogen content are thought to be responsible for this increased tendency of the cells to clump together.

PLASMA ENZYMES. Numerous enzymes (all proteins) occur in plasma. Several of these are of particular importance in diagnosis.

Acid phosphatase is an enzyme that catalyzes the hydrolysis of phosphoric acid esters. It is most active at a rather low pH (3 to 4). The amount in plasma often is increased in cancer of the prostate gland and in certain diseases of the bones. There is recent evidence that many types of cancer are accompanied by an increased level of acid phosphatase in the plasma.

Alkaline phosphatase also catalyzes the hydrolysis of phosphate esters, but its optimal pH lies between 8 and 9. It is elevated in generalized fibrosis of the bones, rickets, and some other diseases of bone. It occurs in bile, and diseases causing obstruction of the bile ducts usually are accompanied by an increased level of the enzyme in the plasma.

Hypophosphatasia is a rare chronic familial disease of children. The disease is associated with an abnormally low level of alkaline phosphatase in the serum and tissues. The characteristic clinical feature is deficient bone formation, with microscopic changes resembling those of rickets (see page 439).

In disease of the pancreas (pancreatitis) various pancreatic enzymes may appear in the blood and urine in increased amounts. (Traces of them are present normally.) When pancreatitis is suspected, it is common hospital practice to test the blood for *amylase*. If this enzyme is present in a concentration greater than normal, the diagnosis of acute pancreatitis is strengthened.

Glutamic oxalacetic aminopherase (transaminase) is an enzyme that catalyzes the transfer of an amino group ($—NH_2$) from glutamic acid to oxalacetic acid.

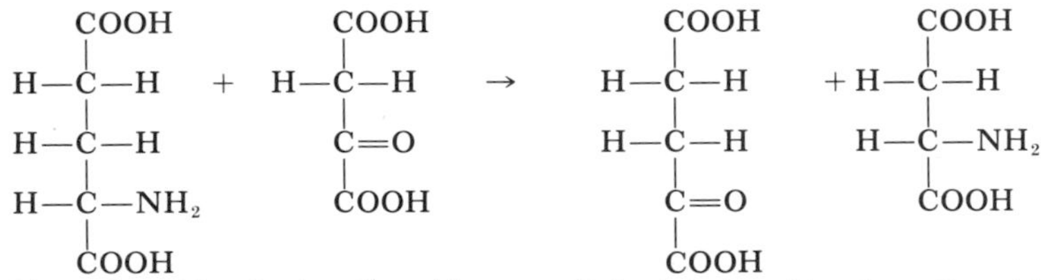

Glutamic acid Oxalacetic acid α-Ketoglutaric acid Aspartic acid

The amount of this enzyme detectable in blood increases from two- to twentyfold after an acute heart attack (myocardial infarction). It increases from twenty- to one hundredfold in the presence of liver disease (hepatitis) caused by toxic or infectious agents. *Lactic dehydrogenase* is another enzyme whose level in the blood increases as a result of acute heart or liver disease (see page 217).

Two enzymes whose level in serum increases following a myocardial infarction (coronary attack) are *creatine phosphokinase* (SCPK) and hydroxybutyrate dehydrogenase (SHBD). SCPK levels increase about fivefold within a few hours and return to normal in three days. SHBD levels increase within 48 hours and remain elevated for two weeks or more.

NON-PROTEIN NITROGEN

The nonprotein nitrogen (npn) of the blood is determined by first removing the blood proteins and then determining all the nitrogen that remains. This nitrogen is present in compounds such as urea, uric acid, creatine, creatinine, ammonium salts, amino acids, and bilirubin. These substances are not secreted at a normal rate in *uremia*. A high nonprotein value thus is a chemical sign of uremia. Normal nonprotein nitrogen values range between 25 and 35 mg per 100 ml of blood.

The chemical determination of the amount of urea in the blood usually is done in such a way that the nitrogen present in urea, rather than urea itself, is determined. The value found is reported as *blood urea nitrogen (bun)*. The normal value is 10 to 15 mg per 100 ml of blood. Like the npn, the bun is elevated in uremia. High values also are found in *Addison's disease*, which is caused by destruction of the outer portion of the adrenal glands.

Another important compound contributing to the nonprotein nitrogen of the blood is *uric acid* (see page 313). The amount normally present in 100 ml of blood is 3 to 6 mg. The level of uric acid is increased in gout (see page 313), toxemias of pregnancy, leukemia, polycythemia, and uremia.

CAUSES OF UREMIA. There are three principal causes of uremia: (1) Disease of the kidney so that this organ is unable to excrete waste products at a normal rate. (2) Dehydration, or excessive loss of water from the body. If this is severe, the kidney is unable to obtain sufficient water to form urine. (3) Severe heart disease, in which the blood pressure falls to such a low value in the kidney capillaries that it is incapable of forcing fluid from the blood into the kidney tubules.

ICTERUS INDEX. Most of the color of jaundiced plasma is from the presence of bilirubin. A rough measure of the concentration of bilirubin in plasma can be made by determining how many times the plasma must be diluted with water or saline solution in order that the color of the diluted material match that of a 0.01 percent solution of potassium dichromate. This dilution factor is known as the *icterus index*. For example, if 1 ml of plasma must be diluted with 24 ml of water, the icterus index of the plasma is 25 (since the volume of the original plasma has been increased 25 times). Average normal values for the icterus index vary from about 4 to 7. When jaundice can be recognized on physical examination of the patient, the icterus index generally is higher than 15. In conditions in which the rate of hemoglobin destruction and consequently of bilirubin formation is below normal, values lower than 4 may be found. For example, a low value may be found in iron deficiency anemia.

VAN DEN BERGH REACTION. When the diazo reagent (a specially prepared mixture of nitrous and sulfanilic acids) is added to plasma taken from a patient with jaundice, a red color is produced. This color is caused by a reaction involving the bilirubin in the plasma. The color may appear almost instantly *(direct prompt van den Bergh test)*. If it does not develop for a number of minutes, the reaction is said to be a *direct delayed van den Bergh test*. Sometimes no color appears unless alcohol is present in the reacting mixture. In this case the reaction is reported as an *indirect van den Bergh test*. Finally, the addition of the diazo reagent to the plasma may result in the appearance of some color, but more color may develop if the mixture is allowed to stand. This result is known as a *biphasic van den Bergh test*.

Plasma from a patient with obstructive jaundice usually gives a direct prompt test, whereas plasma from a patient with hemolytic jaundice ordinarily gives either an indirect test or a direct delayed test. Diphasic reactions are of little help in deciding what type of jaundice the patient has, since such reactions may be given sometimes by either type (obstructive or hemolytic) of jaundiced plasma.

It has been found that the bilirubin responsible for the indirect van den Bergh test is bound to plasma protein but is not otherwise chemically combined. In this form it is rather insoluble in water, and alcohol must be present in order that color formation proceed when the diazo reagent is added. As bilirubin passes through the liver cells into the bile, it is conjugated (combined chemically) with glucuronic acid to form bilirubin monoglucuronide and bilirubin diglucuronide. Small amounts of bilirubin sulfate also are formed. In these forms it is water soluble and will react with the diazo reagent in the absence of alcohol. In obstructive types of jaundice the direct-acting bilirubin in the blood has passed through the liver into the bile, but has found its way back into the blood because of the obstruction to the outflow of bile. Bilirubin is excreted in the urine in obstructive jaundice but not in hemolytic jaundice. In other words, bilirubin cannot be excreted by the kidney except when it is combined with glucuronic or sulfuric acid.

In the rare congenital disease known as *Gilbert's disease*, the enzyme uridine diphosphate glucuronate transferase is lacking from the liver. As a result, bilirubin is not excreted properly, and an intense jaundice results. Babies with this condition may develop staining and damage of parts of the brain (kernicterus).

BLOOD SUGAR LEVEL

The normal sugar of the blood is *glucose (dextrose)*. Its metabolism has been discussed in Chapter 24. In a fasting normal individual the value of the blood glucose level usually is between 70 and 100 mg per 100 ml. Some methods give slightly higher values (up to 120 mg per 100 ml). The most common cause of an elevated fasting blood glucose level is diabetes mellitus (see page 264). Asphyxia, emotional states, and certain diseases of the endocrine (hormone) glands also are accompanied by high levels. Low fasting levels are found in hyperinsulinism (see page 265) and in some types of liver disease.

The *glucose tolerance test* has been described on page 264.

PLASMA LIPIDS

Although lipids are not soluble in water, plasma contains appreciable quantities of them (normally approximately 700 mg per 100 ml). This is explained by the fact that they have been solubilized by combining loosely with various proteins in the α-globulin and β-globulin fractions of the plasma proteins (see page 234). Fats, phospholipids, and sterols are represented.

Cholesterol occurs in blood both as the free compound and as esters. (Both forms are combined loosely with proteins.) The total level of cholesterol varies normally from 150 to 230 mg per 100 ml of plasma. It is increased in nephrosis, hypothyroidism, uncontrolled diabetes mellitus, biliary obstruction, and pregnancy. It is lowered in hyperthyroidism, uremia, and certain infections.

SOME IMPORTANT INORGANIC COMPONENTS

Water is the most abundant compound of the blood, as it is of the body as a whole. Plasma is 90 to 92 percent water, and the red blood cells contain 64 to 65 percent of it. The metabolism of water has been discussed in Chapter 29.

In human blood, *sodium* is found chiefly in the plasma and *potassium*, mainly in the red blood cells. The importance of these elements in the transport of CO_2 has been discussed elsewhere in this chapter, as has the role of sodium in the regulation of the acid-base balance of the blood. The level of plasma sodium normally is 300 to 330 mg per 100 ml (130 to 143 milliequivalents per liter*). The plasma sodium level is elevated in excep-

*Often it is convenient to report the concentrations of electrolytes in blood as milliequivalents per liter. A milliequivalent is the equivalent weight (see page 58) divided by 1,000. In other words, it is the equivalent weight in milligrams rather than in grams. A concentration of 320 mg of sodium per 100 ml can be converted to milliequivalents per liter as follows: First multiply by 10 in order to calculate the milligrams of Na per *liter*. This gives a value of 3,200 mg per liter. Since the valence of Na is 1, and since its atomic weight is 23, then 3,200 mg per liter = 3,200 ÷ 23 = 139 milliequivalents per liter.

tional cases of overactivity of the adrenal glands. It is lowered in Addison's disease (see page 431). Thc normal level of potassium in the plasma is 14 to 20 mg per 100 ml (3.5 to 5.0 milliequivalents per liter). This level is elevated in Addison's disease, uncontrolled diabetes mellitus, uremia, intestinal obstruction, and some acute infections. It is lowered in hyperinsulinism, and in the disease known as familial periodic paralysis.

Calcium and *magnesium* ordinarily are determined in serum since the addition of the usual anticoagulants to blood before the removal of the plasma interferes with the determination. Calcium is not present in the red blood cells. Its normal concentration in serum is 9 to 11.5 mg per 100 ml (4.5 to 5.7 milliequivalents per liter). Its level is elevated in hyperparathyroidism (see page 397), multiple myeloma (see page 376), and in certain diseases of the bones (for example, Paget's disease). Its level is lowered in nephrosis, tetany (see page 343), gluten enteropathy (see page 329), and osteomalacia (see page 440). The level of magnesium in serum is low – 1 to 3 mg per 100 ml (0.8 to 2.5 milliequivalents per liter). It is elevated in hyperparathyroidism and is low in hypoparathyroidism and infantile tetany.

The *inorganic phosphorus* content of plasma normally is 3 to 4 mg per 100 ml (1.9 to 2.6 milliequivalents per liter*) for adults and 4 to 6 mg per 100 ml (2.6 to 3.9 milliequivalents per liter) for children. It is lowered in rickets, gluten enteropathy, and hyperparathyroidism and is increased in hypoparathyroidism, uremia, and nephritis.

Exceedingly small amounts of *iodine* occur in blood. A portion of this is present as part of a protein molecule (see page 390). The level of this "protein-bound iodine" is increased in hyperthyroidism and is decreased in hypothyroidism (see page 391).

The major portion of the iron present in blood has a valence of 2^+ and is combined as a part of the hemoglobin molecule (see page 277). However, normal plasma contains 0.05 to 0.18 mg (50 to 180 μg) of ferric iron (Fe with a valence of 3^+) per 100 ml. This iron is bound to one of the proteins (transferrin) in the plasma globulin fraction of the plasma proteins. The level of plasma iron is low in the anemias because of iron deficiency. It

*Most of the inorganic phosphorus in plasma or serum exists as the ion $HPO_4^{=}$. Since this ion has a valence of 2, the equivalent weight of the phosphorus present is approximately 15.5 (one-half the atomic weight, which is 30.9738). If a sample of plasma contains 3 mg per 100 ml the number of milligrams per liter present is 30. Hence, 3 mg per 100 ml = 30 ÷ 15.5 = approximately 1.9 milliequivalents per liter.

Table 30-4. Enzymes that are deficient in hemolytic diseases

6-Phosphogluconate dehydrogenase	Pyruvate kinase
Glucose-6-phosphate dehydrogenase	Glutathione peroxidase
Glucose phosphate insomerase	Glutathione reductase
Triose phosphate isomerase	Glutathione synthetase
Hexokinase	2,3-Diphosphoglycerate mutase
Adenosine triphosphatse	Phosphoglycerate kinase

is elevated in aplastic anemia (failure of the bone marrow to produce hemoglobin) and in untreated pernicious anemia (see pages 324 and 431).

Hemolytic diseases due to enzymic defect. Hemolytic diseases are characterized by rupture of red blood cells and the appearance of extracellular hemoglobin in the blood. In some cases, this condition is due to an enzymic defect (Table 30-4).

STUDY QUESTIONS

1. What fraction of the human body is blood?
2. What is meant by the term "formed elements?" Plasma?
3. What are erythrocytes? Leukocytes? Thrombocytes? What is the function of each?
4. List several important functions of the blood.
5. How much loosely combined oxygen is present in 1 g of fully oxygenated hemoglobin (oxyhemoglobin)?
6. What force causes oxygen to move from the alveoli of the lungs into the blood?
7. About how much blood passes through the lungs in an hour?
8. Calculate the approximate amount of hemoglobin present in the body.
9. How much loosely bound oxygen is present in 100 ml of arterial blood?
10. What is the oxygen tension of the tissues?
11. List the factors that favor the conversion of oxyhemoglobin to reduced hemoglobin in the tissues.
12. Are most of the potassium ions of the blood in the red blood cells or in the plasma? Most of the sodium ions?
13. Write a series of symbolic equations summarizing the chemical changes that take place when carbon dioxide enters the blood.
14. How do you explain the fact that carbonic anhydrase catalyzes the *formation* of carbonic acid in the tissues and the *breakdown* of carbonic acid in the lung capillaries?
15. What is meant by the term *chloride shift*? Explain why it occurs.
16. About what percentage of the combined carbon dioxide of the blood is transported as carbamate? As free gas?
17. What is the partial pressure (tension) of carbon dioxide in the tissues? In the alveoli of the lungs?
18. What percentage of the bicarbonate of the blood is in the plasma?
19. Which has the greater tendency to combine with potassium ions: reduced hemoglobin or oxyhemoglobin?
20. Approximately what percentage of the free and combined carbon dioxide is removed during the passage of blood through the lungs?
21. Approximately what percentage of the loosely bound oxygen is removed during the passage of the blood through the tissues?
22. What two substances are the most important buffers of the blood?
23. Name some other buffers present in blood.
24. What is acidosis? Alkalosis?
25. What is the alkali reserve?
26. What is meant by CO_2 *combining power*? How is it determined? How does it help in the detection of acidosis?
27. What is the role of the kidney in acid-base balance?
28. What four protein fractions are found in plasma? What is the function of each?
29. For what purpose is immune serum globulin used in medicine?
30. Write symbols for the 4 types of immunoglobulins. Which of them is most abundant in normal serum?
31. What is the usual cause of death in disease characterized by a low level of immunoglobulin?
32. What is C-reactive protein?
33. What are haptoglobins?
34. Name four important causes of edema. Name one condition in which each of these causes is present.
35. Describe how a low level of plasma protein can cause edema. Name some diseases or conditions in which the concentrations of serum albumin and serum globulin are abnormal.
36. Explain why serum albumin is more important in preventing edema than is serum globulin.
37. What are lymphatics? Where does lymph go after it enters the lymphatics?
38. In your own words explain what happens when blood clots.
39. Name some substances that can be used to prevent blood coagulation. How do they work?
40. What is heparin?
41. How do fibrinogen and prothrombin con-

centrations vary in disease? What vitamin is necessary for the formation of prothrombin? What organ makes fibrinogen and prothrombin?
42. Describe how platelets react to an injury to the wall of an artery.
43. Outline one possible cause of coronary occlusion.
44. What is the ESR? What is its significance? Name one *normal* condition in which it is increased.
45. Name one disease in which unusually high blood levels of each of the following occur: acid phosphatase, alkaline phosphatase, amylase.
46. What is meant by npn? Name some compounds that make up the npn. What is the interpretation of a high value for the npn?
47. What is meant by bun? What is the normal value of the bun? How does this value change in uremia?
48. What is uremia? Name three causes of uremia.
49. Name a disease in which each of the following laboratory determinations might be helpful in making a diagnosis: icterus index; van den Bergh test. Explain.
50. What is the most common cause of an elevated fasting blood sugar level?
51. Name some lipids found in blood.
52. What solubilizes the plasma lipids?
53. In what direction does the blood cholesterol level vary from normal in hyperthyroidism? In hypothyroidism?
54. What is the most abundant compound in the blood?
55. What percentage of plasma is water?
56. Name one disease in which the plasma level of each of the following inorganic substances is high and one in which it is low: sodium, potassium, calcium, magnesium, inorganic phosphorus, protein-bound iodine, plasma iron.
57. Are hemolytic diseases ever caused by enzyme deficiencies?

CHAPTER 31

Urine

The waste products of the body are excreted through the skin, the lungs, the kidneys, and in the feces. Water, salts, nitrogenous compounds, and some lipid material are lost through the skin. The lungs excrete water and carbon dioxide. Some metals may be excreted in the feces, which also contain nitrogenous compounds, soaps, and indigestible carbohydrates. The most important organ of excretion is the kidney. We shall find that normally the substances in the urine are mainly inorganic salts and compounds of nitrogen (protein derivatives), but various derivatives of carbohydrates and lipids also can be found in this fluid, particularly in pathological conditions.

FORMATION OF URINE

Blood enters the kidneys by means of the renal arteries. When these arteries enter the kidney, they break up into smaller and smaller branches until thousands of tiny arterioles are formed. Each of these arterioles finally becomes a vessel with thin walls, called a capillary. This capillary coils up to form a *glomerulus,* a mass like a ball of knitting yarn (see Fig. 31-2). A structure called Bowman's capsule surrounds each glomerulus. Passing out from each Bowman's capsule is a small tubule. These small tubules from all parts of the kidney join with each other to form larger tubules, called *collecting tubules*. Finally, the collecting tubules combine to form the *ureter,* a tube that conveys the urine from the kidney to the urinary bladder. Urine passes from the bladder to the outside by means of a single tube, called the *urethra*.

The thin walls of the capillaries that make up the glomerulus act as ultrafilters; that is, all molecules in solution in the blood plasma, except the protein molecules, can pass through the glomerular walls into Bowman's capsule and so into the tubules. The fluid in Bowman's capsule is an *ultrafiltrate*—it has the same composition as blood plasma, except that it is normally free of protein. As this ultrafiltrate passes down the tubule, how-

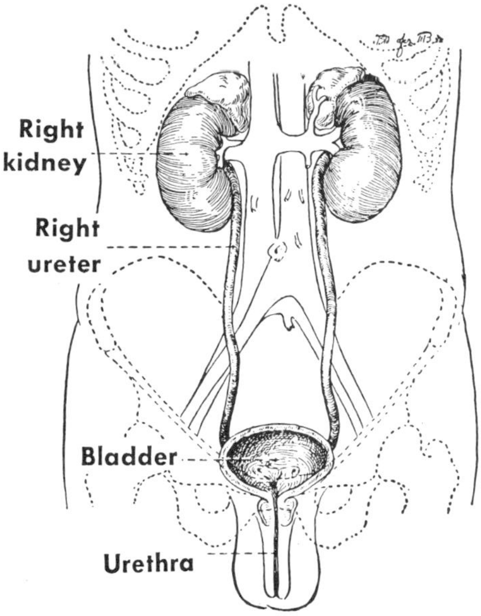

Fig. 31-1. The urinary system in the male. What is the function of this system?

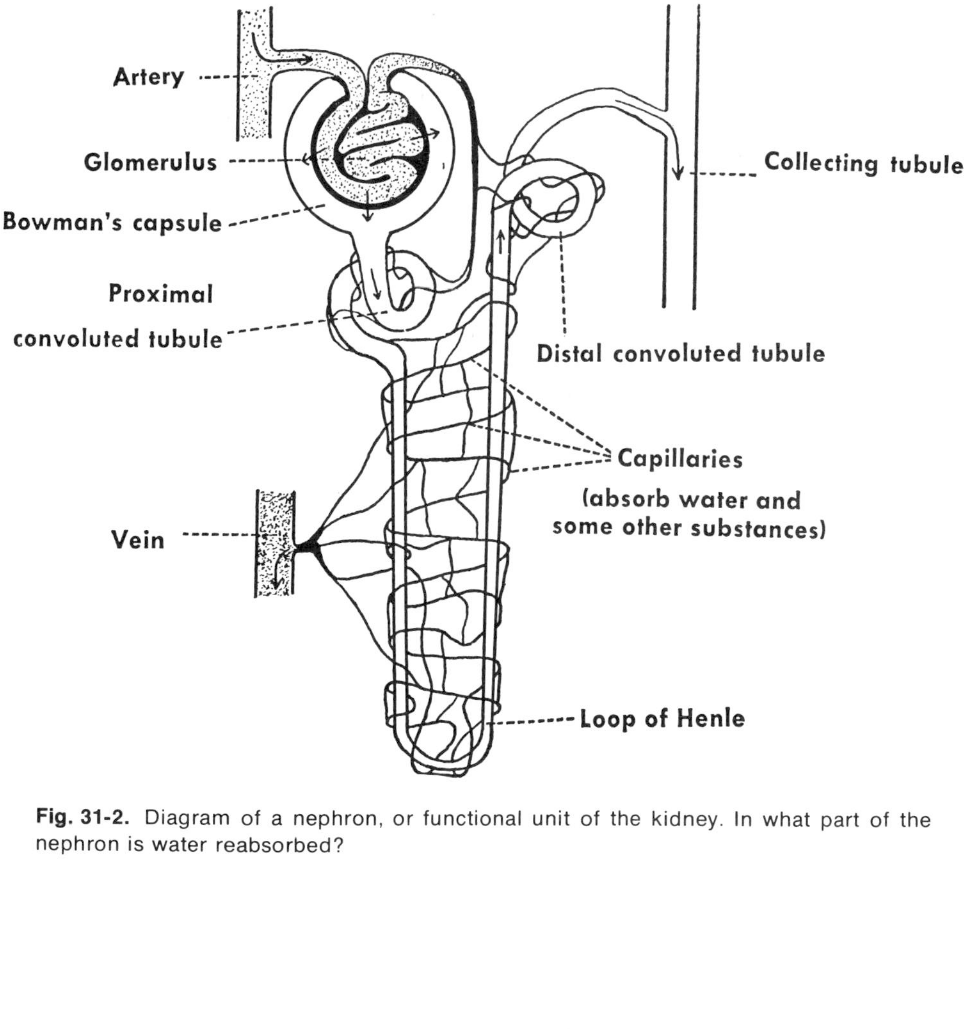

Fig. 31-2. Diagram of a nephron, or functional unit of the kidney. In what part of the nephron is water reabsorbed?

ever, a large proportion of the water, chlorides, and bicarbonates is reabsorbed from the tubules and passes back into the blood. All, or nearly all, the glucose is reabsorbed in this way. Certain substances, such as ammonium salts and hippuric acid, appear to be made in the cells that line the tubules and are secreted directly into the urine by these cells. The urine that reaches the urinary bladder can be represented, then, by the following word equation:

Urine = Glomerular ultrafiltrate − Substances reabsorbed + Substances secreted
in tubules by cells of tubules

The importance of absorption in the tubules is better appreciated when we learn that the volume of glomerular ultrafiltrate for one day amounts to something between 100 and 200 liters. Of this amount only about 1 to 1.5 liters reaches the urinary bladder, the rest being reabsorbed in the tubules.

COLLECTION OF URINE FOR ANALYSIS

The amounts of various substances passing out of the body in the urine vary greatly at different times of the day. If we want to know how much of a given substance is excreted in one day, it is necessary to collect the urine for a twenty-four-hour period. This is desirable, although often not done, even if we only want to know whether or not some abnormal substance is present because this substance may be present only at certain times of the day. The most convenient way to obtain a twenty-four-hour specimen is to discard the first morning voiding and to preserve all the urine pased up to and including the first voiding of the following morning. It is sometimes necessary to obtain the urine of females by catheterization—that is, by inserting a small rubber tube (a catheter) through the urethra and directly into the bladder—in order to avoid contamination of the urine by material from the vagina. If the urine cannot be analyzed immediately, it can be preserved by adding a small crystal of thymol to it or by covering it with a thin layer of toluene, an organic liquid.

VOLUME OF URINE

The volume of urine depends chiefly on the amount of water that the patient drinks. The average twenty-four-hour excretion for men is from 1,000 to 1,500 ml. The figure for women is somewhat lower. From one-third to two-thirds of the water ingested is eliminated in the urine, the remainder leaving the body by way of the skin, lungs, and feces. On a hot day or after violent exercise the loss from the skin may be considerable, whereas almost no water can be lost by this route if the outside air is saturated with moisture.

Oliguria means a decrease in the output of urine; *anuria* means a total lack of urine excretion. In diseases accompanied by fever, oliguria occurs because an increased amount of water is lost from the skin and lungs. It also occurs in diseases of the kidney in which the damaged kidney is unable to form a normal amount of urine. Mercury bichloride damages the kidney and causes oliguria or anuria. If the wrong type of blood is injected into the patient's veins for transfusion, some of the red blood cells disintegrate and release free hemoglobin. This hemoglobin damages the glomerular membrane and escapes into the kidney tubules. Here it may precipitate and "plug up" the tubules, preventing the escape of urine. This results in oliguria or anuria and may lead to death because of the resulting uremia. Anything that causes uremia is likely to cause oliguria or anuria.

Polyuria means an increased flow of urine. The most common cause of polyuria is the ingestion of large quantities of water. Substances such as alcohol that stimulate a flow of urine also cause it. Polyuria is a prominent symptom of diabetes mellitus, in which large quantities of glucose are present in the urine. Diabetes insipidus causes the most striking polyuria of any pathological condition, and there is a case on record in which a patient with this disease excreted 50 liters of urine in one day. Drugs that cause polyuria are called *diuretics*. They are used often in treating diseases accompanied by edema, the idea being to diminish the edema by causing an increased loss of water in the urine.

COLOR OF URINE

Dilute urine has a pale yellow color, while that of concentrated urine is dark brown. The color of an average normal sample is described as amber. A number of pigments occur normally in the urine, the most abundant of them being *urochrome*. Urochrome is thought by some to be formed, along with bilirubin, during the breakdown of hemoglobin. Urobilin is present in small amounts. Since approximately the same amount of urochrome is excreted every day, the color of normal urine depends almost entirely on the urine volume. If this is large, the color is pale yellow; if it is small, the urine is concentrated and the color is brown.

Urine that contains fresh blood has a red color. If the bloody urine has remained for some time in the bladder (as it may do in such conditions as enlargement of the prostate gland, which prevents complete expulsion of the urine), its color is dark brown or black, because of the formation of methemoglobin. Visible blood in the urine is due usually to violent accidents or to cancer, but it may be present in other conditions. The urine of a patient with obstructive jaundice has a brown color from the presence of bilirubin. If urine is shaken, the foam produced is usually white, but in the presence of bile pigment (bilirubin) it is brown. Melanin is present in the urine of some patients with malignant melanoma (melanosarcoma), a type of cancer that is usually fatal; such urine has a black color. Alkaptonuria is a rare disorder characterized by the excretion of homogentisic acid in the urine; such urine is normal in color when freshly voided but turns dark on standing. Various drugs may color the urine, as may also certain pigments found in food (for example, the pigment of beets). Some of the dyes used to color candies are excreted in the urine.

When urine is taken for analysis from a female patient during her menstrual period, care should be taken to avoid mixing menstrual blood with the urine sample.

SPECIFIC GRAVITY OF URINE

The weight of a given volume of urine as compared with the weight of an equal volume of pure water is called the *specific gravity* of the urine. For example, the weight of 1 liter of water is 1,000 g. If a liter of a sample of urine weighs 1,018 g, the specific gravity of the urine is $^{1,018}/_{1,000} = 1.018$. The specific gravity of normal urine varies considerably depending on the amount of dissolved material present, but an average sample ordinarily will have a specific gravity of about 1.018 (1.016 to 1.020). In diabetes insipidus the urine is very dilute, and the specific gravity is close to that of water (1.000). In diabetes mellitus, on the other hand, large amounts of dissolved solids (chiefly glucose) are present, and the specific gravity is higher than normal. The urine of chronic glomerulonephritis has almost the same specific gravity as an ultrafiltrate of blood plasma (1.010). In this condition only a relatively small number of glomeruli are functioning, and the tubules do not concentrate the urine properly. As a result the urine excreted is almost the same in composition as the glomerular filtrate.

REACTION OF URINE

The reaction (acidity or alkalinity) of the urine varies with the diet. Meats tend to make the urine acid, while most vegetables and fruits cause an alkaline reaction. The average pH of urine is between 5.5 and 7; that is, the urine ordinarily is slightly acid. This is because we eath both animal and plant foods (meats and vegetables). The urine of a person who eats only vegetables will have a pH that is higher than 7.

Ketosis causes an acid urine as a rule because of the excretion of acid salts of the ketone bodies. Certain salts that give an acid reaction when dissolved in water, such as ammonium chloride, ammonium nitrate, and sodium biphosphate, are excreted in the urine and cause the pH to be lowered. Salts like sodium bicarbonate cause a rise in the pH of the urine. Some types of bacteria that cause disease in the urinary tract also influence the urinary pH.

The exact pH of urine is seldom determined in ordinary routine urinalysis, but the urine always is tested with indicator papers to see whether it is acid or alkaline.

COMPOSITION OF URINE

The compounds found in normal urine are chiefly inorganic salts and organic nitrogen-containing compounds. The inorganic salts present include the sulfates, chlorides, phosphates, and bicarbonates of sodium, calcium, magnesium, potassium, and ammonium. The most abundant of these salts is sodium chloride. The excretion of this substance amounts to about 10 to 15 g a day. The principal organic compounds of normal urine are as follows:

1. Urea – 25 to 30 g per day
2. Uric acid – about 0.6 g per day
3. Creatinine – about 15 to 25 mg per kg of body weight
4. Small amounts of indican, hippuric acid, and amino acids
5. Various pigments, chiefly urochrome

ABNORMAL COMPONENTS OF URINE

Some abnormal components of urine include glucose, lactose, pentoses, plasma proteins, Bence Jones protein, urobilinogen, indican, and ketone bodies.

GLUCOSE. Under normal circumstances glucose either is absent entirely from urine or is present in such small amounts that a test given with Benedict's solution or with other reagents yields negative results. The causes of glycosuria have been given on page 266.

LACTOSE. Lactose may occur in the urine during pregnancy and lactation. It reduces Benedict's reagent and may be mistaken for glucose. We remember, however, that glucose is destroyed (ferments) when urine con-

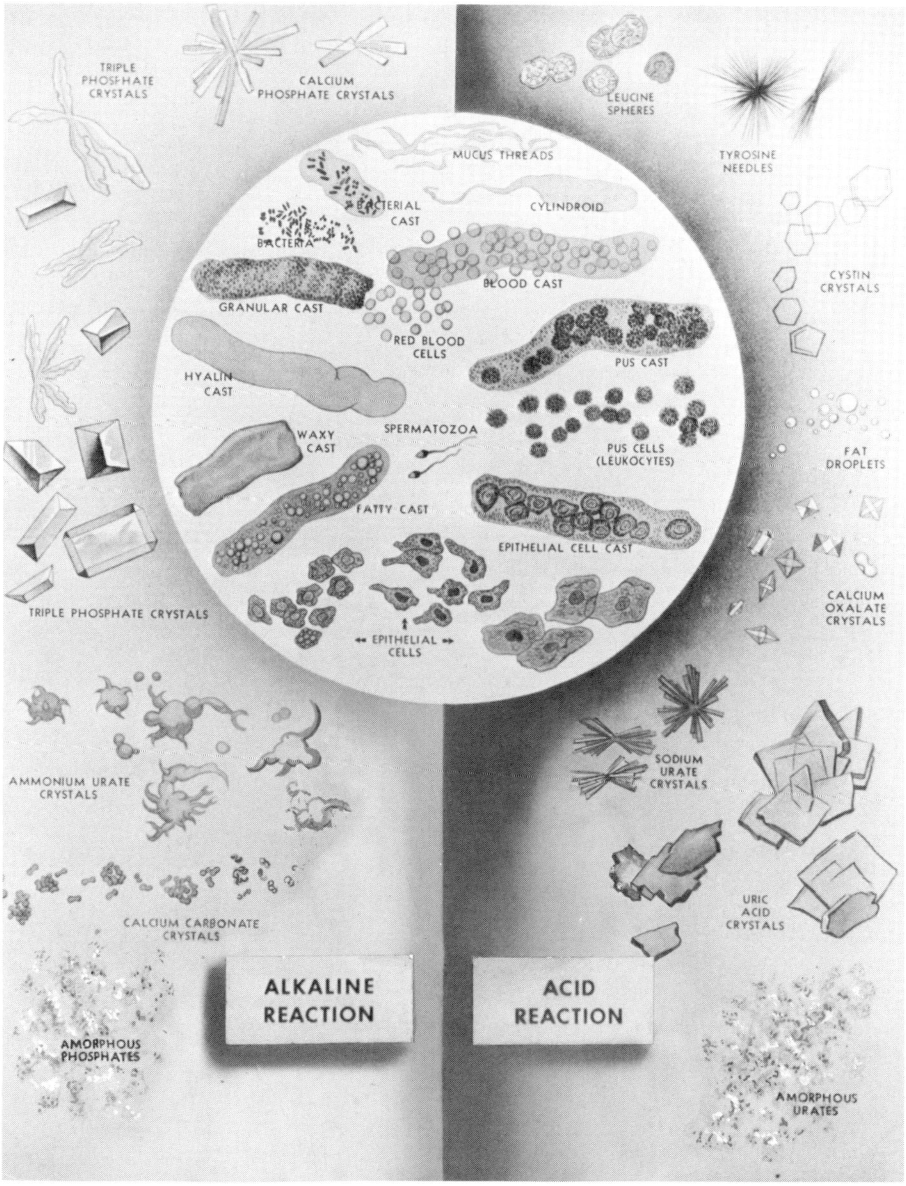

Fig. 31-3. Some structures indicative of disease found by microscopic examination of urine sediment. A few red and white blood cells may be found in normal urine sediment, but large numbers of them indicate disease. What precautions may be required in obtaining urine for examination from some female patients? Why? (Courtesy Merck Sharp & Dohme Division of Merck & Co., Inc.)

taining it is mixed with brewer's yeast, whereas lactose is not. If a urine sample still gives a positive Benedict test after it has been incubated with yeast, we know that some sugar other than glucose (probably lactose) is present.

PENTOSES. Pentoses occasionally are present in the urine. Pentosuria (pentose in the urine) is a rare condition and apparently does not result in harm to the patient. Pentoses reduce Benedict's solution but can be distinguished from glucose with the aid of Bial's reagent (see page 266).

PLASMA PROTEINS. Normally, urine is free from protein except for a small amount of mucin secreted in the urinary tract. Pressure on the renal blood vessels causes some damage to the glomerular membrane, possibly because of the temporary diminution in the blood and oxygen supply, and protein appears in the urine. Certain patients, who are said to have *orthostatic albuminuria,* have protein in the urine unless they lie quietly in bed. Such patients probably have unusual anatomical arrangements of the kidney blood vessels, and these vessels probably are compressed when the patient stands. Protein also occurs in the urine in many infectious diseases, in various types of kidney disease (nephritis, nephrosis, amyloid disease of the kidney, and others), in severe heart disease, in eclampsia (a convulsive condition that is a complication of pregnancy), and in many other conditions. The protein present is usually *albumin,* since this is the plasma protein that has the smallest molecule. If globulin is present also, it is a sign that the damage to the glomerular membrane is more extensive than if albumin alone is found. The presence of protein in the urine is called *proteinuria* or, frequently, *albuminuria.*

The presence of protein is detected most easily by heating a sample of urine. Protein will precipitate if it is present. Phosphates also will precipitate if the urine is alkaline. The addition of acetic acid will dissolve precipitated phosphates but not protein. Other tests for proteinuria are available, but the heat test is the simplest and is most commonly used.

BENCE JONES PROTEIN. This is a peculiar protein that appears in the urine in about 70 percent of cases of multiple myeloma, a disease involving the bone marrow. It is present sometimes in other bone marrow diseases, such as leukemia and cancer. Bence Jones protein has a smaller molecular weight than any of the plasma proteins. It has the peculiar property of precipitating at about 60° C and redissolving again when the urine is boiled (100° C). If the boiling urine is allowed to cool, the protein precipitates again.

Chemically, Bence Jones protein is identical, both structurally and antigenically, with the light chains (κ-chains and λ-chains) of the immunoglobulins (see page 355). Either type of polypeptide may be present in the urine of an individual patient.

URINOBILINOGEN. Less than 3 mg of *urinobilinogen* are found normally in a twenty-four-hour sample of urine. If more than this amount is present, liver damage (or, in some cases, hemolytic jaundice) is suspected (see page 288).

INDICAN. Small amounts of skatole and indole absorbed from the digestive tract are united with sulfuric acid and potassium in the liver to form *indican*. Indican is eliminated in the urine. If excessive putrefaction (bacterial action on proteins) occurs in the intestine, the amount of indican in the urine is increased.

KETONE BODIES. Ketone bodies appear in the urine in any condition that causes ketosis (see page 232). The Rothera test for acetone and acetoacetic acid is performed as follows. Shake a sample of urine with ammonium sulfate until the urine is saturated with this salt. Add a few drops of concentrated ammonium hydroxide solution, followed by a few drops of freshly prepared sodium nitroprusside solution (2 to 10 percent). The test is positive if a pink color develops. A brown color has no significance. This test is more sensitive for acetoacetic acid than for acetone. The Rothera test is negative if performed on normal urine.

URINE SEDIMENT

Most normal samples of urine are clear, although alkaline urines are usually cloudy because of insoluble phosphates. If infections exist in the urinary tract, the urine may be cloudy because it contains many white blood cells (pus cells). All samples of urine, however, deposit some insoluble material when they are allowed to stand or when they are centrifuged.* When this sediment is examined with the microscope, many different crystals and other materials are seen. Several of these have pathological significance. Among these are tyrosine and leucine crystals, cystine crystals, red blood cells, white blood cells, and casts.

TYROSINE AND LEUCINE CRYSTALS. Tyrosine and leucine crystals appear in urine sediment in some severe cases of liver disease. These compounds are amino acids and normally are metabolized in the liver. If the liver is too badly damaged to do this, they appear in the urine. Neither of them is very soluble, and the concentration of the urine in the kidney tubules causes them to precipitate.

CYSTINE CRYSTALS. Cystine crystals are seen in rare instances. Patients that exhibit these crystals in their urine are said to have *cystinuria* (see page 289).

RED BLOOD CELLS. Red blood cells are usually present in very small numbers in the sediment of normal urine. They are increased in number in many diseases of the urinary tract.

WHITE BLOOD CELLS. A few white blood cells are present in normal sediments. Large numbers of these cells indicate that bacterial infection is present in the urinary tract. It must be remembered that white blood cells are present normally in the vagina, and the presence of these cells in the urine of a female patient has little significance unless the urine has been obtained by catheterization.

CASTS. Casts represent particles of protein or other material that have precipitated in the tubules of the kidney. When these particles are expelled from the tubules, they retain their shape and may be regarded as models

*A centrifuge is a machine that causes tubes of urine or other liquids to whirl rapidly; insoluble materials quickly settle to the bottoms of the tubes.

or "casts" of the tubules. Casts may appear in the urine sediment in any of the conditions accompanied by proteinuria.

KIDNEY FUNCTION TESTS. Numerous tests designed to check on the function of the kidneys have been devised. A few of these will be described briefly.

Concentration-dilution test. The patient is not allowed to take any fluids, and the specific gravity of the urine is measured periodically for several hours. If the kidney is normal, the specific gravity should rise to 1.030 or more. The same patient is required to drink a large quantity of water, and the specific gravity of the urine is determined again at regular intervals. The specific gravity should fall until it approaches that of water (1.000). In certain kidney diseases, notably chronic glomerulonephritis and hypertensive kidney disease, the specific gravity may remain close to 1.010 throughout this test.

PSP test. A solution of phenolsulfonphthalein (PSP) is injected into one of the patient's veins. Fifty to 60 percent of the dye should be eliminated in the patient's urine within 2 hours. If the amount eliminated is less than this, the physician suspects that the patient's kidneys are diseased.

Determination of glomerular filtration rate. Certain substances, of which *mannitol* (an alcohol containing six OH groups per molecule) and *inulin* (a polysaccharide that yields fructose on hydrolysis) are examples, escape from the blood and into the urine entirely by glomerular filtration. Moreover, once mannitol or inulin enters the kidney tubule, it does not diffuse back into the blood again.

Suppose a solution of mannitol were injected intravenously into a patient and, during a measured period of time (say, 15 minutes) after this injection, all of the urine formed by the patient were carefully collected, its volume measured, its content of mannitol determined, and the level of mannitol present in the patient's blood plasma determined. Suppose, as an example, that the urine contained 9 mg of mannitol in each milliliter, and that 20 ml of urine were formed. It follows that 180 mg ($20 \times 9 = 180$) of mannitol would have been removed from the blood by glomerular filtration in 15 minutes. Thus, the amount removed ("cleared") from the blood *per minute* during the collection period of fifteen minutes would have been 12 mg ($180 \div 15 = 12$). If the concentration of mannitol present in the blood plasma were 10 mg per 100 ml (that is, 0.1 mg per milliliter), it follows that an amount of mannitol equivalent to that in 120 ml of plasma would have been cleared through the glomerular membrane (since $12 \div 0.1 = 120$). In other words, the *glomerular filtration rate (GFR)* would have been 120 ml per minute for this patient. This is a reasonable normal value. Obviously, patients with diseases in which the kidney glomeruli are damaged will have values lower than normal, since filtration will be less rapid through the thickened glomerular membrane.

Determination of tubular excretory mass. p-Aminohippuric acid (PAH) is a substance that diffuses through capillary walls, including the glomerular walls, with great ease and rapidity. Also, it is excreted readily by the cells of the tubules. Once it has entered the lumen of a tubule, either through the glomerular membrane or from the tubular cells, it is not appreciably reabsorbed. That is, all the PAH entering the kidney tubules from the blood can be assumed to remain in the urine.

Suppose the same patient already used as an example were studied again, this time using PAH instead of mannitol. Larger amounts of PAH than were used in the case of mannitol would have to be used for this measurement since it is necessary to make sure that enough material is presented to the kidney to "saturate" its capacity to secrete the compound. Suppose the urine were found to contain 100 mg of PAH per milliliter and that 20 ml were formed during the 15-minute period. The total amount of PAH excreted during the 15-minute period thus would be 2,000 mg ($20 \times 100 = 2{,}000$). The amount excreted per minute would be $2{,}000/15 = 133$ mg. This represents the total amount of PAH eliminated both by glomerular fitration and by tubular secretion. However, we know from the mannitol measurement that, for this patient, an amount of material equivalent to that present in 120 ml of plasma would have been filtered through the glomerular membrane in 1 minute. If the plasma concentration of PAH were found to be 50 mg per 100 ml, then the amount of PAH in 120 ml must have been $^{120}/_{100} \times 50 = 60$ mg. In other words, 60 mg of the PAH would have been eliminated by glomerular filtration. Obviously, then, the amount eliminated by the tubules would have been 73 mg per minute ($133 - 60 = 73$). Stated in different words, the *tubular excretory mass (Tm)* for this patient would have been 73 mg of PAH per minute. This is an average normal value. In diseases in which the kidney tubules are damaged this value will be decreased.

Determination of minimal renal blood flow. PAH can be used to make one other very useful measurement. If only very small amounts of the material are injected so that the plasma level is approximately 2 mg per 100 ml all of the PAH in the blood that passes through the kidney will be removed and will appear in the urine. Suppose, for example, it were found that the urine collected during a 15-minute period contained 10.5 mg of PAH per milliliter and that the volume collected measured 20 ml. Then the total amount of the compound eliminated during the 15 minutes would have been 210 mg ($10.5 \times 20 = 210$). The average amount eliminated per minute would be $^{210}/_{15} = 14$ mg. Since each milliliter of plasma contained 0.02 mg of PAH (assuming that the concentration found was 2 mg per 100 ml), 700 ml of plasma would be required to furnish 14 mg ($14 \div 0.02 = 700$). Hence, at least 700 ml of *plasma* per minute must have passed through the patient's kidneys during the measurement. This value is referred to as the *minimal renal plasma flow (MRPF).* If it were determined that the hematocrit reading for the patient was 40 percent (that is, that 40 percent of the blood volume represented cells and 60 percent represented plasma), it is possible for us to calculate that 1,167 ml of blood ($700 \div 0.6$) would be the minimal volume of *blood* that must have passed through the patients kidneys during the test. This value is the *minimal renal blood flow (MRBF)* for this patient. Both the MRPF and the MRBF will be lower than normal in diseases in which the blood vessels of the kidneys are damaged or constricted.

KIDNEY AND BLADDER STONES. Urine is a *supersaturated solution* of certain sub-

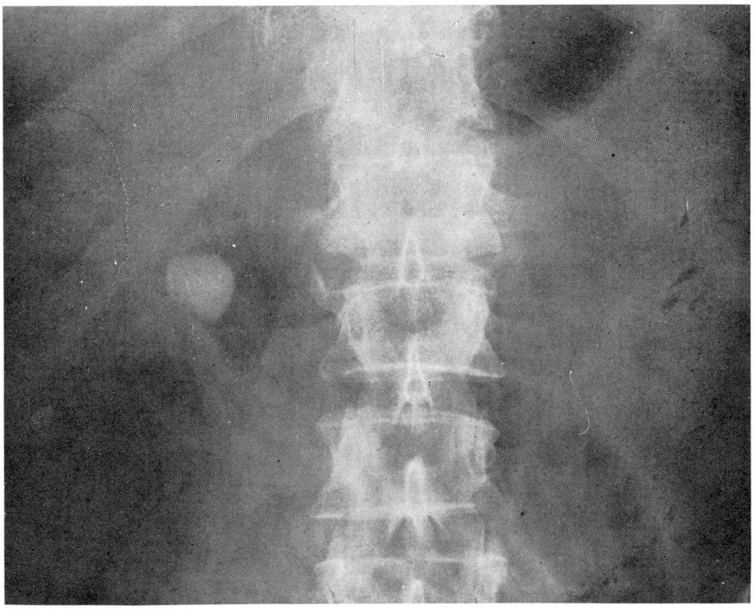

Fig. 31-4. X-ray photograph showing a stone (calculus) in the right kidney. Explain why it can be predicted that this stone contains calcium salts.

stances. For example, it would require about 25 liters of water to dissolve the amount of uric acid present in about 1 liter of urine. It is supposed that the small amount of colloidal material present in the urine helps to keep these materials in solution. This colloidal material probably is chiefly a complex polysaccharide. Under certain circumstances, however, insoluble crystalline or amorphous masses settle out of the urine either in the kidney or in the urinary bladder. These masses, which may be very small or as large as a small orange, are called *kidney stones* (if they occur in the kidney) or *bladder stones* (if they occur in the bladder). They are also known as *calculi.* If the urine is acid, these stones are composed usually of uric acid, salts of uric acid (urates), or calcium oxalate. In alkaline urine the common stones are composed of calcium carbonate, calcium phosphate, or magnesium ammonium phosphate.

STUDY QUESTIONS

1. How are waste products eliminated from the body?
2. Briefly describe the formation of urine by the kidney.
3. What precautions should be observed in collecting urine for examination? Why is it preferable to collect twenty-four–hour samples?
4. Name some factors that affect the volume of urine excreted.
5. What is oliguria? Anuria? Polyuria? Name some conditions in which each of these is found.
6. What are diuretics? Name one use for them in medicine.
7. Name some factors that affect the color of normal urine.
8. What is urochrome?
9. Name one pathological condition that might cause urine to have each of the following colors: red, brown, black. What would you assume might be the cause of a blue-green color in a urine sample?
10. What is meant by specific gravity of urine? What is the average specific gravity of normal urine? How may this specific gravity be raised or lowered if the patient is not suffering from a disease?
11. Name a disease in which the specific gravity of the urine is lower than normal. Name one condition in which it is higher than normal.
12. How do you explain the fact that most samples of urine are slightly acid? How would you test for the reaction of a urine sample?
13. Make a list of the more important inorganic and organic components of the urine. From what type of food are most of the organic urinary compounds derived?
14. Is glucose found normally in the urine when tested with Benedict's reagent? Name five conditions in which the test for glucose in urine is positive.
15. Under what conditions does lactose occur in urine? How can it be distinguished from glucose?
16. How can pentosuria be distinguished from true glycosuria?
17. Name four abnormal conditions in which plasma proteins are found in the urine. How would you test a sample of urine for the presence of proteins? Why is acetic acid used in this test? Does normal urine give a positive test for proteins?
18. Why is albumin found in urine more often than globulin? What is proteinuria? Albuminuria?
19. What is Bence Jones protein? How can it be detected in urine? In what conditions is it most commonly found in the urine? Is it ever found in other conditions?
20. Name three causes of ketosis. How would you test for the presence of acetoacetic acid in urine?
21. What is the significance of an increased excretion of urobilinogen in the urine?
22. What causes an increased elimination of indican in the urine? Explain.
23. What are pus cells? What conclusion would you draw if you found large numbers of them in a urine sediment? Why might you be misled if the patient is a female?
24. What is the significance of tyrosine and leucine crystals in urine sediment? Of cystine crystals?
25. What do you think the finding of red blood cells in urine sediment indicates? Why?
26. What are casts? Name several conditions in which you might expect them to be found in sediment.
27. Briefly describe three kidney function tests.
28. Name some substances that often form kidney stones in acid urine.
29. Name some substances that often form kidney stones in alkaline urine.

CHAPTER 32

Hormones

Scattered throughout the body are isolated groups of cells called *endocrine*, or *ductless, glands*. They are also referred to as *glands of internal secretion*. These glands manufacture substances called *hormones* that are necessary for normal functioning of the body. As their name implies, ductless glands do not have ducts, and hormones pass directly from the cells that manufacture them into the bloodstream. It is generally true that hormones do not affect the cells that make them; instead they are carried by the blood to some other organ or tissue, where they produce their characteristic effects. Most hormones are stimulating substances, and the term hormone is derived from a Greek word meaning "to stimulate." Internal secretions that are depressing are sometimes called *chalones* (Greek, "to depress") instead of hormones.

STEROIDS AND THEIR NOMENCLATURE. Several of the hormones are classified as *steroids*. They all contain the characteristic ring system found in sterols, such as cholesterol.

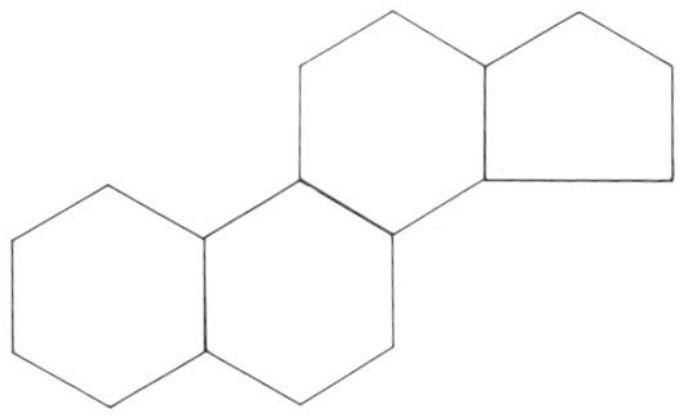

Steroid ring system

A number of synthetic compounds having this same ring structure have been found to have hormonelike activity, and many of them are used as drugs.

The steroid nucleus, in its most complex form (see coprostane, page 167), is numbered as follows:

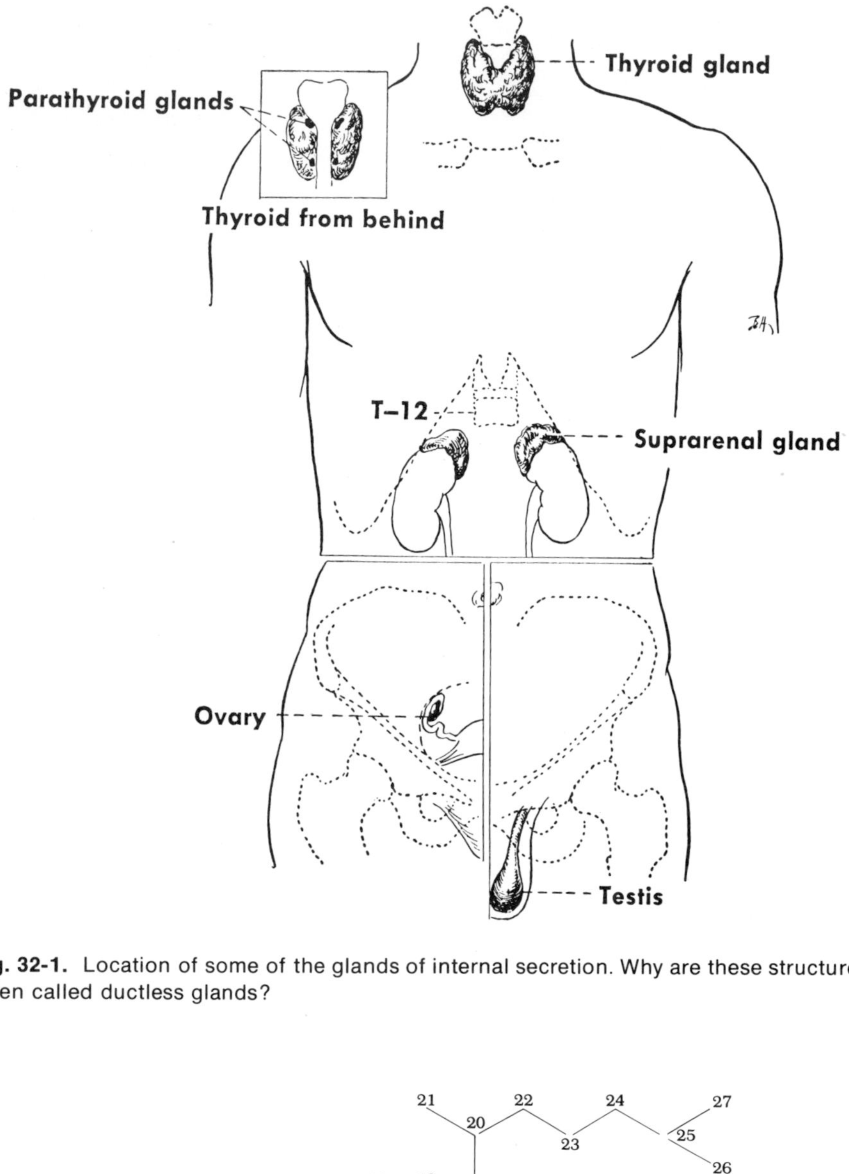

Fig. 32-1. Location of some of the glands of internal secretion. Why are these structures often called ductless glands?

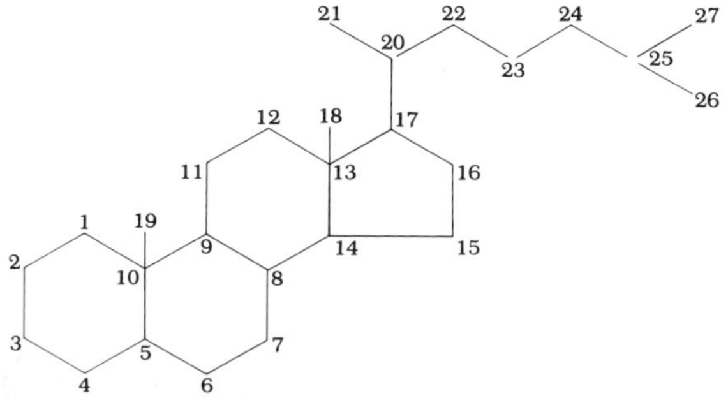

A dotted line in the formulas indicates the α-configuration, meaning that the atom or radical lies below the plane of the paper (see page 167). A solid line denotes the β-configuration, in which the atom or radical projects above the plane of the paper.

The International Union of Pure and Applied Chemistry (IUPAC) has recommended the use of three basic names: estrane, androstane, and pregnane. When double bonds occur in the ring system, the -ane ending becomes -ene. Each of these three structures exists in two basic forms: α- or β-oriented; that is, the hydrogen atom attached at carbon 5 is either α or β. Ordinarily, this orientation is not indicated if it is α for estrane or androstane, or β for pregnane. (Most steroids of interest have these configurations.)

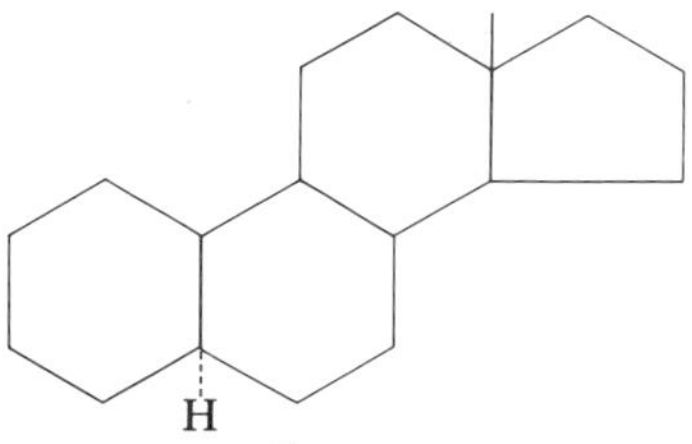

Estrane

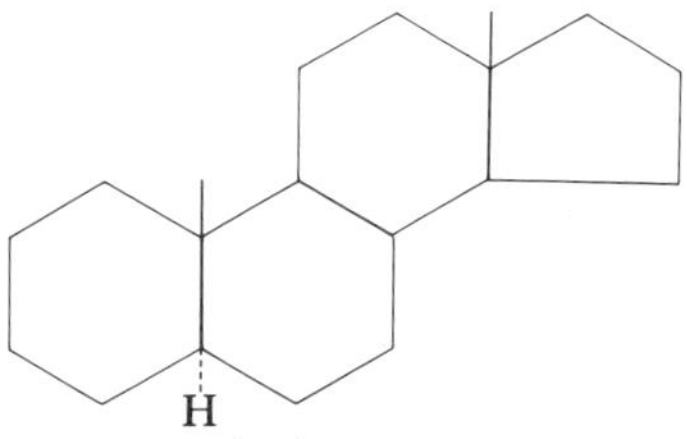

Androstane

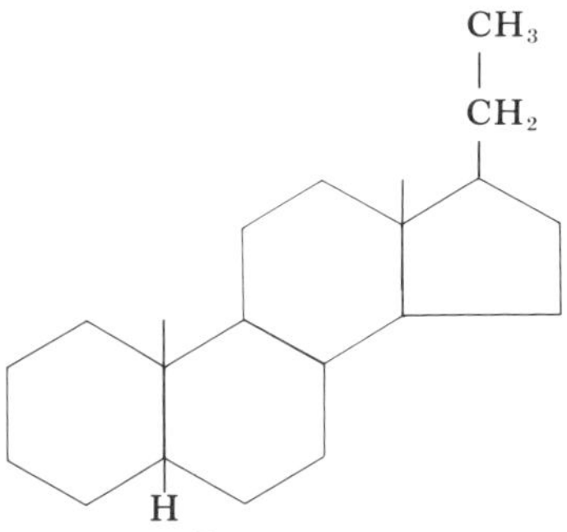

Pregnane

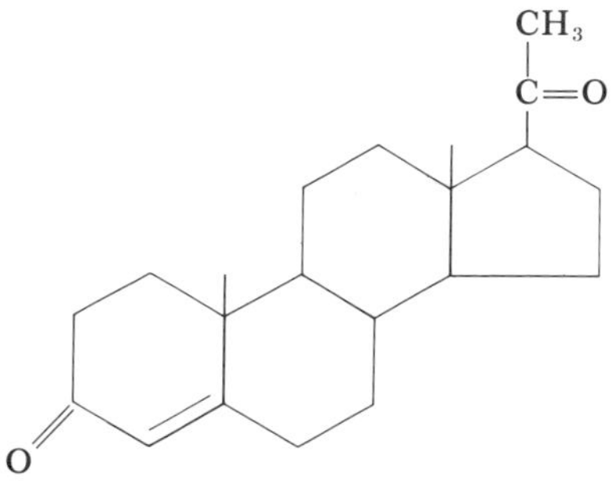

Common name: progesterone
Descriptive name: 3,20-dioxopregn-4-ene

The descriptive name for progesterone indicates that the structure is pregnane with a double bond in the ring system: 3,20 dioxo indicates that oxygen atoms are attached at positions 3 and 20; the -4-ene indicates that the double bond occurs at 4 (that is, between 4 and 5).

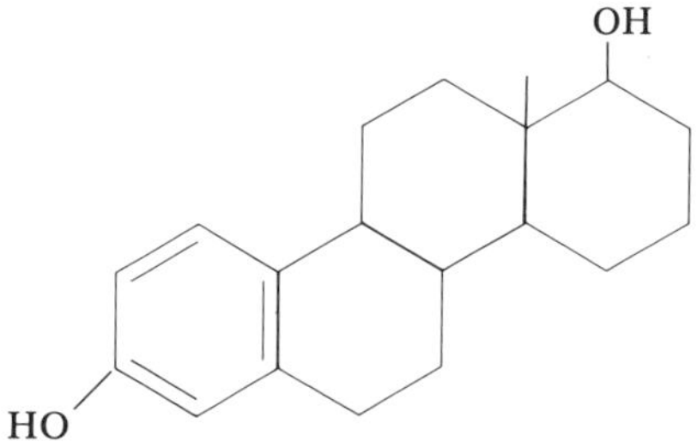

Common name: estradiol
Descriptive name: 3,17 β-dihydroxyestra-1,3,5(10)-triene

The structure is derived from estrane. The 3,17 β-dihydroxy indicates that OH groups occur at the 3 and 17 positions, and that the 17 position has the β-configuration. (The OH at position 3 has only one possible spatial arrangement because it is attached to a carbon to which a double bond is attached. See page 163.) The -1,3,5(10)-triene indicates that there are three double bonds originating at positions

1, 3, and 5; the (10) indicates that the double bond originating at position 5 connects with position 10 and not with position 6.

HORMONES OF THE OVARY

The ovaries are two small almond-shaped structures that contain the ova (eggs) of the female. The ovary does not actually manufacture ova; they are present in immature form at birth, and after the age of puberty one of these immature ova is matured and expelled each month (except during pregnancy, sometimes during lactation, and in abnormal conditions). Ova cease to be expelled after the menopause (change of life).

Shortly before expulsion the ovum is located in a hollow space, called a *follicle*. This follicle is filled with *follicular fluid* and is lined by cells called *follicle cells*. At ovulation the follicle ruptures and the ovum escapes (is expelled) into the body cavity. The follicle then fills with a blood clot, which is replaced in a few days by large cells that have a yellow color. This mass of cells is called the *corpus leuteum* ("yellow body"). If pregnancy does not occur, the corpus luteum is soon replaced by scar tissue, but if the ovum is fertilized, the corpus luteum remains throughout the first trimester (third) of pregnancy.

The hormone made by the follicle cells is called *estradiol*. Apparently this substance can be changed chemically in the body into other substances that are eliminated in the urine. *Estrone* and *estriol* are the most important of these. These three substances exhibit hormonal activity when they are injected into animals; they are known collectively as the *follicular* or

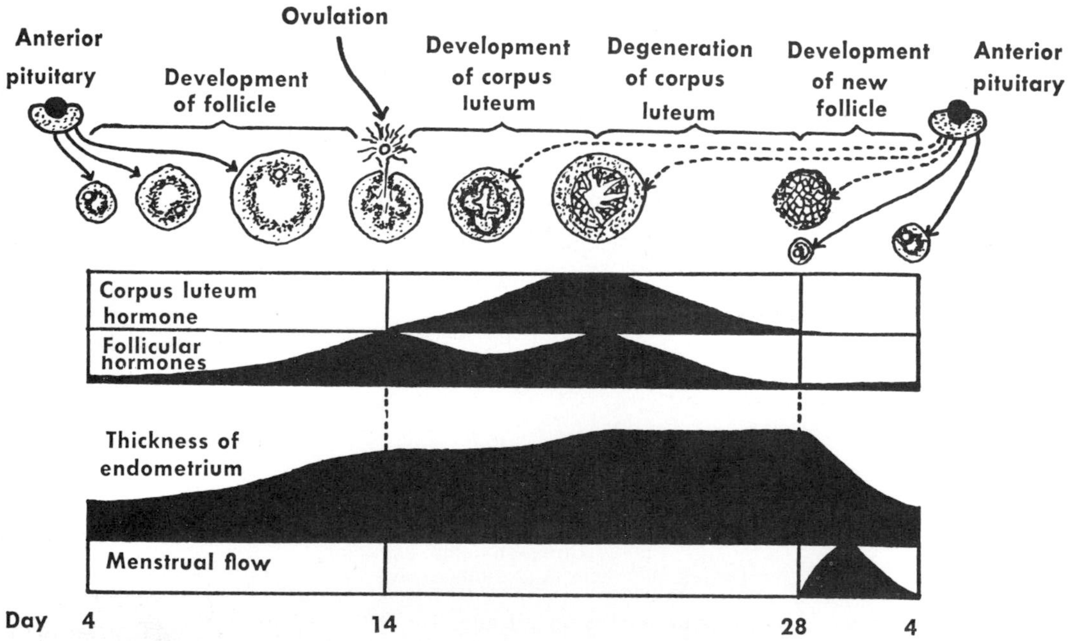

Fig. 32-2. Diagram to show the supposed endocrine control of the uterine endometrium. What two pituitary hormones regulate the production of the ovarian hormones? (Adapted from a drawing in color supplied through courtesy of Parke, Davis & Co.)

estrogenic hormones. The use of the word estrogenic is explained by the fact that these hormones are responsible for the periodic occurrence of estrus (desire on the part of the female for mating) in the lower animals.

The estrogenic hormones are responsible for the development of secondary sex characters – such as growth of the breasts, distribution of the body hair, and changes in the uterus and vagina – at puberty. During menstruation the lining of the uterus (the endometrium) largely sloughs off and is expelled with the menstrual blood. The regeneration of the endometrium that begins after menstruation is caused by the follicular hormones. At about the fourteenth day of the menstrual cycle – ordinarily about 28 days elapse from the beginning of one menstrual period to the beginning of the next – the follicle ruptures and the ovum is expelled. At this time the endometrium is much thicker, and the excretion of follicular hormones in the urine has risen to a peak. After the rupture of the follicle the excretion of these hormones rapidly falls. A second rise occurs before the beginning of the next menstrual period. Presumably this secondary rise results from the production of estrogenic hormones by the corpus luteum.

Compounds having estrogenic activity are known as *estrogens*.

Changes in the endometrium that occur during the second half of the menstrual cycle are caused mainly by *progesterone,* a hormone secreted by the corpus luteum cells. Progesterone causes an engorgement of the endometrium with blood, and, under its influence, the endometrial glands fill with secretion. A certain type of cell, which is used to help form the placenta if pregnancy occurs, develops under progesterone stimulation. In other words, progesterone appears to prepare the endometrium for the nourishment and attachment of the fertilized ovum. If the ovum is not fertilized, the production of both progesterone and estrogenic hormones ceases rather abruptly on about the twenty-third or twenty-fourth day of the menstrual cycle; menstruation follows in 4 or 5 days. This sudden failure on the part of the ovary to manufacture its hormones is responsible for the onset of menstruation.

Progesterone is secreted throughout pregnancy. In some animals, at least, abortion occurs if the corpus luteum is removed before delivery of the fetus.

Cyclic changes also take place in the lining of the vagina. These changes are caused by the follicular hormones. These hormones, progesterone, and a pituitary hormone appear to be responsible for the growth of the mammary glands (breasts) at the time of menstruation and during pregnancy.

Progesterone is changed in the body to a compound called *pregnandiol.* Pregnandiol unites with sodium and glycuronic acid (an organic acid related chemically to glucose) and is then excreted in the urine.

Compounds having biological activity similar to progesterone are known as *progestogens* or *gestogens*.

The accompanying skeleton structural formulas show the close chemical relationship between the ovarian hormones and cholesterol. These formulas are written in such a manner that only the ring systems (composed of carbon atoms) and the characteristic groups are shown.

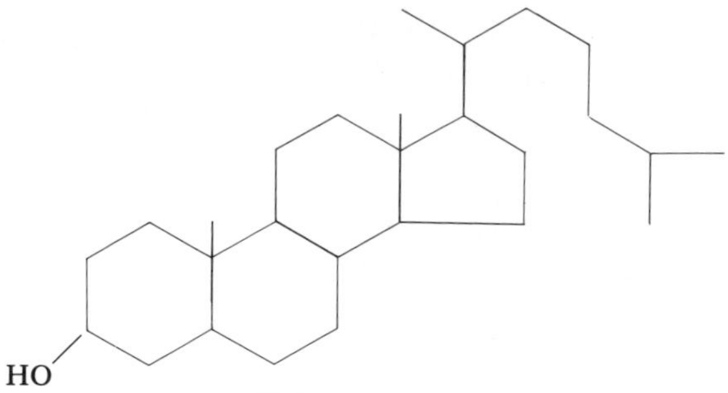

Cholesterol
(A sterol – not a hormone)

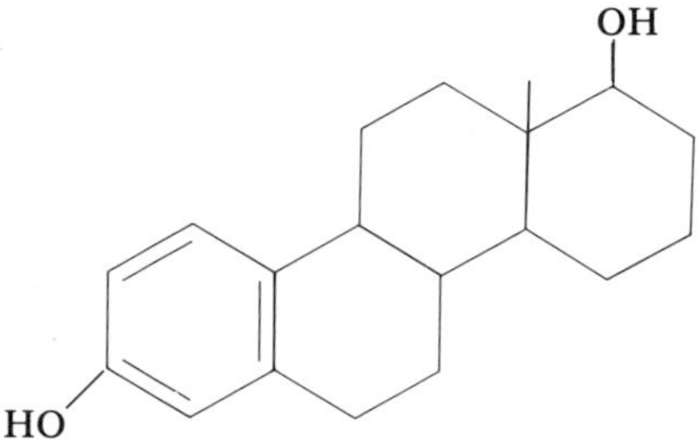

Estradiol
3,17β-dihydroxyestra-1,3,5(10)-triene

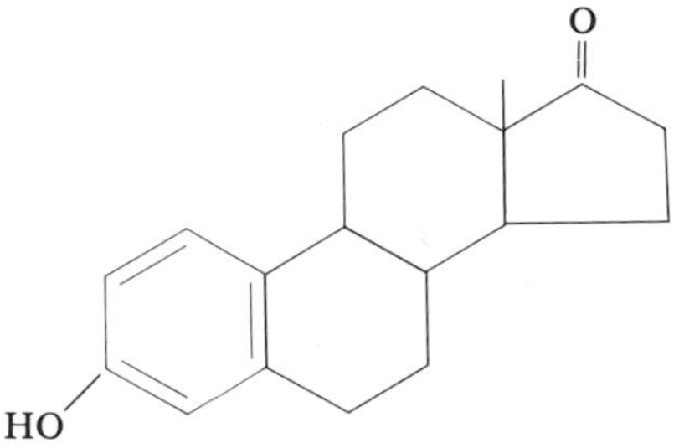

Estrone
3-hydroxy-17-oxoestra-1,3,5(10)-triene

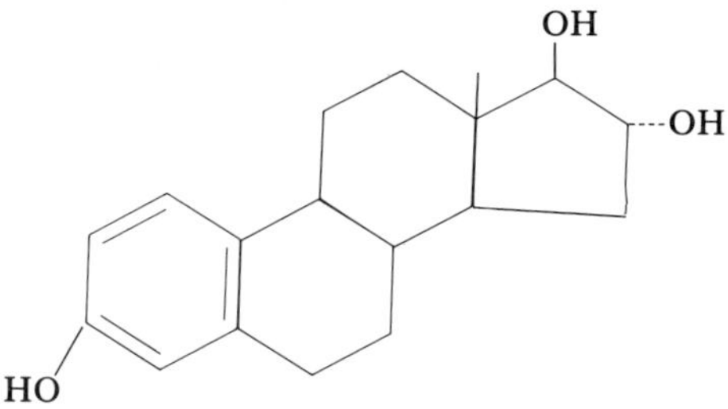

Estriol
3β,16α,17β-trihydroxyestra-1,3,5(10)-triene

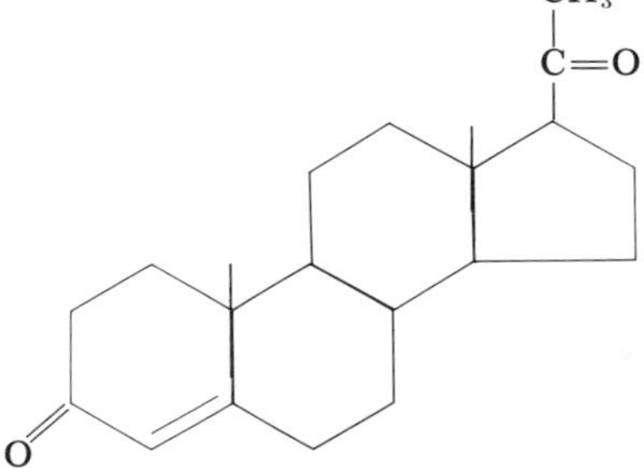

Progesterone
3,20-dioxopregn-4-ene

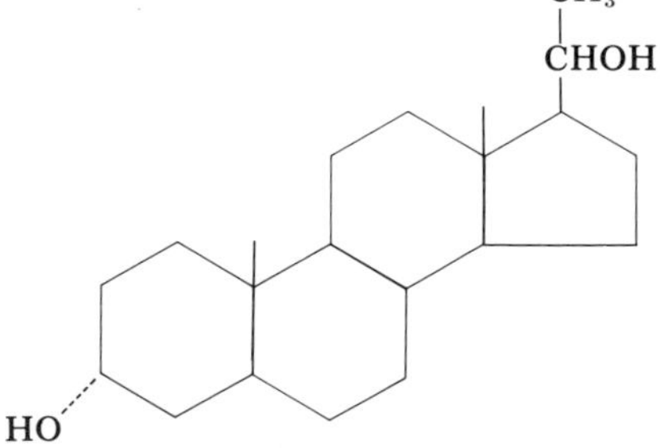

Pregnandiol
3α,20-dihydroxypregnane

It is an interesting finding that follicular hormones occur in the urine of both females and males. Indeed, one of the best natural sources of these

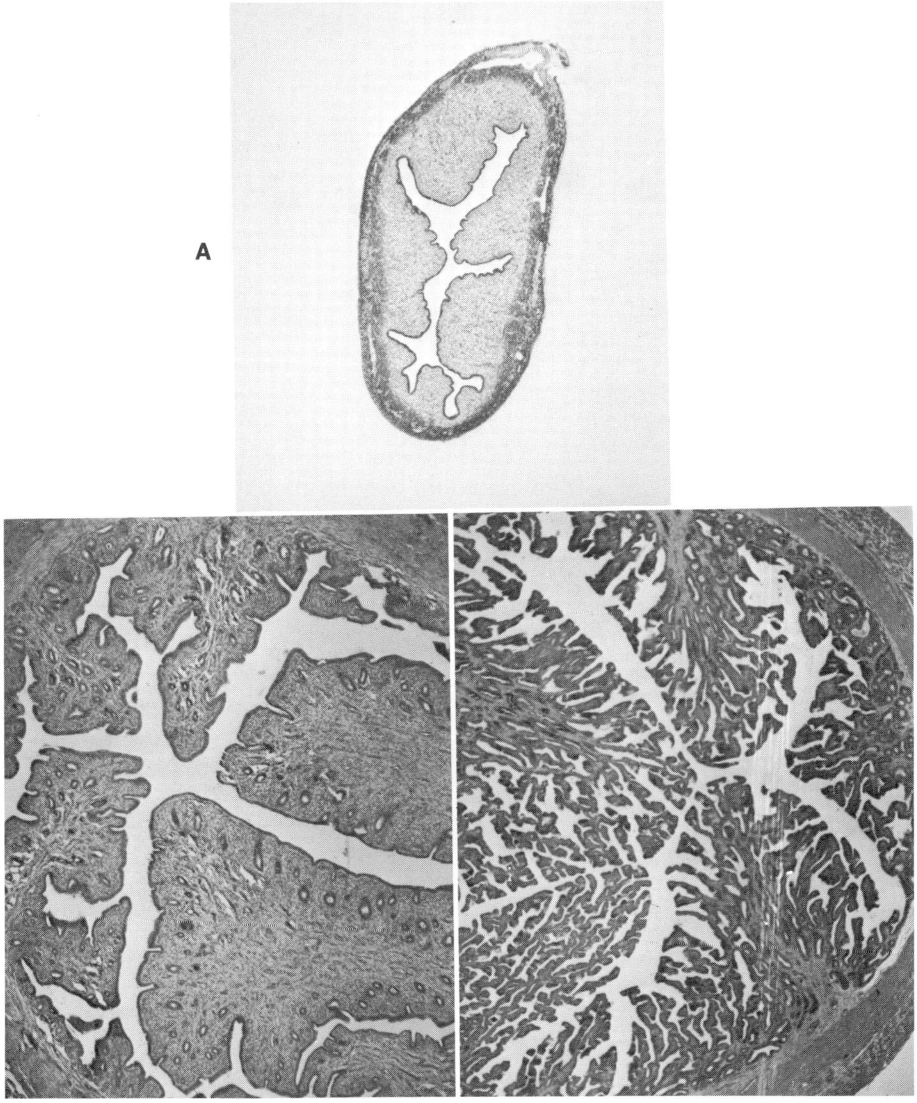

Fig. 32-3. Sections of uteri removed from sexually immature rabbits. **A,** No treatment; **B,** after treatment with an estrogen; **C,** after treatment with a combination of an estrogen and progesterone. How does the action of progesterone on the uterine endometrium differ from that of estrone? (Courtesy Dr. Albert Meli and Dr. John Manning.)

hormones is the urine of the stallion (male horse). Pregnancy urine is also an excellent source.

Stilbestrol (diethylstilbestrol) is a synthetic organic compound that has estrogenic properties. It is active when given by mouth and is widely used in medicine. Several other synthetic compounds also are used in medicine. Estrone sulfate occurs in the urine of horses and is a commonly used form of the hormone.

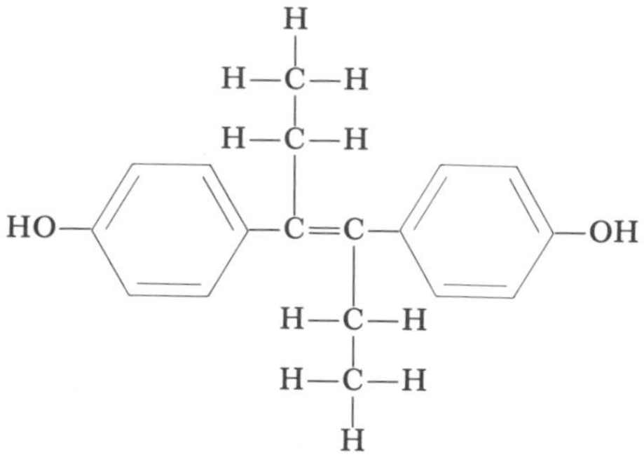

Stilbestrol (diethylstilbestrol)

Relaxin is a hormone made principally, although not exclusively, by the corpus luteum. Its chemical nature does not resemble that of the other hormone of the corpus luteum, progesterone. Although it has not yet been isolated in pure form, the available evidence makes it probable that it is a mixture of two polypeptides having molecular weights between 9,000 and 12,000.

In rodents such as guinea pigs and mice relaxin is secreted in in-

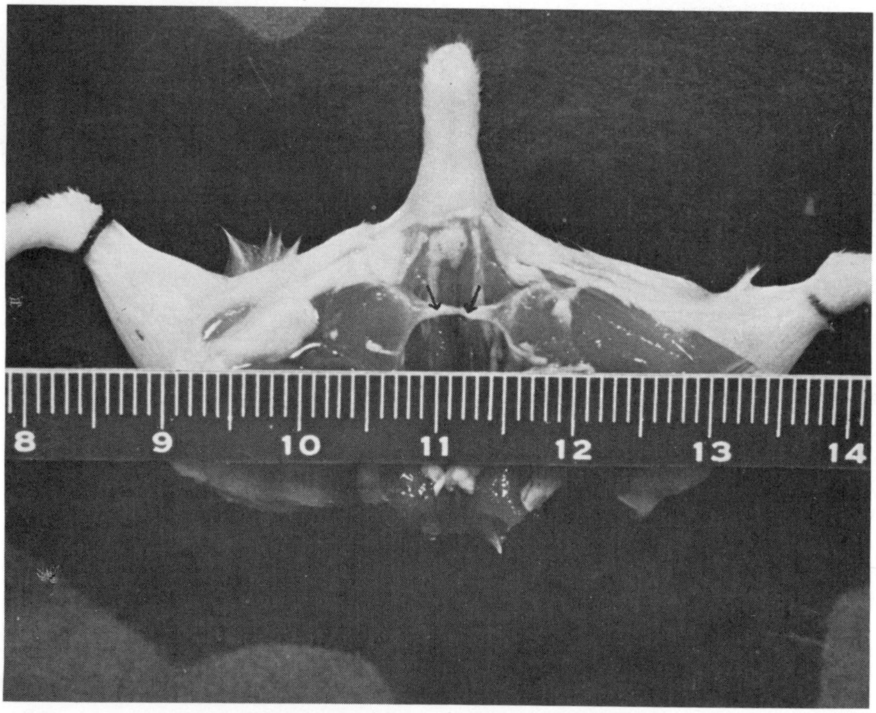

Fig. 32-4. Photograph showing separation of the two halves of the symphysis pubis and corresponding increase in the length of the connective tissue connecting them (arrows), 24 hours after injecting relaxin into a female mouse. Does this hormone occur in the human being? (Courtesy Dr. Robert L. Kroc.)

creasing amounts during pregnancy. The first of its functions to be recognized was its ability to increase the length of the ligaments of the symphysis pubis, which bind together the two halves of the bony pelvis. This serves to increase the size of the birth canal, thus facilitating birth of the young. The hormone also causes softening of the uterine cervix and increases the distensibility of the body of the uterus. It has been reported to induce growth of the mammary gland and to exert anabolic effect on the uterus (that is, to cause an increase in the size, protein content, water content, and glycogen content).

Relaxin is not only found in the pregnant animal. It has been detected in the ovaries and testes of birds; in the blood of female mammals, including human beings; in mammalian testes; in placentas; in the ovaries of elasmobranch fishes; in the ovaries of pregnant sharks; and in the abdominally located testes of the armadillo.

Relaxin does not exert its physiological effects unless sufficient estrogen is present in the animal. Progesterone and related compounds inhibit its activity.

HORMONES OF THE TESTIS

The testes are two oval structures located in the scrotum of the male. In each testis are many coiled ducts; the lining of these ducts manufactures spermatozoa, the male sex cells, which have the power to fertilize a mature ovum. Located between the ducts are large, clear cells, called *interstitial cells*. The interstitial cells manufacture *testosterone*, a male sex hormone. Testosterone apparently is changed in the body to other substances that also have hormonal activity. The most important of these is *androsterone*. So far, testosterone has been obtained only from the testis itself, and androsterone has been isolated only from urine. This causes us to suppose that testosterone is manufactured in the interstitial cells and is later converted to androsterone, which is excreted in the urine. Some testosterone is converted to substances other than androsterone.

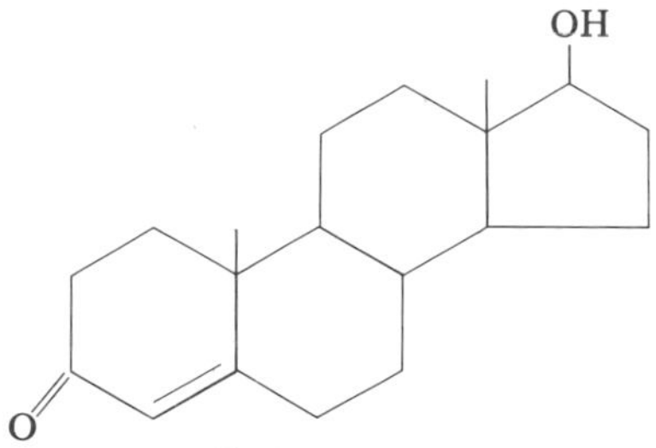

Testosterone
17β-hydroxy-3-oxoandrost-4-ene

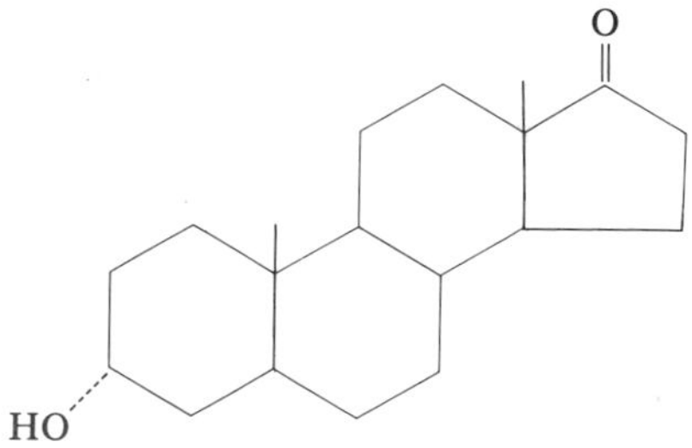

Androsterone
17-oxo-3α-hydroxyandrostane

The male sex hormones are responsible for the development of the secondary sex characters at the time of puberty—that is, the growth of hair on the face and pubic regions, the deepening of the voice, and so on. The normal size and function of the secondary sex glands (prostate gland, seminal vesicles, Cowper's glands) are also under the influence of the male sex hormones. If the testes are removed, these glands become small and cease to function properly.

Male sex hormones are found in the urine of both males and females.

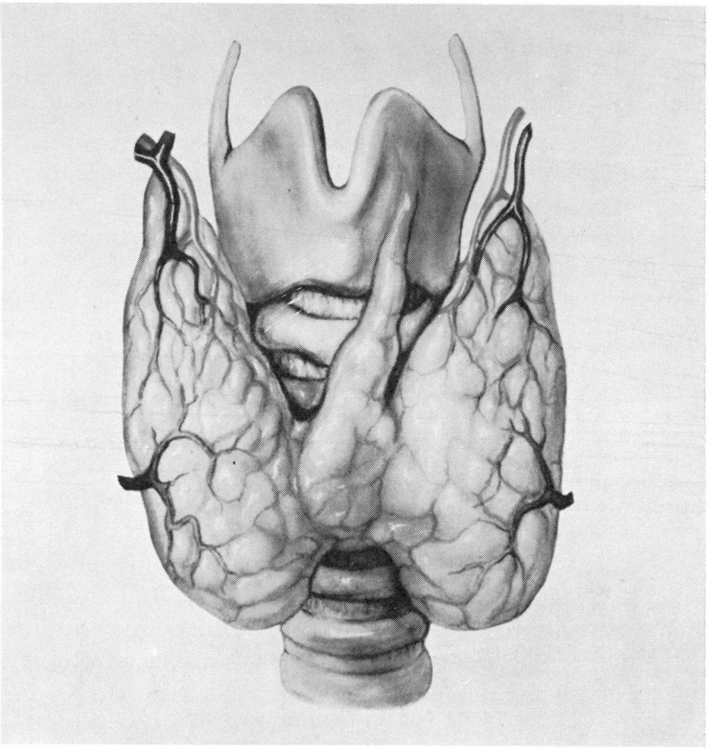

Fig. 32-5. The thyroid gland. What inorganic element is concentrated in this gland? (Courtesy Warner-Chilcott Laboratories.)

Substances having male hormone activity are manufactured by the adrenal cortex (see page 401).

HORMONE OF THE THYROID GLAND

The thyroid gland is situated in the neck just below the larynx (voice box). It consists of two lobes that are connected to each other by means of a strip of tissue called the thyroid isthmus. If the gland is cut open and examined with the microscope, it is found to be filled with small follicles that contain *colloid.* This colloidal material is composed mainly of thyroglobulin (a protein) and water. One of the amino acids contained in this protein is *thyroxine.* This compound is liberated into the blood as a thyroid hormone when thyroglobulin hydrolyzes (that is, breaks down to its amino acids). It combines with a specific protein in the plasma and is transported in the blood as "protein-bound" thyroxine. Thyroxine is 65 percent iodine and is believed to be made from *tyrosine,* another amino acid.

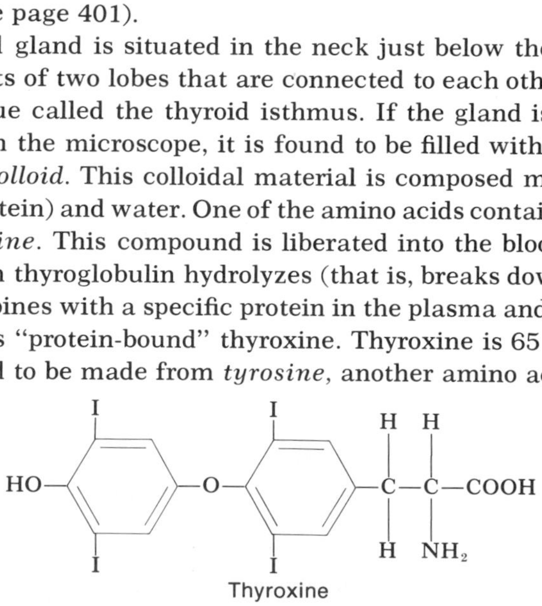

Thyroxine

In recent years it has been found that three other compounds having thyroid-hormone activity exist in the thyroid gland. One of these, 3,5,3′-triiodothyronine, is of special interest because it seems to be several times as active biologically as is thyroxine.

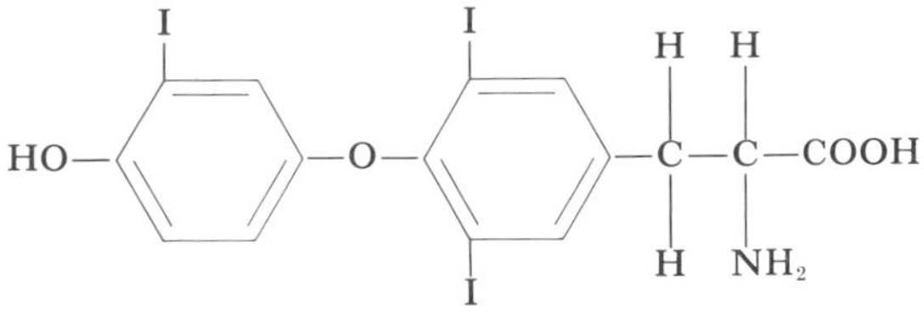

3,5,3′-triiodothyronine

Some scientists have speculated that thyroxine is converted to triiodothyronine in the tissues and that the latter is the true biologically active hormone. There is no direct evidence for this, however. Triiodothyronine probably can diffuse in and out of cells more readily than can thyroxine because it is not tightly bound to a specific plasma protein.

It is the function of thyroid hormones to speed up the rate of metabolism of all the cells of the body. If the thyroid gland is removed, or if it is destroyed by disease, the rate at which chemical reactions take place in the body is slowed up. The patient becomes overweight unless food intake is reduced because food is not burned at a normal rate. The heartbeat is slowed; the thyroid gland is sometimes removed in severe heart disease in order to decrease the amount of work required of the weak heart. Injections of thyroxine speed up metabolism, the patient loses weight unless the food intake is increased, and the heart rate is increased.

Hypothyroidism is a term usually used to indicate a failure on the part of the thyroid gland to manufacture sufficient thyroxine. It may sometimes result from destruction of the thyroid gland by disease and, occasionally, from a congenital absence of this gland (that is, the patient may have been born without a thyroid gland). A rare type of hypothyroidism has been classified as a disease of enzymic defect (see page 215)—that is, certain enzymes required for the synthesis of thyroid hormone are lacking. In other rare diseases of enzymic defect, hypothyroidism may be caused by a lack of transporting protein or by a failure of the tissues to utilize thyroid hormones.

Simple hypothyroidism is most common in regions where the iodine content of the drinking water is low. Patients with simple hypothyroidism are sluggish, have poor appetites, and their mental processes are somewhat slower than normal. In spite of the loss of appetite they tend to be overweight. Women with simple hypothyroidism may have menstrual disorders and may be unable to bear children.

Cretinism is a severe form of hypothyroidism occurring in children. It usually results from a lack of iodine in the diet, but one type *(sporadic cretinism)* is caused by a congenital absence of the thyroid gland. Cretins (patients with cretinism) are not smaller than usual at birth, but their subsequent growth and mental development are greatly retarded. They become dwarfs, with short, broad bodies, wide, flat noses, and coarse, dry hair. The mouth hangs open, the thick tongue tends to protude, and there

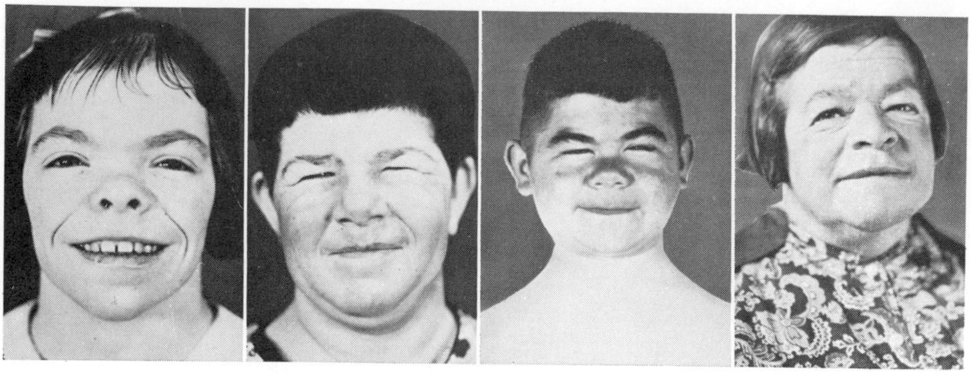

Fig. 32-6. Cretins. Note the close resemblance among these four cretins, all born in America, but descendants of Italian, Canadian, German, and mixed American stock. What is the cause of cretinism? (Courtesy Warner-Chilcott Laboratories.)

is a constant dribbling of saliva. The skin is thick, dry, and inelastic. If the condition continues after puberty, there is a partial failure of sex development. Intelligence is greatly reduced, and many cretins are idiots. Cretins may live to reach old age, but this is uncommon. If treatment with thyroxine or thyroid gland is begun early, the child may become normal, or nearly so. In the type of cretinism caused by lack of iodine, addition of this element to the diet is all that is necessary for the prevention and cure of this condition.

Severe hypothyroidism that occurs in adult life is called *myxedema*. This condition is most common at about 40 years of age and is seen seven times as frequently in women as in men. The tongue becomes thick and dry; the temperature is below normal; and the pulse rate is slow. The skin fills with a thick, protein-containing fluid and becomes thick and dry. Mental processes are often impaired. The patient gains weight in spite of a poor appetite. If the condition is not too severe, it can be controlled by the daily administration of thyroxine, desiccated thryoid (dried thyroid gland), or extracts of thyroid containing thyroglobulin.

Goiter (struma) refers to an enlargement of the thyroid gland. *Simple goiter* (colloid goiter, endemic goiter) is found in regions where the drinking water is low in iodine. Many people in such areas have goiters without any clinical signs of hypothyroidism. Both cretinism and myxedema are usually accompanied by goiter.

Two types of goiter are accompanied by symptoms that are opposite to those of myxedema. Clinically, these types are classified as *hyperthyroidism*.

In *toxic adenoma* the enlargement of the thyroid gland is due to the presence of circumscribed enlargements (tumors) called *adenomas*. Patients with this condition usually have an increased appetite but lose weight in spite of this. Marked nervousness and weakness are present. The patient feels hot, even on a cold day, because of the increased production of heat in the tissues. Excessive sweating and an increased heart rate are

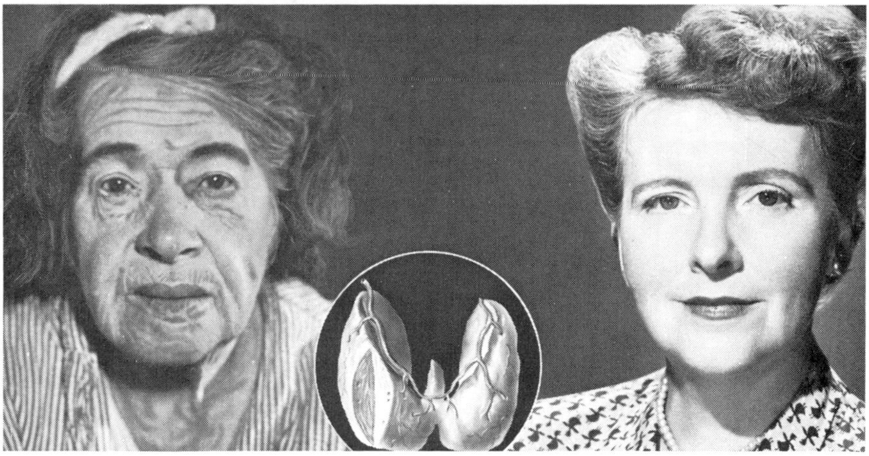

Fig. 32-7. Photograph of a woman with myxedema before and after treatment with thyroid hormone. What is the cause of myxedema? (Courtesy Warner-Chilcott Laboratories.)

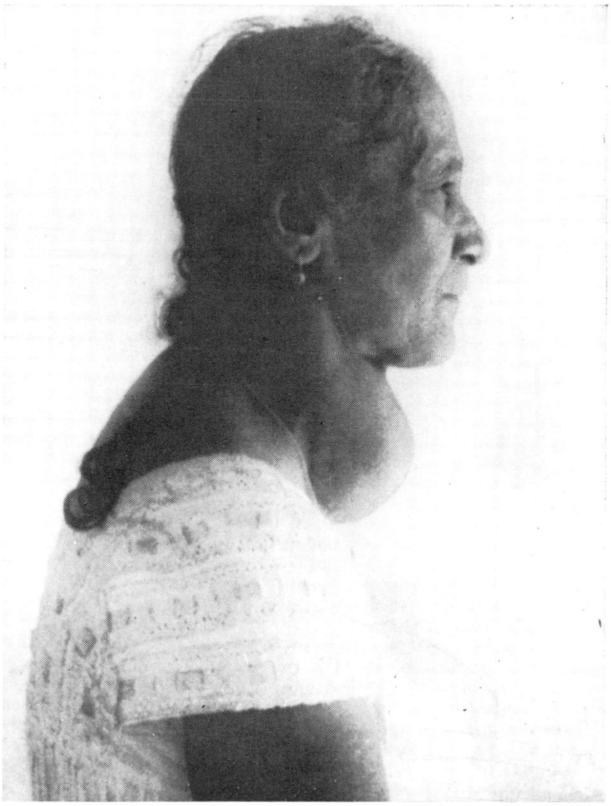

Fig. 32-8. This woman, who has a large goiter, lives in Oaxaca, Mexico. Cretinism afflicts one of every thirty children born in this region of Mexico. Define goiter. (From Mexico's struggle against goiter, Med. World News **4**:76, August 1963.)

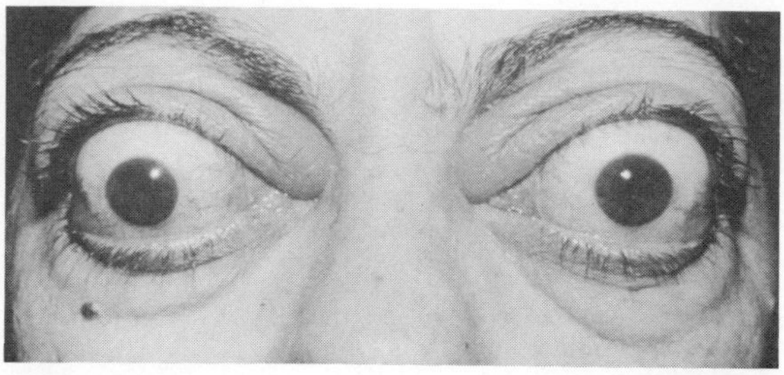

Fig. 32-9. Photograph of a patient with extreme exophthalmos. What does this term mean? (From Haddad, H. M.: Endocrine exophthalmos, J.A.M.A. **199:**559, 1967.)

noticed. These patients have emotional instability, in contrast to the mental dullness that accompanies myxedema. The symptoms of toxic adenoma are usually relieved by surgical removal of a portion of the thyroid gland or by destruction of a part of this gland with x-rays.

Exophthalmic goiter (Graves' disease, Basedow's disease) exhibits a diffuse regular enlargement of the thyroid gland, in contrast to the uneven enlarge of toxic adenoma. The symptoms are much like those of toxic adenoma. Exophthalmos (protusion of the eyeballs) frequently is present. The treatment of this condition is the same as that for the other type of hyperthyroidism.

At the present time we are not certain that clinical hyperthyroidism actually is due primarily to overactivity of the thyroid gland. Many physicians and scientists are of the opinion that it results from oversecretion of the thyrotropic hormone of the pituitary gland (see page 406). It is true that the symptoms observed are the opposite of those observed in hypothyroidism and that the condition can be relieved by removing or destroying a portion of the gland. On the other hand, the symptoms of hyperthyroidism can be relieved temporarily *by giving iodine to the patient*. Indeed, Lugol's solution (a water solution of iodine and potassium iodide) is given to such patients before surgery is performed. The condition is much more common in regions where the drinking water is low in iodine. It has not yet been possible to produce exophthalmos by injecting thyroxine into animals or humans. (Exophthalmos can be produced in animals by injecting the thyrotropic hormone of the pituitary gland; the experiment is more often successful if the thyroid glands have previously been removed from the test animals.)

It has been found that certain organic compounds (some sulfonamides, thiourea, thiouracil, propyl thiouracil, and others) interfere with the production of thyroxine by the thyroid gland, even in the presence of an abundance of iodine. When these substances are administered to laboratory animals or to human beings, the signs and symptoms of underactivity of the thyroid gland appear. Certain of them, especially thiouracil, are used in the therapy of hyperthyrodism (thyroid overactivity).

Another interesting finding is that certain proteins, such as casein and serum albumin, can be made to combine with iodine in such a way that thyroxine is formed in the intact protein molecule. Such iodinated proteins are potent substitutes for the natural hormone of the thyroid. It has been reported that the administration of iodinated casein to milk cows results in an increased yield of milk and butterfat.

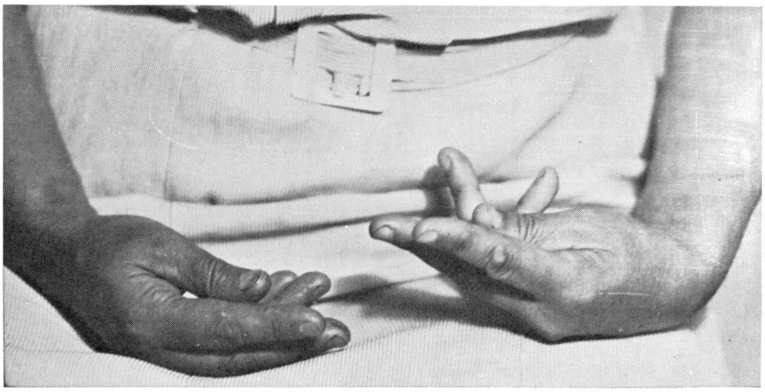

Fig. 32-10. Photograph illustrating parathyroid tetany of the fingers. This tetany of the fingers and hands can often be brought on by compressing the nerve trunks in the upper arm (Trousseau's sign), if the patient is suffering from underactivity of the parathyroid glands. What is one cause of parathyroid underactivity?

Calcitonin is a hormone made in special cells, the C cells, of the thyroid gland. It acts with parathormone and vitamin D (page 438) to regulate the level of calcium ions (and, incidentally, of phosphate ions) in body fluids. When the level of calcium ions is low, parathormone causes a loss of calcium from the bones; when the level becomes too high, calcitonin is secreted and somehow shuts off the release of calcium from bone. It is possible, but unproved, that it helps prevent or retard the occurrence of osteoporosis (see page 441) in old age as well as the loss of calcium from the bones that occurs during extended bed rest and in immobilized fractures. Perhaps it may play a role in the healing of fractures.

The calcitonins made by different animals differ somewhat in chemical composition. Human calcitonin molecules contain 32 combined amino acid residues. The hormone made by the pig has been synthesized.

HORMONE OF THE PARATHYROID GLANDS

The parathyroid glands are four small structures located immediately back of the thyroid gland. Complete removal of these glands results in death. The parathyroid hormone is called *parathormone*. It has been isolated in pure form and is a protein with a molecular weight of 9,500.

It is the function of parathormone to help maintain the level of calcium in the blood and body fluids. Removal of the parathyroids causes a decrease of blood calcium, and the patient dies with tetany (convulsions). This was the cause of death in many of the early operations on the thyroid gland. Injections of parathormone cause an increase in the calcium of the blood and an increased excretion of phosphate in the urine.

The rate of secretion of parathormone is controlled by the concentration of calcium in the circulating blood. When this level falls, hormone is secreted. Parathormone acts on the kidney to decrease the excretion of calcium by increasing its reabsorption by the tubules. It also causes bone cells to change to cells known as osteoclastic cells; these cells break down bone and release calcium and phosphate to the blood. These activities result in

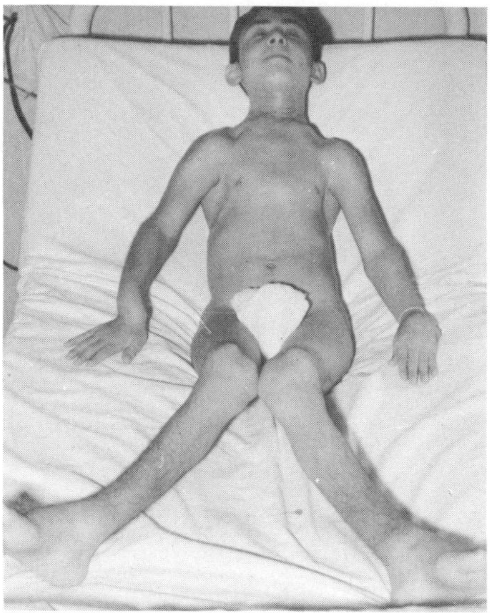

Fig. 32-11. A 15-year old patient with hyperparathyroidism caused by a tumor (adenoma) of a parathyroid gland. Would the level of calcium in his serum probably be normal, low, or high? (From Lomnitz, E., and others: Primary hyperparathyroidism simulating rickets, J. Clin. Endocr. **26:**309, 1966.)

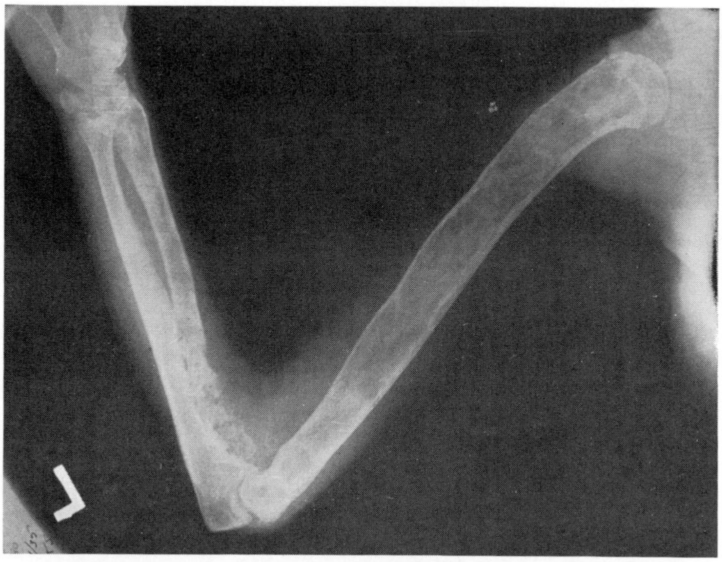

Fig. 32-12. X-ray photograph of bones in a case of osteitis fibrosa cystica. Notice that large areas in the bones do not photograph well. This indicates the presence of cysts, or areas of loss of bone material. What is the usual cause of osteitis fibrosa cystica?

an increase in the calcium level of the body fluids. The hormone also promotes the excretion of phosphate in the urine. This more than offsets the increased phosphate released from bone, and actually leads to a net decrease in the phosphate content of body fluids.

Overactivity of the parathyroid glands is usually caused by adenomas (tumors) of these glands. In this condition the blood calcium level is high and the patient may sometimes fall into *coma*. Decalcification (loss of calcium) of the bones occurs. One type of decalcification, in which many bones are affected, is known as *osteitis fibrosa cystica*. Overactivity of these glands is treated by finding and removing the parathyroid adenoma that is responsible for the increased production of parathormone.

HORMONES OF THE ADRENAL GLANDS

One adrenal ("next to the kidney") gland is perched on top of each kidney. These glands are called also the suprarenal ("above the kidney") glands. Each gland consists of an inner portion, called the *medulla*, and an outer portion, called the *cortex*.

The hormone made by the medulla is called *epinephrine (adrenaline)*. We believe that this compound is made from the amino acid *tyrosine*.

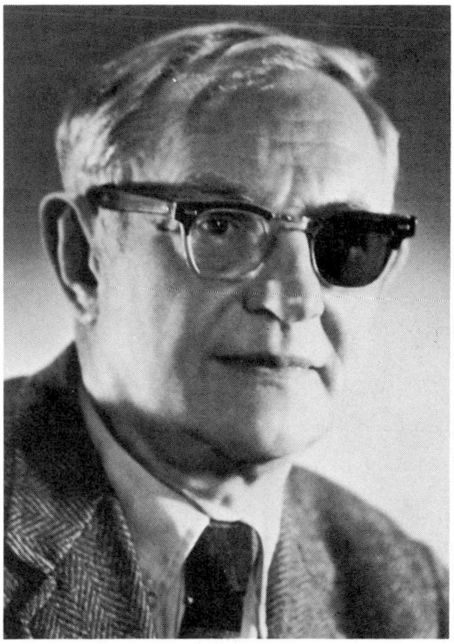

Fig. 32-13. Dr. Julius Axelrod, who shared the Nobel Prize in Medicine or Physiology for 1970 with Swedish scientist, Dr. Ulf S. von Euler, and British scientist, Sir Bernard Katz. The awards were given in recognition of fundamental studies on the chemistry and physiology of nerve impulse transmission. Dr. Axelrod, who did his research at the National Institute of Mental Health, discovered the two ways in which norepinephrine is inactivated after a nerve cell fires off an impulse. This work also led to a better understanding of the mechanism of action of some important drugs. How does norepinephrine differ chemically from epinephrine?

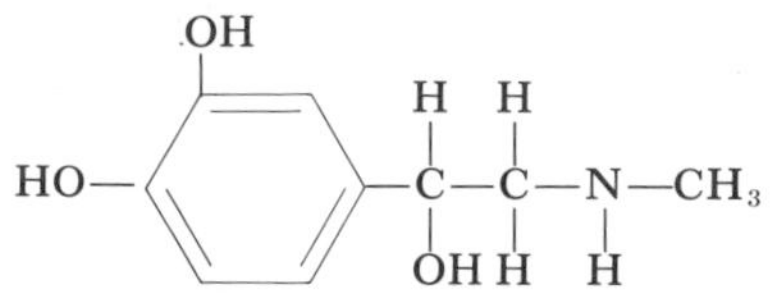

Epinephrine (adrenaline)

The nerves of the body are divided into three systems: the voluntary nervous system, the sympathetic nervous system, and the parasympathetic nervous system. We shall not have space here to describe these systems, but for those who have a knowledge of them, it will be helpful to learn that the effects produced by injecting epinephrine into the body are similar to those that result when the *sympathetic nerves* are stimulated. Indeed, the sympathetic nerve endings secrete a substance known as norepinephrine, noradrenaline, or arterenol. This compound lacks the methyl group ($—CH_3$) present in the molecule of epinephrine. Some of the important effects caused by injecting epinephrine and norepinephrine are:

1. *Elevation of blood pressure.* In conditions where the blood pressure falls to dangerously low levels, epinephrine is used as an emergency drug to raise it until more permanent treatment can be instituted.
2. *Construction of small arterioles.* Epinephrine sometimes is applied to bleeding areas; it helps check the bleeding by constructing the arterioles (small arteries) from which the blood is escaping. The hormone is also frequently mixed with local anesthetics that are injected

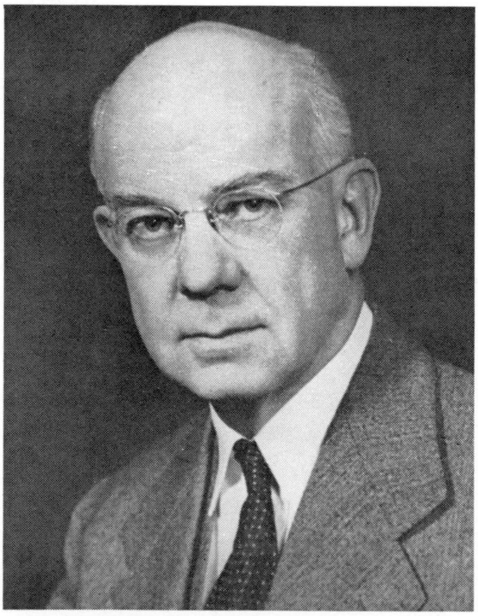

Fig. 32-14. Dr. Edward C. Kendall in 1950 (then at the Mayo Clinic) was awarded the Nobel Prize in medicine or physiology for his work in isolating and characterizing the adrenocortical hormones. What types of disease are relieved by these hormones?

under the skin. By constricting small blood vessels, epinephrine reduces the amount of blood flowing through the area and slows down the diffusion of the anesthetic into the blood stream. This increases the length of time the anesthesia is effective.

3. *Stimulation of the heart muscle.* Epinephrine sometimes is injected directly into the heart muscle in cases where this organ has ceased to beat. This may occur, for example, while the patient is under general anesthesia. If the heart of a newborn baby is not beating, it can sometimes be started with the aid of epinephrine.
4. *Constriction of the blood vessels of the mucous membranes of the nose and a relaxation of the muscles of the bronchi (air tubes leading into the lungs).* These effects make epinephrine useful in treating asthma, a condition accompanied by nasal stuffiness and constriction of the bronchial muscles. Ephedrine, a plant drug, is also used in treating asthma and similar conditions. Ephedrine does not act as quickly as does epinephrine, but its action is more prolonged. Numerous other compounds chemically related to ephedrine are used as drugs.
5. *Rise in blood sugar.* As we have seen in a previous chapter, this rise is due to increased glycogenolysis. Any sudden emotion causes the secretion of epinephrine by the adrenal glands, and this explains why *emotional glycosuria* exists. The sudden rise in blood sugar may exceed the renal threshold, and glucose will then appear in the urine.

Paroxysmal hypertension (intermittent attacks of high blood pressure) may be caused by pheochromocytomas, which are tumors of the adrenal medulla. The increased blood pressure is believed to be caused by an increased production of epinephrine by the tumor.

The *cortex* of the adrenal gland makes several substances that have hormone activity. The structures of these hormones are similar to those of the sex hormones.

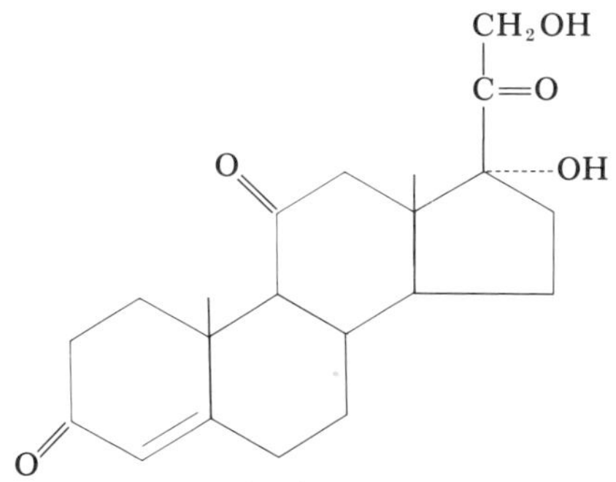

Cortisone
17α,21-dihydroxy-3,11,20-trioxopregn-4-ene

Cortisone (compound E) has been found to give dramatic relief in certain of the so-called collagen diseases (that is, diseases involving the connective tissue of the body). The best known of these in lay circles are rheumatoid arthritis and acute rheumatic fever. Some allergic diseases (for example, allergic asthma and drug reactions) also respond. Unfortunately, these diseases are not cured, and if large doses of the hormone are given for long periods of time, serious toxicity may result.

Cortisol (hydrocortisone, compound F) is the major active steroid secreted by the adrenal cortex of the human. It is more active than is cortisone.

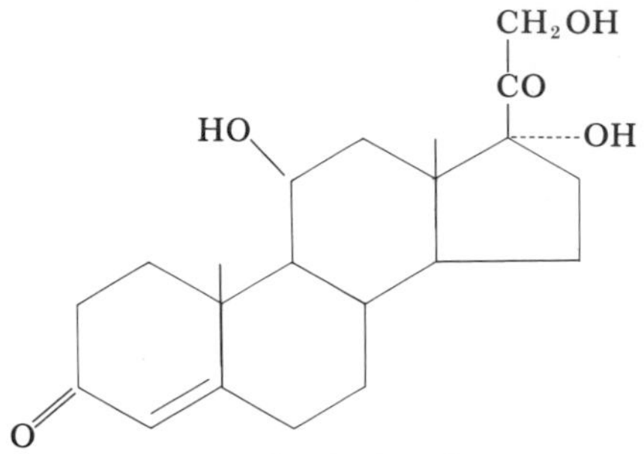

Cortisol
11β,17α,21-trihydroxy-3,20-dioxopregn-4-ene

A number of synthetic steroids having adrenocortical activity have been made. Some of them are many times as active as is cortisol, and several of them are used as drugs for the symptomatic treatment of allergic and collagen diseases.

Complete removal of the cortex of both adrenal glands leads to death unless the animal is treated with a cortical hormone or with special diets. The chemical changes that occur in the body after such removal are numerous and complicated. Some of them are as follows: (1) a loss of sodium chloride from the blood (this salt is excreted in large quantities in the urine), (2) a rise in the level of blood potassium, (3) a rise in the level of blood urea, (4) a fall in the level of blood sugar, (5) a concentration of the blood, that is, a loss of water from the blood to the tissues, and (6) a rise in the level of plasma globulin.

Animals from which the adrenal cortex has been removed can be kept alive either by injecting an active cortical hormone or by giving them diets that are very high in sodium chloride and very low in potassium salts.

Clinically, *hypofunction* (underactivity) of the adrenal cortex causes *Addison's disease*. This disease is accompanied by the foregoing chemical signs. The clinical signs and symptoms include weakness, pigmentation of the skin and mucous membranes, loss of weight, and low blood pressure. Most cases of Addison's disease are caused by tuberculosis of the adrenal cortex. The tuberculous process destroys much of the cortex of both adrenal glands and thus causes hypofunction.

Overactivity of the adrenal cortex *(hyperfunction)* is associated usually with the presence of a cortical tumor or with overdosage with cortisone or ACTH (see page 406). If hyperfunction occurs in childhood, sexual development is hastened, and a child of 6 years may have enlargement of the sex organs and fully developed pubic hair. If the child is a female, the breasts may enlarge and, in some cases, menstruation may begin. Hyperfunction in the adult occurs most commonly in females. The patient becomes more masculine in appearance, the uterus atrophies, menstruation ceases, the breasts decrease in size, the voice deepens, and hair may appear on the face. In the case of adult males, masculine characters are usually accentuated: there is an increase in the size of the sex organs, an increase in the amount of body hair, a deepening of the voice, and so on. In some cases the hyperactive adrenal cortex produces estrogenic steroids, and female characteristics appear.

The adrenal cortex elaborates a large number of compounds related chemically to cortisone and the sex hormones. Some of these (the adrenocortical androgens) have physiological effects resembling those of testosterone and are responsible for some of the clinical signs of overactivity of the gland. The other active substances can be divided into two major groups. The members of one group, of which *desoxycorticosterone (DOCA)* is an example, have marked effects on water and salt metabolism and only small effects on carbohydrate metabolism. Members of the other group, of which *cortisone* is representative, have relatively slight effects on water and salt metabolism but cause a rapid deposition of glycogen in the liver when they are administered to animals from which the adrenals have been removed. (Such animals have almost no glycogen in their livers.) DOCA is useful in treating patients with Addison's disease, but it is of no value in the therapy of arthritis or the other collagen and allergic diseases that respond to cortisone.

The most powerful DOCA-like substance in the adrenal cortex is *aldosterone*. This substance is not secreted in response to ACTH (see page 406). It may play a role in the development of water and salt retention in patients with kidney or heart disease. Rarely, patients secrete abnormally large quantities of aldosterone as a result of an adrenal tumor. Such patients, said to have *primary aldosteronism*, have a type of high blood pressure that usually can be cured by an operation to remove the tumor.

HORMONE OF THE PANCREAS

Insulin, the hormone of the pancreas, is produced in specialized pancreatic cells known as the islands of Langerhans. This hormone has been isolated in pure crystalline form. It is a protein, with a molecular weight of 5,734. The molecule is composed of two polypeptide chains joined together by the disulfide (—S—S—) bridges of two cystine (an amino acid) residues. Its synthesis was reported in 1966. Insulin cannot be given by mouth because it is digested in the stomach and small intestine.

We have already learned that underactivity of the islands of Langerhans causes diabetes mellitus. The blood sugar is high, glucose appears in the urine, and ketosis is present. The glucose tolerance test gives a diabetic type of curve. Patients with this disease are treated by giving them injections of insulin. It will be remembered that this is not a cure for diabetes mellitus and must usually be continued throughout the patient's life. Diabetic persons are more susceptible to infections than are normal people, partly because the high sugar content of their body fluids forms a good medium in which harmful bacteria can grow and multiply.

When a *protamine* (a protein of low molecular weight; see page 269) is mixed with a solution of insulin, a precipitate of *protamine insulin* is formed. Protamine insulin is more slowly absorbed than is regular insulin and is used a great deal now in treating diabetes mellitus. It has the advantage that fewer injections are required; also, there is a constant diffusion of insulin into the blood, which more closely imitates the normal secretion of insulin than does the periodic injection of regular insulin.

Globin insulin is prepared by precipitating insulin with globin (see page

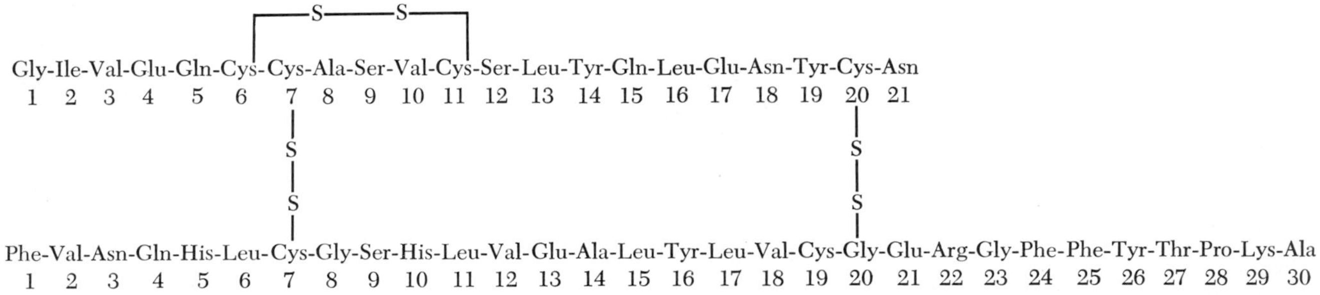

Fig. 32-15. The structure of insulin. (See page 480 for the amino acids and their abbreviations.) Why is insulin inactive when given by mouth?

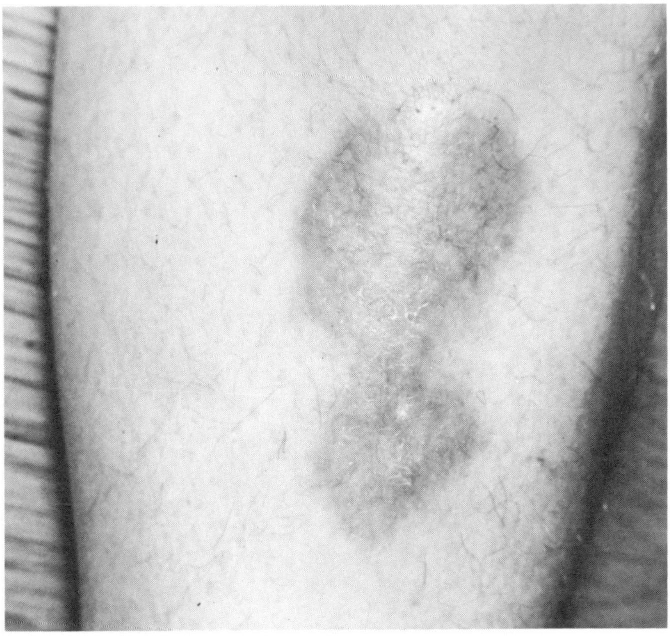

Fig. 32-16. A skin lesion present, usually over the tibia, in some patients with diabetes mellitus or in the prediabetic state. It exibits striking hues of brown, red, yellow, and purple, due to vascular damage. Dermatologists refer to it as necrobiosis lipidoidica diabeticorum. How does juvenile diabetes mellitus often differ from the disease that develops in adult life? (From Halprin, K. M.: Diabetes calling card, J.A.M.A. **198:**175, 1966.)

277). Its duration of action is longer than that of regular insulin but shorter than that of protamine insulin.

Several synthetic substances that cause a lowering of blood sugar are used as therapeutic agents.

Overactivity of the islands of Langerhans *(hyperinsulinism)* causes *hypoglycemia,* or low blood sugar. This is accompanied by periodic attacks of weakness, apprehension, dizziness, fainting, and sometimes convulsions. This condition usually is caused by an adenoma (tumor) of the pancreas.

A *unit of insulin* was originally defined as one-third the amount of insulin required to reduce the level of blood sugar of a 2,000 g fasting rabbit to a point where the rabbit went into convulsions (45 mg of glucose per 100 ml of blood). The unit used at present is about 40 percent stronger than this. One milligram of crystalline insulin is equivalent to from 22 to 27 units.

HORMONES OF THE PITUITARY GLAND

The pituitary gland (hypophysis) is a small structure (weight about 0.5 g) connected to the base of the brain by means of a stalk, called the infundibulum. It consists of three parts: the *anterior lobe,* the *pars intermedia,* and the *posterior lobe.* The anterior lobe has been called the "master gland" of the body because its hormones are necessary for the proper functioning of most of the other endocrine glands and are impor-

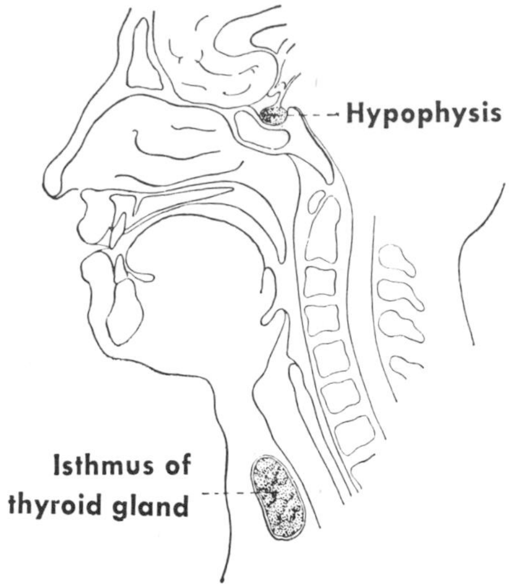

Fig. 32-17. Drawing to show the location of the pituitary gland (hypophysis). Why is the anterior lobe of this gland often called the "master gland" of the body?

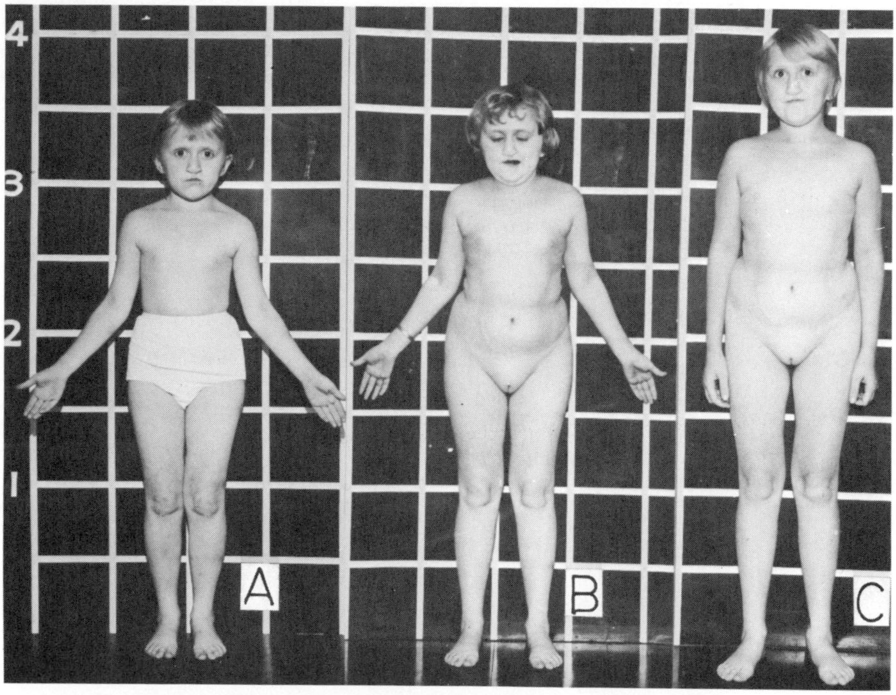

Fig. 32-18. A patient who had a deficiency of growth hormone. **A,** Age 11 years; **B,** age 11 years 8 months, after treatment for 5 months with human growth hormone (HGH or human STH); **C,** age 12 years 8 months, after treatment for 16 months with HGH. Name three other hormones found in the anterior pituitary gland. Are they manufactured there? (From Rosenbloom, A. L.: Growth hormone replacement therapy, J. A. M. A. **198:**364, 1966.)

A

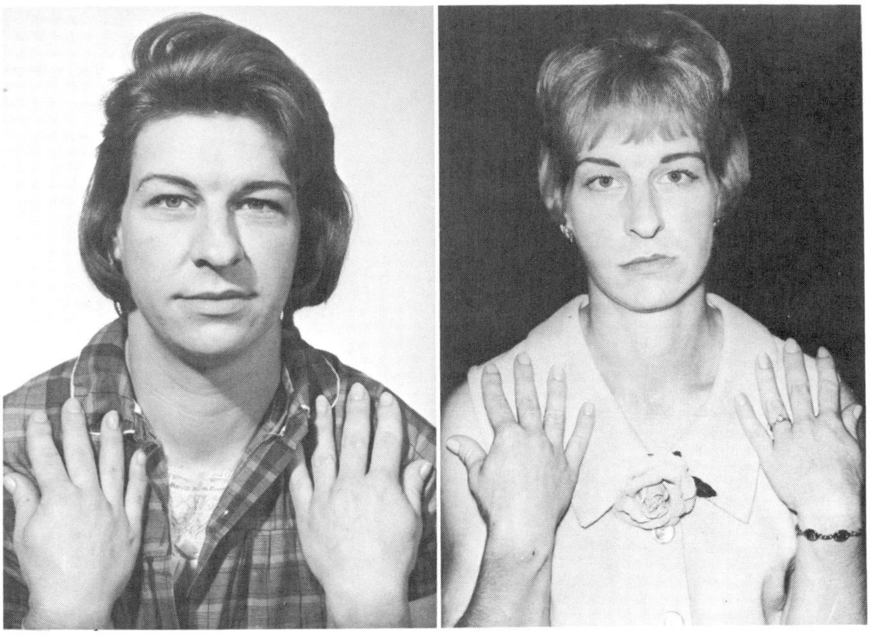

B

Fig. 32-19. A, A 28-year old woman with acromegaly. She was treated by surgical removal of a tumor of the pituitary gland; **B,** same woman, some time after surgery. What is the usual cause of acromegaly? (From Dashe, A. M., and others: Stereotaxic hypophyseal cryosurgery in acromegaly and other disorders, J.A.M.A. **198:**591, 1966.)

tant in the growth processes of the body. The pituitary hormones are proteins or peptides.

GROWTH HORMONE. This anterior lobe hormone formerly was called *phyone* (from a Greek word meaning "I cause to grow"). Lack of this principle causes *dwarfism*. Pituitary dwarfs are frequently perfectly formed but are very small for their age. The familiar circus midgets are examples of this condition. In contrast to cretinism, the intellect is not impaired. In some cases there is a failure of proper sex development.

This hormone is known also as the somatotropic hormone, or STH. Growth hormone of human origin (sometimes abbreviated HGH) also has prolactin (see page 407) activity.

Theoretically it is possible to treat pituitary dwarfs with STH. However, only STH of human or monkey origin has activity for humans. One human pituitary yields only about 5 mg of STH—only enough to treat one dwarf for 1 week. The small size of monkeys makes this animal an impractical source of the hormone.

Overactivity of the anterior lobe is due usually to the presence of an adenoma. If this occurs in childhood, the child grows up to be a giant, and the condition is called *gigantism*. Most circus giants have pituitary adenomas. Overactivity that occurs in adult life causes marked enlargement of the jaw, hands, and feet, and a bowed spine. This condition is called *acromegaly*.

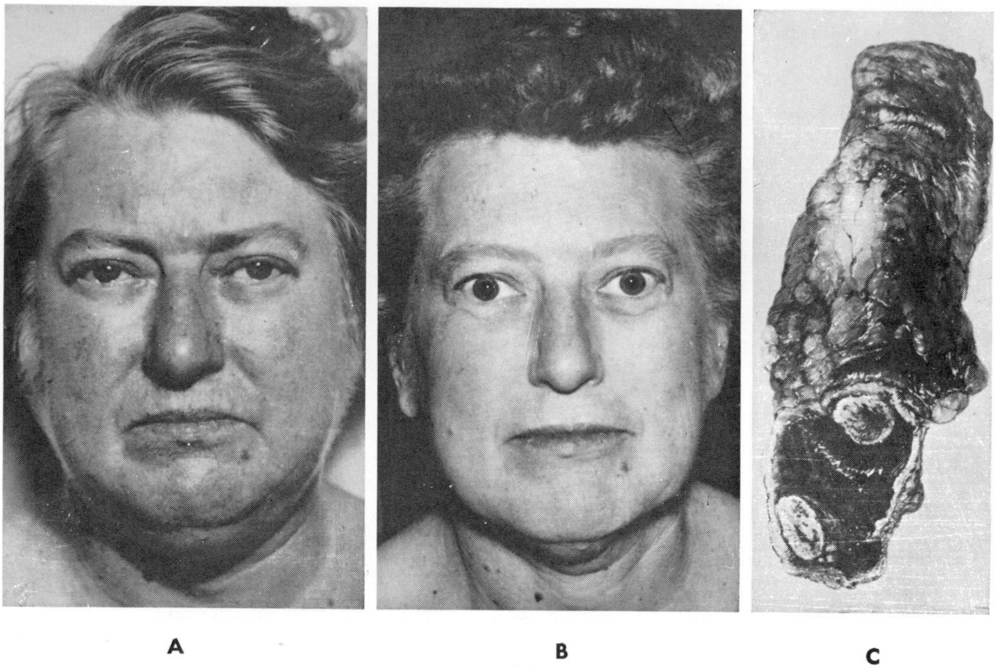

Fig. 32-20. **A,** Female, 45 years of age, who has Cushing's disease as a result of an overgrowth of the cortex of the adrenal gland. **B,** Same patient 8 months after removal of the adrenal glands. She was maintained in good health by giving her cortisol and desoxycorticosterone. **C,** The left adrenal gland removed at operation; it shows diffuse enlargement and a cystic adenoma. Why do you think she was given both cortisol and desoxycorticosterone after the operation? (Courtesy Dr. Peter Forsham; from Lisser, H., and Escamilla, R. F.: Atlas of clinical endocrinology, ed. 2, St. Louis, The C. V. Mosby Co., 1962.)

THYROTROPIC HORMONE. Removal of the anterior lobe of the pituitary gland causes the thyroid gland to become smaller and to cease to produce its hormone in normal amounts. Injection of active extracts of the anterior lobe causes enlargement of this gland. These facts indicate that the anterior lobe of the pituitary gland manufactures a hormone, the *thyrotropic hormone* (TSH, *thyroid stimulating hormone*), that is necessary for proper functioning of the thyroid gland. TSH is a glycoprotein.

ADRENOCORTICOTROPIC HORMONE (ACTH). This hormone stimulates the adrenal cortex, causing it to enlarge and to secrete its hormones. Active preparations cause the secretion of cortisone or biologically similar compounds from the adrenal cortex and are used in medicine in the symptomatic treatment of those diseases for which cortisone is useful (see page 399).

ACTH is a peptide and has been made synthetically in the laboratory.

Cushing's disease may result from oversecretion of, or overdosage with, ACTH or cortisone. Important symptoms are: high blood pressure; a rapidly developing, painful obesity of the face, neck, and trunk; amenorrhea (absence of menstruation) in females; and sexual impotence in males.

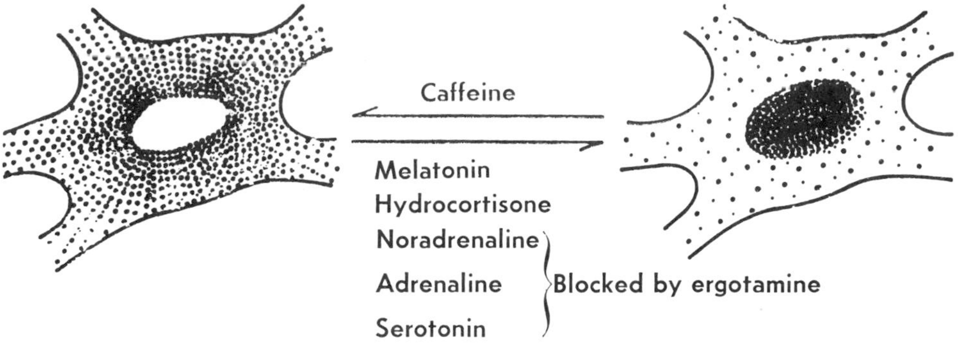

Fig. 32-21. Diagram to show mechanism involved in the darkening and lightening of melanocytes. What pituitary hormone causes darkening of these cells? (Courtesy Dr. Aaron B. Lerner.)

PROLACTIN. This hormone is known also as the *lactogenic hormone.* It has been isolated in crystalline form. Acting with ovarian and adrenocortical hormones, it causes growth of the breast. Prolactin, cortisol, and insulin work together to stimulate the synthesis of milk. In pigeons and doves, who do not make milk, prolactin stimulates the formation of a milk-like material by cells in a structure known as the crop: this material is used as food by the young birds.

GONADOTROPIC HORMONES. One of these factors is called the *follicle-stimulating hormone* (FSH). The other pituitary gonadotropic factor is the *luteinizing hormone* (LH), known also as the *interstitial cell-stimulating hormone* (ICSH). FSH stimulates growth of the follicles of the ovary in the female, and in the male causes growth of the cells that manufacture the spermatozoa. Both FSH and LH appear to be necessary for the secretion of estrogenic hormones. LH induces ovulation. It also stimulates growth of the interstitial cells of the testis and ovary. In the male these interstitial cells secrete the male sex hormones. The interstitial cells of the female are not believed to secrete hormones. LH takes part in initiating growth of the corpus luteum and in causing the secretion of progestrone. Both FSH and LH are glycoproteins.

The melanophore-stimulating hormones, abbreviated MSH, are found throughout the pituitary, but are most concentrated in the pars intermedia. (An older name for these substances is intermedin.) MSH has been made synthetically. It consists of two active peptides, α-MSH and β-MSH. These substances cause the pigment granules in pigmented skin cells to migrate from a zone close to the nucleus toward the periphery (outside) of the cell. This causes the skin to darken in color. There is evidence that an increased amount of MSH is released by the pituitary gland when the adrenal cortex is underactive. This probably explains why the skin darkens in Addison's disease (see page 400). Another suggestion is that the darkening is caused by secretion of ACTH. The ACTH molecule (a peptide) contains within its long peptide chain a sequence of amino acid residues that is very similar to that of MSH. ACTH has some melanocyte-stimulating properties.

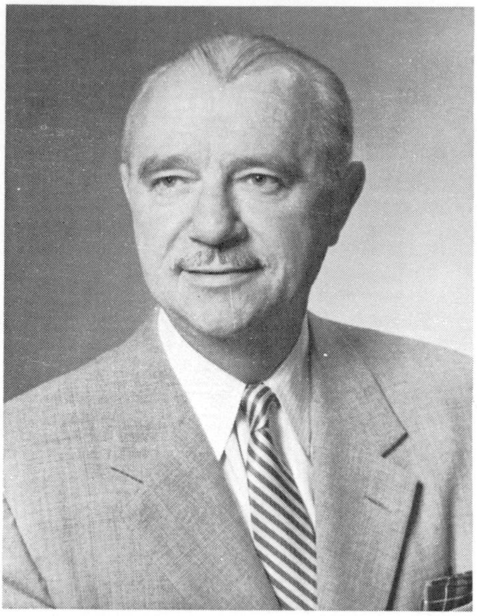

Fig. 32-22. Dr. Vincent du Vigneaud, then at Cornell Medical College, was awarded the Nobel Prize in chemistry in 1955 for successfully synthesizing oxytocin. He and his collaborators later synthesized vasopressin. How do the biological activities of these two substances differ?

The *posterior lobe* of the pituitary gland stores 2 hormones that are made in cells in the hypothalamus, the part of the brain to which the pituitary is attached. They migrate into the posterior lobe by way of axons (nerve processes) orginating in the hypothalamus. One of these, *oxytocin*, has an *oxytocic* effect; that is, it causes a contraction of the muscles of the uterus. It is used in obstetrics after the birth of the child and the placenta; the contraction of the uterine muscles that it causes helps to stop uterine bleeding. The other hormone, *vasopressin*, causes a rise of blood pressure and is sometimes called the *pressor substance*. Extracts containing both oxytocin and vasopressin are called *Pituitrin*.

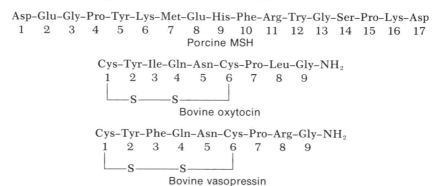

Asp–Glu–Gly–Pro–Tyr–Lys–Met–Glu–His–Phe–Arg–Try–Gly–Ser–Pro–Lys–Asp
1 2 3 4 5 6 7 8 9 10 11 12 13 14 15 16 17
Porcine MSH

Cys–Tyr–Ile–Gln–Asn–Cys–Pro–Leu–Gly–NH_2
1 2 3 4 5 6 7 8 9
└S——S┘ (disulfide bridge between 1 and 6)
Bovine oxytocin

Cys–Tyr–Phe–Gln–Asn–Cys–Pro–Arg–Gly–NH_2
1 2 3 4 5 6 7 8 9
└S——S┘ (disulfide bridge between 1 and 6)
Bovine vasopressin

Oxytocin has at least five physiological activities:

1. It causes contraction of the uterus.

2. It brings about a release of milk in mammals (the so-called milk-letdown effect).
3. It lowers blood pressure in birds. This effect is the basis of the usual method of bioassay of the hormone.
4. It causes a slight rise in blood pressure in mammals.
5. It causes an increased flow of urine in mammals.

In the hypothalamic region of the brain, just above the area where the optic nerves (sensory nerves from the eyes) cross, there is a small group of nerve cells called the *supraoptic nucleus*. Extending from this nucleus down the infundibulum (stalk connecting the pituitary to the brain) and into the pituitary gland is a group of nerve fibers called the *supraoptic tract*. Injury or disease of any portion of this nucleus or tract causes *diabetes insipidus*, a disorder that has been described in previous chapters (see pages 336 and 373). The disease is caused also by removal of the posterior lobe. Strangely, diabetes insidipus cannot be produced by any of these procedures in the absence of the anterior lobe. Injection of vasopressin relieves this condition. This is not a curative procedure, and injections must be given at regular intervals. It is a curious but unexplained fact that if the patient is under the influence of an anesthetic, vasopressin *increases, rather than diminishes,* the elimination of water in the urine.

Vasopressin is also referred to as the *antidiuretic hormone (ADH)*. When the plasma becomes hypertonic (too low in water content), sensitive cells in the hypothalamus shrink and send out impulses that cause the release of ADH from the posterior pituitary and also send signals that cause the sensation of thirst in higher brain centers. The released ADH then decreases the loss of water in the urine. When the plasma becomes hypotonic (too much water), the same hypothalamic cells swell (since they have a higher osmotic pressure than the plasma) and inhibit the release of ADH. Emotional stress, morphine, barbiturates, and pain stimulate release of ADH; cold, alcohol, carbon dioxide, and some drugs inhibit its release, resulting in an increased flow of urine.

DISEASES OF ENZYMIC DEFECT INVOLVING ANTERIOR PITUITARY HORMONES. The following are diseases that involve defects of the anterior pituitary hormones.

Isolated deficiency of ACTH. Some of these patients are deeply pigmented. They exhibit signs and symptoms of adrenal cortical insufficiency: weakness, fatigue, weight loss, anorexia (loss of apetite), nausea, vomiting, low blood sugar, low blood pressure. They can be treated successfully with ACTH, which is available commercially as a drug.

Isolated deficiency of TSH. These patients have numerous and bizarre symptoms, not always immediately suggestive of thyroid underactivity. Some of these are weakness, angina pectoris (periodic pains in the chest), mental lassitude (laziness), intolerance to cold, polyuria (increased flow of urine), polydipsia (increased thirst), weakness on fasting, and dizzy spells. Not all patients exhibit all of these symptoms. TSH can be used as a therapeutic agent; it is available commercially.

Isolated deficiency of STH. Only a few patients with STH deficiency have been studied. They have ranged in age from 1 year to 76 years. All were dwarfs. They exhibited marked hypoglycemia (see page 265) after fasting.

Isolated gonadotropin deficiency. These patients do not develop normally sexually. Growth and development are normal prior to puberty. Gonadotropins cannot be detected in the urine.

OTHER FACTORS

An *anterior-pituitary-like hormone* is found in the urine of pregnant women. It is known commonly as *chorionic gonadotropin*. Apparently it is produced by the placenta. This substance causes maturation of the follicles, hemorrhage into the follicles, and the formation of a corpus luteum. The ovum is not expelled but is retained in the corpus luteum. The presence of this substance is the basis for a common test for pregnancy. Twenty milliliters of urine from the patient are injected into the vein of a female rabbit. The ovaries of the rabbit are examined 36 to 48 hours later. The presence of hemorrhagic (blood-filled) follicles indicates that the patient is pregnant. This test is the Friedman modification of a similar test devised by Aschheim and Zondek.

Toads and frogs also are used in testing for pregnancy. The Hogben test, using female South African clawed toads, is positive if eggs are deposited 8 to 16 hours after 1 ml of urine from the patient is injected into the dorsal lymph sac. The male South American toad and the North American male frog also can be used. Urine is injected into the dorsal lymph sac. If the test is positive, spermatozoa appear in the animal's urine within 2 to 4 hours.

Animal tests for pregnancy usually do not become positive until about 40 days after the last menstrual period.

Gonadotropic hormones (pregnant mare serum: PMS) occur in the serum of pregnant mares, and preparations of such serum formerly were used in clinical medicine as a source of this type of hormone (for example, in the treatment of undescended testes or deficiency of estrogenic hormones). Unfortunately, many patients become refractory (no longer respond) to PMS after a short course of treatment.

Hydatiform moles are large tumors of the uterus that sometimes develop from retained fragments of the placenta after delivery or abortion. They resemble clusters of grapes. Sometimes they change to *chorionepithelioma*, a type of cancer that is usually fatal. Both hydatiform moles and chorionepitheliomas give positive Friedman tests; if the patient is known not to be pregnant, the presence of these tumors is suspected when the pregnancy test is positive.

The *pineal gland* in the brain makes a substance known as *melatonin* (5-hydroxyindole-3-acetic acid). Melatonin reverses the action of MSH and causes a lightening of the color of pigment cells.

HORMONES OF THE HYPOTHALAMUS

In addition to oxytocin and vasopressin, cells in the hypothalamus manufacture at least seven hormones that regulate the release of hormones from the pituitary. Five of them cause release; two inhibit release. A network of blood vessels connects the hypothalamus with the pituitary; these seven hormones are transported by this network. The hormones are:

1. ACTH-releasing hormone, CRH
2. LH-releasing hormone, LH-RH or LRH
3. FSH-releasing hormone, FSH-RH or FRH
4. TSH-releasing hormone, TRH
5. STH-releasing hormone, SRH or GRH (G for "growth hormone")
6. Prolactin release-inhibiting hormone, PRIH

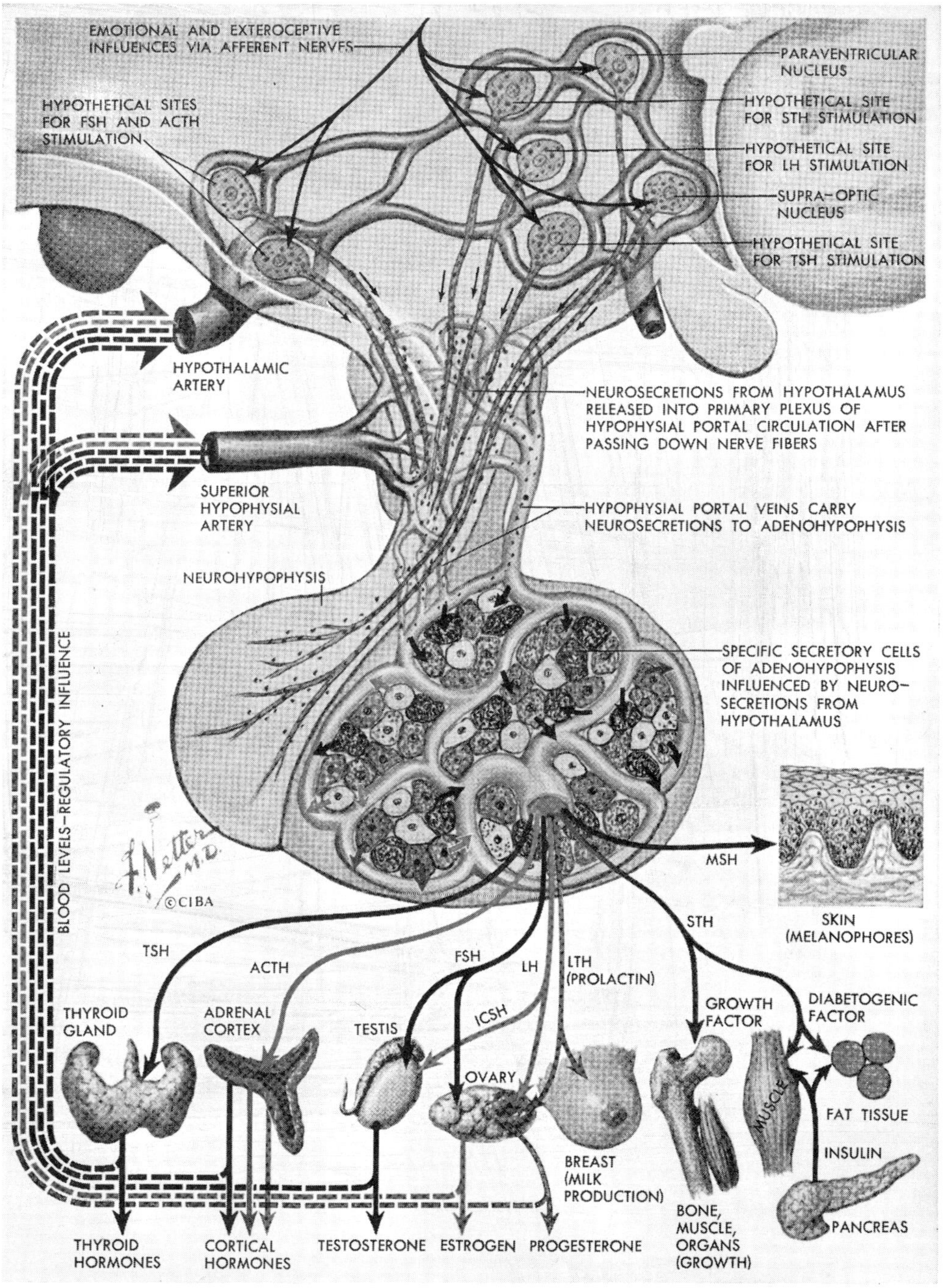

Fig. 32-23. Drawing illustrating interrelationships among the hypothalamus, the pituitary gland, and target organs. How does the hypothalamus influence the secretion of pituitary hormones? (From the CIBA collection of medical illustrations by Dr. Frank H. Netter. Copyright CIBA.)

7. MSH release-inhibiting hormone, MRIH

TRH has been synthesized in the laboratory. It is a tripeptide composed of cyclized glutamic acid, histidine, and proline: the —COOH group of the terminal proline has been replaced by $—CONH_2$.

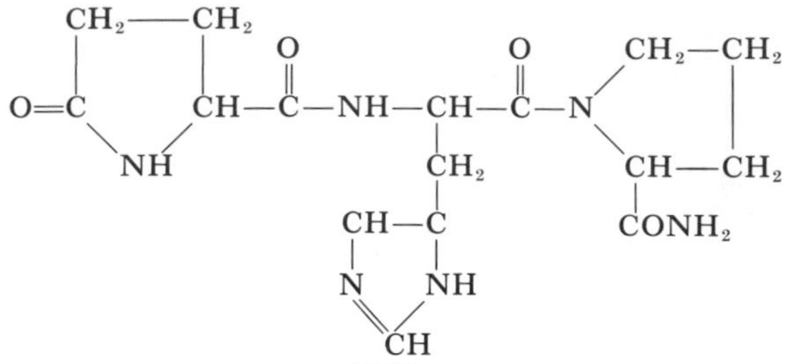

TRH

In June 1971, the isolation and determination of the structure of a single hormone from pigs that has the biologic activity of both LH–RH and FSH–RH was announced at a meeting of the Endocrine Society. About one-half million hypothalamus glands were required to obtain enough material for study. The work was done at the Veterans Administration Hospital in New Orleans, Tulane University Medical Center, and Abbott Laboratories. One microgram of this hormone is enough to stimulate a human pituitary body to release both LH and FSH. Its structure is:

$$\text{Glu–His–Tyr–Ser–Tyr–Gly–Leu–Arg–Pro–Gly–NH}_2$$

Some scientists refer to these hormones as *factors* and accordingly use different abbreviations (CRF instead of CRH, for example).

HORMONE OF THE THYMUS GLAND

The thymus is a structure that has two lobes and is located in the upper part of the chest, in front of the aorta. At birth, the gland in the human weighs about 13 g. It increases in size gradually and weighs about 20 to 35 g at puberty. After this it slowly atrophies.

Most of our knowledge about the function of the thymus has been gained since 1961. Scientists had been unable to note any particular effect when it was removed from animals, but in 1961 it was found that when the gland was removed from mice immediately after birth, lymphocytes failed to appear in normal numbers in the lymph nodes, spleen, and Peyer's patches (in the intestine). These mice also became stunted and died at an early age.

There are two important immunological systems that operate in the body. One system involves plasma cells and germinal centers of lymphocytes in the lymph nodes. These cells are capable of producing antibodies (immunoglobulins) that circulate in the bloodstream. The other system involves small lymphocytes that can become sensitized as a result of exposure to an antigen. This second immunological system is responsible for so-called delayed hypersensitivity reactions such as rejection of skin grafts and transplanted organs, and certain diseases. The first system is important as a defense against microbial diseases and other disorders in which antibodies appear in the blood.

The thymus and a hormone (thymosin) produced by it are required for activation of the delayed hypersensitivity system. Small lymphocytes of the system migrate from the thymus to other regions of the body. In the presence of thymosin, these cells are capable of becoming sensitized when are exposed to an appropriate antigen.

The other immunological system seems to be activated in very young individuals by lymphoepithelial tissue present in the intestine.

The seeding (migration) and activation processes occur during a relatively short period of time—perhaps 2 months in the mouse—after which the thymus atrophies without harm to the animal.

HORMONES AS CONTRACEPTIVE AGENTS. Balanced mixtures of an estrogen and a progestogen (synthetic compound having progesterone-like activity) are used (usually in tablet form) for contraception. The woman takes one tablet each day, beginning on the fifth to seventh day after menstruation. One tablet is taken daily for 20 or 21 days. This mixture inhibits the production of hormones by the pituitary, and ovulation does not occur (see page 384). When the woman stops taking the tablets, uterine bleeding (menstruation) soon follows, indicating that she is not pregnant (see page 385).

In some cases, only the estrogen is taken during the first 10 or 15 days, and the mixture during the second 5 or 10. Here, inhibition of the pituitary is due almost entirely to the estrogen.

RENIN MECHANISM

The pulse pressure (difference between the highest and lowest arterial pressures during one heartbeat) of the kidney arteries can be reduced by appropriate surgical procedures in experimental animals. One such procedure involves placing a metal clamp around the renal artery in such a way that the vessel is partly, but not completely, occluded. The same effect can be obtained by wrapping the kidney with a sheet of cellophane, silk, or cotton. This latter procedure causes the formation of scar tissue around the kidney; this hard, fibrous tissue contracts and "squeezes" the kidney arteries. When the arterial pulse pressure in the kidney is reduced by either of the methods, the animal develops hypertension (high blood pressure). The sequence of biochemical events leading to this development of hypertension appears to be as follows: As a result of the lowered pulse pressure, the kidney cells produce and release into the blood a protein known as *renin*.* Renin appears to be an enzyme, and it catalyzes the formation of a polypeptide, *angiotensin I* from one of the serum globulins *(angiotensinogen)*. Angiotensin I is converted to a substance known as angiotensin II in the presence of an enzyme present in plasma. Angiotensin II is thought to be the substance actually responsible for the rise of blood pressure. Angiotensin I contains 10 amino acid residues and is sometimes called the decapeptide. Angiotensin II (the octapeptide) contains 8 amino acid residues. Substances capable of inactivating both renin and angiotensin are present in blood and other tissues. One type of hypertension in human beings is caused by kidney disease.

Renin is produced in cells located immediately adjacent to the arterioles that

*Do not confuse the enzyme *renin (rē′ nĭn)* with the digestive enzyme *rennin (rĕn′ nĭn)*.

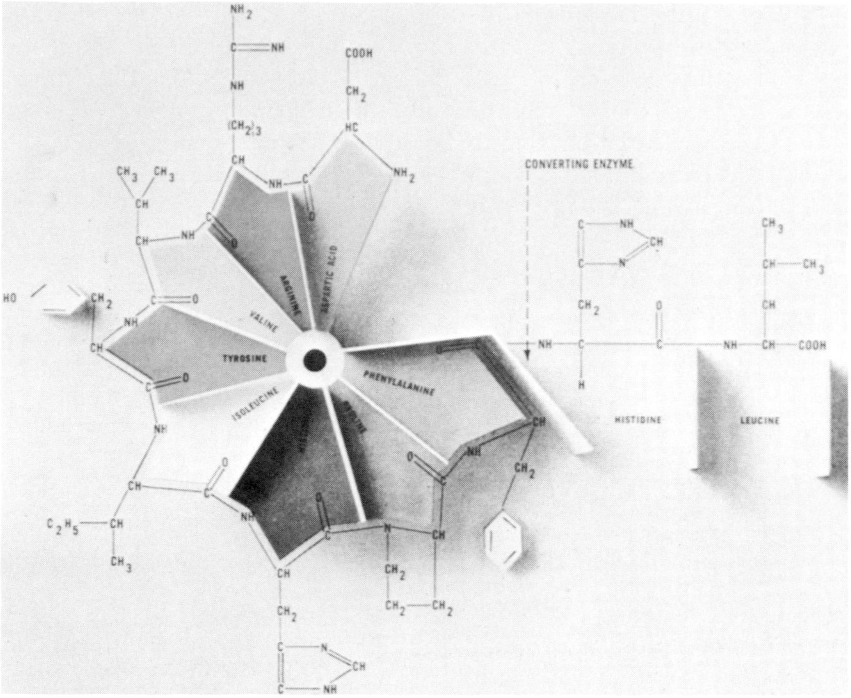

Fig. 32-24. Chemical structure of angiotensin showing the splitting off of histidyl leucine from the decapeptide by the converting enzyme to yield the active octapeptide. What biologic activity has angiotensin? (Courtesy Merck Sharp & Dohme Seminar.)

enter the glomeruli (see page 370). According to one theory, when the muscular walls of these arterioles relax as a result of a lowered blood volume and pressure, the release of renin is stimulated, and angiotensin II is formed in the plasma. In addition to its property of raising blood pressure, this substance stimulates the release of aldosterone (see page 401) from the adrenal cortex. Aldosterone, in turn, causes an increased retention of sodium chloride in the body fluids, including the blood (as a result of increased absorption of this salt from the kidney tubules; see page 372). This increases the volume of fluid (blood) in the blood vessels (both as a result of the increased osmotic pressure [see page 61] and as a result of the extra water required to dissolve the sodium chloride), and the release of renin by the kidney cells is suppressed. This, then, is a mechanism for regulating blood volume. Also, the increased blood volume produced by aldosterone causes an increase in blood pressure. Thus both angiotensin II and aldosterone play a role in the regulation of blood pressure.

STUDY QUESTIONS

1. What names are given to the glands that manufacture hormones? How do these glands differ from those that manufacture the digestive enzymes?
2. What are hormones? Chalones?
3. What three substances are the basis of the IUPAC system for naming steroids?
4. Name three follicular hormones. Which of these is believed to be made by the follicle cells?
5. What hormones are responsible for the changes that occur at puberty in the female? In the male?
6. What are the effects of the follicular hormones on the endometrium? What is the function of progesterone? Where is progesterone made?

7. What hormones cause cyclic changes in the vagina? Increase in the size of the breasts?
8. What is the fate of the corpus luteum if pregnancy does not occur? If pregnancy does occur? How is pregnancy affected if the corpus luteum is removed before delivery?
9. What excretion product is formed from progesterone in the body?
10. Name two good sources of follicular hormones. What is stilbestrol?
11. Name two male sex hormones. What cells manufacture testosterone? What are the functions of this hormone?
12. What halogen is needed to manufacture thyroxine? From what amino acid is this hormone made?
13. What is the function of thyroxine?
14. What is cretinism? Myxedema? Simple hypothyroidism? How are they treated?
15. What is a goiter?
16. What is toxic adenoma? Exophthalmic goiter? How are these conditions treated?
17. What is parathormone? What is its function? What is the treatment for osteitis fibrosa cystica?
18. What is the chemical nature of calcitonin?
19. What is the potential usefulness of calcitonin as a therapeutic agent?
20. What hormone is secreted by the medulla of the adrenal gland? Name five effects produced by an injection of this substance. Why are these effects useful in medicine?
21. How do pheochromocytomas cause paroxysmal hypertension?
22. Name some effects produced by removal of adrenal glands.
23. How can animals that have no adrenal cortex be kept alive? How do you think a patient with Addison's disease should be treated? What is the usual cause of this disease?
24. Discuss the symptoms that are usually produced by overactivity of the adrenal cortex.
25. What is the chemical nature of insulin? What cells manufacture it?
26. What are believed to be the functions of insulin (review Chapter 24)?
27. What is protamine insulin? What advantages does it have over ordinary insulin?
28. Give one reason why diabetic patients are more susceptible to infections that are normal people.
29. What is the usual cause of hyperinsulinism?
30. What is a unit of insulin?
31. Why is the anterior lobe of the pituitary gland called the "master gland"? List the hormones elaborated by this lobe.
32. What is the cause of pituitary dwarfism? Of gigantism? What is acromegaly? What is its cause?
33. What are the gonadotropic hormones? What are their functions in the female? In the male? How is the secretion of these hormones influenced by the follicular hormones?
34. Name 3 anterior pituitary hormones involved in diseases of enzymic defect.
35. What is the anterior-pituitary-like hormone? What effects are produced by injection of this hormone? What cells produce it?
36. Describe the Friedman test for pregnancy. In what conditions, other than pregnancy, is this test useful as a diagnostic procedure?
37. What is MSH?
38. Name the hormones stored by the posterior lobe of the pituitary gland. Give one effect produced by injecting each of these. Which of these do you imagine is present in highest physiological concentration in "obstetrical" Pituitrin?
39. What is the cause of diabetes insipidus? What substance is used in its treatment.
40. Describe Cushing's syndrome. What is believed to be its cause?
41. What role does the hypothalamus play in the physiology of the pituitary?
42. Describe the functions of the thymus.
43. Explain how a mixture of an estrogen and a progestogen can be used to prevent conception.
44. Give a brief discussion of the renin mechanism.

CHAPTER 33

Vitamins

Vitamins resemble hormones in many ways. Like the hormones, they are carried by the bloodstream to the various tissues of the body, which they influence, only small amounts of them being required to produce amazingly important effects. There is one important difference: *vitamins, or their provitamins, must be present in the diet, or must be made by bacteria in the intestinal tract.* The body is unable to make some of the vitamins; other vitamins can be made only from certain specific substances, called *provitamins,* that are present in balanced diets.

Early in this century it was realized that certain factors other than proteins, fats, carbohydrates, and inorganic salts must be included in the diet in order to secure correct nutrition. Dr. Casimir Funk believed these substances were organic amines, and, since they were necessary for life, he called them "vitamines" (vital amines). We have since learned that most of the vitamins do not have amino groups and have dropped the final "e." Also, there is a growing tendency to drop the vitamin terminology altogether and to designate the vitamin by an appropriate chemical name. The use of letters to designate the vitamins does serve a couple of useful purposes, however. The vitamins of the B family, or complex, often occur together in foods. In this group, a subscript number indicates a different vitamin: vitamins B_1 and B_2 differ both chemically and in biological function. In all other cases, the subscript denotes different chemical forms of the *same* vitamin: vitamins A_1 and A_2 are slightly different chemically but they have the *same* biological activity. There is only one vitamin C and thus a subscript number is unnecessary. Also, there are gaps in the letter nomenclature. The B complex vitamins proved to be essential for the human are B_1, B_2, B_6, and B_{12}. (Niacin and folic acid also are members of this complex, but we no longer use the letter terminology for them.) Vitamins A, C, D, E, and K are required vitamins, but F, G, H, I, and J are missing from the list. Historically, these missing names were applied to concentrates thought to contain new vitamins. In most cases, this proved to be wrong; in some cases duplicate names, now discarded, were used for the same vitamins. Vitamins A, D, E, and K are fat soluble: they do not dissolve in water. Vitamin C and members of the B complex are water soluble, but do not dissolve in fat.

VITAMIN A

PRO-VITAMINS

Carotenoid pigments are a class of colored substances made by plants. Some of these pigments—among them, α-carotene, β-carotene, γ-carotene, and cryptoxanthin—can be converted into vitamin A by animals. As far as we know, plants cannot make vitamin A itself. On the other hand, *only plants* can make the pigments necessary for the production of the vitamin by animals. Theoretically, one molecule of β-carotene can be converted to two molecules of vitamin A, and one molecule of each of the other three provitamins mentioned can yield one molecule of the vitamin. Actual experiments indicate, however, that β-carotene is only one-half as active as vitamin A when ordinary diets are fed.

CHEMICAL NATURE OF VITAMIN A

Vitamin A is a fat-soluble substance—that is, it dissolves in fats and in fat solvents but not in water. It has been isolated in pure crystalline form and has also been synthesized (made artificially) in the chemical laboratory. Crystalline vitamin A melts at 64° C.

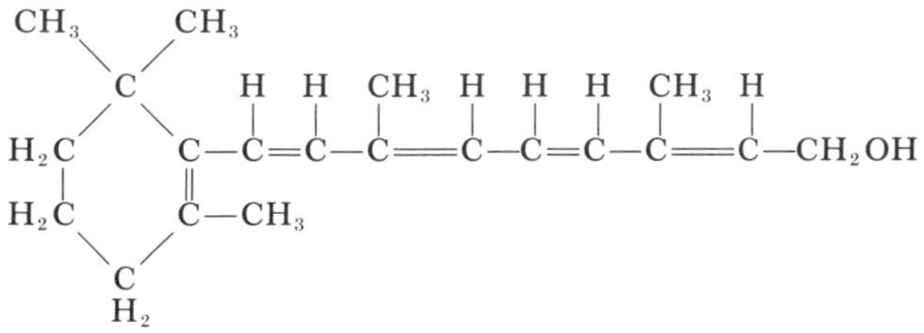

Vitamin A
(Retinol or vitamin A_1)

It has been found that the vitamin present in the livers of fresh-water fish differs slightly from the substance described above. This second substance, called dehydroretinol, or vitamin A_2, has the same physiological activity as vitamin A_1.

Vitamin A is fairly stable to heat, and the vitamin A potency of foods is not decreased very much by normal cooking and canning procedures.

VITAMIN A DEFICIENCY

Vitamin A deficiency results in failure of growth, atrophy and keratinization of epithelial tissues, night blindness, and defective formation of teeth.

FAILURE OF GROWTH. The discovery of vitamin A was due directly to the finding that animals failed to grow on diets that were low in certain animal fats. This failure of growth is not specific for any one of the vitamins, however, and almost all vitamin deficiency diseases are accompanied by it.

ATROPHY AND KERATINIZATION OF EPITHELIAL TISSUES. The epithelial tissues affected by vitamin A deficiency include the lacrimal glands (which make the tears), the conjunctiva (membrane that covers the front of the eyeball and lines the eyelids), the cornea (transparent portion of the eyeball), the salivary glands, the respiratory tract, the digestive tract, the genitourinary tract, and certain ductless glands. The surfaces of these structures *atrophy,* or shrink, and new cells appear that are hard and resemble the outer layer of the skin. Since the outer skin layers contain keratin, a scleroprotein, this formation of skinlike cells is called *keratinization.*

A condition in which the cornea becomes cloudy and thus unable to transmit light as well as it does normally is called *xerophthalmia.* The cause of this condition is vitamin A deficiency. The keratinization accompanying the vitamin lack lowers the resistance of the cornea, and bacteria are able to grow and multiply in the corneal tissue. Xerophthalmia is thus not entirely a deficiency disease. Rather, it is a bacterial infection superimposed on the changes accompanying the vitamin deficiency. The disease occurs most commonly in young boys and is a major public health problem in many parts of the world, especially in rapidly growing urban centers in the Far East. Ironically, plants rich in vitamin A activity grow, or will grow, in these areas, but the people will not eat them. Also, vitamin A is cheap: five cents will buy enough at United States prices to supply the entire annual requirement of a single human being.

The *skin* is an important epithelial structure. If vitamin A deficiency is severe, the skin of adult patients becomes rough and dry and presents a "tanned" appearance. Many of the sweat glands are destroyed, and a skin rash appears. This skin condition has been called *follicular hyperkeratosis.* Topical preparations containing vitamin A are used to treat some skin disorders. Changes in the salivary glands and tear ducts may cause them to become partially dry; this causes dryness of the mouth and eyes. Digestion and absorption of food may be adversely affected by changes in the mucous membrane of the gastrointestinal tract. In the genitourinary tract, similar

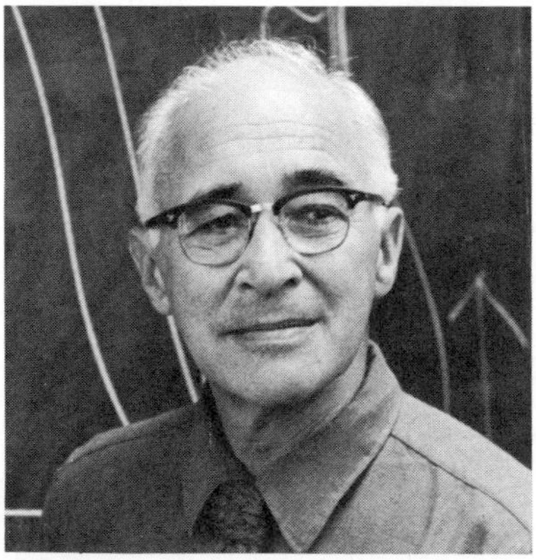

Fig. 33-1. Dr. George Wald of Harvard University won the Nobel Prize in physiology or medicine in 1967 for his pioneering work in elucidating the chemical events that occur when the retina is exposed to light. What vitamin is intimately involved in these changes?

changes sometimes cause failure of reproduction and predisposition to kidney and bladder stones.

NIGHT BLINDNESS (NYCTALOPIA). The inner lining of the eyeball is called the *retina*. The retina contains two types of cells that receive light energy and that are, therefore, necessary for sight. One type, the *cones*, is used to see and distinguish colors. The other cells, the *rods*, do not distinguish colors but are sensitive to small amounts of light and are responsible for vision in dim light. This explains why all colors appear gray if viewed by starlight. The rods contain a pigment, *visual purple (rhodopsin)*, that is necessary for their function. Visual purple is formed *by the chemical union of vitamin A aldehyde (retinal), and a protein(opsin)*. One of the first symptoms of vitamin A deficiency is *night blindness*, or inability to see in a dim light. This results from the failure of visual purple production so that the rods are unable to function.

When rhodopsin is exposed to light, a complicated series of reactions takes place. The most important ones are indicated in the following diagram.

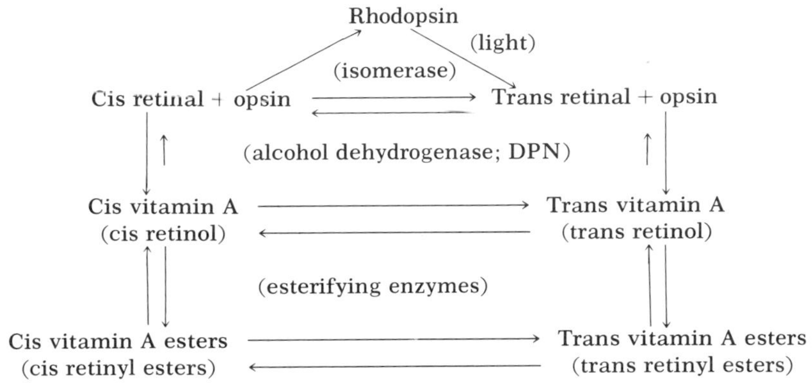

The prefixes cis and trans indicate that retinal and retinol exist in 2 isomeric forms. Cis retinal has the same chemical and structural formula as does trans retinal, but the way in which the molecules of each are twisted or bent in space differs (see page 161). The action of light in vision is to cause a change from the cis to the trans configuration of the combined retinal of the visual pigments (rhodopsin and others that will be mentioned). The other reactions of the cycle are independent of light and will occur in the dark.

The rod pigment in fresh-water fish (formed by the chemical union of vitamin A_2 aldehyde [$retinal_2$] and opsin) is known as *porphyropsin*.

Retinal pigments also occur in the cones. They are formed by the union of retinal opsins (which are proteins) with retinal and are known as *iodopsins* (if $retinal_1$ is involved) or as *cyanopsins* (if $retinal_2$ is involved). The 3 normal cone pigments are sensitive, respectively, to blue, green, and red light. They differ from each other in the chemistry of their opsins. The series of reactions that occurs when they are exposed to light is similar to that already diagrammed for rhodopsin.

About 1 percent of men lack the cone pigment sensitive to red and thus are red-blind. Approximately 2 percent of men are green-blind. Both of these conditions are extremely rare in women. Blue-blindness is very rare and is not sex-linked. It occurs in about 1 in 20,000 people, 40 percent of whom are women.

All of these symptoms of vitamin A deficiency (except those due to permanent damage, such as that caused by severe xerophthalmia) are rapidly cured by administration of the vitamin. The night blindness apparently disappears within a few hours after treatment is started; healing of epithelial structures begins in five or six days. A gain in weight is also noticed in less than a week after therapy is begun.

STORAGE OF VITAMIN A IN THE BODY

The normal adult has an amazing ability to store vitamin A. Laboratory animals can store enough in a week to last for several months. Approximately 95 percent of this stored vitamin is present in the liver. It is important to remember that the amount stored in a newborn infant is proportionally much less than that stored in the normal adult. This is true even when the mother has been given large amounts of vitamin A before delivery. Some pediatricians (physicians who specialize in the care of children) give babies vitamin A from the first week of life, but many of them feel that this is unnecessary at least for several months. Milk, the food of the infant, is an excellent source of the vitamin if the mother's diet is adequate. The first milk produced by the mother is five to ten times richer in vitamin A than is cow's milk, but after a few months of nursing the mother's milk and cow's milk contain about the same amounts.

ABSORPTION OF VITAMIN A

Most of the vitamin A given by mouth is absorbed within three to five hours. Carotene absorption is a little slower (seven to eight hours). Bile is not necessary for the absorption of vitamin A itself, but the carotenes cannot be absorbed in the absence of this material. This fact is worth remembering in connection with diseases in which bile does not reach the small intestine in normal amounts (obstructive jaundice, certain liver diseases, bile duct fistula). Vitamin A and its provitamins, like the fats, pass directly from the intestine into the lymph stream and are then carried through the thoracic duct to the bloodstream.

Mineral oil, a common laxative, has been shown to inhibit the absorption of the carotenes, but it does not affect the absorption of the active vitamin. Patients who are constantly taking mineral oil, therefore, must depend on sources of vitamin A other than plant foods (which contain only provitamins).

HYPERVITAMINOSIS A. This condition, although rare, is a recognized clinical syndrome. Usually there is a history of ingestion of large amounts of the vitamin for a long period of time – six to fifteen months. A thickening of the outer layers of the bones occurs, and hard, tender lumps can be felt in the extremities. Enlargement of the liver is common, and some patients exhibit jaundice, dry pigmented skin, loss of hair, and fissures of the lips. Symptoms subside rapidly after administration of the vitamin is discontinued – sometimes within seventy-two hours. The overgrowths of bone disappear over a period of several months.

Hypervitaminosis A usually is not observed unless the patient has been taking as much as 50,000 units of vitamin A daily for a long time.

In young children the clinical picture is somewhat different. There is a tenderness over the long bones, itching skin rashes, general irritability, loss of hair, weight loss, and loss of appetite. The child may be reluctant to stand and to walk. The ends of the long bones may be enlarged sufficiently to be palpable. The lips are dry and scaly, and bleeding may occur in fissures located at their corners.

Acute vitamin A poisoning in the infant is characterized by vomiting, hydrocephalus ("water on the brain") with bulging of the anterior fontanelle, insomnia, and agitation. Symptoms subside promptly, usually within twenty-four hours, after withdrawal of the vitamin.

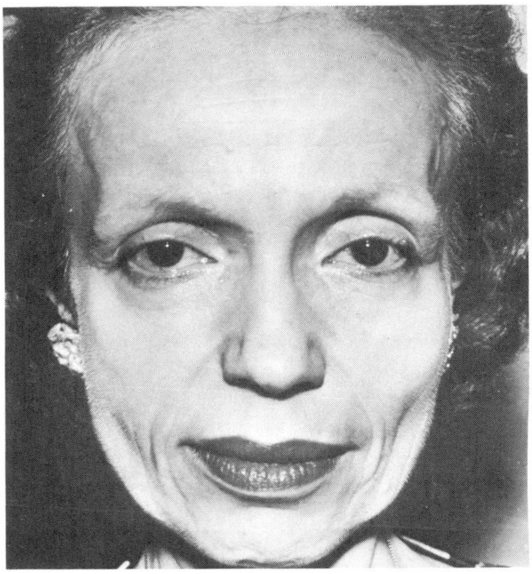

Fig. 33-2. Patient who had chronic hypervitaminosis A, as a result of ingesting 600,000 units of vitamin A daily for 3 years. What are some of the signs and symptoms of this condition? (From Di Benedetto, R. J.: Chronic hypervitaminosis A in an adult, J.A.M.A. **201**:700, 1967.)

Hypervitaminosis A has been caused by overzealous mothers who gave their children excessive amounts of vitamin A because of an erroneous belief that "if a little is good, more is better." Occasionally children have swallowed large amounts in the form of liquid concentrates or capsules. Some adults have the disease because excessive vitamin A has been used in treating skin disorders. Some have taken large amounts "to prevent colds."

If foods (such as carrots) that contain relatively large amounts of the provitamin, carotene, are eaten in large amounts for a time, *carotenemia* (increased level of carotene in the blood) may result. The skin assumes a yellow color. The condition is not dangerous and soon disappears if the patient stops eating the causative food. This disorder readily is differentiated from jaundice: the white of the eyes are stained in jaundice but not in carotenemia.

STANDARDIZATION AND REQUIREMENTS OF VITAMIN A

The international unit (IU) of vitamin A is defined as the vitamin activity equivalent to 0.0006 mg of crystalline β-carotene or 0.0003 mg of pure retinol. The following are recommended daily intakes:

1. For *adults,* 5,000 IU daily. This amount would be obtained in a diet that contained all of the following: 1 pint of whole milk, 1 egg, 1 ounce of butter, and an average serving of a green, leafy vegetable.
2. For *infants,* 1,500 IU daily and for *children* one to 18 years of age, 2,000 to 5,000 IU daily. More than this would be furnished by a diet containing all of the following: 3 g of cod-liver oil, 1 quart of milk, 1 egg, and servings of butter and green, leafy vegetables suited to the size of the child.
3. For *pregnant* and *nursing women,* at least 6,000 to 8,000 IU daily. A diet that offered all of these – 1 teaspoonful of cod-liver oil, 1 quart of milk, 1 egg, 1 ounce of cheese, and 1 serving of a green, leafy vegetable – would contain approximately this amount.

SOURCES OF VITAMIN A

Food sources of vitamin A are usually rated as *fair* (20 to 99 units per 100 g), *good* (100 to 999 units per 100 g), or *excellent* (1,000 to 10,000

Table 33-1. Some food sources of vitamin A

Excellent sources	Good sources
Apricots	Asparagus
Beef liver	Bananas
Butter	Beans, green
Carrots	Beef fat
Cheese, cream	Cabbage
Collards	Ice cream
Cream	Kidney
Eggs	Oranges
Fish roe	Peas, green
Parsley	Tomatoes
Spinach	Watermelon
Sweet potatoes	Whole milk

units per 100 g). In plant foods there seems to be a close agreement between the greenness of the plant and its vitamin A content. We cannot yet explain this because the green color of plants is due to chlorophyll and not to the provitamins of vitamin A. As an example, the outer green leaves of lettuce may contain thirty to forty times as much vitamin A provitamin as the nearly colorless "heart." Carotenes have yellow colors, and the yellow color of some plants is correlated with their vitamin activity. Carrots and sweet potatoes (yams), for example, are excellent sources of vitamin A. Yellow corn, which contains cryptoxanthin, is a much better source than is white corn. Eggs, milk, and milk products are the most important animal food sources of the vitamin.

Foods that have been dried show considerable loss of vitamin activity. Prolonged cooking at temperatures above the boiling point of water (100° C) also causes a loss of activity.

VITAMIN B COMPLEX

Thiamine (vitamin B_1)

CHEMICAL NATURE OF THIAMINE

Thiamine, or vitamin B_1, has been called *aneurin* by some authors. This compound was made in the laboratory by Dr. R. R. Williams and his colleagues in 1936.

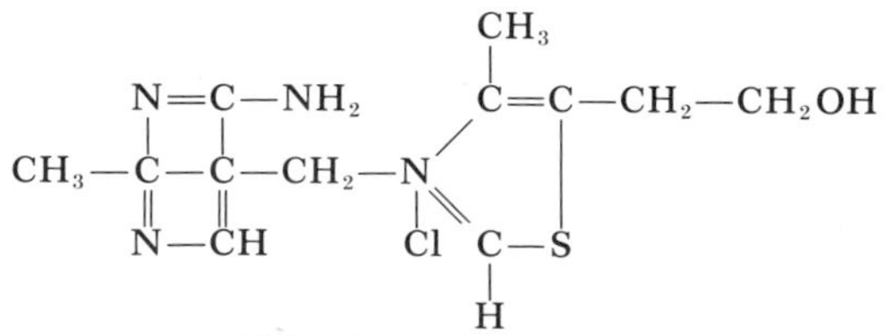

Thiamine hydrochloride

Thiamine is a white crystalline compound. Since it contains a free amino (NH_2) group, it can react with acids to form salts. Thiamine hydrochloride, the salt produced by allowing thiamine to react with hydrochloric

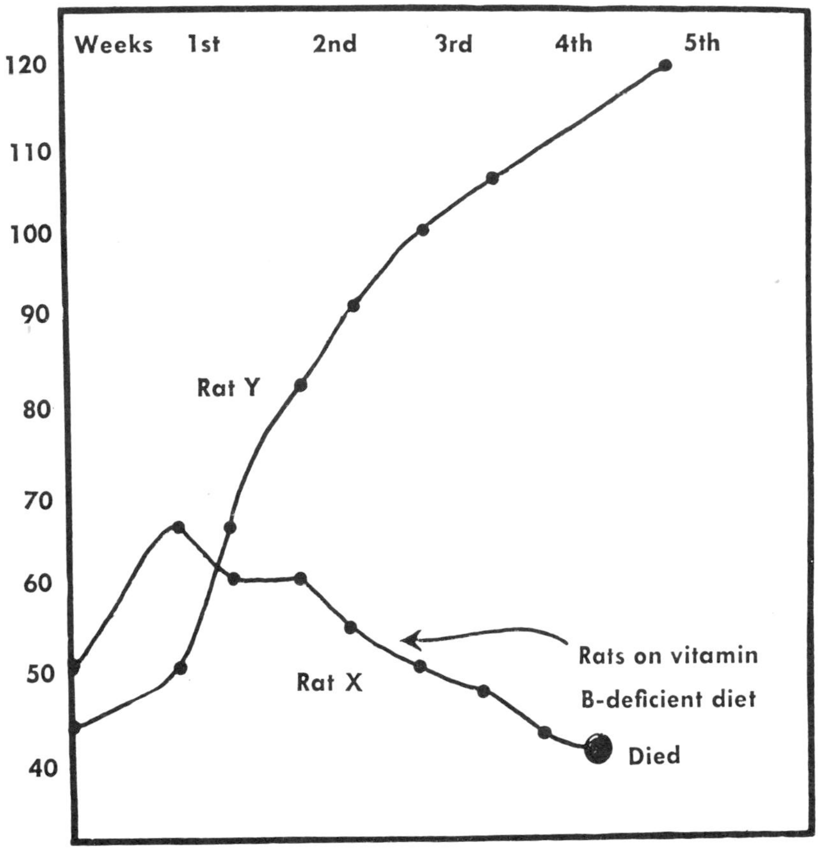

Fig. 33-3. Chart to show the effect of a deficiency of the vitamin B complex on growth. Is failure of growth characteristic of a particular vitamin deficiency, or are nearly all vitamin deficiencies accompanied by it? (Courtesy Mead Johnson & Co.)

acid, is more soluble than thiamine itself and is usually used in medicine. The vitamin is insoluble in fats and fat solvents and is classed as a water-soluble vitamin. It is destroyed by moist heat but is stable to heat when it is dry.

THIAMINE DEFICIENCY

Thiamine deficiency results in beriberi, other types of polyneuritis, failure of growth, anorexia, failure of lactation, and the Wernicke-Korsakoff syndrome.

Beriberi. This disease is most common in the Orient, where polished rice and fish are the chief articles of diet. The most outstanding symptom is *polyneuritis,* a disease in which the sheaths surrounding the nerves that supply many of the muscles of the body degenerate and decompose. Pain along the course of these nerves when pressure is applied is common, and the muscles supplied by these diseased nerves become paralyzed and atrophy from disuse. The heart enlarges, and the usual cause of death in beriberi is heart failure. One type of the disease, known as *wet* beriberi, is accompanied by marked edema. If edema is not present the disease is called *dry beriberi.*

OTHER TYPES OF POLYNEURITIS. It seems probable that the polyneuritis that may accompany chronic alcoholism, pregnancy, diabetes mellitus, and improper nutrition is really caused by thiamine deficiency. The administration of thiamine hydrochloride often cures these types of polyneuritis.

FAILURE OF GROWTH. As we have already learned, most vitamin deficiencies are accompanied by this symptom.

ANOREXIA. Anorexia, or loss of appetite, is a prominent feature of thiamine deficiency. It seems unlikely, however, that thiamine will stimulate the appetite of patients who are not suffering from a deficiency of this vitamin.

FAILURE OF LACTATION (MILK PRODUCTION). In animals, at least, thiamine is said to be necessary for the production of milk by the nursing mother. The amount of thiamine required for normal lactation is thought to be four or five times that needed for normal growth.

WERNICKE-KORSAKOFF SYNDROME. This syndrome first was described by Carl Wernicke in 1881. It is characterized by an ataxic gait, paralysis of eye movements, and mental disturbance. The mental disturbance usually is the type known as Korsakoff's psychosis, in which memory is disturbed out of all proportion to other intellectual functions. The administration of thiamine can improve dramatically the psychosis, although recovery is not always complete. Mild ataxia and abnormal eye movements may persist for months or years.

THIAMINE PYROPHOSPHATE AS A COENZYME

Thiamine combines in the tissues with two molecules of phosphoric acid to form the coenzyme *thiamine pyrophosphate.* This coenzyme is required for a number of metabolic reactions. Among them are:

1. The decarboxylation of α-keto acids to form aldehydes
2. The oxidative decarboxylation of α-keto acids to form carboxylic acids
3. The conversion of α-keto acids to organic phosphates and to formate

ABSORPTION AND STORAGE OF THIAMINE

Thiamine is easily absorbed from both the small and the large intestine. The largest amounts of the vitamin present in the tissues of normal animals are found in the liver, kidneys, and heart; it is supposed that excess

Table 33-2. Some sources of thiamine

More than 3 mg per 100 g	0.3 to 3 mg per 100 g	0.08 to 0.3 mg per 100 g	Less than 0.08 mg per 100 g
Brewer's yeast	Asparagus	Beef	Cheese
	Baker's yeast	Brown rice	Egg white
	Kidney beans	Cabbage	White flour, wheat
	Peanuts	Corn	White rice
	Soybeans	Egg yolk	Whole milk
	Whole wheat	Potatoes	

thiamine is stored in these organs. The body's ability to store this substance is limited, however, and deficiency symptoms appear ordinarily in from ten to thirty days after the removal of thiamine from the diet. Thiamine is found in the urine, and it has been claimed that a daily excretion of less than 0.04 mg is chemical evidence of thiamine deficiency.

REQUIREMENTS OF THIAMINE

The recommended daily intake for infants is 0.2 to 0.6 mg and for normal children and adults is 0.7 to 1.5 mg, depending on age. During pregnancy and lactation an additional 0.1 mg and 0.5 mg, respectively, should be provided.

SOURCES OF THIAMINE

The richest source of thiamine yet found is brewer's yeast. Vegetables and fruits have a comparatively low content of the vitamin. Legumes, nuts, and whole grains are good sources. Good animal sources include eggs and meat. Milk is not as rich in thiamine as are eggs and meat, but it is an important source because the amount of it consumed each day is large.

Boiling foods for as long as an hour does not result in appreciable chemical loss of the vitamin. We must remember, however, that thiamine is soluble in water, and a considerable portion of it may go into solution in the cooking water and be lost. Very little loss occurs in canning procedures, and the loss resulting from the evaporation and drying of milk is not significant.

Riboflavin

CHEMICAL NATURE OF RIBOFLAVIN

Riboflavin, vitamin B_2, when pure, exists as orange-yellow, needle-shaped crystals. It is slightly soluble in water and in alcohol. It is not easily destroyed by heat, but it becomes inactive if it is exposed to visible light for long periods. On hydrolysis it yields a pentose (ribose) and a dye (flavin).

RIBOFLAVIN IN NUTRITION

Storage of riboflavin in the body is limited. Deficiency does not endanger life or lead to serious disease in the human. The healing of wounds, even minor ones, is delayed. Cheilosis (a red, denuded area along the line of closure of the lips) and angular stomatitis (cracking of the skin at the corners of the mouth) appear. Seborrheic dermatitis (a greasy skin disorder), glossitis (a swollen, reddened tongue), and cracks along the edges of the nose may be noted. Small extra blood vessels invade the cornea; the eyes burn and itch. Riboflavin is *not* the only cause of these conditions, however. When riboflavin deficiency does occur, usually it accompanies deficiencies of other members of the vitamin B complex and protein.

Table 33-3. Some sources of riboflavin

More than 7 mg per 100 g	0.2 to 1.2 mg per 100 g	0.01 to 0.06 mg per 100 g
Liver	Beef, lean	Bananas
Yeast	Cheese	Carrots
	Eggs	Milk
	Spinach	Oranges
	Turnip greens	Potatoes
	Wheat germ	Tomatoes

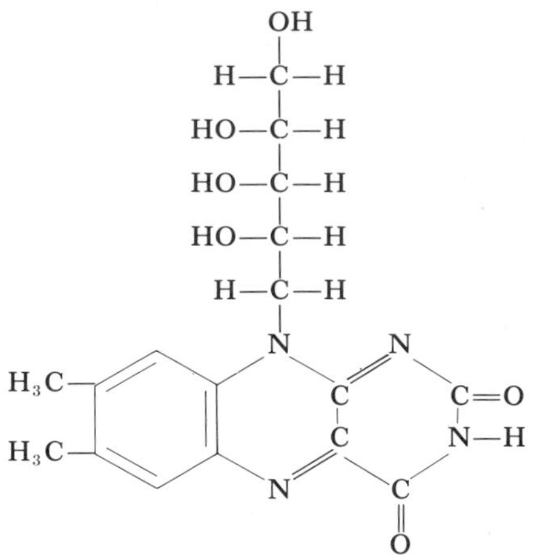

Riboflavin

SUGGESTED REQUIREMENTS OF RIBOFLAVIN It has been estimated that human beings require 0.4 to 2.0 mg daily.

COENZYME FORMS OF RIBOFLAVIN Riboflavin forms two coenzymes in the tissues: flavine mononucleotide and flavine-adenine dinucleotide. They serve as agents for the transfer of hydrogen between nicotinic acid-coenzymes (NADH and NADPH; see pages 212 and 215) and the cytochromes (see page 213). They form only a small part of the electron transport system found in the mitochondria (see page 213). The overall effect of this system is to transfer hydrogen from a substrate to molecular oxygen, forming water.

NIACIN AND NIACINAMIDE

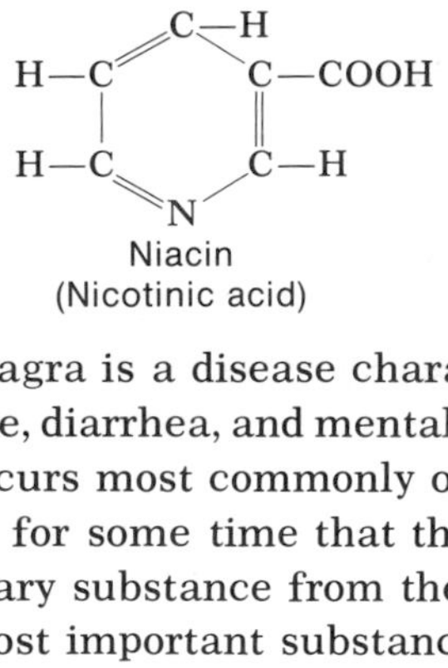

Niacin
(Nicotinic acid)

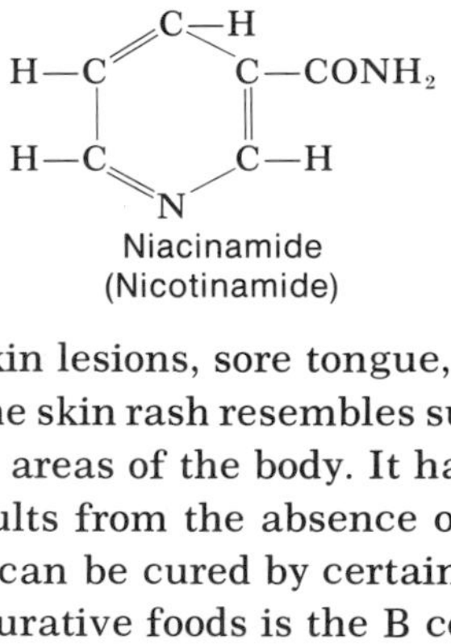

Niacinamide
(Nicotinamide)

PELLAGRA Pellagra is a disease characterized by skin lesions, sore tongue, loss of appetite, diarrhea, and mental symptoms. The skin rash resembles sunburn and occurs most commonly on the exposed areas of the body. It has been known for some time that this disease results from the absence of some necessary substance from the diet since it can be cured by certain foods. The most important substance present in curative foods is the B complex vitamin, *niacin*. *Niacinamide* also is active. But tryptophan, an essential amino acid (see page 281) can be converted to niacin in the body and thus also is effective. In humans, 60 mg of tryptophan are required to yield 1 mg of niacin in the body. Pellagra commonly is found in populations who eat corn (maize) as a major item of the diet. Corn is low in both niacin and tryptophan. Moreover, as much as 80 to 90 percent of the niacin in corn, rice, wheat, and barley is present in a chemically bound, inactive form.

Large doses (several hundredfold greater than the nutritional requirement) of niacin, given daily, have been used to lower the cholesterol and triglyceride levels of the blood. This is intended to minimize the occurrence

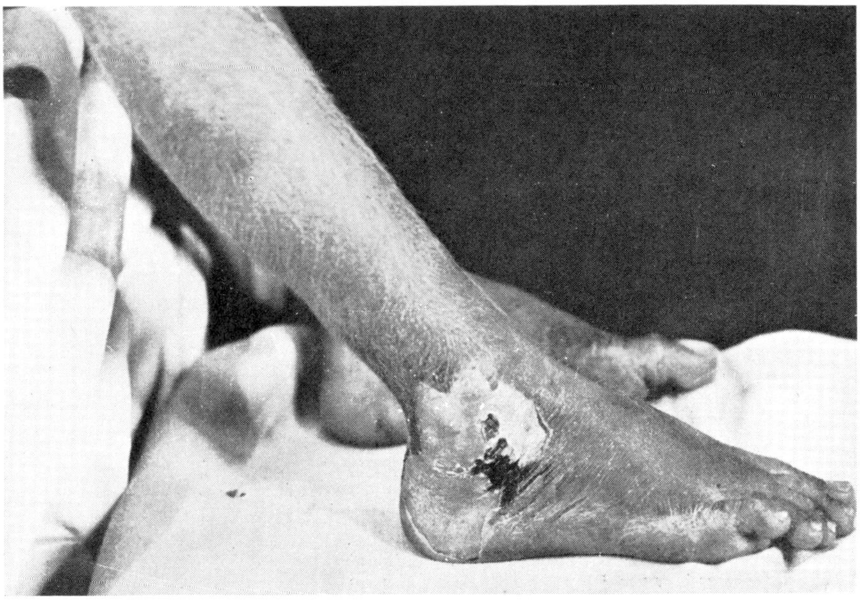

Fig. 33-4. Subsiding inflammation and hyperpigmentation in pellagra. What is thought to be the cause of this disease? (Courtesy Dr. Walter B. Shelley.)

Table 33-4. The efficiency of some foods in curing pellagra

No value	Slight value	Fair value	Good value
Beans, navy	Beans, green	Beans, kidney	Meat
Corn meal	Butter	Cabbage	Buttermilk
Lard	Carrots	Egg yolk	Collards
Onions	Cottonseed meal	Evaporated milk	Liver
Potatoes	Lettuce	Mustard greens	Peas, green
Prunes, dried	Turnips	Peas, dried green	Tomato juice
Rolled oats	Whole wheat	Spinach	Turnip greens
			Yeast

of coronary heart attacks and strokes. These large doses cause distressing side effects—flushing of the skin, with itching and a feeling of heat. Niacinamide does not cause these side effects, but it is ineffective in lowering blood lipids levels.

COENZYME FORMS OF NICOTINAMIDE

Niacinamide is a constituent of two important coenzymes:

1. Nicotinamide adenine dinucleotide and its reduced form (NAD^+ and NADH; see page 212).
2. Nicotinamide adenine dinucleotide phosphate and its reduced form ($NADP^+$ and NADPH; see page 215).

SOURCES AND REQUIREMENTS

Meat, beans, peanuts, and peas are good sources of niacin. Corn, rice, and most fruits and vegetables are poor sources. The National Research Council lists its recommended daily dosage in *niacin equivalents*. Since each 60 mg of tryptophan in the diet is equivalent to 1 mg of nonbound niacin, a sample of food containing 60 mg of tryptophan and 1 mg of available niacin supplies *two* niacin equivalents. The Council suggests 6.6 niacin equivalents per 1,000 Calories of food intake and not less than 13 niacin equivalents for intakes less than 2,000 Calories. This translates to 5 mg equivalents daily for young infants; 20 for 18-year-old males; 13 to 17 for adults; 15 and 20, respectively, during pregnancy and lactation.

Pyridoxine

Pyridoxine (vitamin B_6) is a white odorless compound with a slightly bitter taste. It dissolves readily in water and alcohol and is slightly soluble in ether and chloroform.

This factor is essential for the normal nutrition of rats, pigs, dogs, chicks, and many microorganisms. The first definite description of pyridoxine deficiency in the human was published in 1954. A batch of commercially prepared baby food was overheated during manufacture. Babies that were fed this formula had convulsions, irritability, and disordered behavior. These symptoms disappeared when the defective food was replaced by a formula containing adequate pyridoxine. The affected infants had some stores of pyridoxine when they were born. Even though the deficient diet was started soon after birth, symptoms did not appear for six to eight weeks. Pyridoxine is required for reactions involving amino acids in the body. It is interesting to note that the symptoms of deficiency disappeared when the babies were fed a diet devoid of protein; they returned when protein was restored. Pyridoxine acts quickly—improvement was evident within minutes after it was given to the affected babies. Also, the infants did not suffer any permanent damage as a result of the temporary deficiency.

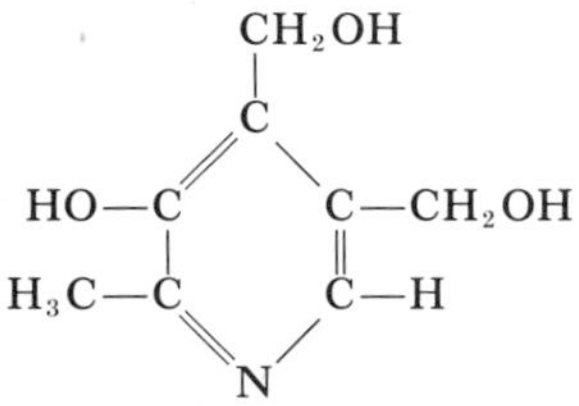

Pyridoxine

Pyridoxine-deficient monkeys develop malocclusions and caries of the teeth. A type of arteriosclerosis also develops in the walls of their arteries. One possible explanation for the development of caries (tooth decay) is as follows: Two types of lactobacilli are in the mouth. One of these requires pyridoxine for growth and does not produce harmful amounts of acid. The other type can synthesize its own pyridoxine and produce sufficient acid to cause caries. When insufficient pyridoxine is supplied to the animal (or, presumably, to the human) the acid-producing type of lactobacillus grows at the expense of the type requiring pyridoxine. The acid thus produced then erodes the teeth, producing caries.

Pyridoxine appears to be necessary for the synthesis of protein (and, hence, of tissue) in the body. It has been found that hamsters born of

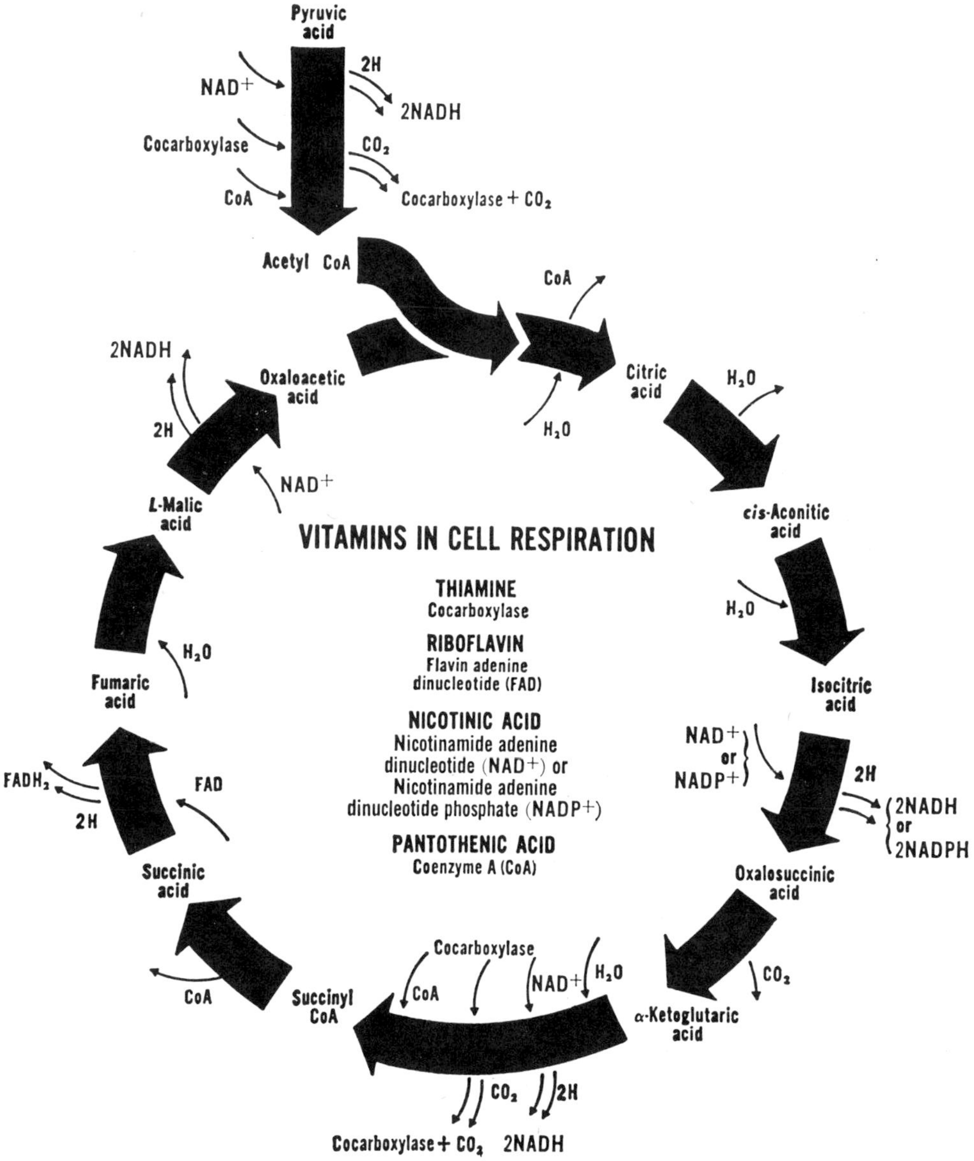

Fig. 33-5. Coenzyme forms of certain vitamins are essential to a basic cycle of energy-transfer reactions in cell respiration. This cycle, called the citric acid, or Krebs', cycle, is a final common metabolic pathway that, by using simple products of carbohydrate, fat, and protein catabolism, produces carbon dioxide and water. What is a coenzyme? (Courtesy Parke, Davis & Co.)

mothers who were fed pyridoxine-deficient diets at a critical period during pregnancy developed cleft palates. This might have been caused by a failure of protein synthesis at a time when the two sides of the palate normally would have fused.

Pyridoxal and pyridoxamine are compounds that can be prepared from pyridoxine by relatively simple procedures.

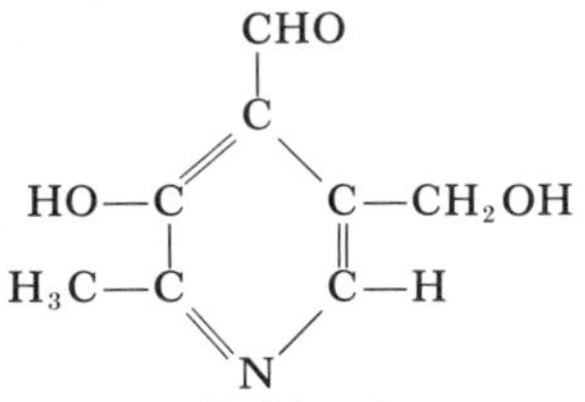

Pyridoxal

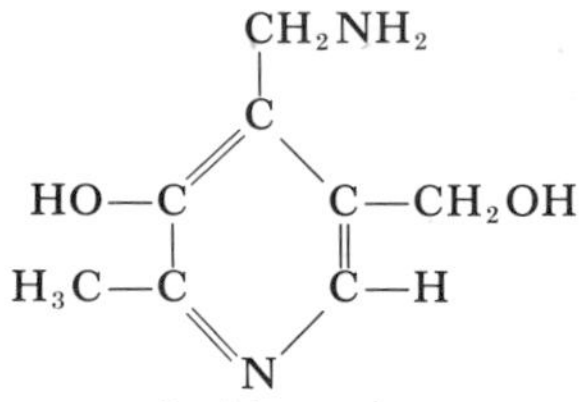

Pyridoxamine

Pyridoxal and pyridoxamine can replace pyridoxine in animal diets and in bacterial culture media. Indeed, it seems very probable that pyridoxal is the active form of the vitamin.

THE COENZYME OF PYRIDOXINE

The coenzyme of which pyridoxine is a constituent is *pyridoxal phosphate*. It is important in nonoxidative transformations of amino acids. The following are examples of reactions in which it participates:

1. The enzymatic decarboxylation (loss of CO_2) of amino acids
2. Transamination reactions (see page 364)
3. The cleavage of the amino acid tryptophan to indole, pyruvic acid, and ammonia

SOURCES AND REQUIREMENTS

Liver, kidney, other meats, corn, wheat, and yeast are good sources of pyridoxine. Only limited amounts are found in milk, eggs, and vegetables. The nutritional need varies with the protein intake. The recommended daily intakes range from 0.2 mg for young infants to 2 mg for adults. The suggested intake during pregnancy and lactation is 2.5 mg.

Vitamin B_{12} (cyanocobalamin)

This member of the vitamin B complex was isolated in 1948. It is specific in the treatment of pernicious anemia (see page 324). There is evidence that it may increase the appetite and growth rate of undernourished children. Vitamin B_{12}, particularly when it is used in combination with certain antibiotics, increases food intake, growth, and efficiency of protein utilization in mice, rats, chicks, and pigs. The injection of only 0.001 mg daily into some patients with pernicious anemia will abolish the signs and symptoms of the disease. Vitamin B_{12} exists as a large organic molecule containing cobalt and phosphorus. The natural form has a cyanide radical (—CN) attached to the cobalt atom.

The lining of the stomach and duodenum elaborates a substance that enhances the absorption of vitamin B_{12} from the gastrointestinal tract. This substance is known as the *intrinsic factor* (see page 324). Patients with pernicious anemia do not make intrinsic factor in adequate quantity, with the result that insufficient vitamin B_{12} is absorbed from food sources.

Thomas Addison, a member of the staff of Guy's Hospital, London, first described pernicious anemia (Addisonian anemia) in 1849. The red blood cells are abnormally large in size and low in number. The disorder develops insidiously; the patient loses weight and becomes weak. In about 40 percent of untreated cases neurological signs appear: numbness and tingling of the extremities, stiffness of the arms and legs, and difficulty in walking, especially in the dark. The disease, which causes death in two to three years if untreated, is rare. Approximately 6,000 Americans died of it annually before it was discovered in 1926 that eating ½ to 1 pound of lightly cooked liver controlled, though it did not cure, the disease. Thus, even though there is little or no intrinsic factor available to patients with pernicious anemia, they can absorb vitamin B_{12} given by mouth (the so-called extrinsic factor in liver) if enough is supplied.

PROPERTIES

Vitamin B_{12}, whose chemical name is *cyanocobalamin,* is freely soluble in water. It contains 4 percent cobalt. Other closely related substances have vitamin activity; one of them is hydroxycobalamin. The vitamin is stored in the liver for long periods of time and the liver of a healthy adult contains enough to last for more than two years. Some other anemias (such as those associated with pregnancy, gastrointestinal diseases, and surgical removal of the stomach) respond to administration of the vitamin. It is used in treating cirrhosis of the liver.

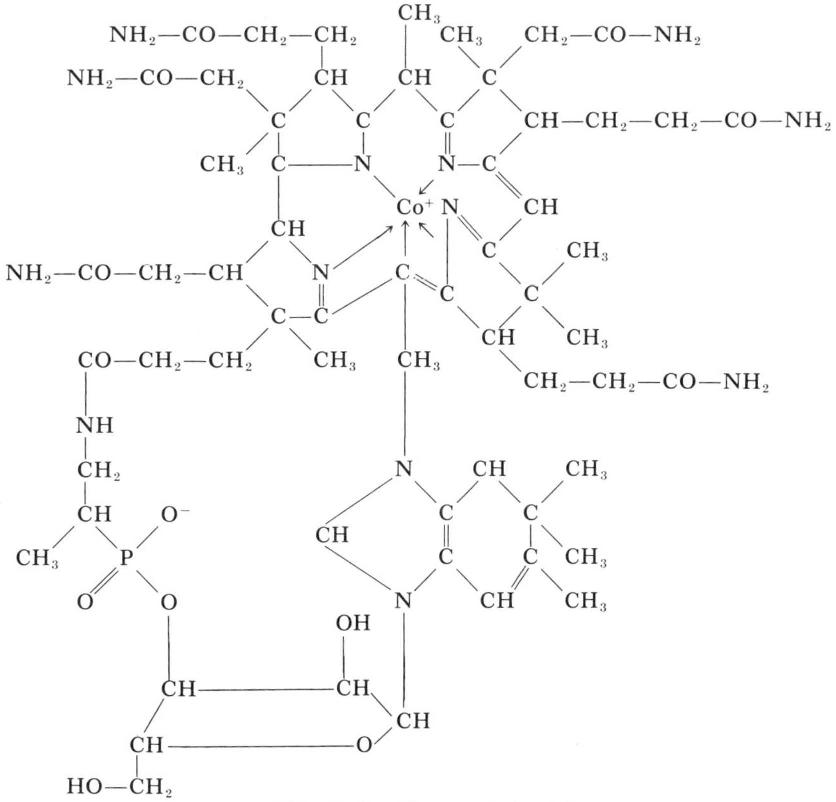

Vitamin B_{12} (Cyanocobalamin)

METABOLIC ROLE OF CYANOCOBALAMIN

Cyanocobalamin is known to be a constituent of several complex coenzymes in the tissues. The vitamin, presumably in the form of these coenzymes, is required for a number of important metabolic reactions:

1. Reactions involving the metabolism of single carbon-containing units, such as active methyl groups and formate. This type of reaction is involved, for example, in the biosynthesis of the amino acid methionine (see page 292) and of choline (see page 292). Another example is the reduction of formate (HCOO—) to form the methyl group of thymine (see page 298).
2. The biosynthesis of amino acids

SOURCES AND REQUIREMENTS

Vitamin B_{12} has the distinction of being the only known vitamin that does not occur naturally in plant foods, though it is made by some microorganisms. Most vegetarians get a modest supply by drinking milk, but definite manifestations of dietary deficiency have been found in strict vegetarians in India and great Britain. Some of the microorganisms that contaminate foods may be sources of the vitamin. The National Research Council suggests a daily intake of 5 μg (0.005 mg) for adults, an amount thought to allow a considerable margin of safety. The best food sources are liver, kidney, meat, eggs, milk, and cheese.

Folic acid

DISCOVERY AND BIOLOGICAL PROPERTIES

A type of anemia sometimes observed in pregnant women was reported in 1931 to be of nutritional origin by Dr. Lucy Wills, who was working in Bombay, India. She fed the diet commonly eaten by her patients (mainly white bread and polished rice) to monkeys and reproduced the disease. She found also that a yeast preparation cured the disorder. In 1941 investigators in America cured a dietary anemia in chicks by feeding an extract of spinach. In the same year, the curative substance was isolated; it proved to be *pteroylglutamic acid,* now known more commonly as *folic acid* or *folacin.** Folic acid is useful in the treatment (and prevention) of certain anemias, all characterized by abnormally large red blood cells. Usually these anemias are associated with malnutrition, pregnancy, or gastrointestinal disorders. Folic acid and vitamin B_{12} are used together in the treatment of cirrhosis of the liver. Relatively large intakes of folic acid, even in the absence of vitamin B_{12}, prevent the signs and symptoms of pernicious anemia except—and this is an important exception—the late symptoms caused by degeneration in the nervous system. Thus, if people taking excessive amounts of the vitamin develop pernicious anemia, the disease will not be recognized until actual or potential crippling neurological changes appear. For this reason the amount of folic acid in the recommended daily dose of nonprescription vitamin preparations is limited to 0.4 mg of folic acid by a regulation of the Food and Drug Administration.

CHEMISTRY

Folic acid is one of a group of substances with the same biological activity. A very active member of this group, *folinic acid,* is formed from

*These names come from the Latin word, *folium,* meaning leaf, because folic acid occurs in green leafy vegetables such as spinach.

folic acid in the body. The vitamin is soluble in water and is a member of the vitamin B complex.

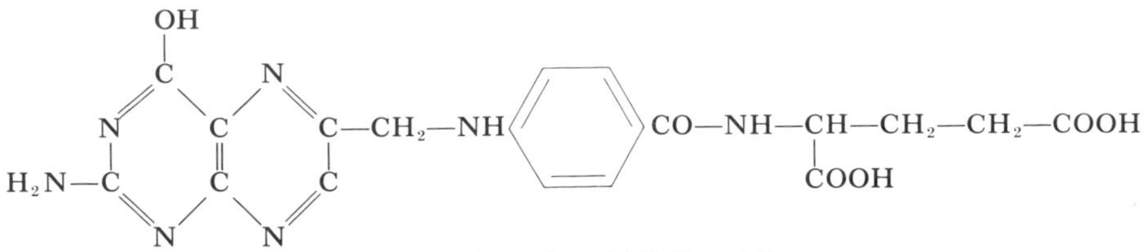

Pteroylglutamic acid (folic acid)

FOLIC ACID COENZYMES

Several important coenzymes containing folic acid participate in metabolism by controlling the transfer of the single carbon of formate ($HCOO^-$) or formaldehyde (HCHO) from one molecule to another. The reactions for which these coenzymes are necessary include:

1. The conversion of the amino acid glycine to the amino acid serine
2. The methylation of ethanolamine to form choline
3. The methylation of homocysteine to form the amino acid methionine
4. The methylation of nicotinamide to form N′-methylnicotinamide
5. The methylation of a pyrimidine derivative to form the pyrimidine thymine
6. The introduction of C-2 and C-8 into the purine molecule
7. The introduction of one of the carbon atoms into the ring present in the amino acid histidine

SOURCES AND REQUIREMENTS

Good food sources of folic acid include green leafy vegetables, liver, and kidney. Eggs, milk, poultry, and fruits are poor sources. The National Research Council recommends daily intakes of 0.05 to 0.1 mg for infants, 0.1 to 0.4 mg for children, 0.4 mg for adults, 0.8 mg during pregnancy, and 0.5 mg during lactation. The average good American diet supplies an amount of folic acid and related active substances equivalent to about 0.6 mg of pure folic acid per day.

P-AMINOBENZOIC ACID. This compound is one of the hydrolytic products of folic acid. It has the interesting property of counteracting the activity of the sulfonamide drugs. This has led to the hypothesis that these drugs owe their bacteriostatic properties to their chemical similarity to p-aminobenzoic acid. It is supposed that because of this structural similarity, they can attach themselves to some bacterial enzyme required in the metabolism of p-aminobenzoic acid. They are sufficiently different from the latter compound, however, to prevent any further metabolic change. If this hypothesis is correct, sulfonamide drugs prevent the growth of bacteria by blocking the utilization of p-aminobenzoic acid. In the presence of large quantities of p-aminobenzoic acid the sulfonamide is forced away from the enzyme by mass action; this explains why it can reverse the bacterial inhibition caused by the sulfonamides.

The finding that p-aminobenzoic acid occurs in combined form in folic acid makes it possible that the compound is active in metabolism only in this combined form.

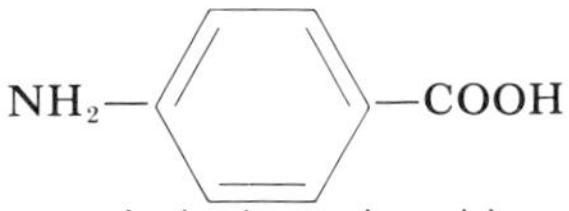

p-Aminobenzoic acid

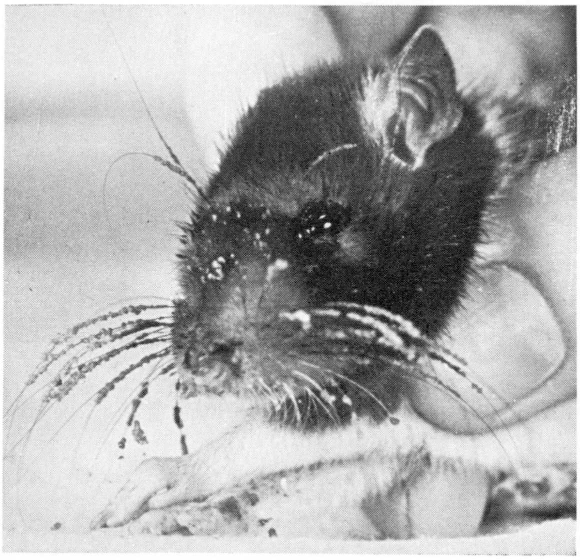

Fig. 33-6. The so-called bloody whisker condition. Rats on diets deficient in pantothenic acid frequently develop this appearance. The phrase "bloody whisker" is inaccurate, since the deposit on the whiskers is composed of porphyrins (pigments related chemically to heme). They are secreted from glands located in the nose region. (Courtesy Albert R. Latven and Dr. L. D. Wright.)

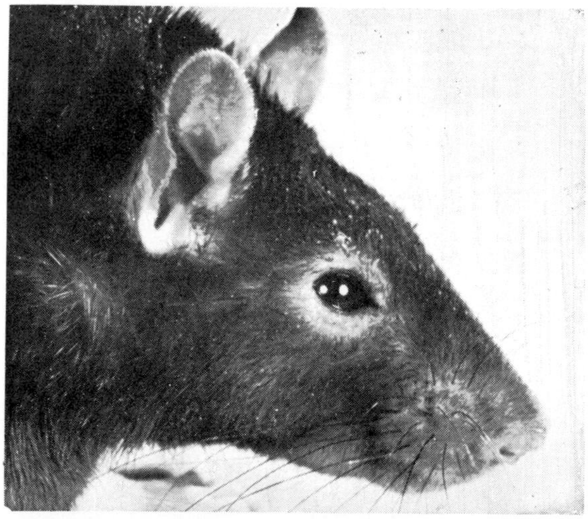

Fig. 33-7. The "spectacled eye" condition. This has been ascribed to inositol deficiency by some authors and to biotin deficiency by others. (Courtesy Albert R. Latven and Dr. L. D. Wright.)

Other members of the vitamin B complex

Other water-soluble vitamins, classified as members of the vitamin B complex, are required by animals. They have not been shown to be required nutrients for human beings, however, and thus the National Research Council has not listed daily allowances for them. The list includes *pantothenic acid, biotin, inositol,* and, sometimes, *choline* (see page 292).

ASCORBIC ACID (VITAMIN C)

CHEMICAL NATURE OF ASCORBIC ACID *Asorbic acid* ("against scurvy acid"), or vitamin C, has also been called *cevitamic acid.* It is a white crystalline substance and is soluble in water. It is also soluble in alcohol and acetone but is insoluble in most other fat solvents. This substance has been isolated in pure form and has been made artificially in the laboratory.

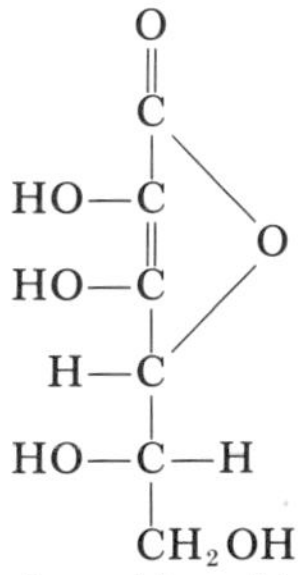

Ascorbic acid

Ascorbic acid is a strong reducing agent and is destroyed by heat in the presence of oxygen. Alkalies and copper salts catalyze its destruction by oxidation.

DEFICIENCY OF ASCORBIC ACID A deficiency of ascorbic acid results in scurvy and "asymptomatic scurvy" and also markedly affects the teeth. The normal value of the ascorbic acid of the blood ranges from 0.5 to 2 mg in 100 ml. In patients who have definite scurvy the amount present is only 0 to 0.15 mg per 100 ml. If the blood ascorbic acid is between 0.15 and 0.5 mg per 100 ml, the patient is said to have "asymptomatic scurvy."

The cells that make up the body tissues are cemented together by a material called the *intercellular substance.* This substance is not formed in the absence of asorbic acid, and most of the symptoms of scurvy, the deficiency disease prevented by this vitamin, result from a lack of this substance. It has been suggested also that ascorbic acid may be necessary for some of the oxidations and reductions that take place in the body.

SCURVY. Scurvy is caused by severe ascorbic acid deficiency. In this disease the bones become thin and porous, the ends of the long bones become flared, and a characteristic dense line can be seen in the ends of the long bones with the aid of x-ray photographs. The gums become swollen and boggy and bleed easily. In severe types of this disease muscular weakness is marked. Small pinpoint areas of bleeding (petechiae) occur in mucous membranes, in the skin, and around the eyes. Joint pain may be severe, from filling of the joint cavities with blood. Atrophy (shrinking) of the bone marrow is common, and, since the bone marrow makes hemo-

A

B

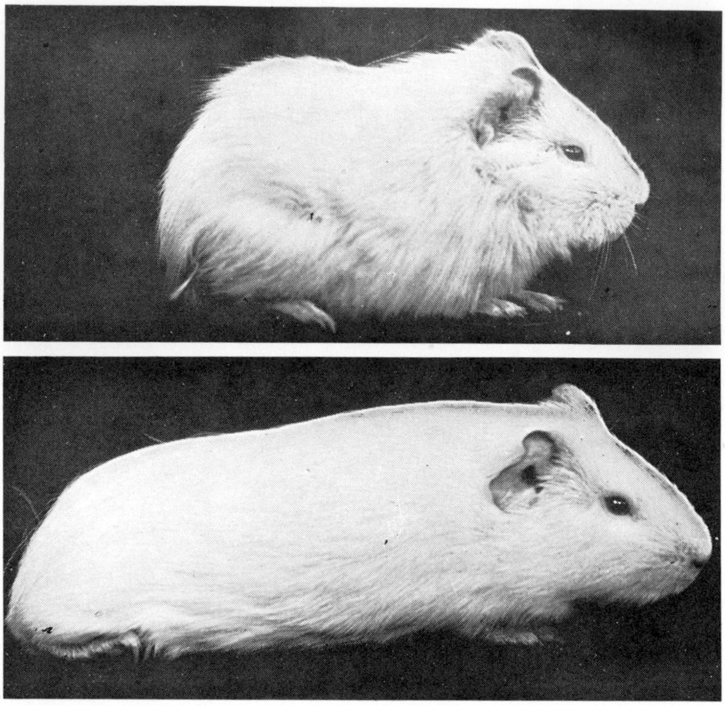

Fig. 33-8. A, Ascorbic acid deficiency in the guinea pig; **B,** guinea pig cured of scurvy by adding ascorbic acid to the deficient diet. Why is the guinea pig chosen as a test animal in studying ascorbic acid deficiency? (Courtesy Mead Johnson & Co.)

globin and red blood cells, this causes anemia. A failure of growth (children) or a loss of weight (adults) is a prominent feature.

"ASYMPTOMATIC SCURVY." Patients with "asymptomatic scurvy" (scurvy without symptoms) have none of the symptoms just described except perhaps a slow growth rate and a tendency to show petechiae. Wound and fracture healing is said to be slower than normal if the ascorbic acid intake of the patient is inadequate.

TEETH DEFECTS. The teeth are markedly affected by ascorbic acid deficiency. The dentin slowly disappears and that which is left becomes porous. Small amounts of abnormal new material, called osteodentin, may be formed. The gums may bleed easily. The cement is affected as well as the dentin, and, in animals at least, defects appear in the enamel.

ASCORBIC ACID DEFICIENCY IN ANIMALS

As far as we know, the only animals that require ascorbic acid in the diet are primates (including man), guinea pigs, fruit-eating bats, and the red-vented bulbul bird. All other laboratory animals can make this substance in their bodies and do not require it in the diet. Guinea pigs have been used in most of the animal experiments concerned with vitamin C.

REQUIREMENTS OF ASCORBIC ACID

The estimated requirements of ascorbic acid are summarized as follows:

1. For *infants,* 35 mg daily. The milk of normal mothers contains from 8 to 15 mg of ascorbic acid in each 100 ml. Breast-fed infants, there-

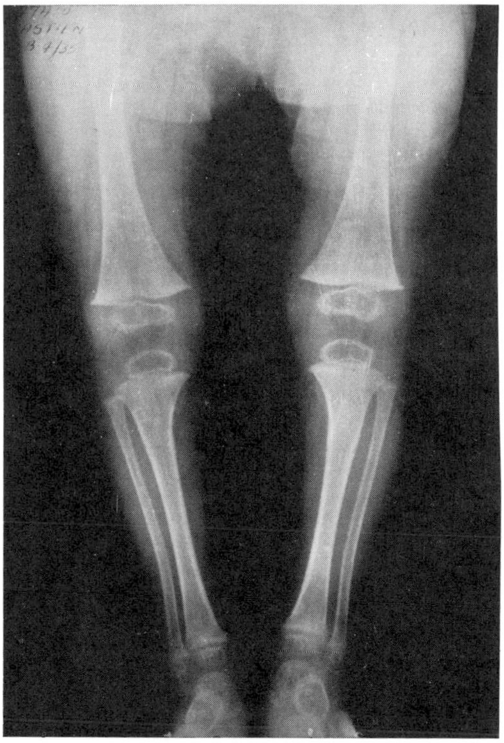

Fig. 33-9. X-ray photograph of the legs of a patient with infantile scurvy. Notice the increased density at the ends of the bones and the flaring ends of the long bones. What chemical substance prevents scurvy?

fore, receive from 20 to 40 mg daily from the time of birth. Raw cow's or goat's milk, however, contains only about 2 mg, and pasteurized milk, only 0.3 to 1 mg per 100 ml. Only a small amount is present in sweetened condensed milk, and evaporated milk contains almost none. These figures explain why many pediatricians give extra ascorbic acid (usually in the form of orange juice) to infants, often starting after the first few days of life. This practice is particularly important if the baby is not receiving normal breast milk.

2. For *children*, from 40 to 55 mg daily.
3. For *adults*, 40 to 60 mg daily.
4. For *women* during *pregnancy* and *lactation*, 60 mg daily.

FOOD SOURCES OF ASCORBIC ACID

Vitamin C is especially abundant in citrus fruits (oranges, lemons, limes, grapefruit, tangerines), raw or canned tomatoes, fresh strawberries, green peppers, and raw cabbage. Green leafy vegetables, if properly prepared, also have relatively large amounts. Dry cereals, legumes, meats, eggs, and dairy products contain only small amounts of the vitamin.

Ascorbic acid is readily destroyed by prolonged boiling. Green vegetables may lose 90 percent of their activity after immersion in boiling water for as long as an hour. The practice of adding baking soda to cooking water to

Table 33-5. Ascorbic acid content of some foods

0 to 5 mg per 100 g	5 to 25 mg per 100 g	25 to 100 mg per 100 g	100 to 250 mg per 100 g
Apples	Asparagus	Brussels sprouts	Parsley
Beef, cooked	Beans, green	Grapefruit juice	Green peppers
Beets	Corn, sweet	Lemon juice	Red peppers
Blackberries	Cranberries	Lime juice	
Butter	Gooseberries	Mustard greens	
Carrots	Lettuce	Orange juice	
Cucumbers	Peas, green	Spinach	
Eggs	Pineapple	Tomato juice	
Milk	Tomatoes	Turnip greens	

enhance the green color of vegetables increases the loss of ascorbic acid. Copper utensils should not be used for cooking because copper is a catalyst for the oxidation of vitamin C. Since the vitamin is soluble in water, some of it undoubtedly is lost in the water used in cooking. Drying, aging, and storing foods causes a loss of activity.

VITAMIN D

CHEMICAL NATURE OF VITAMIN D

There is evidence that at least ten different forms of vitamin D exist. Only two of them are known to occur in the foods and drugs commonly used in medicine and nutrition as sources of the vitamin. These two can be formed by exposing *ergosterol* and *7-dehydrocholesterol* to ultraviolet radiant energy. Ergosterol is a sterol found in yeast and molds. 7-Dehydrocholesterol, also a sterol, has been found in the skins of animals, and the vitamin formed from it *(activated 7-dehydrocholesterol,* or *vitamin* D_3) occurs in various fish-liver oils (tuna-liver oil, halibut-liver oil). When ergosterol is irradiated, several products are formed. One of these is an active vitamin D and is called *calciferol, activated ergosterol,* or *vitamin* D_2. The mixture of substances formed by ergosterol irradiation, including calciferol, is called *viosterol.*

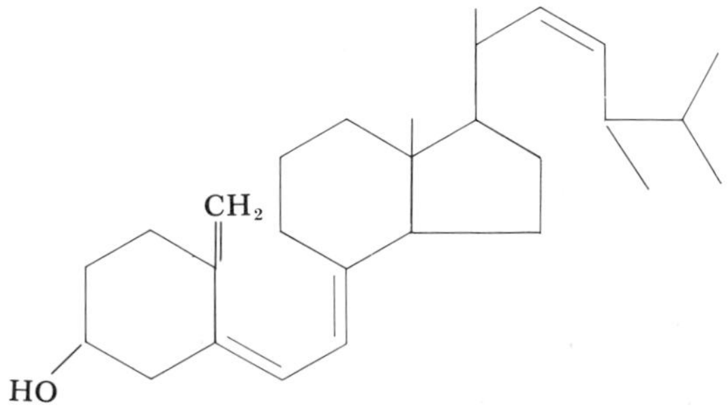

Activated ergosterol
(Calciferol, vitamin D_2)

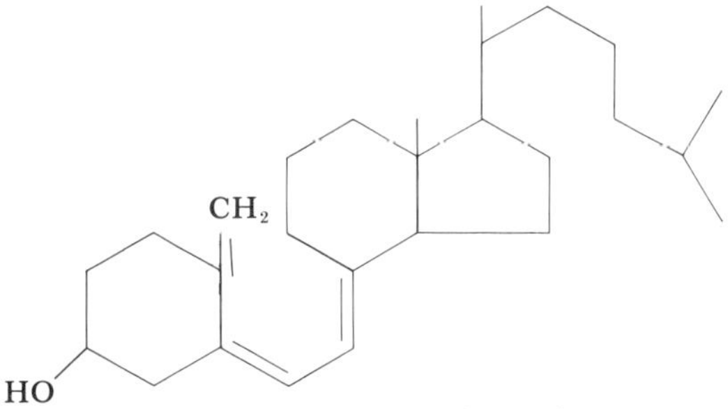

Activated 7-dehydrocholesterol
(Vitamin D_3)

Vitamin D_3 is converted to 25-hydroxycholecalciferol (25-hydroxy vitamin D_3) in the body. This compound is more active biologically than is vitamin D_3 itself.

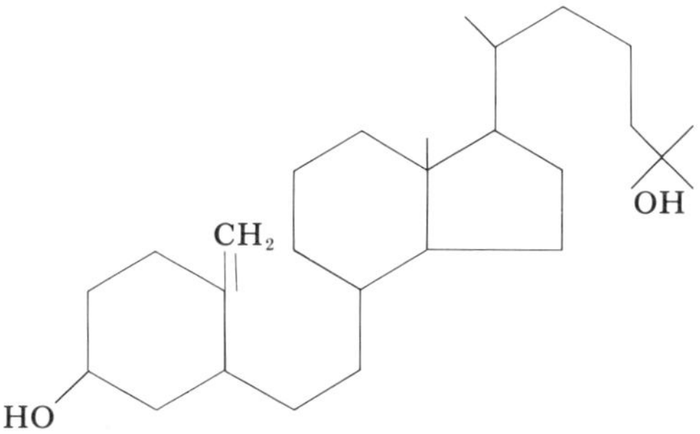

25-Hydroxycholecalciferol

FUNCTION OF VITAMIN D

If optimal levels of calcium and phosphate are not maintained in body fluids, formation of bone ceases. Since a portion of the bones is constantly breaking down, it is necessary that replacement occur promptly. It is the function of vitamin D, working in concert with the hormone of the parathyroid gland (see page 395), to maintain an adequate level of calcium and phosphate. Normally, calcium is excreted from the body mainly in the feces; phosphate is excreted mainly in the urine. Vitamin D reduces the excretion of each, thus promoting their retention in the body. When vitamin D is administered to chicks with rickets, a protein known as calcium-binding protein appears in the intestinal mucosa. Presumably this protein combines loosely with calcium and enhances its absorption into the body. The binding capacity of the protein is about 1 atom of calcium per molecule (molecular weight is 25,000 to 28,000) of protein. One function of vitamin D, then, is to cause the production of this protein. Thus the vitamin promotes the absorption of calcium from the intestine; when phosphate is present in the intestine in normal relationship to calcium (approximately $C:P = 1$), phosphate absorption accompanies the absorption of calcium. It also plays a role in the constant relocation of old, and deposition of new, apatite (see page 318) in growing bones.

DEFICIENCY OF VITAMIN D

Deficiency of vitamin D results in rickets, osteoporosis, and infantile tetany; the teeth may also be affected.

Rickets. This disease is caused by a deficiency of vitamin D. The shaft of a long bone is called the *diaphysis,* and the end of the bone is the *epiphysis.* Between the diaphysis and the epiphysis is a narrow band of

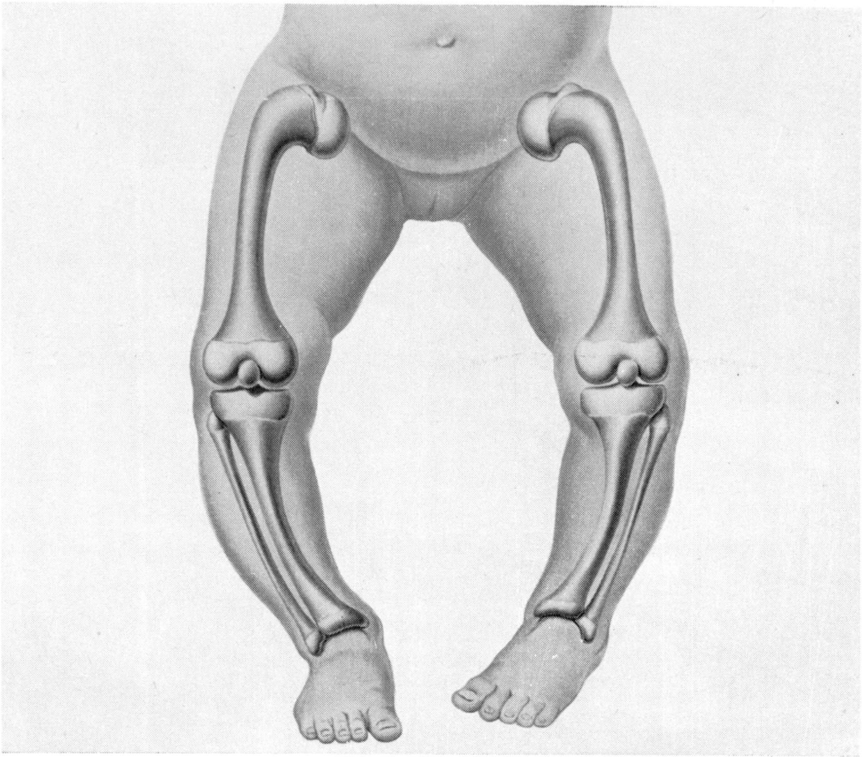

Fig. 33-10. Drawing to show typical appearance of leg bones in rickets. What causes this disease? (Courtesy Warner-Chilcott Laboratories.)

cartilage called the *epiphyseal line*. In rickets the epiphyseal cartilage continues to grow, but *it is not converted into bone*. In x-ray photographs the epiphyseal line appears to be widened. This overgrowth of rather soft cartilage at the ends of long bones causes enlargement of the wrists, knees, and ankles, and knobby enlargements where the ribs join the breast bone, or strenum. (These knobs are called the "rachitic rosary.") In addition to this, bone formation is impaired; the bones are soft and bend easily, which causes deformities of the spine and pelvis, bowlegs, deformities of the ribs, and craniotabes (softening of the skull). Blood phosphate is lower than normal, blood calcium is usually normal, and the phosphatase level of the blood is increased. Infants with rickets are irritable and fail to grow at a normal rate. Muscle tone seems to be lowered, and a bulging abdomen resulting partly from the relaxed muscles, is usually present.

Deficiency symptoms are rare in older children and adults. This suggests that the requirement of vitamin D is low in these age groups. Occasionally "late rickets" is observed in older children. Adult rickets, or *osteomalacia*, is a rare condition. Since growth of the bones ceases before adult life, osteomalacia does not cause bulging of the joints, but the bones soften, and marked deformities may appear. This disease is most common in women after repeated pregnancies.

INFANTILE TETANY. One type of *spasmophilia,* or *infantile tetany,* may result when the vitamin D content of the diet is low. Spasmophilia is characterized by hyperirritability. Sudden noises, sudden movements, or even touching the patient may cause convulsions. The level of blood calcium is low in this condition.

TEETH DEFECTS. Vitamin D deficiency causes a failure of proper formation of the dentin and enamel of the teeth. Abnormalities of the jaws from rickets may also produce considerable difficulty in later years because of improper eruption and spacing of the teeth.

VITAMIN D BINDING GLOBULIN. A specific vitamin D binding globulin exists in the serum of the rat, and presumably in other animals. This globulin transports vitamin D to various tissues of the body. It has a much greater affinity for vitamin D_3 than for other forms of the vitamin.

HYPERVITAMINOSIS D

Occasionally, the ingestion of only four or five times the ordinary amount of vitamin D for long periods of time may cause toxicity. It has been reported, for example, that an intake of 1,800 units or more daily slows the growth of the liver, decreases appetite, and reduces the retention of calcium and phosphate by the body.

More commonly, toxic effects are seen in adults who have received 100,000 or more units daily for several months and in children who have received as much as 40,000 units daily. The clinical picture resembles hyperactivity of the parathyroid hormone (see page 397): nausea, loss of appetite, diarrhea, vomiting, drowsiness, headache, polyuria (increased urine output), and polydipsia (thirst). The levels of calcium and phosphate in plasma are elevated. Depositions of calcium may occur in the heart, blood vessels, lungs, renal tubules, and other soft tissues. Similar deposits may be found in the bones in the cervical, subscapular, elbow, and wrist areas. Osteoporosis (a thinning of the bones, but with the maintenance of a normal ratio of calcified to soft tissue) develops as a result of increased activity of osteoclasts (bone cells that dissolve bone, releasing calcium and phosphate to the body fluids).

Hypervitaminosis D usually is reversible if withdrawal of vitamin D occurs promptly after signs and symptoms are observed.

STANDARDIZATION AND REQUIREMENTS OF VITAMIN D

The international unit (IU) of vitamin D is equivalent to 0.000025 mg of crystalline calciferol. It is estimated that full-term babies should receive 400 IU daily, and premature infants should receive twice this amount until a normal rate of growth is attained. Four hundred IU also is an adequate intake for children. The requirement for adults has not been determined with any degree of accuracy and, indeed, most experts think that adults can maintain good health even when vitamin D is lacking entirely from the diet. It has been recommended that 400 units a day be given to women during pregnancy and lactation.

SOURCES OF VITAMIN D

The richest sources of vitamin D are the *fish-liver oils* (cod-liver oil, 100 IU per gram; blue fin tuna-liver oil, 40,000 IU per gram) and *viosterol* (10,000 IU per gram). Food sources of the vitamin are scarce. It is probably absent from nearly all plant foods except those that have been irradiated with ultraviolet light. Salmon, sardines, and herring are the richest animal

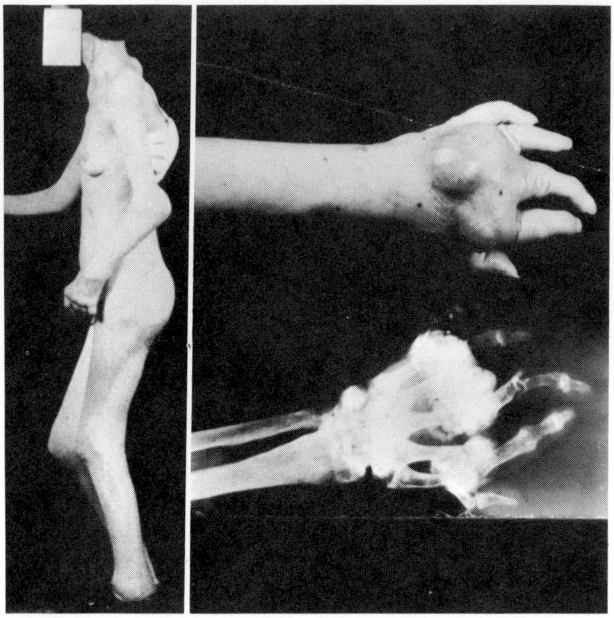

Fig. 33-11. Hypervitaminosis D in a patient with severe rheumatoid arthritis. Note swellings in the cervical, subscapular, elbow, and wrist areas. These swellings are caused by deposition of amorphous calcium phosphate in these regions. Photograph on the lower right is a radiograph of the hand of this patient. Why would you guess she had taken many times the physiological dose of vitamin D? (Courtesy Dr. F. Albright; from Moldawer, M.: Hypercalcemia, Med. Sci. **6**:377, 1959.)

sources; eggs rank next in importance; and milk and meat products contain small amounts of the vitamin. The scarcity of this vitamin in foods explains why it is so necessary that it be added to the diets of infants and children. It is now common practice to fortify milk and many foods by the addition of vitamin D during manufacture.

Vitamin D is formed in the body if the skin is exposed to ultraviolet light. Outdoor play in the summer causes significant increases in the vitamin D content of the body, but the low ultraviolet content of the rays of the winter sun, together with the necessity for additional clothing in the winter, means that outdoor exposure is not an efficient year-round procedure for increasing the body stores of the "sunshine vitamin."

VITAMIN E

CHEMICAL NATURE OF VITAMIN E

Several different substances are known to have vitamin E activity. The most active of these has been named *α-tocopherol* (from the Greek: *tokos,* childbirth; *pher,* to carry; and *ol* indicates that the compound is an alcohol). β-Tocopherol, γ-tocopherol, δ-tocopherol, neotocopherol, and cumotocopherol are less active forms of the vitamin. These compounds are oily yellow liquids.

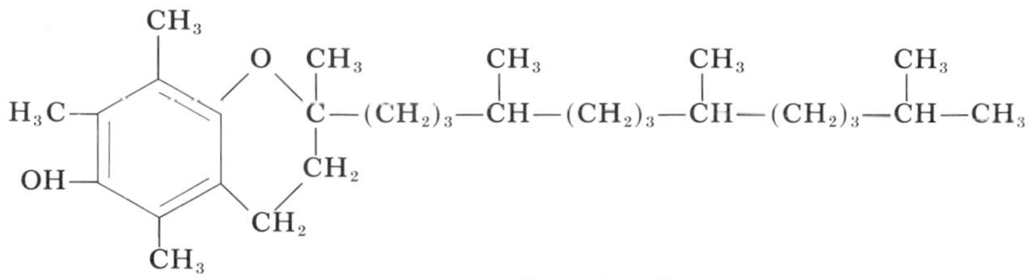

α-Tocopherol

METABOLIC ROLE OF VITAMIN E

Vitamin E acts as a general antioxidant in the body. That is, it protects body fats and some enzymes from destruction by chemical oxidation. In its absence, red blood cells are destroyed by peroxides formed in metabolism, and anemia results.

The signs and symptoms of deficiency vary somewhat in different animals. The vitamin was discovered in studies with rats. In these animals there is a partial failure of reproduction because of absorption of the fetuses. (This explains the choice of the term tocopherol.) In other animals, however, this is not observed. The first symptoms are principally muscular weakness, anemia, and pigmentation of body fats. In poultry, signs of damage to the brain and nervous system occur early. In prolonged severe deficiency, there is actual damage to the liver and heart with eventual death. Rats also exhibit these features if deficiency is prolonged.

At birth, the content of tocopherol in human infants is low. If they do not ingest adequate amounts of vitamin E, the signs and symptoms noted in deficient animals eventually will appear.

Infants receiving large amounts of polyunsaturated fats exhibit edema, skin lesions, and elevated blood platelet counts. These difficulties are overcome rapidly by giving α-tocopherol daily.

REQUIREMENTS AND SOURCES

The National Research Council suggests a daily intake equivalent to 5 mg of α-tocopherol for infants, 10 to 20 mg for children, and 25 to 30 mg for adults. Wheat germ oil is the richest source yet found. Many other plant oils (cottonseed oil, palm oil, corn oil) also contain the vitamin. The green leaves of vegetables (lettuce, spinach, watercress) are good sources. Egg yolk and meat are animal sources. Very little vitamin E is found in milk.

VITAMIN K

CHEMICAL NATURE OF VITAMIN K

The name vitamin K (Koagulations-vitamin in the Danish language) was proposed by H. Dam, of Copenhagen, in 1935. This substance is soluble in fat solvents, but it is neither a fat nor a sterol. It is not easily destroyed by heat but quickly loses its activity in alkaline solution.

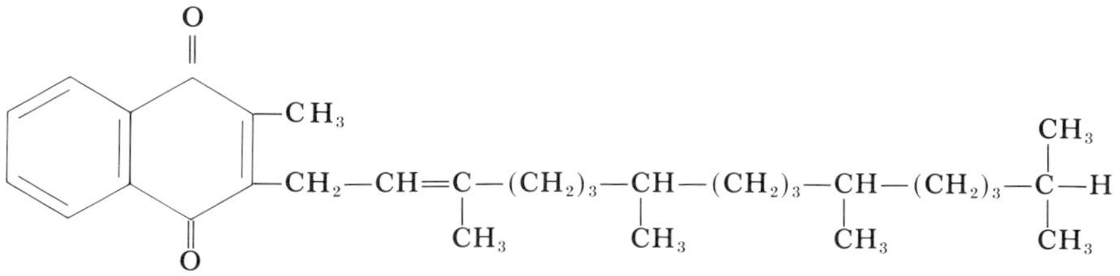

Vitamin K_1 (phytonadione)

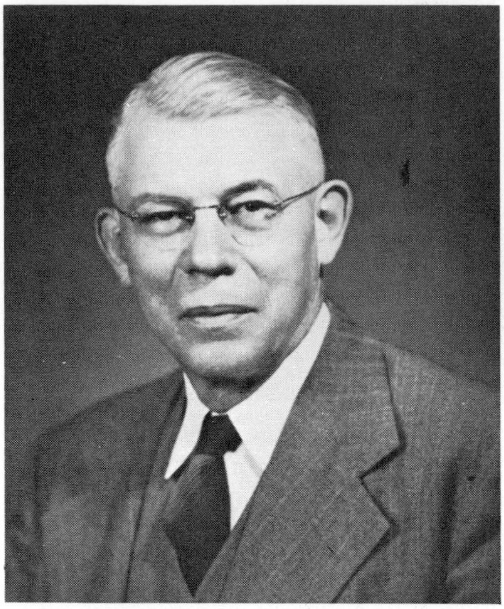

Fig. 33-12. Dr. Edward A. Doisy, Sr., of St. Louis University, received the Nobel Prize in medicine or physiology in 1943 for the synthesis of vitamin K. Dr. Doisy has made many very important contributions in the field of endocrinology. Can you think of a medicinal use for natural vitamin K?

Another form of vitamin K, known as vitamin K_2, is made by intestinal bacteria. A number of synthetic substances having vitamin K activity have been prepared in the chemical laboratory. One of the most active of these synthetic compounds is *menadione*.

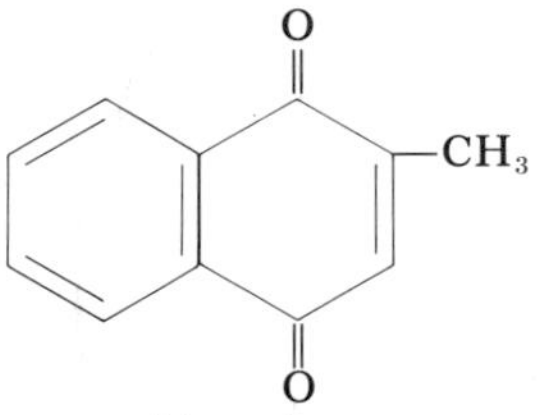

Menadione

FUNCTION OF VITAMIN K

Vitamin K is necessary for the formation of several factors necessary for blood clotting (prothrombin; factors VII, IX, and X; see page 361). It cannot be absorbed from the intestinal tract in the absence of bile.

USE OF VITAMIN K IN HUMAN PATHOLOGY

In conditions in which bile does not enter the small intestine in normal amounts (obstructive jaundice and biliary fistula) a tendency to bleed for long periods of time after slight injury or operations develops. Analysis of the blood shows that the prothrombin level is low in these patients. This tendency to bleed can be cured and the prothrombin level can be raised to normal by giving bile daily *for several weeks*. It can be cured *in a few days* if both bile and vitamin K are given or if vitamin K without bile is injected into the muscles or bloodstream of the patient. These observations lead us to believe that the chief cause of the tendency to bleed in obstructive jaundice is the low amount of prothrombin and other clotting factors in the blood and that the cause of these low levels is the absence of vitamin K from the tissues. This does not mean that the diet is deficient in the vitamin but rather that vitamin K cannot pass from the intestine into the body of the patient without the assistance of bile.

It should be remarked that vitamin K lack may not be the only cause of a low blood prothrombin level. This protein appears to be manufactured by the liver. In some liver diseases the prothrombin level will be low even though there is no lack of vitamin K.

Some infants are born with subnormal levels of prothrombin. These infants bleed readily and may die because of brain hemorrhage. But this condition is rare—perhaps once in 800 births—and it is not always caused by a deficiency of vitamin K. The vitamin usually is administered if abnormal bleeding occurs between the second and fifth day after birth. An emulsion of vitamin K_1 can be injected intravenously into patients who have a tendency to bleed as a result of overdosage with Dicumarol or similar drugs (see page 363).

SOURCES OF VITAMIN K The best known sources of vitamin K are alfalfa, hog-liver oil, cabbage, hemp seed, and spinach. There is no established nutritional requirement. Bacteria in the intestine normally produce it in adequate amounts.

STUDY QUESTIONS

1. In what ways do vitamins resemble hormones? In what way do they differ from hormones?
2. What was the origin of the term "vitamin"?
3. What substances are provitamins of vitamin A? Can animals make these substances? Can plants make vitamin A?
4. What organ converts carotenes to vitamin A?
5. Is vitamin A soluble in water? In fats? In fat solvents?
6. What is vitamin A_2?
7. List four results of vitamin A deficiency.
8. What is meant by atrophy? By keratinization?
9. What is xerophthalmia?
10. Explain why lack of vitamin A causes night blindness.
11. What organ stores vitamin A?
12. Why is it important to give infants vitamin A, especially if cow's milk is used as the chief article of diet?
13. Why are patients with obstructive jaundice particularly likely to develop symptoms of vitamin A deficiency?
14. What is the effect of mineral oil on the absorption of vitamin A from the intestine?
15. What is an international unit of vitamin A? How many such units per day are believed to be necessary for adults? For children? For pregnant and nursing women?
16. Is there any relationship between the color of plants and their vitamin A potency? Explain.
17. Is vitamin A easily destroyed by ordinary cooking procedures?
18. Name ten sources of vitamin A.
19. What is the clinical picture of hypervitaminosis A?
20. Are the members of the vitamin B complex water soluble or fat soluble?
21. What is the chemical name for vitamin B_1? How is it affected by heat?
22. Name five results of thiamine deficiency.
23. What is beriberi?
24. Name one metabolic reaction for which thiamine pyrophosphate is required.
25. How long after removal of thiamine from the diet do deficiency symptoms appear?
26. How many milligrams of thiamine are required daily by adults? By children? By pregnant and nursing women?
27. Name ten sources of thiamine in the diet. Is much thiamine lost in cooking procedures?
28. What sugar is produced by the hydrolysis of riboflavin?
29. List some signs of riboflavin deficiency. If these signs appear, can riboflavin deficiency be diagnosed with certainty?
30. What is the function of the coenzymes that are formed from riboflavin?

31. What is the estimated daily requirement of riboflavin in the diet?
32. What important coenzymes are formed from nicotinamide in the tissues?
33. What disease is prevented and cured by niacin? What are the outstanding symptoms of this disease?
34. Name ten foods that are efficient in curing pellagra.
35. What is a niacin equivalent? Explain.
36. What symptoms are produced by large doses of niacin? For what purpose are such large doses prescribed?
37. Discuss the importance of pyridoxine in nutrition.
38. Name one function of pyridoxal phosphate.
39. Name some good food sources of pyridoxine. How much is required daily?
40. For what purpose is vitamin B_{12} used in medicine?
41. What is the chemical name of vitamin B_{12}?
42. What is distinctive about the occurrence of vitamin B_{12} in foods?
43. What is the suggested daily intake of vitamin B_{12}? Name some food sources.
44. Give some examples illustrating the metabolic roles of the coenzymes of vitamin B_{12}.
45. What is the chemical name of folic acid? What is folacin?
46. For what purposes is folic acid used in medicine?
47. Name a few metabolic reactions that require folic acid coenzymes.
48. List some food sources of folic acid. What is the suggested daily requirement of it?
49. What chemical relationship has p-aminobenzoic acid to folic acid? How does it affect the biological activity of sulfonamide drugs?
50. Name a few substances that are vitamins for animals, although perhaps not for humans.
51. What are two chemical names for vitamin C? Is this substance soluble in water or in fats?
52. What is the function of ascorbic acid?
53. Name three results of ascorbic acid deficiency. What is scurvy?
54. What animals require ascorbic acid in the diet?
55. What is the estimated daily requirement of ascorbic acid for infants? For children? For adults? For pregnant and nursing women?
56. Why is it especially important to give ascorbic acid to infants not receiving breast milk?
57. Name ten food sources of ascorbic acid.
58. Is there any danger of destroying ascorbic acid in cooking procedures? Why does sodium bicarbonate catalyze the destruction of the vitamin? Why should copper cooking utensils not be used if prevention of ascorbic acid destruction is desired?
59. One hundred milliliters of orange juice contains about 50 mg of ascorbic acid. How many teaspoonfuls of orange juice would be required to furnish sufficient ascorbic acid for a week-old infant for one day?
60. How many different forms of vitamin D are believed to exist? What two vitamin D provitamins are of most importance in medicine?
61. What is calciferol? Vitamin D_3? Vitamin D_2? Viosterol?
62. What is the function of vitamin D?
63. Name four possible results of vitamin D deficiency.
64. What is the function of calcium-binding protein?
65. What is late rickets? Osteomalacia? Infantile tetany? How can you explain the fact that osteomalacia is most common in women after repeated pregnancies?
66. What is the effect of vitamin D deficiency on the teeth?
67. What is hypervitaminosis D?
68. Which form of vitamin D is most readily bound to vitamin D binding globulin?
69. What is an international unit of vitamin D? What is the estimated daily requirement of this vitamin for full-term infants? For premature infants? For children? For adults? For women during pregnancy and lactation?
70. Name five sources of vitamin D. Is this vitamin present in most plants?
71. Explain how exposing the body to ultraviolet light reduces the amount of vitamin D required in the diet.
72. How many natural substances are known to have vitamin E activity? What name has been given to the most active of these?
73. List some signs of vitamin E deficiency.
74. Name five sources of vitamin E.
75. Is vitamin K soluble in fats or in water? Is it a fat? Is it a sterol?
76. What is the function of vitamin K?
77. Of what use is vitamin K in treating human disease?
78. What is the relationship of bile to vitamin K deficiency symptoms?
79. Why is vitamin K sometimes injected intravenously?

CHAPTER 34

Introduction to nutrition

We spend many millions of dollars each year for food. Most people know surprisingly little about the materials that this money buys. However, this much can be said in defense of the general public: Even the experts in the fields of nutrition have gained most of their knowledge from the experimental work of the last 65 years. At the beginning of this century it was supposed that we needed food only to supply the body with carbohydrate, fat, protein, inorganic salts, and water. Now we know that this conception was much too simple. It is the function of the diet to supply us with numerous compounds—not all of which probably are yet known—that are absolutely essential for the life and well-being of the body. In short, a plentiful supply of food is no guarantee that nutrition is adequate. As Dr. L. S. Palmer has said, "It is literally possible to starve with a full stomach."

Foods can be classified into four major groups. If foods from each group are eaten regularly, and if caloric requirements are met, the diet probably will be adequate. These groups are:

1. *Milk group.* Milk, cheese, ice cream, products made with whole or skimmed milk.
2. *Meat group.* Beef, veal, lamb, pork, poultry, fish, seafood, eggs. *Alternates:* dry beans, dry peas, nuts, peanut butter.
3. *Vegetables and fruits.*
4. *Breads and cereals.*

It is possible that nutritionists will recommend changes in these basic groups when we learn more about the relationship of diet to coronary heart disease, the major cause of death in the United States. Future recommendations—made now by many physicians for certain of their patients—may involve a somewhat lower intake of fat, an increase in the ratio of polyunsaturated to saturated dietary fat, and a reduction in the intake of foods high in cholesterol and sucrose.

A table listing the National Research Council's recommended daily allowances of nutrients is included in the Appendix.

BASAL METABOLISM The heat eliminated from the body at rest, when no digestion is taking place and the body temperature is normal, is a measure of the *basal metabolism*. This basal metabolism represents, as nearly as we can measure it, the least amount of energy required for existence. We might expect that an adult who weighed twice as much as another adult of the same age would eliminate twice as much heat in a given time, but this is not the case. We find that the elimination of heat depends much more on the *surface area* of the body than on the body weight. The number of large calories of heat eliminated from each square meter of body surface in one hour (under the basal conditions listed in the first sentence in this paragraph) is called the *basal metabolic rate* (BMR). The basal metabolic rate is highest in infancy and gradually declines thereafter throughout life. As somebody has said, "We begin to die in early childhood." Some average normal values are given in Table 34-1. It will be noticed that the normal values for males are slightly higher than the values for females.

Clinically, the basal metabolic rate is usually reported as percent above or below normal. For example, we see that the average normal basal metabolic rate for a woman 50 years old is 33.4 large calories per square meter per hour (Table 34-1). Suppose a woman patient, 50 years old, actually has

Table 34-1. BMR at various ages—calories per square meter per hour

Age (years)	Males	Females	Age (years)	Males	Females
3	60.1	54.5	26	38.2	35.0
4	57.9	49.9	27	38.0	35.0
5	56.3	53.0	28	37.8	35.0
6	54.0	51.2	29	37.7	35.0
7	52.3	49.7	30	37.6	35.0
8	50.8	48.0	31	37.4	35.0
9	49.5	46.2	32	37.2	34.9
10	47.7	44.9	33	37.1	34.9
11	46.5	44.1	34	37.0	34.9
12	45.3	42.0	35	36.9	34.8
13	44.5	40.5	36	36.8	34.7
14	43.8	39.2	37	36.7	34.6
15	43.7	38.3	38	36.7	34.5
16	42.9	37.7	39	36.6	34.4
17	41.9	36.2	40	36.5	34.3
18	40.5	35.7	45	36.3	33.9
19	40.1	35.4	50	36.0	33.4
20	39.8	35.3	55	35.4	32.9
21	39.4	35.2	60	34.8	32.4
22	39.2	35.2	65	34.0	31.8
23	39.0	35.2	70	33.1	31.3
24	38.7	35.1	75+	31.8	31.1
25	38.4	35.1			

From DuBois, E. F. 1968. In *Metabolism*, Federation of American Societies for Experimental Biology, Bethesda, Md., p. 345.

a basal metabolic rate of 40.5 large calories per square meter per hour. This value is higher than normal, and in terms of percent is:

$$\frac{40.5 - 33.4}{33.4} \times 100 = \frac{7.1}{33.4} \times 100 = 21$$

This would be reported as +21 percent. If the basal metabolic rate is lower than normal, a minus sign is used. The basal metabolic rate is not ordinarily considered abnormal unless it differs by more than 10 to 15 percent from the standard value.

The heat eliminated from the body can be measured either directly or indirectly. In the direct method the patient is placed in an insulated box, or small room, and the rise in temperature over a measured interval of time is determined. This method is expensive and cumbersome, however, and is used only for certain experimental purposes. In the indirect method we determine how much protein, fat, and carbohydrate the patient has burned up during a given time and calculate the heat production from this. To determine this accurately, we must know the amount of nitrogen (combined in molecules) eliminated in the feces and urine, the amount of oxygen used, and the amount of carbon dioxide eliminated in a given time period. For clinical purposes, however, it is customary to measure only the amount of *oxygen* the patient breathes during a measured time interval (usually six minutes). The patient must have a normal temperature, must not have eaten for at least twelve hours, and must have rested quitely in bed for half an hour just before the test. Under these circumstances it is assumed that each liter of oxygen (measured at 0° C and 760 mm of mercury atmospheric pressure) used by the patient is equivalent to 4.8 large calories of heat liberated.

Thyroxine, the hormone of the thyroid gland, regulates the rate of metabolism, and the determination of the basal metabolic rate is particularly valuable as an aid in diagnosing diseases of the thyroid gland. It is low in cretinism, myxedema, and simple hypothyroidism. It is high in exophthalmic goiter and toxic adenoma. The basal metabolic rate is frequently elevated during pregnancy, in leukemia (a disease characterized by abnormal white blood cells), in polycythemia vera, also known as erythremia (characterized by abnormally large numbers of red cells in the blood; its cause is unknown), and in overactivity of the pituitary gland. It is usually low in nephrosis (a disease in which large quantities of protein are lost in the urine), anemias, wasting diseases, and in underactivity of the pituitary gland.

ENERGY REQUIREMENT

In calculating diets, it is convenient to divide the energy requirement of the diet into two parts: (1) Sufficient energy must be provided to satisfy the *basal metabolic requirements*. This might also be called the *energy of maintenance*. It represents the energy required to maintain the circulation of the blood, respiration, secretion, excretion, muscle tone, and so on. (2) The energy required for muscular work (activity) must be provided.

Suppose we want to calculate the daily calorie requirement of a young woman 25 years of age. In order to calculate her basal requirement we

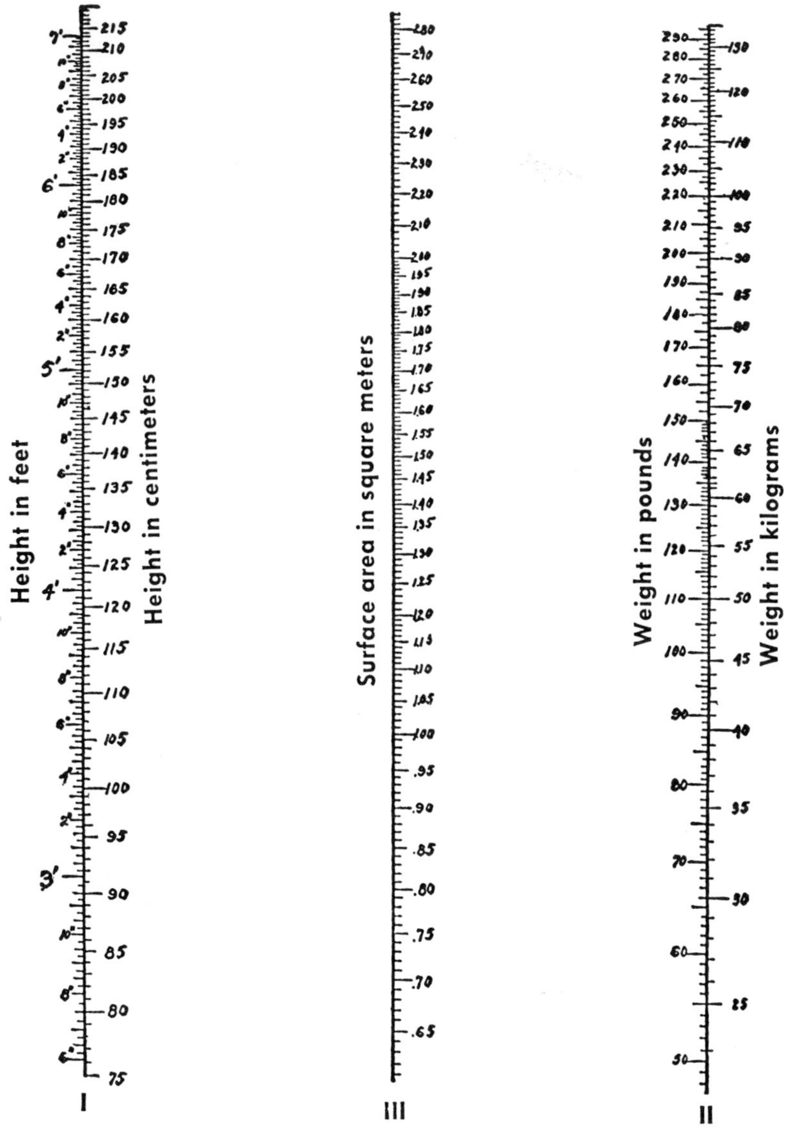

Fig. 34-1. DuBois body surface chart (as prepared by Boothby and Sandiford of the Mayo Clinic) for determining body surface area. Connect the correct height (column **I**) with the correct weight (column **II**) by means of a straight edge. The intersection of the straight edge with column **III** gives the surface area. What is your surface area?

Table 34-2. Average daily energy requirement per kilogram of body weight

Age	Large calories per kg
1 year	100
2 years	90
5 years	80
9 years	70
13 years	65
17 years	50
Adult, no exercise	33
Adult, light exercise	37
Adult, moderate exercise	43
Adult, hard labor	47

Table 34-3. Approximate energy expenditures in calories per hour above basal

Activity	Man: age, 40 yr; wt, 150 lb; ht, 5 ft 9 in; basal calories, 65 per hr	Woman: age, 40 yr; wt, 132 lb; ht, 5 ft 6 in; basal calories, 56.5 per hr
Awake, lying still	12	11
Sitting, at rest	35	31
Standing, relaxed	40	35
Ironing, standing	50	43
Dressing and undressing	53	47
Vacuum-cleaning rug, 2 ft/sec	70	62
Sewing	70	62
Typewriting rapidly	75	66
Driving a car	98	86
Light exercise	105	93
Walking slowly (2.6 mph)	135	119
Scrubbing floors	158	139
Sweeping	158	139
Mopping	214	189
Moderate exercise	225	198
Making beds	310	265
Vigorous exercise	365	340
Swimming	435	383
Jogging (5.3 mph)	505	445
Heavy exercise	535	472
Walking up steps	1,015	895
Walking down steps	346	314

must known her surface area. The surface area of human beings was first determined by covering the body with adhesive tape, removing the tape, and measuring the area used. Now we can refer to a standard table or chart (see Fig. 34-1) that tells us the surface area corresponding to any given height and weight; or, we can calculate by means of the DuBois formula:

$$A = W^{0.425} \times H^{0.725} \times 71.84^{*}$$

*This equation can also be expressed in logarithmic form as follows: $\log A = 0.425 \log W + 0.725 \log H + \log 71.84$.

Table 34-4. Content of protein, carbohydrate, and fat, and average caloric value of some common foods

Food	Average serving in g	Protein in g	Carbo-hydrate in g	Fat in g	Total large calories per serving
		Fruits			
Apple	100	0.4	14.2	0.5	65
Grapefruit	100	0.6	12.2	0.1	50
Orange	100	0.8	11.6	0.2	50
Strawberries	100	1.0	7.4	0.6	40
		Vegetables			
Asparagus	50	0.9	1.6	0.1	10
Beans, baked	100	6.9	19.6	2.5	130
Beans, green	100	2.3	7.4	0.3	40
Beans, lima, green	100	7.5	23.5	0.8	130
Brussels sprouts	100	4.2	8.0	0.5	55
Cabbage	30	0.5	1.7	0.1	10
Celery	50	0.6	1.7	0.05	10
Corn	100	3.7	20.5	1.2	110
Cucumber	60	0.5	1.9	0.1	10
Lettuce	50	0.6	1.5	0.2	10
Onions	10	0.2	1.0	0.03	5
Peas, green	100	7.0	17.0	0.5	100
Potatoes, sweet	100	1.8	27.4	0.7	125
Potatoes, white	150	3.3	27.6	0.2	125
Radish	35	0.5	2.0	0.04	10
		Cereals			
Bread, white (1 slice)	30	2.8	15.9	0.4	80
Bread, whole wheat	30	2.9	14.9	0.3	75
Macaroni	25	3.4	18.5	0.1	90
Oatmeal	25	4.0	16.9	0.2	100
		Nuts			
Almonds	15	3.2	2.6	8.2	100
Brazil nuts	15	2.6	1.1	10.0	105
Coconut, dry	15	0.9	4.7	8.6	100
Peanuts	15	3.9	3.7	5.8	80
Pecans	15	1.7	2.0	10.7	85
		Meats and poultry products			
Bacon	30	3.2	–	19.4	190
Beef, liver	100	20.4	2.5	16.3	150
Beef, steak	100	18.9	–	18.5	240
Chicken	100	21.5	–	2.5	110
Duck	100	18.0	–	19.0	245
Eggs, two	100	13.4	–	10.5	150
Fish, cod	100	11.1	–	0.2	45
Fish, sardines in oil	100	19.2	–	25.5	315
Fish, white fish	100	22.9	–	6.5	150
Ham	100	19.8	–	20.8	265
Pork, chops	75	12.5	–	22.6	255
Pork, sausage	75	9.8	0.8	33.1	300
Veal, cutlet	100	17.8	1.5	16.0	220

Table 34-4. Content of protein, carbohydrate, and fat, and average caloric value of some common foods—cont'd

Food	Average serving in g	Protein in g	Carbo-hydrate in g	Fat in g	Total large calories per serving
		Dairy products			
Butter	10	0.06	–	8.2	75
Cheese, American	25	7.2	0.08	9.0	110
Cream, sweet	15	0.4	0.7	2.8	30
Ice cream	100	4.0	20.0	14.0	220
Milk, skim	250	8.5	12.8	0.8	95
Milk, whole	250	8.3	12.5	10.0	170
		Miscellaneous			
Apple pie	200	3.2	64.0	18.2	430
Marmalade, orange	10	0.06	8.5	0.01	35
Sponge cake	100	11.8	62.0	7.5	360
Sugar, 1 teaspoonful	5	–	5.0	–	20

A is the area in square meters, W is the weight in kilograms, and H is the height in centimeters. We shall suppose our subject weighs 49 kg (108 pounds) and is 162 cm (5 feet, 4 inches) tall. Reference to Fig. 34-1 (or use of the DuBois formula) tells us that her surface area is 1.5 square meters. Table 34-1 informs us that she can be expected to produce 35.1 large calories per hour per square meter of body surface. Therefore, the total heat production under basal conditions will be $1.5 \times 35.1 = 52.7$ large calories per hour. In twenty-four hours the basal heat production and, therefore, the basal energy requirement, will be $24 \times 52.7 = 1{,}265$ large calories. Now, we must add the energy required for the voluntary movement of muscles—that is, for activity. This energy will vary considerably, depending on the individual's occupation. For office workers, professional workers (doctors, dentists, lawyers, nurses, dental hygienists), and for housewives the energy required will usually vary between 500 and 1,000 large calories per day. A man who spends most of the day digging a ditch may require as much as 4,000 calories above his basal requirement. We shall suppose that the young lady of our example is a nurse and requires probably about 600 large calories daily for the performance of work. Her total energy requirement for the day will be:

$$1{,}265 + 600 = 1{,}865 \text{ large calories}$$

PROTEIN REQUIREMENT

The amount of protein required each day will depend on several factors. Growing children obviously need proportionally more than do adults because they are growing and are building new cells at a rapid rate. If the diet contains insufficient carbohydrate and fat to supply energy, protein will be burned and the protein requirement will thereby increase. In general, larger amounts of plant proteins will be required than animal proteins because many plant proteins are inadequate—that is, they do not contain sufficient amounts of all the essential amino acids (see page 281). The protein requirement is increased in wasting diseases and in diseases in which large amounts of protein are lost in the urine (for example, in nephrosis).

Experiments with normal adults on diets low in protein but containing an abundance of carbohydrate and lipid indicate that the normal daily loss of protein from the tissues is approximately 20 to 35 g. Since so many factors can increase the protein demand, however, and particularly since only a part of the protein in the diet is adequate from a nutritional point of view, *it seems safest to include at least 55 to 65 g of protein in the daily ration of normal adults.* This amount would be more than supplied by one egg, one glass of milk, 20 g of cheese (two-thirds ounce), and 120 g of fish or meat one-fourth pound).

It was formerly supposed that high protein diets might predispose to diseases of the kidneys and heart. This idea has been abandoned by most clinicians. The diet of the Eskimos may contain as much as 500 g of protein per day, yet the incidence of kidney and heart disease among them is no higher than among other people. Men have lived for a year on an exclusive meat diet with no apparent deleterious results.

MINERAL (INORGANIC) REQUIREMENT

Inorganic elements and compounds* required daily by human beings include calcium, phosphorus, iron, copper, iodine, fluorine, sulfur and other elements in trace amounts.

CALCIUM AND PHOSPHORUS. The daily requirement of calcium is estimated to be about 0.8 g for adults, 1.2 g for pregnant women, and 1 g for growing children. The phosphorus requirement for both children and adults is probably about 0.8 to 1.4 g each day. All of these values apply only if the intake of vitamin D is adequate. Phosphorus deficiency is rare when there is no vitamin D deficiency because phosphorus compounds are present in nearly every food we eat.

A diet containing a high percentage of acid-forming foods (meats, bread) favors the absorption of calcium from the intestinal tract. At the same time, however, it may increase the elimination of calcium salts in the urine. If the diet contains a large amount of bulk-producing foods (fruits, vegetables) the absorption of calcium may be slightly impaired. In the presence of adequate amounts of vitamin D, probably both the above factors can be disregarded in computing diets.

IRON AND COPPER. Menstruation, pregnancy, lactation, and hemorrhage (bleeding) cause a loss of iron from the body, and this iron must be replaced. If it is not, *anemia* (low amount of hemoglobin in the blood) will result. About 400 mg of iron are present in the body at birth; in the adult body, this has increased to about 4,000 mg (4 g). The loss of iron from the adult body is very small (except in the conditions mentioned above), and it is generally agreed that 10 to 15 mg per day in the diet is sufficient. As a matter of fact, only a portion of the iron in the food is absorbed, and the actual amount that gains entrance into the body is much smaller than 10 mg.

*Also review Chapter 29.

Table 34-5. Amounts of different foods required to supply approximately 1 gram of calcium and 1 gram of phosphorus

Food	Amount to supply 1 g of Ca		Amount to supply 1 g of P	
Almonds	1 lb	0.4 kg	0.5 lb	227 g
Bananas	24 lb	10.9 kg	6.5 lb	3 kg
Beef, steak	18 lb	8.2 kg	1 lb	0.4 kg
Bread, white	8 lb	3.6 kg	2.5 lb	1.1 kg
Bread, whole wheat	4.5 lb	2 kg	1 lb	0.4 kg
Cauliflower	2 lb	0.9 kg	4 lb	1.8 kg
Cheese, American	3.5 oz	100 g	5 oz	150 g
Corn, fresh	37 lb	16.8 kg	2 lb	0.9 kg
Fish, cod	18 lb	8.2 kg	2 lb	0.9 kg
Milk	1.5 pt	750 ml	1 qt	1,000 ml
Peanuts	3 lb	1.4 kg	0.5 lb	227 g
Turnip tops	1 lb	0.4 kg	3 lb	1.4 kg

Table 34-6. Amounts of various foods required to furnish 15 mg of iron

Almonds	13 oz	370 g	Mushrooms	1 lb	450 g
Beans, baked	1 lb	450 g	Mustard greens	6 oz	180 g
Beans, dry	6 oz	180 g	Oatmeal	14 oz	400 g
Beans, lima, dry	5 oz	150 g	Oysters	12 oz	350 g
Beef, brains	10 oz	290 g	Parsley	3 oz	90 g
Beef, liver	7 oz	210 g	Peanuts	26 oz	700 g
Beef, steak	17 oz	480 g	Peas, dry	8 oz	225 g
Brazil nuts	13 oz	370 g	Pecans	20 oz	600 g
Bread, whole wheat	1 lb	450 g	Pistachios	7 oz	210 g
Butter	17 lb	8 kg	Spinach	14 oz	400 g
Chard	1 lb	450 g	Turnip tops	6 oz	180 g
Cheese, American	38 oz	1.1 kg	Veal, cutlet	17 oz	480 g
Dandelion	8 oz	225 g	Walnuts, black	9 oz	260 g
Eggs (12)	17 oz	480 g	Walnuts, English	26 oz	700 g
Milk	14 pt	7 l	Watercress	7 oz	210 g

During pregnancy and lactation, 15 mg daily is believed to be a sufficient amount.

The infant is born with enough iron to last about six months. Since milk contains only about 1 or 2 mg per liter (quart, approximately), extra iron must be added to the infant's diet after the first few months. During the growing period the amount of hemoglobin in the body increases rapidly, and about 200 mg of iron are needed for hemoglobin synthesis during the first year of life. For older children, 100 to 200 mg will be required each year until the age of puberty, after which 200 to 400 mg per year will be required until adult growth is reached. Since only a portion of the iron in the diet is absorbed, the preschool child probably should receive about 15 mg of iron daily in his food.

It is known that copper is necessary for the formation of hemoglobin.

Presumably it acts as a catalyst because no copper is present in the hemoglobin molecule. Only traces of this element are necessary, however, and it seems unlikely that any ordinary diet will fail to have a sufficient amount of it. Copper deficiency has been observed in starving infants treated with supposedly adequate diets. After 64 to 108 days, during which they gained weight and strength, they developed fragile bones, severe anemia, and a low level of neutrophils in the blood. The deficiency was reversed by feeding them 135 to 170 μg of copper daily.

IODINE. Vegetables grown in regions where plentiful amounts of iodine occur in the surface water contain much more iodine than the same variety of vegetables grown in iodine-deficient regions. There are many more cases of thyroid gland disease and goiter in the states bordering the Great Lakes than in the southern states, for example, simply because the Great Lakes and their tributaries contain extremely small amounts of iodine.

It has been estimated that 25 to 100 μg of iodine daily will prevent hypothyroidism. Iodized salt, which contains 0.01 percent potassium iodide, easily supplies this quantity. Broccoli, clams, seafood, butter, beans, corn, and spinach are amount the best food sources of iodine. It must be remembered, however, that the iodine content of vegetables grown in different localities varies widely.

FLUORINE. Optimal amounts of fluorine (as fluoride) in the drinking water inhibit tooth decay, but excessive amounts cause mottled enamel. The amount of fluorine in foods is extremely low, and there is no danger of producing mottled enamel unless the drinking water contains excessive amounts of the element.

OTHER ELEMENTS. It is known that manganese, zinc, cobalt, and potassium, are necessary for normal nutrition in animals. They are necessary for normal growth, for activation of enzymes, and for proper functioning of the nervous system. The human requirement of these elements is unknown, but it is probable that the average diet contains adequate amounts of them. The sulfur requirement of the diet will be adequate if the protein intake is adequate. The symptoms of magnesium deficiency, which is extremely rare, include muscular weakness, depression, dizziness, and occasional convulsions and painful muscular cramping (tetany). The element is widespread in foods and it is unlikely that a dietary deficiency will occur. The recommended daily allowance is 350 mg daily for men and 300 mg for women. Zinc deficiency has been described elsewhere (page 343).

LIPID REQUIREMENT

During World War I it was found that diets very low in lipid resulted in early fatigue, reduced capacity for doing heavy work, and loss of appetite. It is generally supposed that about one-third of the calories of the diet should be supplied by lipid (chiefly, fats). Diets that are extremely low in fat are unpalatable to most people in this country.

Three of the unsaturated fatty acids found in lipids—*linoleic acid, linolenic acid,* and *arachidonic acid*—are known to be necessary in the diet of white rats. If one or more of these acids is not present in the diet, the rats fails to grow; they develop scaly areas on their tails, have blood in the urine, and die. We are not yet sure that human beings need these substances.

However, it has been reported that some cases of infantile eczema (a skin disease) have been cured by giving these acids in the form of corn oil or raw linseed oil. It has also been stated that the administration of these acids improves the resistance of human beings to colds and allergic conditions.

Choline, one of the hydrolytic products of lecithins, is known to be essential for normal fat metabolism in laboratory animals (see p. 226). Normal diets contain lecithins, and, as far as we know, true choline deficiency is not found in human beings.

ACID AND ALKALINE EFFECTS OF FOODS

When proteins are burned in the body, some of the normal end products are acids (uric acid, phosphoric acid, sulfuric acid). These acids combine with metals to form salts and are eliminated in the urine. Foods rich in protein (meat, eggs, bread) are called acid-forming foods.

Fruits and vegetables are called alkali-forming foods. They contain salts of metals, such as sodium, potassium, calcium, and magnesium. These salts are largely organic; the nonmetal portions of them are burned to carbon dioxide and water in the body. The metals that remain combine either with the acids formed in protein metabolism or with carbon dioxide and water to form bicarbonates. Cranberries, plums, and prunes contain benzoic acid, which is not burned in the body; these fruits are, therefore, acid forming.

KETOGENIC AND ANTI-KETOGENIC DIETS

Foods that can form ketone bodies in the body are called *ketogenic foods*. Foods that can form glycogen oppose ketosis and are called *antiketogenic foods*. All the carbohydrate, 0.58 (58 percent) of the protein, and 0.1 (10 percent) of the fat (the glycerol portion of the fat molecule) present in the diet may be regarded as antiketogenic. Nine-tenths (90 percent) of the fat (the fatty acid part of the fat molecule) and about 0.24 (24 percent) of the protein are regarded as ketogenic.

Ketogenic diets are sometimes used in the treatment of infections in the urinary tract and in the treatment of epilepsy.

RESIDUE AND WATER IN THE DIET

Water and residue (material that is not digested) are needed in the diet to ensure elimination of waste products from the body. Water has many other important functions as well (see Chapter 29). A normal adult probably needs about 3 or 4 liters (approximately 3 or 4 quarts) of water each day. About half of this amount is present in the daily intake of food; the other half is taken into the digestive tract as free water.

Many individuals suffer from constipation unless the diet contains a certain amount of residue. Most of the residue present in the diet is in the form of cellulose, the "woody" framework of plants. Residue is furnished by fruits and vegetables (Table 34-7). Raw fruits may cause diarrhea in some cases, but almost everyone can eat cooked fruits without unpleasant symptoms. Patients with constipation are usually instructed to eat fruits with every meal and to eat liberal amounts of green cooked vegetables with the noon and evening meal.

If the patient has diarrhea, on the other hand, a low-residue diet is desirable. Such patients should avoid coarse breads and cereals, raw fruits,

Table 34-7. Fruits and vegetables high in residue

Fruits high in residue	Vegetables high in residue
Applesauce	Beets
Apricots	Carrots
Baked apples	Cauliflower
Peach sauce	Greens
Pear sauce	Peas
Prunes	Spinach
Rhubarb	String beans

and raw vegetables. Cooked fruits and vegetables should be strained or passed through a sieve to remove most of the residue. Spices, vinegar, greasy foods, and rich desserts also increase the activity of the intestinal tract and are omitted from the diet in the treatment of diarrhea.

DIET IN PREGNANCY AND LACTATION

It is obvious that the diet of the pregnant woman should contain extra amounts of minerals, protein, and vitamins. Extra calcium, phosphorus, iron, and iodine can be supplied by increasing the daily allowance of foods rich in these elements or by giving them in some other form. The vitamin requirements in pregnancy have been given in Chapter 33. Extra protein is needed to build tissues in the fetus, to form the placenta, and to allow for the increased size of maternal structures (such as the uterus and breasts). Probably 100 g of protein daily is sufficient, provided it is of good nutritional quality. If the diet is well balanced and contains a quart of milk, an egg, and a liberal serving of meat each day, the protein intake will be adequate. The basal metabolic rate increases during the latter half of pregnancy, but the extra energy required is largely compensated for by decreased muscular activity. The average energy requirement during pregnancy is about 2,400 large calories daily.

During lactation the mother loses a considerable amount of materials in the milk and stores a certain amount in addition to this. During the latter months of breast feeding 600 or more large calories may be lost each day in the milk. Ordinarily, the caloric demands of the mother can be taken care of by allowing, in addition to the mother's own requirement, 150 large calories per kg of the baby's body weight during the first three months; 125 large calories during the second three months; and about 100 large calories during the third three months. To ensure that the mother receives enough extra protein, she should be supplied with two extra calories of protein for each calorie lost in the milk. Each liter of human milk contains about 0.3 g of calcium, and extra calcium in the form of milk, cheese, and eggs should be present in the diet. At least 2 liters (approximately 2 quarts) of water, in addition to that contained in the food, is a desirable daily intake. Extra amounts of iron will prevent the anemia that sometimes complicates lactation.

NUTRITION IN INFANCY AND CHILDHOOD

Infant nutrition really begins during fetal life, and the diet recommended for the pregnant women is equally important for the mother and for the unborn child. Most evidence indicates that the human fetus is en-

Table 34-8. Daily calorie distribution of the diet of infants

	Infant, 1 month (3.8 kg)	Infant, 1 year (10 kg)
Basal requirement	210 large calories	550 large calories
Growth	170 large calories	150 large calories
Activity	80 large calories	160 large calories
Lost in excreta	40 large calories	100 large calories
Total	500 large calories	960 large calories

Table 34-9. Average daily caloric requirements of infants

Age (months)	Weight (kg)	Weight (lb)	Large calories
1	3.8	8.4	500
2	4.7	10.3	600
3	5.4	11.9	670
4	6.2	13.6	720
5	6.7	14.8	760
6	7.3	16.1	800
7	7.8	17.2	830
8	8.3	18.3	860
9	8.8	19.4	880
10	9.2	20.2	910
11	9.6	21.1	935
12	10.0	22.0	960

tirely parasitic and will take nearly everything it requires for nutrition from the mother, even if this depletes her tissues.

The intake of food is proportionally higher in infancy and childhood than in adult life because the materials necessary for growth must be supplied and because the basal metabolism is higher. The daily calorie distribution of the diet of infants is summarized in Table 34-8. It will be noticed that the caloric requirement for growth declines from about 45 large calories per kg during the first month to about 15 large calories per kg at one year. The requirement for activity is variable; vigorous crying may increase it as much as 40 percent. The average total requirement for infants is given in Table 34-9.

Most of the protein in human milk is lactalbumin, a nearly perfect protein from a nutritional point of view. If this type of milk constitutes the infant's major food, 2 to 2.5 g of protein per kg of body weight will be a sufficient daily allowance. If cow's milk is used, this allowance should be increased to 3 to 3.5 g. Cow's milk contains some lactalbumin, but the majority of its protein is casein. Retarded growth, feeble musculature, poor circulation, and perhaps edema are indicative of insufficient protein in the diet.

The body of the infant is about 12 percent fat. If the infant is breast fed, about half the calories are supplied as fat. This high a percentage of fat is not necessary in artificial diets, however, and most of them contain enough fat to make up approximately one-third of the calories.

Even young infants can digest sugars other than lactose (milk sugar), and the carbohydrate in artificial diets is often partly supplied in the form of sucrose (cane sugar). If too little carbohydrate is present, the needed calories must be made up mainly with protein. This is difficult. On the other hand, too much carbohydrate may lead to excessive fermentation in the lower intestine, causing diarrhea. This is especially evident in the presence of infections.

Nursing infants receive about 125 to 150 ml of water per kg of body weight per day. If the protein intake is high, more water will be required. Symptoms of dehydration ordinarily are not present unless the water intake is reduced below 35 to 60 ml per kg daily.

Artificial formulas for infant feeding are usually made from cow's milk. This milk contains more protein and less carbohydrate than does human milk. It is customary, therefore, to dilute the milk somewhat in order to decrease the content of protein, and sugar is added to increase the carbohydrate content.

Some infants suffer from skin or digestive disorders if fed on cow's milk. Such infants often are able to tolerate goat's milk.

The vitamin requirement in infancy and childhood has been discussed in Chapter 33.

REDUCING DIETS

Obesity (fatness) interferes with activity and increases the work of the heart. Since fat is an excellent heat insulator, it also interferes with body temperature regulation. It has been stated that a fat man of early adult age has only one chance in three of living as long as a lean man of the same age.

One pound of body fat is equivalent to approximately 4,050 large calories. However, when body fat is lost as a result of dietary restriction, there is also some loss of water and other substances. In calculating the loss of weight caused by dietary restriction, it is more accurate to assume a loss of 1 lb. of body weight as a result of a deficit of 3,500 large calories of food.

A good reducing diet necessarily is low in calories, but it should contain all the necessary nutrients. "Fad" diets low in both calories and nutrients do cause a loss of weight, but both the diet and the weight loss are tempo-

Table 34-10. Average composition of milk (100 ml)

Source	Protein (g)	Carbo-hydrate (g)	Fat (g)	Ash (g)	Calcium (g)	Phos-phorus (g)	Iron (mg)	Large calo-ries
Cow	3.3	5.0	4.0	0.7	0.12	0.09	0.24	69
Cow, evaporated	8.7	10.2	8.2	1.5	0.25	0.2	0.53	150
Cow, dried	26.1	38.0	26.5	6.0	0.92	0.71	1.5	495
Goat	4.3	4.5	4.8	0.8	0.13	0.1	—	98
Human	1.5	6.8	3.3	0.2	0.034	0.015	—	63

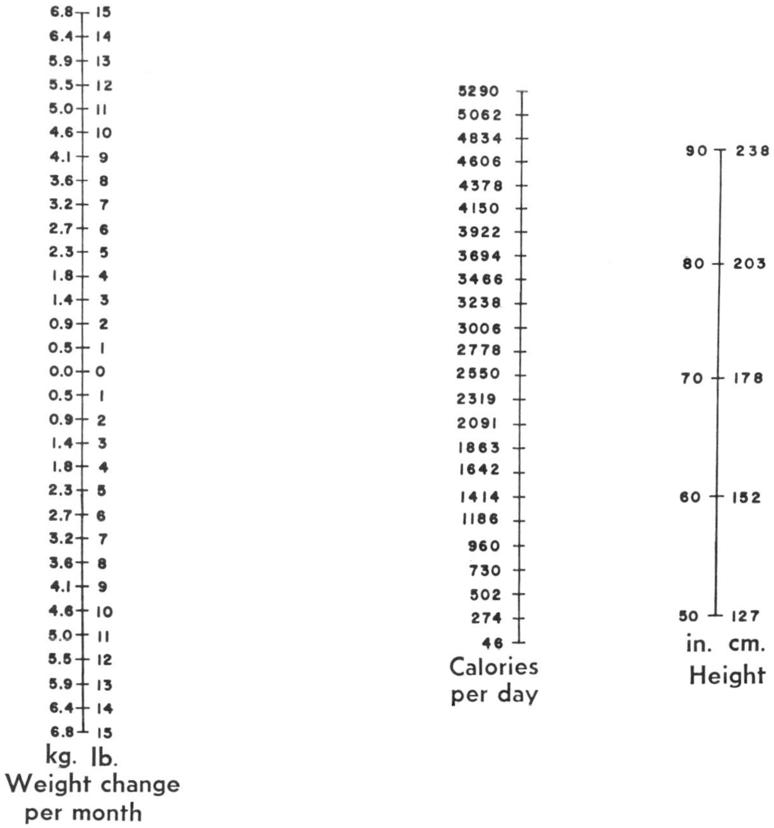

Fig. 34-2. Nomogram for calculating weight-changing diets. Select the patient's height along the right margin and the weight loss or gain desired per month along the left margin. The line connecting these two points crosses the calorie line at the desired caloric allowance. How many calories per day should be eaten by a nurse 60 inches tall who wishes to lose 10 pounds per month? (Courtesy Dr. Ralph J. Slonim, Jr.)

rary, whereas the problem—obesity—may persist for a lifetime. A good diet plan is the exchange system of dietary control. It was devised by a joint committee representing the American Diabetes Association, the American Dietetic Association, and the Public Health Service.* Foods are divided into six basic "exchange" groups. Each food in a group is assumed to be approximately equal in nutritional value to the other foods in the group.

The best time for patients on reducing diets to weigh themselves is first thing in the morning (without clothing and with an empty bladder). At other times body weight varies with the intake of food and with water loss and intake. Insensible water loss (see page 335) and urinary excretion can result in a loss of 1 to 2.5 lbs. during the night. Patients on reducing diets often store water at times and daily weights may be misleading. It is a good plan to record body weight once each week.

*Journal of the American Dietetic Association **26:**575, 1950.

Table 34-11. Food exchange groups*

List 1. Milk exchanges.

Whole	1 cup	(Cream portion of whole milk equals two fat exchanges. One cup of whole milk equals 1 cup of skim milk plus two fat exchanges.)
Skim milk	1 cup	
Buttermilk	1 cup	
Evaporated milk	1/2 cup	
Posdered skim milk	1/4 cup	
Yogurt, plain	1 cup	

List 2. Vegetable exchanges (as served plain, without fat seasoning or dressing). (Any fat used is taken from fat exchange allowance.)

Group A. (Use as desired. Negligible carbohydrate, protein, and fat in amounts commonly eaten.)

Asparagus	Greens	Mushrooms
Bak choi, Gai choi	Beet greens	Okra
Bamboo shoots	Chard	Peppers (Bell, Chili, etc.)
Broccoli	Collards	Radishes
Brussel sprouts	Kale	Sauerkraut
Cabbage	Mustard	String Beans, young
Cauliflower	Spinach	Summer squash
Celery	Turnip greens	Tomatoes
Chicory		Watercress
Chinese cabbage	Salad greens	Parsley
Cucumbers	Lettuces	Pimientoes
Escarole, endive		
Eggplant		

Group B. (1/2 cup equals one serving)

Artichoke (1 medium)	Peas, green	Squash, winter
Beets	Pumpkin	Turnip
Carrots	Rutabaga	
Onions		

List 3. Fruit exchanges (unsweetened—fresh, frozen, canned, cooked). (One exchange is portion indicated by each fruit.)

Berries	
Blackberries	1 cup
Blueberries	2/3 cup
Raspberries	3/4 cup
Strawberries	1 cup
Citrus fruits	
Grapefruit	1/2 small
Grapefruit juice	1/2 cup
Orange	1 small
Orange juice	1/2 cup
Tangerine	1 large
Melons	
Cantaloupe	1/4 med.
Honeydew	1/8 med.
Watermelon	1/2 center slice

Dried fruits	
Apricots	4 halves
Dates	2
Figs	1 small
Prunes	2 medium
Raisins	2 tablespoons

Others	
Apple	1 small
Apple Juice	1/3 cup
Applesauce	1/2 cup
Apricots (fresh)	2 med.
Banana	1/2 small
Cherries	10 large
Fig (fresh)	1
Grapes	12 med.
Grape Juice	1/4 cup
Peach	1 medium
Pear	1 small
Pineapple	1/2 cup, 1 slice
Pineapple juice	1/3 cup
Plums	2 medium
Prunes (fresh)	2
Prune juice	1/4 cup

*From Williams, S. R.: Nutrition and diet therapy, St. Louis, 1969, The C. V. Mosby Co.

Table 34-11. Food exchange groups* — cont'd

List 4. Bread exchanges (equivalent portions indicated by each item).

Bread		Cereal	
Bagel	$\frac{1}{2}$	Cereal, cooked	$\frac{1}{2}$ cup
Biscuit, roll (2 in. diam.)	1	Cereal, dry (flakes, puffed)	$\frac{3}{4}$ cup
Bread (white or dark)	1 slice	Flour	$2\frac{1}{2}$ tablespoons
Cornbread ($1\frac{1}{2}$ in. cube)	1	Rice, grits (cooked)	$\frac{1}{2}$ cup
Frankfurter roll	1 small	Corn	$\frac{1}{3}$ cup
Hamburger roll	$\frac{1}{2}$ large	Spaghetti, macaroni, noodles (cooked)	$\frac{1}{2}$ cup
Crackers		Vegetables, and other	
Animal	8	Baked beans, no pork	$\frac{1}{4}$ cup
Graham ($2\frac{1}{2}$ in. square)	2	Beans, peas, dried, cooked	$\frac{1}{2}$ cup
Oyster	$\frac{1}{2}$ cup	Corn on the cob	$\frac{1}{2}$ large ear, 1 small ear
Round, thin ($\frac{1}{2}$ in. diam.)	6–8		
Saltines (2 in square)	5	Popcorn (popped)	1 cup
Soda ($2\frac{1}{2}$ in. square)	3	Parsnips	$\frac{2}{3}$ cup
Matzos (6 in. diam.)	1 piece	Potatoes, white	1 small
Muffin (2 in. diam.)	1	Potatoes, mashed white	$\frac{1}{2}$ cup
Melba thins	4	Potatoes, sweet or yams	$\frac{1}{4}$ cup
Pretzels (22 per lb.)	1 med.	Sponge cake, plain ($1\frac{1}{2}$ in. cube)	
Pretzel sticks (av. thin)	14	Ice cream, vanilla (omit 2 fat exch.)	$\frac{1}{2}$ cup
		Ice milk, vanilla	$\frac{1}{2}$ cup

List 5. Meat exchanges (all items refer to cooked weight).

Lean meat, poultry	1 ounce	Fish	
Cold cuts ($4\frac{1}{2}$ in. × $\frac{1}{8}$ in.)	1 slice	Cod, halibut	1 oz.
Frankfurter (8–9/lb.)	1	Salmon, tuna, crab, lobster	$\frac{1}{4}$ cup
Egg	1	Shrimp, clams, oysters, etc.	5 small
Cheese, cheddar type	1 ounce	Sardines	3 medium
Cheese, cottage	$\frac{1}{4}$ cup	Scallops (12 pcs. per lb.)	1 large
Sausage (3 in. × $\frac{1}{2}$ in.)	2	Peanut butter (limit 1 exch. per day)	2 tablespoons

List 6. Fat exchanges

Avocado (4 in. diam.)	$\frac{1}{8}$	French dressing	1 tablespoon
Bacon, crisp	1 slice	Half and half (10% cream and milk)	4 tablespoons
Butter or margerine	1 teaspoon	Mayonnaise	1 teaspoon
Cream, light (20%)	2 tablespoons	Nuts	6 small
Cream, heavy (40%)	1 tablespoon	Oil or cooking fat	1 teaspoon
Cream cheese	1 tablespoon	Olives	5 small
Cheese spreads	1 tablespoon	Sour cream	2 tablespoons

Miscellaneous foods allowed as desired (negligible carbohydrate, protein, fat).

Artificial sweeteners	Gelatin, plain	Rennet tablets, plain
Bouillion, fat-free	Lemon	Rhubarb
Broth, clear	Mustard	Spices
Coffee	Pepper	Tea
Cranberries, unsweetened	Pickle, dill and sour	Vinegar
Catsup		

Table 34-12. Weight reduction diets using the exchange system of dietary control*

Food exchange group*	Approx. measure	800 calories	1,000 calories	1,200 calories	1,500 calories
	Total number of exchanges per day				
Milk (nonfat)	1 cup	2	2	2	2
Vegetable A	As desired	Free	Free	Free	Free
Vegetable B	½ cup	1	1	1	1
Fruit	Varies	3	3	3	4
Bread	1 slice	1	3	4	4
Meat	1 ounce	6	6	7	9
Fat	1 teaspoon	1	1	2	4
	Distribution of food exchanges				
Breakfast					
Fruit		1	1	1	1
Meat		1	1	1	1
Bread		1	1	1	1
Fat		1	1	1	1
Lunch and dinner					
Meat		2 to 3	2 to 3	3	4
Vegetable A		Any	Any	Any	Any
Vegetable B (either meal)		1	1	1	1
Bread		0	1	1 to 2	1 to 2
Fat		0	0	0 to 1	1 to 2
Fruit		1	1	1	1 to 2
Milk		1	1	1	1

*From Williams, S. R.: Nutrition and diet therapy, St. Louis, 1969, The C. V. Mosby Co.

THE SATIETY AND FEEDING CENTERS

The *satiety center* is a small region located in the ventromedial portion of the hypothalamus. (One such center is present on each side of the brain.) If it is removed surgically from a laboratory animal, the animal eats almost constantly and becomes extremely obese. On the other hand, if an electrode is implanted in it and a small current is applied to the electrode, an animal that is eating hungrily will cease eating immediately.

Another small area (one on each side of the brain) located in the lateral portion of the hypothalamus is known as the *feeding center*. When it is stimulated, a satiated animal (that is, an animal that has eaten all the food it cares to ingest) immediately will resume eating. If it is removed surgically, the animal ceases to eat or to drink water.

Some physiological mechanism (perhaps changes in the glucose level of the plasma) stimulates the feeding center periodically, and the animal ingests food. The satiety center acts as a brake to inhibit the feeding center when enough food has been ingested.

What stimulates the satiety centers to exert their braking action? Probably there are a number of mechanisms involved. The one that has received most experimental attention has to do with the catabolism of glucose by the satiety centers. The entire brain utilizes glucose in preference to protein and fat as a source of energy, but it cannot store it very long. In the intervals between feeding periods, the level of glucose in the brain de-

Table 34-13. Desirable weights for men and women aged 25 years and over (nude weight in pounds)*

Height		Small frame	Medium frame	Large frame
		Men		
Feet	inches			
5	1	104–112	110–121	118–133
5	2	107–115	113–125	121–136
5	3	110–118	116–128	124–140
5	4	113–121	119–131	127–144
5	5	116–125	122–135	130–148
5	6	120–129	126–139	134–153
5	7	124–133	130–144	139–158
5	8	128–137	134–148	143–162
5	9	132–142	138–152	147–166
5	10	136–146	142–157	151–171
5	11	140–150	146–162	156–176
6	0	144–154	150–167	160–181
6	1	148–159	154–172	165–186
6	2	152–163	159–177	170–191
6	3	156–167	164–182	174–196
		Women		
4	8	87–93	91–102	99–114
4	9	89–96	93–105	101–117
4	10	91–99	96–108	104–120
4	11	94–102	99–111	107–123
5	0	97–105	102–114	110–126
5	1	100–108	105–117	113–129
5	2	103–111	108–121	116–133
5	3	106–114	111–125	120–137
5	4	109–118	115–130	124–141
5	5	113–122	119–134	128–145
5	6	117–126	123–138	132–149
5	7	121–130	127–142	136–153
5	8	125–135	131–146	140–158
5	9	129–139	135–150	144–163
5	10	133–143	139–154	148–168

*Modified from figures published by the Metropolitan Life Insurance Company. Their figures included shoes and indoor clothing. Figures in this table have been calculated by subtracting 1 inch from men's height and 2 inches from women's height; it was assumed that men's indoor clothing weighs 8 lbs and that women's indoor clothing weighs 5 lbs.

creases. Only the intake of food will replenish it. It is postulated that the satiety centers use relatively more glucose than does the remainder of the brain. When it is actively burning glucose during and following a meal, it is an effective brake that inhibits the feeding centers. When the supply of glucose in the satiety centers is not adequate, it ceases to be a brake, and the constantly activated feeding centers somehow create the desire to eat.

This mechanism presumably ceases to function during starvation, at least in the human. If hospitalized individuals are fed diets very low in calories (less than 500 large calories per day), the sensation of hunger dis-

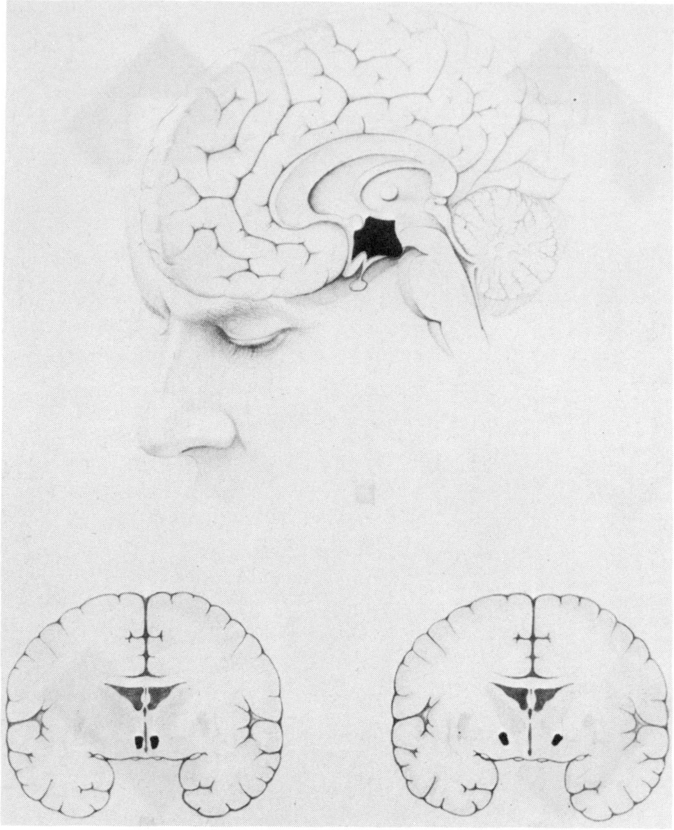

Fig. 34-3. **A,** The approximate location of the hypothalamus; **B,** the satiety center; **C,** the feeding center. What happens if the satiety center of an animal is removed? (Courtesy Warner-Chilcott Laboratories.)

appears after three days or so. It does not return even if the diet is maintained for several months.

It is probable that some of the drugs used to curb appetite actually work by stimulating the satiety center. Others may inhibit the feeding center.

KWASHIORKOR AND MARASMUS

In large areas of Africa, Asia, and Latin America millions of people, most of them children, suffer from protein deficiency. When adequate calories are ingested, but very little protein, the nutritional disease known as *kwashiorkor** results. Another disorder, *marasmus,* results when the diet is low both in protein and in calories. Marasmus is most common in children below one year of age. Kwashiorkor usually occurs during the second and third years of life. In many cases the clinical picture suggests a condition intermediate between the kwashiorkor and true marasmus. This condition is referred to as *marasmic kwashiorkor.*

*The term kwashiorkor first was used by a tribe in Ghana. It means "deposed child"—in other words, a child "removed from health."

A 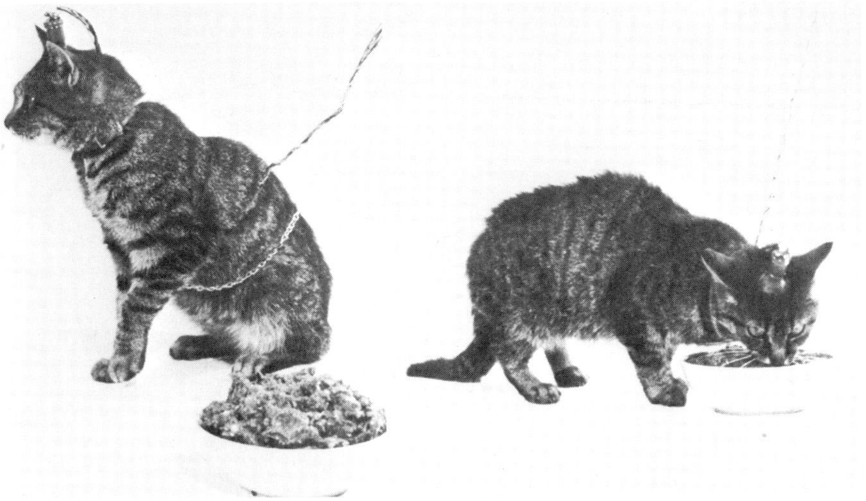 B

Fig. 34-4. A, The cat, with a small electrode implanted in his feeding center, has eaten his fill and is satiated; **B,** when a weak electric current is applied through the electrode, the cat immediately rushes over to the dish of food and eats as though starved. How would a hungry cat act if his satiety center were stimulated? (Courtesy Dr. Jane Frances Emele, Warner-Lambert Research Institute.)

In true kwashiorkor there is desquamation, hyperpigmentation, and keratosis of the skin. Pitting edema is present. The hair becomes loosened so that it can be pulled out without pain; sometimes it falls out spontaneously. It becomes lighter in color. Patients exhibit a mixture of apathy and irritability. Loss of appetite and diarrhea are common. A loss of muscle tone often is observed.

The appearance of the victim of kwashiorkor is not easily forgotten by those who have seen children stricken with this disorder. The piercing eyes, bloated belly, and matchstick legs are characteristic. In the advanced form of the disorder, the child resists any interference, even feeding.

In maramus the predominant signs are a virtual lack of subcutaneous fat, extreme muscular wasting, and marked retardation in growth and development. An infant with marasmus "looks like a living skeleton," or a dried-up old man.

A child with kwashiorkor should be treated by giving him a diet that provides 3 to 5 g of protein of good biological quality per kilogram of body weight per day. Milk is an excellent source of such protein. Often, however, it is unavailable, and good results can be obtained with suitable mixtures of plant foods. Other foods are added gradually, so that the child should be receiving a varied, adequate diet by the second or third week of treatment. Usually, an intake of 150 large calories per kilogram of body weight, assuming adequate protein, is satisfactory. In marasmus, or marasmic

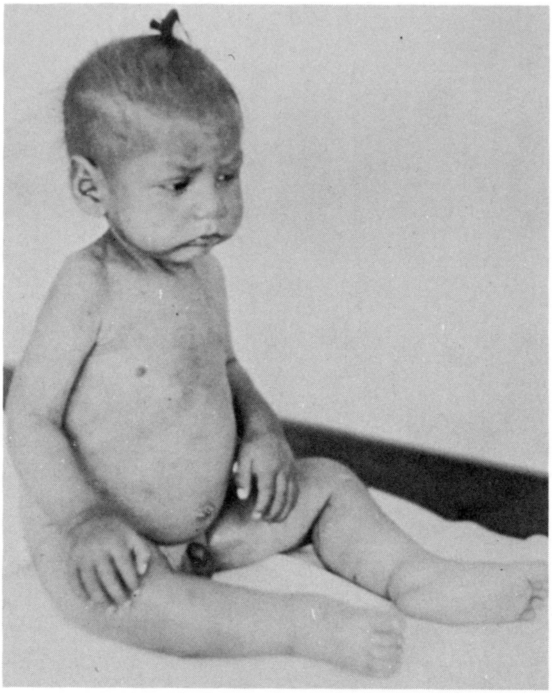

Fig. 34-5. A child (1 year and 10 months old) with kwashiokor. What is the cause of this condition? (Courtesy Dr. George Graham, Anglo-American Clinic, Lima, Peru.)

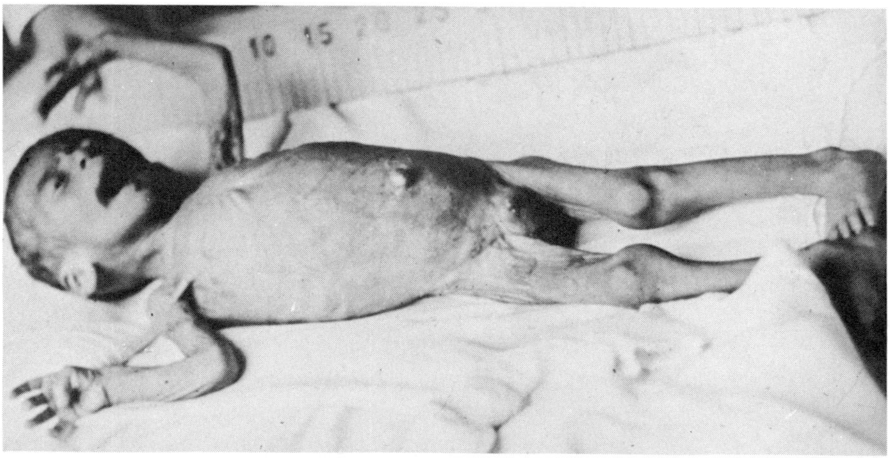

Fig. 34-6. This child, who at 8 months of age weighs only 3.5 kg (7.7 lb.), has marasmus. How does marasmus differ from kwashiokor? (Courtesy Dr. George Graham, Anglo-American Clinic, Lima, Peru.)

kwashiorkor, more calories than this may be necessary after the first two or three weeks of treatment.

During the first few days of treatment it is customary to give an antibiotic or a sulfonamide, or both, to prevent infection, which is a high risk in these patients.

DIET AND CORONARY HEART DISEASE

More Americans die of heart disease each year than from any other cause. Various surveys conducted throughout the world make it probable that the incidence of coronary heart disease is related to the diet. Diets supplying more than 450 mg of cholesterol daily and containing a ratio of polyunsaturated to saturated fatty acids lower than about 1 : 1 cause and maintain relatively high levels of cholesterol and triglycerides (fats) in the plasma. Monounsaturated fatty acids do not affect these levels. Large intakes of sucrose, though not starch, do not affect cholesterol levels but do increase the level of triglycerides. The atheromatous plaques in the coronary arteries that usually precede clinical manifestations of the disease are rich in these lipids. Men with a level of cholesterol of 260 mg per 100 ml of serum have three times the chance of a heart attack as do men with levels below 200 mg per 100 ml.

Although it is not known *with certainty* that modifying the diet will decrease the risk of coronary heart attacks, many physicians believe that it will. The recommended dietary modifications are summarized in the following statements taken from a pamphlet published by the American Heart Association.*

To control your intake of cholesterol-rich foods:

Eat no more than three egg yolks a week, including eggs used in cooking.

Limit your use of shellfish and organ meats.

To control the amount and type of fat you eat:

In most of your meat meals for the week, use fish, chicken, turkey, and veal; and limit beef, lamb, pork, and ham to five moderate-sized portions per week.

Choose lean cuts of meat, trim visible fat, and discard the fat that cooks out of the meat.

Avoid deep fat frying; use cooking methods that help to remove fat—baking, boiling, broiling, roasting, stewing.

Restrict your use of fatty "luncheon" and "variety" meats like sausages and salami.

Instead of butter and other cooking fats that are solid or completely hydrogenated, use liquid vegetable oils and margarines that are rich in polyunsaturated fats.

Instead of whole milk and cheeses made from whole milk and cream, use skimmed milk and skimmed milk cheeses.

The diet summarized in Table 34-14 is a slight modification of a diet published by Sue Rodwell Williams in *Nutrition and Diet Therapy.*

*The Way To A Man's Heart, American Heart Association, 44 East 23rd Street, New York, N. Y. 10010.

Table 34-14. Controlled fat diet—high polyunsaturated fatty acids diet*

	Foods allowed	*Foods not allowed*
Soups	Bouillon cubes, vegetables and broths from which fat has been removed. Cream soups made with nonfat milk	Meat soups, commercial cream soups and cream soups made with whole milk or cream
Meat, fish, poultry	One or two servings daily (not to exceed a total of 4 oz.) lean muscle meat, broiled or roasted; beef, veal, lamb, pork, chicken, turkey, lean ham, organ meats (all visible fat should be trimmed from meat); all fish and shell fish	Bacon, pork sausage, luncheon meat, dried meat, and all fatty cuts of meat; weiners, fish roe, duck, goose, skin of poultry, and T. V. dinners
Milk and milk products	At least one pint nonfat milk or nonfat buttermilk daily; nonfat cottage cheese, Sap Sago cheese	Whole milk and cream; all cheeses (except nonfat cottage cheese), ice cream, imitation ice cream (except that containing safflower oil), ice milk, sour cream, commercial yogurt
Eggs	Not more than three per week.	
Vegetables	All raw or cooked as tolerated (leafy green and yellow vegetables are good sources of vitamin A)	No restrictions
Fruits	All raw, cooked, dried, frozen or canned; use citrus or tomato daily; fruit juices	Avocado and olives
Salads	Any fruit, vegetable, and gelatin salad	
Cereals	All cooked and dry cereals; serve with nonfat milk or fruit; macaroni, noodles, spaghetti, and rice	
Breads	Whole wheat rye, enriched white, French bread, English muffins graham crackers, saltine crackers	Commercial pancakes, waffles, coffee cakes, muffins, doughnuts and all other quick breads made with whole milk and fat; biscuit mixes and other commercial mixes, cheese crackers, pretzels
Desserts	Fruits, tapioca, cornstarch, rice, Junket puddings all made with non-fat milk and without egg yolks; fruit whips made with egg whites, gelatin desserts, angle food cake, sherbet, water ices, and special imitation ice cream containing vegetable safflower oil; cake and cookies made with nonfat milk, oil, and egg white; fruit pie (pastry made with oil)	Omit desserts and candies made with whole milk, cream, egg yolk, chocolate, cocoa butter, coconut, hydrogenated shortenings, butter and other animal fats

*Modified from Williams, S. R.: Nutrition and diet therapy, St. Louis, 1969, The C. V. Mosby Co.

Table 34-14. Controlled fat diet—high polyunsaturated fatty acids diet*—cont'd

Concentrated fats	Corn oil, soybean oil, cotton seed oil, sesame oil, safflower oil, sunflower oil, walnuts and other nuts except cashew and those commercially fried or roasted Margarine made from above oils Commercial French and Italian salad dressing if not made with olive oil Gravy may be made from bouillon cubes, or fat-free meat stock thickened with flour and add oil if desired Freshly ground or old fashioned peanut butter	Butter, chocolate, coconut oil, hydrogenated fats and shortenings, cashew nuts; mineral oil, olive oil, margarine, except as specified; commercial salad dressings, except as listed; hydrogenated peanut butter; gravy, except as specified
Sweets	Jelly, jam, honey, hard candy, and sugar	
Beverages	Tea, coffee, or coffee substitutes; tomato juice, fruit juice, cocoa prepared with non-fat milk	Beverages containing chocolate, ice cream, ice milk, eggs, whole milk or cream

If the diet is also to be high in unsaturated fat it should include liberal amounts of:

1. Oils allowed which can be incorporated in salad dressings, or added to soups, to nonfat milk, to cereal, to vegetables
2. Walnuts, almonds, Brazil nuts, Filberts, pecans
3. Extra margarine containing some untreated vegetable oil in or on foods

STUDY QUESTIONS

1. What is the function of the diet?
2. List the factors that must be thought of in planning adequate diets.
3. What is meant by basal metabolism? Define basal metabolic rate.
4. What is the influence of age on the BMR? Which sex has the higher BMR at a given age?
5. What is the average normal BMR for a person of your age and sex? What is your surface area?
6. How is the BMR usually reported clinically? If a girl 15 years old has a measured BMR of 45 large calories per square meter per hour, how would this be reported clinically?
7. Explain the difference between the direct and indirect methods of measuring the heat eliminated from the body. What is measured in the usual clinical determination of the BMR?
8. Name several conditions in which the BMR is higher than normal. Name several in which it is lower than normal.
9. Calculate the daily energy requirement of a man 30 years old who weighs 160 pounds and is 5 feet, 10 inches tall. Assume moderate exercise.
10. An average doughnut supplies 175 large calories of energy. How many doughnuts would be required to supply your total energy requirement for one day?
11. Why do children need proportionally more protein than do adults?
12. What are essential amino acids? Adequate proteins? Why is it desirable to have animal protein in the diet?
13. How much protein should adult diets contain per day? Why do we need protein?
14. Do high-protein diets predispose to diseases of the kidneys and heart? What reasons can you give for your answer?
15. Choose your diet for one day from Table 34-4. Calculate the number of grams of protein, fat, and carbohydrate consumed. Calculate the caloric value of the food consumed. Estimate the amounts of calcium, phosphorus, and iron consumed.

16. What is the daily requirement of calcium? Of phosphorus? How much milk would be necessary to supply each of these amounts.
17. Name some causes of loss of iron from the body. How much iron should be present in the food eaten in one day by an adult? By a preschool child? By a pregnant woman?
18. How much iron is present in a quart of milk? Why must extra iron be added to the diet of an infant 6 months old?
19. What is the function of copper in nutrition?
20. What daily intake of iodine will prevent hypothyroidism? How much KI or NaI is present in most samples of iodized salt?
21. Name some other inorganic substances that are necessary in nutrition.
22. What unsaturated fatty acids are necessary for the normal functioning and nutrition of rats? What evidence suggests that they may be necessary in human nutrition?
23. What is the role of choline in nutrition?
24. What fraction of the total calories of the diet should be supplied in the form of lipid?
25. What types of food are acid-forming in the body? Alkali-forming?
26. What fruits are acid-forming? If lemons are alkali-forming in the body, how do you account for the fact that they taste sour?
27. What types of disease are sometimes treated with ketogenic diets?
28. What is the nutritional importance of residue? How is constipation treated with diet? How is diarrhea treated with diet?
29. Name some foods of high residue value. Name some of low residue value.
30. How much water does an average normal adult require per day? How much of this is present in the food he eats?
31. What is the average total energy requirement of an infant 1 month old? One year old? What percentage of the food ingested by infants is lost in the excreta?
32. What is the recommended daily protein intake for infants? Why is it higher if cow's milk, rather than human milk, is used?
33. How is the diet modified in pregnancy? In lactation?
34. Why is it undesirable to have either very low or very high levels of carbohydrate in the diets of infants?
35. How low may the water intake of infants be before dehydration results?
36. Make up an infant formula using goat's milk. Adjust the protein content, carbohydrate content, and caloric value as close to those of human milk as possible.
37. Name several disadvantages of obesity. Make a menu for a reducing diet for one day. Calculate its caloric value.
38. What is the satiety center? What is its function?
39. What happens to an animal if the feeding centers are removed surgically?
40. What is kwashiorkor? Describe the appearance of a child with this disorder. How is it treated?
41. How does marasmus differ from kwashiorkor?
42. What dietary modifications are thought to be useful in the prophylaxis of coronary heart disease?

Appendix

Table 2. Food and Nutrition Board, National Academy of Sciences—National Research maintenance of good nutrition of practically all healthy people in the U. S. A.

Age[2] (years)	Weight (kg)	Weight (lbs)	Height (cm)	Height (in)	kcal	Protein (mg)	Fat-soluble vitamins: Vitamin A activity (IU)	Vitamin D (IU)	Vitamin E activity (mg)
Infants									
0–1/6	4	9	55	22	kg × 120	kg × 2.2[5]	1,500	400	5
1/6–1/2	7	15	63	25	kg × 110	kg × 2.0[5]	1,500	400	5
1/2–1	9	20	72	28	kg × 100	kg × 1.8[5]	1,500	400	5
Children									
1–2	12	26	81	32	1,100	25	2,000	400	10
2–3	14	31	91	36	1,250	25	2,000	400	10
3–4	16	35	100	39	1,400	30	2,000	400	10
4–6	19	42	110	43	1,600	30	2,500	400	10
6–8	23	51	121	48	2,000	35	3,500	400	15
8–10	28	62	131	52	2,200	40	3,500	400	15
Males									
10–12	35	77	140	55	2,500	45	4,500	400	20
12–14	43	95	151	59	2,700	50	5,000	400	20
14–18	59	130	170	67	3,000	60	5,000	400	25
18–22	67	147	175	69	2,800	60	5,000	400	30
22–35	70	154	175	69	2,800	65	5,000	–	30
35–55	70	154	173	68	2,600	65	5,000	–	30
55–75+	70	154	171	67	2,400	65	5,000	–	30
Females									
10–12	35	77	142	56	2,250	50	4,500	400	20
12–14	44	97	154	61	2,300	55	5,000	400	25
14–16	52	114	157	62	2,400	55	5,000	400	25
16–18	54	119	160	63	2,300	55	5,000	400	25
18–22	58	128	163	64	2,000	55	5,000	400	25
22–35	58	128	163	64	2,000	55	5,000	–	25
35–55	58	128	160	63	1,850	55	5,000	–	25
55–75+	58	128	157	62	1,700	55	5,000	–	25
Pregnancy					+200	65	6,000	400	30
Lactation					+1,000	75	8,000	400	30

[1]The allowance levels are intended to cover individual variations among most normal persons as they live in the of common foods, providing other nutrients for which human requirements have been less well defined.
[2]Entries on lines for age range 22–35 years represent the reference man and woman at age 22. All other entries represent
[3]The folacin allowances refer to dietary sources as determined by *Lactobacillus casei* assay. Pure forms of folacin
[4]Niacin equivalents include dietary sources of the vitamin itself plus 1 mg equivalent for each 60 mg of dietary tryptophan.
[5]Assumes protein equivalent to human milk. For proteins not 100 percent utilized factors should be increased

Council recommended daily dietary allowances[1] (revised 1968). Designed for the

Water-soluble vitamins							Minerals				
Ascorbic acid (mg)	Folacin[3] (mg)	Niacin (mg equiv)[4]	Ribo-flavin (mg)	Thia-mine (mg)	Vitamin B_6 (mg)	Vitamin B_{12} (μg)	Calcium (g)	Phos-phorus (g)	Iodine (μg)	Iron (mg)	Mag-nesium (mg)
35	0.05	8	0.4	0.2	0.2	1.0	0.4	0.2	25	6	40
35	0.05	7	0.5	0.4	0.3	1.5	0.5	0.4	40	10	60
35	0.1	8	0.6	0.5	0.4	2.0	0.6	0.5	45	15	70
40	0.1	8	0.6	0.6	0.5	2.0	0.7	0.7	55	15	100
40	0.2	8	0.7	0.6	0.6	2.5	0.8	0.8	60	15	150
40	0.2	9	0.8	0.7	0.7	3	0.8	0.8	70	10	200
40	0.2	11	0.9	0.8	0.9	4	0.8	0.8	80	10	200
40	0.2	13	1.1	1.0	1.0	4	0.9	0.9	100	10	250
40	0.3	15	1.2	1.1	1.2	5	1.0	1.0	110	10	250
40	0.4	17	1.3	1.3	1.4	5	1.2	1.2	125	10	300
45	0.4	18	1.4	1.4	1.6	5	1.4	1.4	135	18	350
55	0.4	20	1.5	1.5	1.8	5	1.4	1.4	150	18	400
60	0.4	18	1.6	1.4	2.0	5	0.8	0.8	140	10	400
60	0.4	18	1.7	1.4	2.0	5	0.8	0.8	140	10	350
60	0.4	17	1.7	1.3	2.0	5	0.8	0.8	125	10	350
60	0.4	14	1.7	1.2	2.0	6	0.8	0.8	110	10	350
40	0.4	15	1.3	1.1	1.4	5	1.2	1.2	110	18	300
50	0.4	15	1.4	1.2	1.6	5	1.3	1.3	115	18	350
50	0.4	16	1.4	1.2	1.8	5	1.3	1.3	120	18	350
50	0.4	15	1.5	1.2	2.0	5	1.3	1.3	115	18	350
55	0.4	13	1.5	1.0	2.0	5	0.8	0.8	100	18	350
55	0.4	13	1.5	1.0	2.0	5	0.8	0.8	100	18	300
55	0.4	13	1.5	1.0	2.0	5	0.8	0.8	90	18	300
55	0.4	13	1.5	1.0	2.0	6	0.8	0.8	80	10	300
60	0.8	15	1.8	+0.1	2.5	8	+0.4	+0.4	125	18	450
60	0.5	20	2.0	+0.5	2.5	6	+0.5	+0.5	150	18	450

United States under usual environmental stresses. The recommended allowances can be attained with a variety

allowances for the midpoint of the specified age range.
may be effective in doses less than 1/4 of the RDA.

proportionately.

Table 3. Common organic radicals*

Listed below are the names and formulas of radicals frequently referred to in organic chemistry; included are suffixes used in naming important groups

acetamido, $CH_3\overset{O}{\overset{\|}{C}}—\overset{H}{N}—$

acetonyl, $CH_3COCH_2—$

acetoxy, $CH_3—\overset{O}{\overset{\|}{C}}O—$

acetyl, $CH_3—\overset{O}{\overset{\|}{C}}—$

-al, name ending for aldehydes

alkoxy, RO—(R = any alkyl radical)

allyl, $CH_2{=}CH—CH_2—$

amino, $H_2N—$

amyl = pentyl

-ane, name ending for saturated aliphatic hydrocarbons

anilino, $C_6H_5NH—$

arseno, —As=As—

-ase, name ending for enzymes

azo, —N=N—

azoxy, —N(O)N—

benzamido, $C_6H_5\overset{O}{\overset{\|}{C}}—\overset{H}{N}—$

benzoxy = benzoyloxy

benzoyl, $C_6H_5\overset{O}{\overset{\|}{C}}—$

benzoyloxy, $C_6H_5\overset{O}{\overset{\|}{C}}—O—$

benzyl, $C_6H_5CH_2—$

benzylidene, $C_6H_5\overset{H}{C}{=}$

benzylidyne, $C_6H_5C\lessgtr$

biphenylene, $C_6H_4 \cdot C_6H_4—$

bromo, Br—

butyl, $CH_3(CH_2)_3—$

isobutyl $(CH_3)_2\overset{H}{C}—CH_2—$

sec-butyl, $CH_3CH_2(CH_3)\overset{H}{C}—$

tert-butyl, $(CH_3)_3C—$

butyryl, $CH_3(CH_2)_2\overset{O}{\overset{\|}{C}}—$

carbamido = ureido

carbamyl, $NH_2\overset{O}{\overset{\|}{C}}—$

carbonyl, $>C{=}O$

carboxy, $—\overset{O}{\overset{\|}{C}}—OH$

chloro, Cl—

cinnamyl, $C_6H_5\overset{H}{C}{=}\overset{H}{C}—CH_2—$

cinnamylidene, $C_6H_5\overset{H}{C}{=}\overset{H}{C}—\overset{H}{C}{=}$

crotonyl, $CH_3—\overset{H}{C}{=}\overset{H}{C}—\overset{O}{\overset{\|}{C}}—$

cyano, $—C{\equiv}N$

cyclobutyl, $\underline{CH_2—CH_2—CH_2\overset{H}{C}}—$

cyclohexy, $\underline{CH_2(CH_2)_4\overset{H}{C}}—$

diazo, —N=N— or N≡N=

diazoamino, $R—N{=}N—\overset{H}{N}—$

diene, name ending for diolefins

diol, name ending for dihydroxyalcohols

-ene, name ending for unsaturated olefins or aromatic hydrocarbons

epoxy, —O— (to different atoms already united in some other way)

ethene = ethylene

ethoxy, $C_2H_5O—$

ethyl, $C_2H_5—$

ethylene, $—C_2H_4—$

ethylidene, $CH_3—\overset{H}{C}{=}$

ethynyl, $HC{\equiv}C—$

fluoro, F—

*Courtesy Merck & Co., Inc.

Table 3. Common organic radicals—cont'd

Listed below are the names and formulas of radicals frequently referred to in organic chemistry; included are suffixes used in naming important groups

formyl, $HC(=O)—$

furfuryl, $\overline{OCH{=}CHCH{=}C}—CH_2—$

glyceryl, $—CH_2—CH(—)—CH_2—$

glycolyl, $HOCH_2—C(=O)—$

glycyl, $NH_2CH_2C(=O)—$

heptyl, $CH_3(CH_2)_5CH_2—$

hexyl, $CH_3(CH_2)_4CH_2—$

hydrazo, $—NH—NH—$(to different atoms)

hydroxy, $—OH$

-idene, added to any radical usually means a double bond at point of attachment

imino (imido), $=NH$

-in, name ending for glycosides, glycerides

-ine, name ending for basic compounds, alkaloids

iodo, $I—$

iodoxy, $—IO_2$

keto, $O=$(in generic sense)

leucyl, $(CH_3)_2CH—CH_2CH(NH_2)—C(=O)—$

malonyl, $CH_2(C(=O)—)_2$

mercapto, $HS—$

methene = methylene

metoxy, $CH_3O—$

methyl, $CH_3—$

methylene, $CH_2=$

methylidyne, $CH\equiv$

naphthyl, $—(C_{10}H_7)$ (α or β)

nitro, $—NO_2$

nitroso, $—NO$

octyl, $CH_3(CH_2)_6CH_2—$

-ol, name ending for alcohols, phenols

-ole, name ending for phenolic ethers

-one, name ending for ketone or quinone

-ose, name ending for sugar

oxalyl, $—COCO—$

pentyl, $CH_3(CH_2)_3CH_2—$

phenacyl, $C_6H_5COCH_2—$

phenoxy, $C_6H_5O—$

phenylene, $C_6H_4=$(o, m, p)

picryl, (2, 4, 6) $(NO_2)_3C_6H_2—$

propenyl, $CH_3—HC=CH—$

propionyl, $CH_3CH_2C(=O)—$

propyl, $CH_3CH_2CH_2—$

isopropyl $(CH_3)_2CH—$

propylene, $CH_3—CH(—)—CH_2—$

salicyl, $HOC_6H_4CH_2—$(O)

succinyl, $CH_2—C(=O)—$ / $CH_2—C(=O)—$

sulfinyl, $—SO—$

sulfo, $(HO)O_2S$

sulfonyl, $—SO_2—$

thio, $—S—$

tolyl, $CH_3C_6H_4—$(o, m, p)

trimethylene, $—CH_2CH_2CH_2—$

ureido, $H_2NC(=O)—NH—$

valeryl, $—CH_3(CH_2)_3C(=O)—$

vinyl, $CH_2=CH—$

vinylene, $—CH=CH—$

xylyl, (6 isomers) $(CH_3)_2C_6H_3—$

-yl, name ending for radicals

-yne, name ending for acetylenes

Table 4. Amino acids commonly found in proteins

Common name	Chemical name	Formula	Short-hand symbol
Glycine	Aminoacetic acid	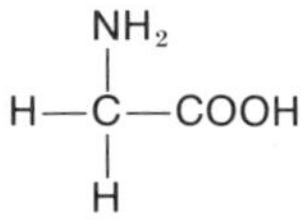 $\begin{array}{c} NH_2 \\ \vert \\ H-C-COOH \\ \vert \\ H \end{array}$	Gly
Alanine	α-Aminopropi-onic acid	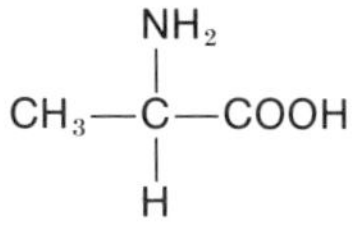 $\begin{array}{c} NH_2 \\ \vert \\ CH_3-C-COOH \\ \vert \\ H \end{array}$	Ala
Valine	α-Aminoiso-valeric acid	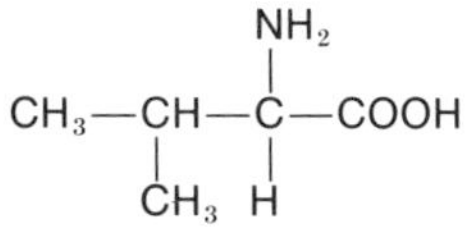 $\begin{array}{c} NH_2 \\ \vert \\ CH_3-CH-C-COOH \\ \vert\qquad\vert \\ CH_3\ \ H \end{array}$	Val
Leucine	α-Aminoiso-caproic acid	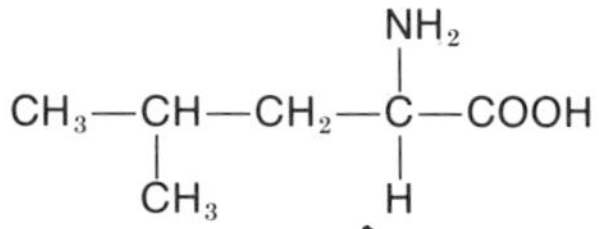 $\begin{array}{c} NH_2 \\ \vert \\ CH_3-CH-CH_2-C-COOH \\ \vert\qquad\qquad\vert \\ CH_3\qquad\ \ H \end{array}$	Leu
Isoleucine	α-Amino-β-methylvaleric acid	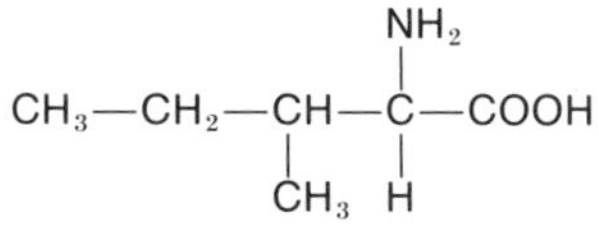 $\begin{array}{c} NH_2 \\ \vert \\ CH_3-CH_2-CH-C-COOH \\ \vert\qquad\vert \\ CH_3\ \ H \end{array}$	Ile
Serine	α-Amino-β-hydroxypro-pionic acid	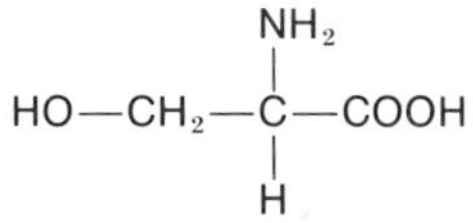 $\begin{array}{c} NH_2 \\ \vert \\ HO-CH_2-C-COOH \\ \vert \\ H \end{array}$	Ser
Threonine	α-Amino-β-hydroxy-n-butyric acid	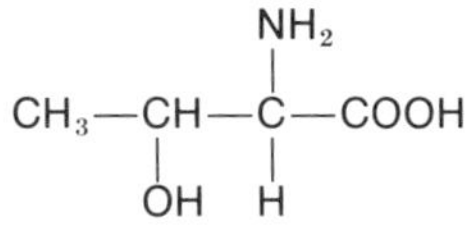 $\begin{array}{c} NH_2 \\ \vert \\ CH_3-CH-C-COOH \\ \vert\qquad\vert \\ OH\ \ H \end{array}$	Thr
Phenylalanine	α-Amino-β-phenylpropi-onic acid	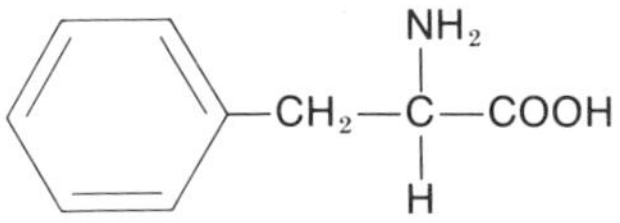 $C_6H_5-CH_2-\underset{\underset{H}{\vert}}{\overset{\overset{NH_2}{\vert}}{C}}-COOH$	Phe
Tyrosine	α-Amino-β-(p-hydroxy-phenyl) pro-pionic acid	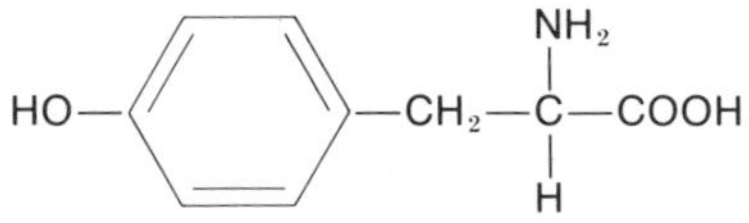 $HO-C_6H_4-CH_2-\underset{\underset{H}{\vert}}{\overset{\overset{NH_2}{\vert}}{C}}-COOH$	Tyr

Table 4. Amino acids commonly found in proteins–cont.

Common name	Chemical name	Formula	Shorthand symbol
Tryptophan	α-Amino-β-indolepropionic acid	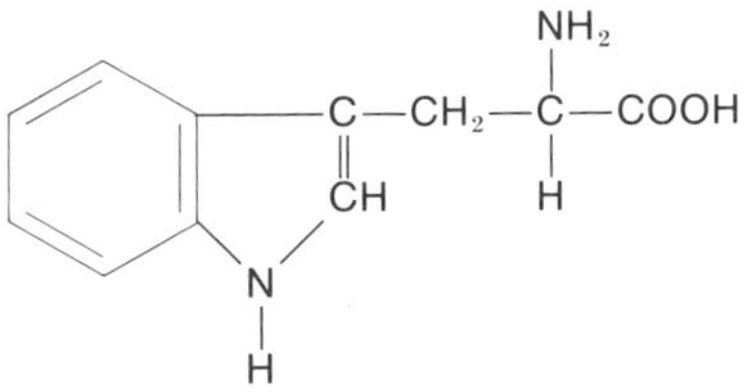	Trp
Cystine	*di* (α-Amino-β-thiopropionic acid)	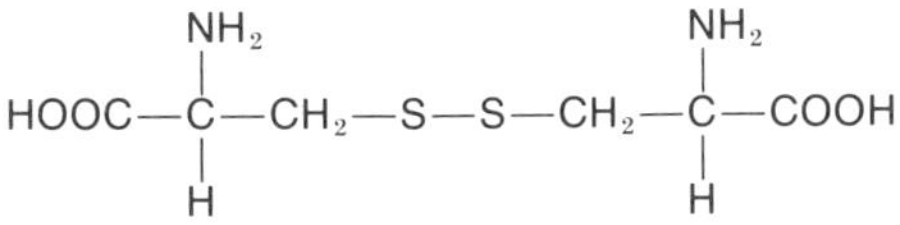	Cys Cys
Cysteine	α-Amino-β-thiopropionic acid	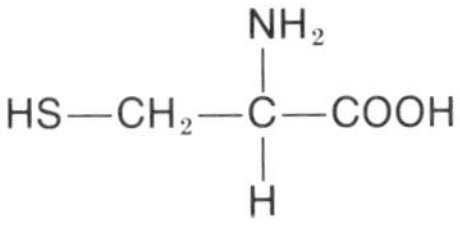	Cys
Methionine	α-Amino-γ-methylthio-*n*-butyric acid	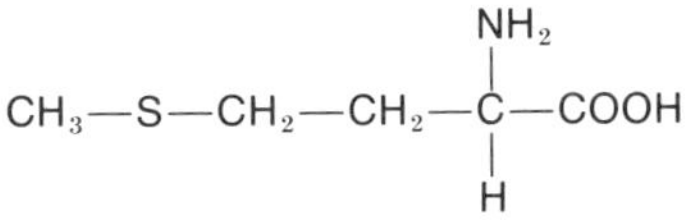	Met
Proline	Pyrrolidine-2-carboxylic acid	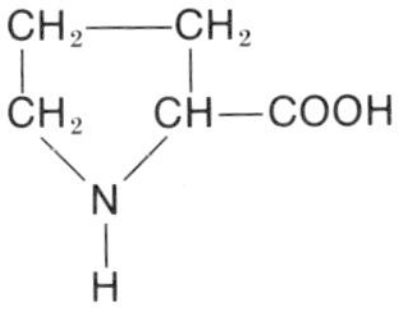	Pro
Hydroxyproline	4-Hydroxypyrrolidine-2-carboxylic acid	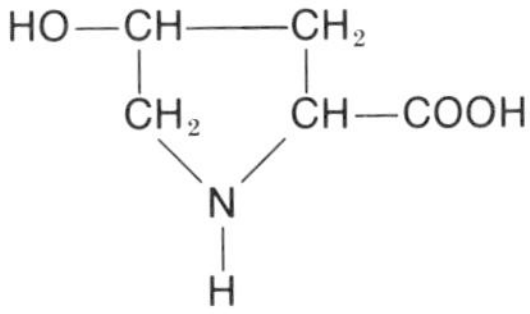	Hyp
Aspartic acid	α-Aminosuccinic acid	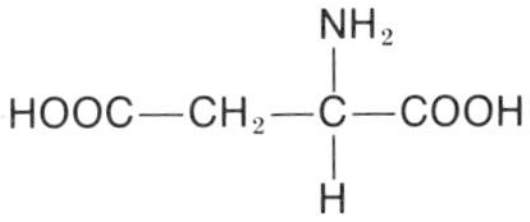	Asp
Glutamic acid	α-Aminoglutaric acid	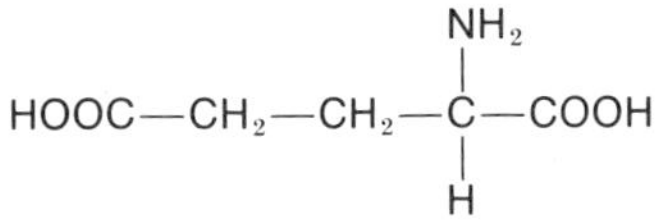	Glu

Continued.

Table 4. Amino acids commonly found in proteins — cont'd

Common name	Chemical name	Formula	Short-hand symbol
Glutamine	α-Amino-glutaramide	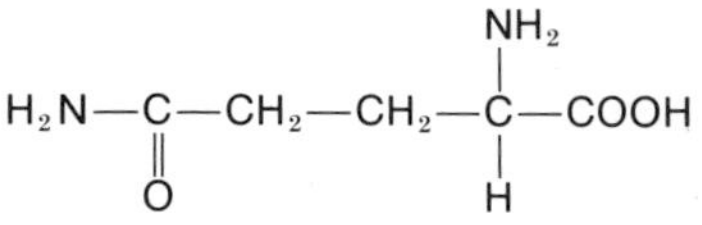 $H_2N-\underset{\underset{O}{\parallel}}{C}-CH_2-CH_2-\underset{\underset{H}{\mid}}{\overset{\overset{NH_2}{\mid}}{C}}-COOH$	Gln
Histidine	α-Amino-β-imidazole-propionic acid	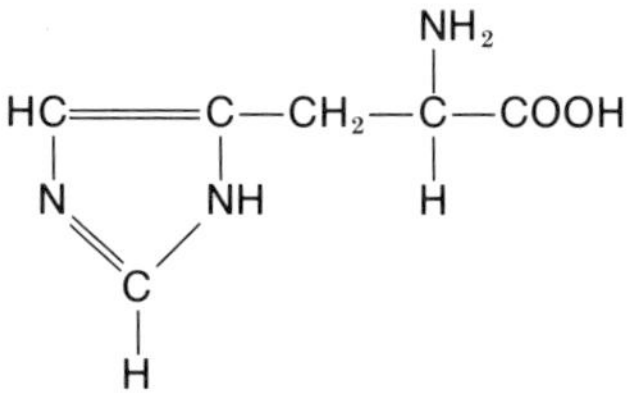 $\underset{\underset{\underset{\underset{H}{\mid}}{C}}{N \diagdown \diagup NH}}{HC}\!=\!\!=\!\!C-CH_2-\underset{\underset{H}{\mid}}{\overset{\overset{NH_2}{\mid}}{C}}-COOH$	His
Arginine	α-Amino-δ-guanido-valeric acid	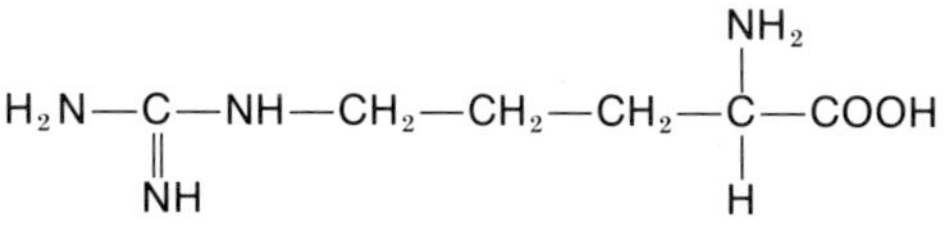 $H_2N-\underset{\underset{NH}{\parallel}}{C}-NH-CH_2-CH_2-CH_2-\underset{\underset{H}{\mid}}{\overset{\overset{NH_2}{\mid}}{C}}-COOH$	Arg
Asparagine	α-Aminosuc-cinamide	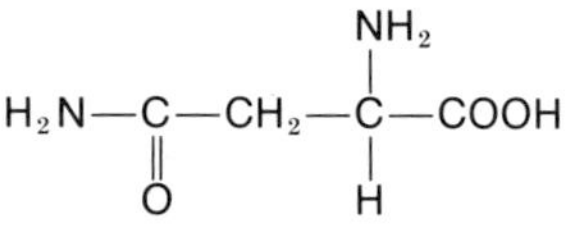 $H_2N-\underset{\underset{O}{\parallel}}{C}-CH_2-\underset{\underset{H}{\mid}}{\overset{\overset{NH_2}{\mid}}{C}}-COOH$	Asn
Lysine	α,ε-Diamino-caproic acid	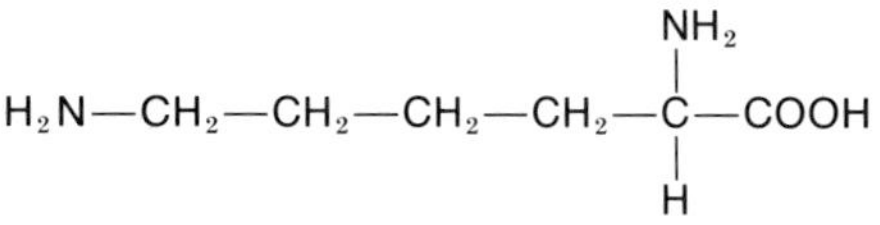 $H_2N-CH_2-CH_2-CH_2-CH_2-\underset{\underset{H}{\mid}}{\overset{\overset{NH_2}{\mid}}{C}}-COOH$	Lys
Hydroxylysine	α,ε-Diamino-δ-hydroxy-caproic acid	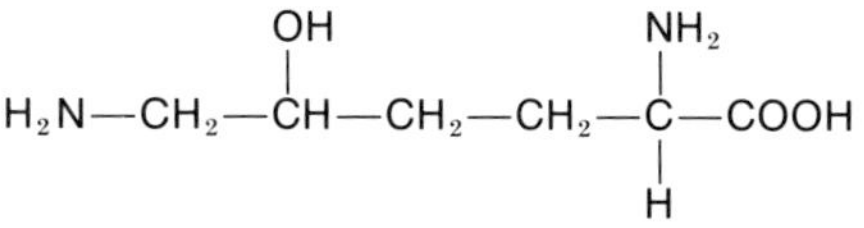 $H_2N-CH_2-\underset{\underset{}{}}{\overset{\overset{OH}{\mid}}{CH}}-CH_2-CH_2-\underset{\underset{H}{\mid}}{\overset{\overset{NH_2}{\mid}}{C}}-COOH$	Hyl

Index

H